Sport and Exercise for Health and Performance

Sport and Exercise for Health and Performance

Guest Editor

Shaher A.I. Shalfawi

MDPI

Basel • Beijing • Wuhan • Barcelona • Belgrade • Novi Sad • Cluj • Manchester

Guest Editor
Shaher A.I. Shalfawi
Department of Education and
Sports Science
University of Stavanger
Stavanger
Norway

Editorial Office
MDPI AG
Grosspeteranlage 5
4052 Basel, Switzerland

This is a reprint of the Special Issue, published open access by the journal *International Journal of Environmental Research and Public Health* (ISSN 1660-4601), freely accessible at: https://www.mdpi.com/journal/ijerph/special_issues/Sport_Exercise_Health_Performance.

For citation purposes, cite each article independently as indicated on the article page online and as indicated below:

Lastname, A.A.; Lastname, B.B. Article Title. *Journal Name* **Year**, *Volume Number*, Page Range.

ISBN 978-3-7258-3855-4 (Hbk)
ISBN 978-3-7258-3856-1 (PDF)
https://doi.org/10.3390/books978-3-7258-3856-1

Contents

About the Editor

Shaher A.I. Shalfawi

Shaher A.I. Shalfawi is an accomplished sports scientist and educator with a distinguished career in physical performance and sports science. Holding a Ph.D. in sport science and performance from the Norwegian School of Sport Sciences, Shalfawi currently serves as an Associate Professor at the University of Stavanger, where he contributes his expertise to advancing research and education in physical performance and public health. Before joining the University of Stavanger, Dr. Shalfawi gained diverse experience as a Researcher and Scientific Assistant at the Norwegian School of Sport Sciences and the Norwegian Olympic Committee and Federation of Sports. These roles underscored his dedication to bridging academic research with practical applications in sports. Shalfawi's qualifications are extensive, including a Ph.D. in physical performance, a master's degree in coaching and sports psychology, and a bachelor's degree in physical education. He also possesses certifications as a Certified Strength and Conditioning Specialist with distinction (CSCS,*D) and a Registered Strength and Conditioning Coach (RSCC) in the USA. Notably, he was honored with the Young Investigator Award in 2017 by the University of Stavanger. His research focuses on the physical performance of high-performance athletes, the validation of test methods and equipment, athlete capacity profiling, and exploring sports' metabolic and physical work demands. Shalfawi is also committed to public health, with a particular interest in women's health. Shalfawi's career reflects a seamless integration of scholarly excellence, practical application, and a commitment to advancing knowledge in sports science and performance. His work continues to inspire and elevate the field of sports science.

Preface

Since the 1980s, research has repeatedly highlighted a critical concern within the realm of physical activity and sports: the heightened risks of sudden death and severe injuries during both organized sports and regular training. These events are most prevalent among specific populations—athletes returning to sports after periods of inactivity, individuals starting or transitioning into physical activity routines, those moving from lower-intensity activities to more demanding levels, and especially adolescents navigating the complexities of puberty. These risks are further influenced by biological sex, adding a layer of complexity to our understanding of health and safety in physical activity.

Despite the volume of data suggesting these risks, a gap remains in the literature concerning the best practices for mitigating these dangers. Methodological studies—both quantitative and qualitative—that aim to outline and evaluate effective strategies for safe participation in physical activity are still lacking.

This reprint aims to make a significant contribution to the field by exploring a broad spectrum of interconnected areas that can directly influence the safety and effectiveness of training regimens. Another key focus is the role of relational coordination between individuals, trainers, administrators, health personnel, clubs, and other stakeholders. Effective communication and coordination across these entities are critical to ensuring a safe environment for all participants.

This reprint encompasses a wide range of studies. It aims to promote better practices among athletes, coaches, scientists, educators, and healthcare professionals. By addressing the various facets of health risk assessment, management, and prevention, this compilation of research strives to optimize the practice of physical activity while prioritizing health, safety, and performance.

The research presented in this reprint will hopefully stimulate further inquiry and contribute to the development of strategies for safely engaging in physical activity across different age groups, sexes, and performance levels.

Shaher A.I. Shalfawi
Guest Editor

International Journal of
Environmental Research and Public Health

MDPI

Article

Bayesian Estimation of Correlation between Measures of Blood Pressure Indices, Aerobic Capacity and Resting Heart Rate Variability Using Markov Chain Monte Carlo Simulation and 95% High Density Interval in Female School Teachers

Shaher A. I. Shalfawi

Department of Education and Sports Science, University of Stavanger, 4036 Stavanger, Norway; shaher.shalfawi@uis.no

Received: 8 July 2020; Accepted: 13 September 2020; Published: 16 September 2020

Abstract: Background: Several explanations regarding the disparity observed in the literature with regard to heart rate variability (HRV) and its association with performance parameters have been proposed: the time of day when the recording was conducted, the condition (i.e., rest, active, post activity) and the mathematical and physiological relationships that could have influenced the results. A notable observation about early studies is that they all followed the frequentist approach to data analyses. Therefore, in an attempt to explain the disparity observed in the literature, the primary purpose of this study was to estimate the association between measures of HRV indices, aerobic performance parameters and blood pressure indices using the Bayesian estimation of correlation on simulated data using Markov Chain Monte Carlo (MCMC) and the equal probability of the 95% high density interval (95% HDI). Methods: The within-subjects with a one-group pretest experimental design was chosen to investigate the relationship between baseline measures of HRV (rest; independent variable), myocardial work (rate–pressure product (RPP)), mean arterial pressure (MAP) and aerobic performance parameters. The study participants were eight local female schoolteachers aged 54.1 ± 6.5 years (mean ± SD), with a body mass of 70.6 ± 11.5 kg and a height of 164.5 ± 6.5 cm. Their HRV data were analyzed in R package, and the Bayesian estimation of correlation was calculated employing the Bayesian hierarchical model that uses MCMC simulation integrated in the JAGS package. Results: The Bayesian estimation of correlation using MCMC simulation reproduced and supported the findings reported regarding norms and the within-HRV-indices associations. The results of the Bayesian estimation showed a possible association (regardless of the strength) between pNN50% and MAP (*rho* = 0.671; 95% HDI = 0.928–0.004), MeanRR (ms) and RPP (*rho* = −0.68; 95% HDI = −0.064–−0.935), SDNN (ms) and RPP (*rho* = 0.672; 95% HDI = 0.918–0.001), LF (ms^2) and RPP (*rho* = 0.733; 95% HDI = 0.935–0.118) and SD2 and RPP (*rho* = 0.692; 95% HDI = 0.939–0.055). Conclusions: The Bayesian estimation of correlation with 95% HDI on MCMC simulated data is a new technique for data analysis in sport science and seems to provide a more robust approach to allocating credibility through a meaningful mathematical model. However, the 95% HDI found in this study, accompanied by the theoretical explanations regarding the dynamics between the parasympathetic nervous system and the sympathetic nervous system in relation to different recording conditions (supine, reactivation, rest), recording systems, time of day (morning, evening, sleep etc.) and age of participants, suggests that the association between measures of HRV indices and aerobic performance parameters has yet to be explicated.

Keywords: psychophysiology health; rate-pressure product; mean arterial blood pressure; MCMC; data simulation

1. Introduction

Heart rate variability (HRV) research has been intensified due to the significant relationship observed between cardiovascular mortality and the autonomic nervous system [1,2]. This has led to establishing a work group called the "Task Force", involving scientists and researchers from both the European Society of Cardiology and the North American Society for Pacing and Electrophysiology in 1996 [3] with the aim of developing the standards for HRV research. The objectives of the task force were to develop the definitions and terms of HRV, identify standard measurement methods, define how HRV correlates with human physiology, describe how the measures are practiced clinically and identify needed research [3]. A search on pubmed.gov using the term "heart rate variability" yielded 39,743 results for studies investigating HRV from a wide variety of disciplines since the task force report was published to date. The HRV is a reflection of the change in the time interval between successive heartbeats [1,3,4]. This inter-beat interval (IBI) has been shown to be influenced by the autonomic nervous system and more specifically, parasympathetic nervous system (PNS) activities and sympathetic nervous system (SNS) activities [3,5,6]. This is because the heart is controlled by both the higher brain center and the cardiovascular control area [1,7]. The PNS is believed to be mediated by the fluctuations of vagal-cardiac nerve [1] and its activity is higher during rest, which contributes to slower heart rate observed in healthy people, and is associated with a respiratory frequency of about 0.15 to 0.4 Hz [1,3,6,7]. The SNS activities have been reported to increase with increased activity (stress) and corresponds to a respiratory frequency range between 0.04 and 0.15 Hz [1,3,4,6,7]. Therefore, the interaction between the two frequencies suggests that the low frequency (i.e., 0.04 and 0.15 Hz) represents both SNS and PNS branches [3,4,6,7]. Due to this dynamic relationship, it is expected that PNS activities (depending on the physical and psychological state of the person) may or may not be associated with SNS activities [6]. Therefore, researchers have pointed out the importance of being careful when interpreting HRV results [3,4,6,8].

The task force report in 1996 was the first robust guide for conducting HRV research [3]. Nevertheless, the task force left many elements regarding the research process open for other researchers to develop. After this report, Berntson et al. [1] were the first to provide the most robust guidelines regarding HRV research process. Thereafter, researchers provided improved guidelines to follow [4,5,9,10]. All these studies provided guides regarding the HRV data collection, analyses and cleaning, calculation and reporting [1,3–5,8–10]. However, the studies agreed that HRV can be analyzed using three domains: the first is based on the statistical method concerned with IBI time series (i.e., time domain); the second is the frequency domain, reported to divide the heart rhythm oscillations into 4 bands; the third is the nonlinear indices (Poincaré plot) (Table 1).

The availability of recording systems and techniques such as photoplethysmography [11], IBI recording [12] and (gold standard) electrocardiography (ECG) [3,4,7] made the recording of HRV noninvasive and accessible. The advancement in technology allowed researchers to use accessible systems, such as heart rate monitors, to record IBI to be able to assess their athletes' HRV. For example, in 2005, Kingsley et al. [12] compared Polar 810s with Reynolds digital ambulatory ECG. They found that Polar 810s produced similar results to the ECG recording during rest and exercise at any relative intensity. In 2009, Nunan et al. [13] reinvestigated the validity and reliability of the Polar 810s using simultaneous recording with CardioPerfect 12-lead ECG module in the resting supine position. Their results indicated a high validity and reliability of the Polar 810s. In 2016, Hernando et al. [14] validated the Polar RS800 for HRV analysis during rest and exercise, the results of the study showing a valid and reliable recording during rest with some variation during exercise. Similar results were reported in 2017 by Cassirame et al. [15], who conducted a study examining the accuracy of the Garmin 920XT HRM compared to the standard ECG recording. They did not report differences in HRV analysis in resting supine position, whereas differences were observed in the exercise condition. These studies confirm the importance of carefully choosing the recording conditions in relation to the purpose of the study for the results to be comparable [3,4].

Table 1. The three heart rate variability (HRV) domains.

Time Domain		
SDNN	Standard deviation of all Normal–Normal intervals in a time series	SDNN indicate total variability [3,7,8]
RMSSD	The root mean square of successive differences	RMSSD and pNN50 (%) reflects vagal tone/PNS activities [4,7,10]
pNN50 (%)	Percent of successive intervals with a difference greater that 50 ms compared to previous interval	
Frequency Domain		
HF	High-frequency band (i.e., 0.15 to 0.4 Hz)	HF reflects vagal tone/PNS activities [4,8,10]
LF	Low-frequency (LF) band (i.e., 0.04 and 0.15 Hz)	LF reflects baroreceptor activity at rest (vagal influenced) and SNS activities during stress [3,4,8,10]
VLF	Very-low-frequency (VLF) band (i.e., 0.0033 to 0.04 Hz)	VLF and ULF reflect long-term thermo- and hormonal regulation mechanisms [3,10]
ULF	Ultra-low-frequency (ULF) band (i.e., <0.0033 Hz)	
Poincaré Plot		
SD1	Standard descriptor 1	SD1 reflects fast IBI variability which is a reflection of PNS activities to the heart [4,7]
SD2	Standard descriptor 2	SD2 reflects the long-term IBI variability, which represents both SNS and PSN activities [4,7]

Note: Both VLF and ULF physiological explanations are less defined and, therefore, are not usually included in the HRV reporting. PNS = parasympathetic nervous system; SNS = sympathetic nervous system; IBI = inter-beat interval.

The ventricular contraction and relaxation are a continues process in a cardiac cycle and the systolic and diastolic blood pressure (BP) are measured during these contractions and relaxations, respectively [10]. The heart continuously pumps blood to different parts of the body and the rate of pumps per minute depends on the body need (i.e., relaxing, during exercise, before and after meals, standing, walking etc.). Body needs have been categorized into "physiological and pathological, neuropsychological, lifestyle, non-modifiable and environmental factors [16]." However, the heart muscle is influenced by the medulla, which is responsible for transmitting the signals coming from the PNS and SNS to the heart [17]. Research shows that an increase in SNS activities increases heart rate, and an increase in PNS activities slows heart rate [1,3,10,17]. Therefore, the ventricular contraction and relaxation is connected to relatively balanced PNS and SNS activities, which are linked to the HRV indices. This can be illustrated by the process of inhaling and exhaling during breathing; during inhaling, heart rate (HR) increases and BP rises and vice versa during exhaling [6]. Hence, the change in BP is continuous and indicates that the body systems function as a regulator to maintain a homeostasis state [18]. Therefore, an increase in BP would implicate a decrease in heart rate and vascular tone and vice versa [6]. This relationship between PNS and SNS (i.e., the source of HRV) and BP has been extensively studied and is well documented [6,10,16,18–24]. Since HR depends on the person state and the IBI varies accordingly, it was expected that HRV indices would be related to the ability of the heart to pump the needed amount of blood per minute to carry the needed amount of oxygen and deliver it to the working tissues via the cardiovascular system [25]. Hence, several researchers investigated this relationship, and a brief review of the published reports indicates a disparity in the reported results (Table 2).

Table 2. A brief review of the literature showing the disparity in the reported results.

Study (Date)	Focus	Findings
De Meersman [26] (year 1993)	Compared different age groups on both $VO2_{max}$ and HRV (assessed by the percent change in mean HR).	(a) Results showed that the participants with higher $VO2_{max}$ have a higher value of HRV.
Melanson and Freedson [27] (year 2001)	Effect of a 12-week endurance training on resting heart rate variability in sedentary adult males.	(a) Increase in $VO2_{peak}$, no change in resting HR, increase in RMSSD and pNN50 after 12 weeks of training, but not during, compared to the baseline. (b) No effect on LF (nu) and only the training group had elevated HF power compared to the baseline. (c) No marked correlations were observed between HRV indices and $VO2_{peak}$ except for HRV indices after 16 weeks of training.
Catai et al. [28] (year 2002)	Effects of aerobic exercise training on heart rate variability during wakefulness and sleep and cardiorespiratory responses of young and middle-aged healthy men.	(a) Exercise training increased $VO2_{peak}$ in all participants with no marked changes observed in HRV indices.
Kouidi et al. [29] (year 2002)	Effect of athletic training on time domain HRV indices.	(a) A relationship between aerobic capacity and time domain HRV indices on athletes training in the long-distance group but not on athletes from the sprint track group, the field weight events group and the control group. They concluded that HRV modulation depends on the exercise training pattern.
Marocolo et al. [30] (year 2007)	Effect of aerobic training program on the electrical remodeling of heart high-frequency components.	(a) Positive correlation between HRV indices and $VO2_{max}$; however, the root mean squared voltage of total (a variable from the signal-averaged ECG) was the only independent predictor of $VO2_{max}$.
Schmitt et al. [31] (year 2008)	Altitude, heart rate variability and aerobic capacities.	(a) No relationship between changes in HRV and $VO2_{max}$. (b) The increase in VO2 and power at the respiratory compensation point was accompanied by decreased PNS activities. (c) The changes in HRV parameters and the changes in VO2 and power at the respiratory compensation point had a statistically significant relationship.
Grant et al. [32] (year 2009)	Relationship between exercise capacity and heart rate variability.	(a) Relationship between $VO2_{max}$ and HRV indices showed different results in relation to measuring position. (b) LF (nu) and LF/HF correlated with $VO2_{max}$ when HRV was recorded in the supine resting position. (c) RMSSD, pNN50, SD1, LF (nu), HF (ms^2) and LF/HF were correlated with $VO2_{max}$ when HRV was recorded in a standing position.

Table 2. *Cont.*

Study (Date)	Focus	Findings
Leite et al. [33] (year 2015)	Correlation between heart rate variability indexes and aerobic physiological variables.	(a) A moderate but statistically significant relationship between HRV and aerobic capacity in patients with chronic obstructive pulmonary disease.
Flatt and Esco [34] (year 2016)	Evaluating individual raining adaptation with smartphone-derived heart rate variability in a collegiate female soccer team.	(a) A statistically significant large relationship between change in RMSSD (expressed as a coefficient of variation) and Yo-Yo IR1 test performance. (b) No statistically significant relationship was observed between mean change of RMSSD and Yo-Yo IR1 test performance.
Flatt et al. [35] (year 2017)	Individual heart rate variability responses to preseason training in high level female soccer players.	(a) Inverse, very large, relationship between mean weekly changes in RMSSD and changes in daily and weekly training loads. (b) Positive and large relationship between mean weekly changes in RMSSD and both fatigue and soreness.
Materko [36] (year 2018)	Stratification of the level of aerobic fitness based on heart rate variability parameters in adult males at rest.	(a) The group with higher $VO2_{max}$ also had higher HRV. (b) Only pNN50 was among the HRV indices, together with Cardiac-Deceleration Rate, that was able to predict $VO2_{max}$
Materko et al. [37] (year 2018)	Maximum oxygen uptake prediction model based on heart rate variability parameters.	(a) Small to moderate relationship between measures of HRV indices (i.e., RMSSD, pNN50, HF and LF/HF) and $VO2_{max}$ (b) Only pNN50 was among the HRV indices, together with mean HR and Cardiac-Deceleration Rate, that was able to predict $VO2_{max}$
Phoemsapthawee et al. [38] (year 2019)	Clarifying the casual link between body composition, aerobic fitness and the alterations in cardiac autonomic modulation after a 12-week exercise training.	(a) Improvement in $VO2_{peak}$ after the training period in the exercise group. (b) Increased PNS indices and reduced SNS indices at rest. (c) Statistically significant relationship between changes in $VO2_{peak}$ and HRV indices. (d) Only SD1/SD2 ratio gave a statistically significant explanation for the changes in $VO2_{peak}$

$VO2_{peak}$, $VO2_{max}$ = highest rate of oxygen consumption measured during incremental exercise.

Several explanations regarding the disparity observed (Table 2) in the literature could be hypothesized; among others, the time of day when the recording was conducted and the condition (i.e., rest, active, post activity). Vitale et al. [39] concluded that the human circadian rhythms could potentially differ during the time of day. The task force indicated that mathematical and physiological relationships could influence the results [3]. Observing all the studies presented earlier, one can note that all mentioned studies followed the frequentist approach to data analyses. To the best of the author's knowledge, no studies to date have investigated the relationship between measures of HRV indices and aerobic capacity using the Bayesian approach to data analyses. Therefore, in an attempt to explain the disparity observed in the literature, the primary purpose of this study was to estimate the association between measures of HRV indices, aerobic performance and blood pressure indices employing the Bayesian estimation of correlation and the equal probability of the 95% high density interval (HDI) on a simulated data. To assure the suitability of the data, a secondary aim was to compare the data produced to the norms and to investigate the estimation of the association within the HRV indices in comparison to those reported.

2. Materials and Methods

2.1. Study Design

It is well documented that BP and respiration affect the measurements of HRV [5,9]. To avoid the interindividual differences in HRV measures caused by BP and respiration, the within-subjects experimental design has been shown to be the optimal experimental design in HRV studies, giving a further increased statistical power when using a small sample size [4,5,9]. Therefore, this study followed these recommendations, and the within-subjects with a one-group pretest experimental design was chosen to investigate the relationship between baseline measures of HRV (rest; independent variable), myocardial work (rate–pressure product (RPP)), mean arterial pressure (MAP) and aerobic capacity performances on female schoolteachers over 30 years old [4,9].

2.2. Participants

Twelve local female schoolteachers aged 53.9 ± 5.7 years (mean ± SD), with a body mass of 71.8 ± 10.1 kg and a height of 164.4 ± 6.2 cm, volunteered to participate in the present study. To be able to compare the results with the norms reported in the literature [40], the participants had to be females ≥30 years old, not consume medication that might influence their results at the time of the study, be free from injuries and illness and complete the testing procedure. After the initial consultation with the participants, two participants reported that they were on BP medication; therefore, those two participants' measures were excluded from the study. Furthermore, two participants did not complete the testing procedure, leaving this study with 8 female schoolteachers aged 54.1 ± 6.5 years (mean ± SD), with a body mass of 70.6 ± 11.5 kg and a height of 164.5 ± 6.5 cm. In addition to their everyday teaching at schools, the participants conducted circuit training with the same instructor twice a week. Written informed consent was obtained from all participants after a verbal and written explanation of the experimental design and potential risks associated with participating in the study. The study was conducted in accordance with the Helsinki Declaration and the Norwegian National Committees for Research Ethics. This study was approved by the Norwegian center for research data (id: 738807).

2.3. Procedure and Instruments

2.3.1. Anthropometry

Participants were asked not to have intense physical training the day before the experiment day and not to consume food for a minimum of 2 h prior to the testing. Then, upon their admission to the laboratory, height and body mass were recorded using a wall mounted Seca stadiometer model 222 and Seca flat digital scale model 877, respectively (Seca Medical Measuring Systems and Scales, Hamburg, Germany).

2.3.2. Blood Pressure

Blood pressure was measured manually using a Reister stethoscope (model: Anestophon) and sphygmomanometer (model: Big Ben; Rudolf Riester GmbH, Jungingen, Germany). All BP instruments were tested and approved by the British and Irish Hypertension Society (BHS) Validation Service [41]. Blood pressure was assessed according to the recommendations described in Kallioinen et al. [42]. Systolic and diastolic pressures together with HR were noted. Baseline RPP (RPP = heart rate x systolic arterial pressure) and MAP (MAP = ((Systolic blood pressure − Diastolic blood pressure) ÷ 3) + Diastolic blood pressure) were then estimated [19,24].

2.3.3. HRV Data Acquisition

Garmin 920XT (Garmin Ltd., Olathe, KS, USA) was used to record HRV in the resting supine position prior to the aerobic capacity test. The Garmin 920XT has been reported to have high HRV accuracy compared to ECG measurements when recording at rest in the supine position [15]. Prior to measuring HRV, Garmin HRM-Tri was placed around the center of the chest and below the level of the breasts. Garmin HRM-Tri uses ANT+ technology to transfer heart rate measures to the Garmin 920XT using a 2.4 GHz ANT wireless communication protocol. To measure Short-Term HRV (5 min), the Garmin 920XT was preprogramed to record for 10 min. The 10 min recording was chosen to ensure that the participants had enough time to acclimatize to the recording environment [4], and to record enough data points to be able achieve a clean 5 min of HRV recording [1,3,43]. To ensure comparability of results across studies and laboratories, the short-term (5 min) recording was adopted in line with the task force recommendations [3].

2.3.4. Aerobic Capacity Test

The mask size for each participant was chosen to insure headspace correction, and the Vyntus CPX gas analyzer (Model: versatile JAEGER; Vyaire medical, Hoechberg, Germany) was calibrated using the fully automated 2-point gas calibration of the O_2/CO_2, through a special Twin Tube sample line combined with a fresh air flush system [44]. The participants were tested on a motorized treadmill (Ergo ELG 55) that was connected to a programmable external WOODWAY User-System version 2.0 (Woodway GmbH, Weilam Rhein, Germany). The modified Bruce continuous incremental test protocol was used to test the participants [45]. The test continued until the participant could no longer continue the test (to exhaustion). Allometrically scaled [45,46] peak VO2 ($VO2_{peak}{}^{\wedge 0.67}$), respiratory exchange ratio (RER), breaths per minute (BPM), maximum heartrate (HR_{max}) and time to exhaustion were recorded using the breath-by-breath method powered by Vyaire's SentrySuite software (Vyaire medical, Hoechberg, Germany). The following criteria had to be met for the measures to be accepted: (i) VO2 plateaued despite increased exercise intensity and (ii) RER > 1.0. Further methodological details are provided in the supplementary materials (S1: methodological details).

2.4. *HRV Data Management*

The IBI time series was retrieved from Garmin 920XT through Garmin connect by downloading the Garmin FIT file. The Garmin FIT file was thereafter imported to Kubios Standard HRV version 3.3 (Kuopio Oy, Finland) for further analysis. The analysis was conducted according to the recommendations [3,6] with a smooth priors detrending method and a sampling frequency of 500 Hz.

2.4.1. Artifact Identification

To be able to obtain a clean short-term 5 min of IBI time series, the last 6 min of the recording was exported from Kubios to a text file for artifact identification. If the last 6 min of the recording had ≥5% artifact, the HRV data of the participant were disqualified from further analysis. Artifacts were first visually inspected [3], then the IBI time series was examined for artifacts using the Berntson et al. [43] artifact detection algorithm, which is based on a real estimation of the distribution of IBI differences from the individual participants' IBI data. Then, percentile-based distribution indices were applied, and a removal of the artifact from the first and fourth quartile was carried out to calculate an estimate of the overall artifact-free standard deviation leading to a final calculation of the IBI threshold criterion for the difference between IBI to identify the artifact. This procedure was carried out automatically using ARTiiFACT tool version 2.13 (University of Würzburg, Würzburg, Germany) [47]. The artifact was identified and manually deleted from the IBI data series [43,47]. In their report, the task force [3] recommended reporting the number of data points edited and analyzed; therefore, Table 3 represents the artefact identification based on 6 min and the final number of data points analyzed based on 5 min.

Table 3. Identification and deletion of the artefact based on the last 6 recorded minutes and the number of the final data points used in HRV analysis.

	Based on the Last 6 min			Based on 5 min
Participant Number	Total Data Point	Artifact	Percentage	Total Data Point Analyzed
P. 1	392	17	4.3	333
P. 2	445	0	0.0	369
P. 3	434	0	0.0	363
P. 4	396	1	0.3	329
P. 5	457	4	0.9	383
P. 6	391	2	0.5	324
P. 7	420	0	0.0	349
P. 8	369	2	0.5	309

2.4.2. Measurements of HRV Indices

The cleaned IBI data were then imported to Kubios in order to calculate measures of HRV indices. From the time domain method, MeanRR (ms), SDNN (ms), RMSSD (ms) and pNN50 (%) were estimated. From the frequency domain method, HF (0.15–0.4 Hz) and LF (0.04–0.15 Hz) in absolute values of power (ms^2) and normalized units (HF or LF/(HF+LF) × 100) were estimated. From the nonlinear (Poincaré plot) method, SD1 and SD2 were estimated [3,6,7]. To standardize and advance the field of study, source data and all calculations of HRV are provided (S1: Source data and all calculations of HRV).

2.5. Statistical Analysis

The data were prepared for analyses using Microsoft Excel for office 365 version 16 (Microsoft, Redmond, WA, USA). Thereafter, all statistical analyses were conducted using R package version 3.5.3 (R Core Team, Vienna, Austria) and RStudio version 1.2.5033 (RStudio Team, Boston, MA, USA). The Bayesian estimation of correlation (Bayesian reallocation of credibility across possibilities also known as the Bayes' rule) was calculated using the Bayesian hierarchical model with Markov Chain Monte Carlo (MCMC) simulation as a part of the model, which is integrated in JAGS package version 4.3.0 (Martyn Plummer, international agency for research on cancer, Lyon, France). However, the Bayes' rule dictates that the Bayesian estimated correlation has equal probability to fall at any point within the 95% HDI. Therefore, an estimated coefficient (*rho* = median) would not be enough evidence of association if the 95% HDI overlapped zero [48,49]. The R code (S1: The R code) provides the complete script, including the model specification and the graphics commands adapted from and adjusted after Kruschke [49]. The MCMC simulation was carried out by running 3 "chains", 500 "adapt" steps, 500 steps to "burn-in" and 10th place as a number of "thin" with 20,000 samples to save for each variable in this study [49]. To apply the model [49–51], the data should be reasonably normally distributed and not be too kurtotic [49]. Therefore, the data were explored through a histogram plot, and the normality of distribution was tested using Shapiro–Wilk's test, Skewness and Kurtosis (the p value for the Shapiro–Wilk's test was set to $p \leq 0.05$). For the data to be considered too kurtotic, the kurtosis should exceed ± 3 [52]. The descriptive statistics were reported as Bayesian estimated median ± 95% HDI and standard deviations (SD) ± 95% HDI of the estimated SD median for all the participants on all recorded variables in this study (Table 4). Furthermore, to be able to make an intuitive decision regarding the size of the Bayesian estimation of correlation, Cohen's effect size for correlation was adapted, where a correlation of 0.1–0.29, 0.3–0.49 and >0.5 were classified as small, medium and large, respectively [53]. Due to the small sample size, the data produced by the MCMC simulation had to pass several criteria: Firstly, retrospective power analysis using "Posterior predictive checks (PPC)", which is described in details in [49,54]. The code for the model check is embedded within the R code (S1: The R code). However, the PPC was qualitatively assessed visually by examining the model and the actual data collected. The figures (S1: The complete correlation figures) show that the superimposed ellipses from the model on the scatter plot of the data effectively contain the data giving a good indication that the model fits the data produced in this study. Secondly, the values of the MCMC chain had to meet the criteria of representativeness and accuracy by examining the convergence of the MCMC algorithm which was checked visually (trace plot and density plot) and numerically (potential scale factor, effective sample size and Monte Carlo standard error) using the approach described by [49] (Figure 1; S1: methodological details). Thirdly, the data produced, should be in line with the data reported in the literature regarding the norms of measuring (see Section 4.1.). Fourthly, the relationships between indices of HRV produced in this study should be comparable to the relationships between HRV indices reported in the literature, as it has been shown that this relationship is very stable and remains stable because the SNS and PNS change dynamically.

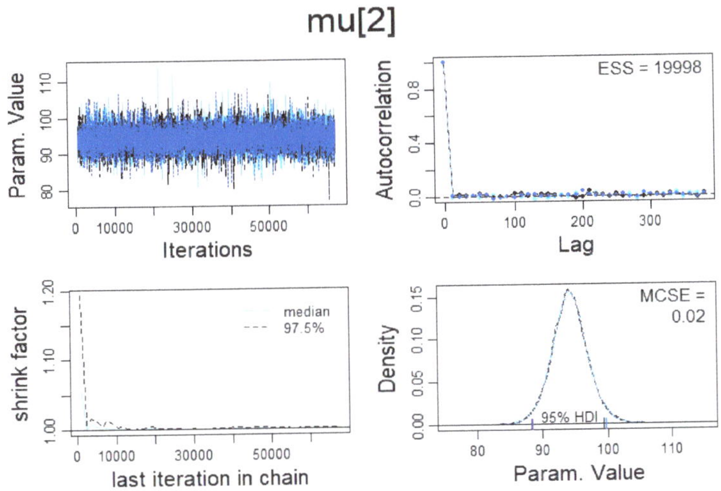

Figure 1. Example of representativeness and accuracy checks by examining the convergence of the Markov Chain Monte Carlo (MCMC) algorithm (the figure describes the convergence diagnostics for the variable MAP).

3. Results

3.1. Sample Characteristics

Examining the normality of distribution using Shapiro–Wilk's test, Skewness and Kurtosis (Table 4), it was found that all variables were approximately normally distributed except for BPM. Therefore, BPM were log transformed and a second examination of normality indicated an approximately normally distributed BPM (Table 4). The data were found to not exceed the kurtosis threshold of ±3 [52]. Sample characteristics are presented in Table 4.

3.2. The Relationship within HRV Indices

The results from the estimated Bayesian correlation between time, frequency and nonlinear domains indicate a clear relationship between SDNN (ms) and LF ms^2 (*rho* = 0.9) with a higher probability (95% HDI) that the true correlation falls between *rho* = 0.568 and *rho* = 0.982. Similar results can be observed between SDNN (ms) and SD2 (Table 5). Furthermore, a relationship with a high probability that the correlation is large between RMSSD (ms) with HF ms^2 and SD1 was detected (Table 5). Similar results can be observed for the pNN50 (%) relationship with HF ms^2 and SD1 (Table 5). The results further show a clear indication of a large correlation between SD1 and HF ms^2 and between SD2 and LF ms^2 (Table 5).

Table 4. Bayesian estimated mean and SD ± HDI, Shapiro–Wilk's test, Skewness and Kurtosis of the raw data.

Variable	Mean ± (95% HDI)	SD ± (95% HDI)	Shapiro–Wilk's Test (Sig.)	Skewness	Kurtosis
Mean HR (bpm)	69.3 (65.5–73.1)	4.93 (3.11–8.78)	0.870	0.17	−1.14
Min HR (bpm)	64.5 (61.3–67.5)	3.91 (2.46–7.06)	0.811	−0.11	−1.08
Max HR (bpm)	76 (71.2–81)	6.13 (4.01–11.3)	0.979	0.00	0.92
MeanRR (ms)	873 (824–924)	58.7 (40.1–111)	0.896	0.06	−1.09
SDNN (ms)	28.9 (20.4–37.1)	9.93 (6.59–18.5)	0.911	0.24	−0.22
RMSSD (ms)	23.8 (17.4–30.8)	8.17 (5.23–14.8)	0.185	0.09	−2.18
pNN50 (%)	5.34 (1.11–9.51)	5.22 (3.39–9.48)	0.132	0.49	−1.64
HF (ms^2)	179 (92.2–273)	110 (73.2–205)	0.677	0.56	−0.73
LF (ms^2)	696 (244–1150)	552 (354–1010)	0.255	1.36	2.34
HF (n.u)	28.2 (13.1–42.9)	18.6 (11.6–33.1)	0.158	1.22	1.65
LF (n.u)	71.7 (57.5–87.2)	17.7 (11.8–33.5)	0.170	−1.19	1.57
SD1	17 (12.3–21.8)	5.68 (3.84–10.7)	0.181	0.09	−2.19
SD2	36.6 (25.6–48)	13.5 (8.81–25.1)	0.734	0.29	0.35
RPP (mmHg/min)	9330 (8210–10,400)	1320 (893–2480)	0.333	0.83	1.05
MAP (mmHg)	94.4 (88.6–99.9)	6.98 (4.48–12.5)	0.090	1.52	2.30
$VO2_{peak}{}^{-67}$	123 (105–140)	21.2 (13.6–38.6)	0.167	0.37	−1.75
RER	1.13 (1.06–1.19)	0.08 (0.05–0.15)	0.920	−0.00	−1.02
BPM	41.5 (34.4–48.4)	8.49 (5.7–15.9)	0.047 * (Nor. 0.097)	1.26 (Nor. 1.10)	0.28 (Nor. −0.18)
HRmax (bpm)	170 (165–176)	6.29 (4.17–11.7)	0.791	−0.01	1.01
Time to exhaustion (s)	842 (718–956)	140 (91.3–261)	0.192	−0.89	0.19

MeanRR = average time for successive heart beats; SDNN = standard deviation of all Normal–Normal intervals; RMSSD = root mean square of SDs between successive N–N intervals; pNN50 = percent of successive intervals with a difference greater that 50 ms compared to previous interval; HF = high frequency; LF = low frequency; SD1 = standard descriptor 1; SD2 = standard descriptor 2; RPP = rate-pressure product; MAP = mean arterial blood pressure; RER = respiratory exchange ratio; BPM = breaths per minute; HRmax = maximum heartrate during exercise; Nor. = calculation after transforming the data that were not observed to follow normality; HDI = high density interval; * = $p \leq 0.05$.

Table 5. Correlation matrix between HRV measures from time domain, frequency domain and nonlinear domain.

Variable		HF (ms^2)	LF (ms^2)	HF (n.u)	LF (n.u)	SD1	SD2
MeanRR (ms)	*rho*	0.357	−0.465	0.324	−0.332	0.231	−0.393
	Upper 95% HDI	0.793	0.284	0.802	0.394	0.799	0.32
	Lower 95% HDI	−0.378	−0.85	−0.392	−0.803	−0.397	−0.824
SDNN (ms)	*rho*	0.651	0.9	−0.702	0.653	0.765	0.918
	Upper 95% HDI	0.923	0.982	−0.074	0.932	0.954	0.987
	Lower 95% HDI	0.041	0.568	−0.937	0.065	0.235	0.654
RMSSD (ms)	*rho*	0.9	0.716	−0.177	0.269	0.92	0.721
	Upper 95% HDI	0.982	0.943	0.464	0.767	0.987	0.947
	Lower 95% HDI	0.567	0.093	−0.752	−0.464	0.665	0.141
pNN50 (%)	*rho*	0.896	0.749	−0.307	0.282	0.907	0.785
	Upper 95% HDI	0.984	0.946	0.42	0.778	0.98	0.953
	Lower 95% HDI	0.574	0.146	−0.781	−0.416	0.588	0.23
SD1	*rho*	0.895	0.691	−0.146	0.179		
	Upper 95% HDI	0.982	0.94	0.483	0.724		
	Lower 95% HDI	0.582	0.1	−0.742	−0.507		
SD2	*rho*	0.605	0.893	−0.731	0.724		
	Upper 95% HDI	0.901	0.98	−0.137	0.942		
	Lower 95% HDI	−0.083	0.575	−0.94	0.135		

3.3. The Relationship between Measures of HRV Indices and Measurments of Blood Pressure Indices and Aerobic Capacity Performance

The results from the correlation between measures of HRV and measurements of blood pressure and aerobic capacity performance (Table 6) indicate a high probability (95% HDI) of a relationship between MeanRR and RPP (Figure 2A), SDNN (ms) and RPP (Figure 2B), pNN50 and MAP (Figure 2C), LF (ms^2) and RPP (Figure 2D) and finally SD2 and RPP (Figure 2E). The complete correlation figures are provided in the supplementary materials (S1. The complete correlation figures).

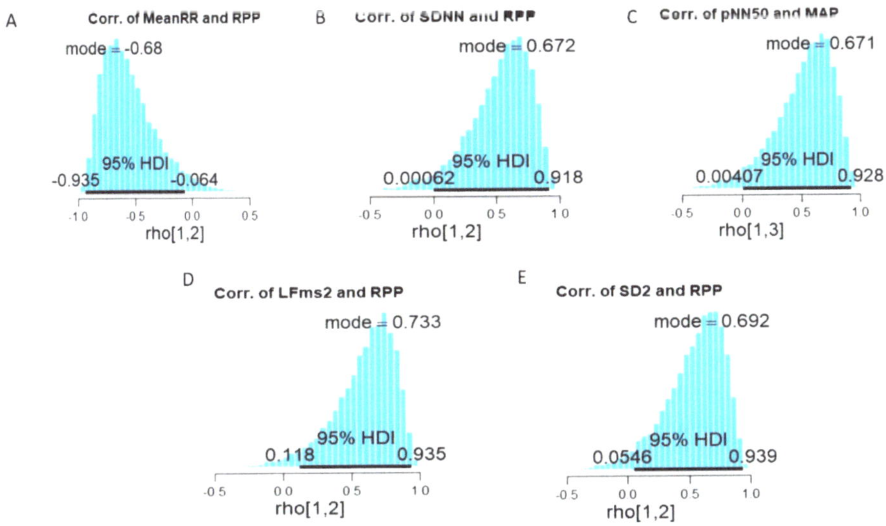

Figure 2. The probability of association between MeanRR and RPP (**A**), SDNN (ms) and RPP (**B**), pNN50 and MAP (**C**), LF (ms^2) and RPP (**D**), SD2 and RPP (**E**).

Table 6. Correlation matrix between HRV measures from time domain, frequency domain and nonlinear domain.

Variable		RPP	MAP	PeakVO2	BPM	HRmax	Time
MeanRR (ms)	*rho*	−0.68	0.134	0.44	0.050	−0.144	0.464
	Upper 95% HDI	−0.064	0.676	0.858	0.655	0.563	0.853
	Lower 95% HDI	−0.935	−0.564	−0.251	−0.601	−0.682	−0.249
SDNN (ms)	*rho*	0.672	0.578	0.132	−0.195	0.488	−0.398
	Upper 95% HDI	0.918	0.89	0.724	0.423	0.863	0.344
	Lower 95% HDI	0.001	−0.12	−0.521	−0.778	−0.216	−0.819
RMSSD (ms)	*rho*	0.366	0.605	0.419	−0.209	0.668	−0.221
	Upper 95% HDI	0.83	0.912	0.843	0.488	0.91	0.415
	Lower 95% HDI	−0.319	−0.058	−0.278	−0.737	−0.044	−0.788
pNN50 (%)	*rho*	0.376	0.671	0.423	−0.237	0.629	−0.37
	Upper 95% HDI	0.827	0.928	0.833	0.432	0.907	0.36
	Lower 95% HDI	−0.31	0.004	−0.323	−0.765	−0.056	−0.805
HF (ms^2)	*rho*	0.303	0.639	0.461	−0.153	0.626	−0.295
	Upper 95% HDI	0.782	0.924	0.858	0.481	0.917	0.412
	Lower 95% HDI	−0.426	−0.017	−0.257	−0.74	−0.06	−0.787
LF (ms^2)	*rho*	0.733	0.629	0.031	−0.227	0.41	−0.323
	Upper 95% HDI	0.935	0.904	0.624	0.434	0.819	0.371
	Lower 95% HDI	0.118	−0.095	−0.624	−0.772	−0.328	−0.81
HF (n.u)	*rho*	−0.346	−0.177	−0.157	−0.061	−0.089	−0.023
	Upper 95% HDI	0.388	0.477	0.496	0.641	0.558	0.613
	Lower 95% HDI	−0.8	−0.757	−0.729	−0.615	−0.702	−0.647
LF (n.u)	*rho*	0.345	0.246	0.16	0.011	0.064	−0.009
	Upper 95% HDI	0.804	0.748	0.719	0.633	0.683	0.616
	Lower 95% HDI	−0.379	−0.471	−0.528	−0.624	−0.559	−0.638
SD1	*rho*	0.362	0.599	0.473	−0.217	0.652	−0.303
	Upper 95% HDI	0.825	0.909	0.856	0.497	0.916	0.426
	Lower 95% HDI	−0.344	−0.064	−0.28	−0.747	−0.055	−0.782
SD2	*rho*	0.692	0.551	0.078	−0.242	0.481	−0.403
	Upper 95% HDI	0.939	0.906	0.672	0.42	0.852	0.326
	Lower 95% HDI	0.055	−0.134	−0.578	−0.785	−0.265	−0.824

4. Discussion

The primary purpose of the present study was to use the Bayesian estimation of correlation to estimate the association between measures of HRV indices, aerobic performance and blood pressure indices using MCMC simulation in an attempt to explain the conflicting results reported in the literature by qualitatively comparing the reported results with the Bayesian estimated results. Hence, to assure the validity of the data presented in this study, a secondary aim was to compare the data produced to the reported norms and to investigate the estimation of the association within the HRV indices in comparison to those reported. The main finding in this study was that the simulation of 20,000 samples to produce the posterior possible association resulted in similar data that were within the reported norms. Furthermore, the association within the HRV indices is in line with what has been reported in the literature. Hence, the Bayesian estimation of correlation using MCMC simulation reproduced and supported the findings reported regarding the norms and within the HRV indices associations. Furthermore, the results of the Bayesian estimation showed that the association between HRV indices and aerobic performance parameters was unclear, indicated by the estimated *rho*, which has an equal chance to fall within the 95% HDI. Finally, a confirmed probability of association between HRV indices (PNS & SNS) and RPP was observed, and a trivial probability of association between pNN50 (%) and MAP at resting condition were also detected.

4.1. Measures of HRV Indices Compared to Norms

At the time of the task force report, there had been no comprehensive investigation regarding HRV indices, and the reported normal values were based on a few studies reporting both long and short term recordings [3]. The approximate values reported for the short-term recording (5 min) were for the LF ms^2 = 1170 ± 416, HF ms^2 = 975 ± 203, LF nu = 54 ± 4 and HF nu = 29 ± 3 [3]. It should be noted that the task force report did not account for age, sex, environment and recording condition (supine (rest), reactivation (during training) and rest (post activation)). Therefore, the normal values from the task force report could be considered incomparable to currently available studies. The most recent comprehensive HRV indices normal values were reported by Nunan et al. [40]. They investigated 3141 studies for suitability and concluded that from these, 44 studies were suitable (based on the task force guidelines) for further analysis with a total number of 21,438 participants. The study [40] accounted for age, sex, environment, recording condition and was based on short-term recordings (5 min). Furthermore, another investigation examining the Nunan et al. [40] study was conducted by Shaffer and Ginsberg [6]. It indicated that the participants reported on in the Nunan et al. [40] study had a minimum age of 40 years and were classified based on their sex. Therefore, the author of the present study feels that the Nunan et al. [40] study would be the most appropriate study for comparison with the results from this study. Based on the most credible value reported in Table 4, all participants of this study were within the normal range for MeanRR (873 ± 59 ms compared to the normal value range 785–1160 ms), SDNN (29 ± 10 ms compared to the normal value range 32–93 ms), RMSSD (24 ± 8 ms compared to the normal value range 19–75 ms), LF (ms^2) (696 ± 552 ms^2 compared to the normal value range 193–1009 ms^2), LF (nu) (72 ± 18 nu compared to the normal value range 30–65 nu), HF (ms^2) (179 ± 110 ms^2 compared to the normal value range 83–3630 ms^2) and HF (nu) (28 ± 19 nu compared to the normal value range 16–60 nu). Despite the fact that the measured variables in this study fall within the reported norms, the values were lower in this study compared to the norms data. This could be due to the participants in this study being older (53.9 ± 5.7 years) compared to those reported in Nunan et al. [40] (40 years old) and the different systems used for recording HRV. Research suggests that older people tend to have lower HRV indices values compared to younger people [2,6,7]. However, further research is needed to address the norms of HRV based on age, sex, environment and testing condition. For this reason, the source data are attached to this report (S1: Source data and all calculations of HRV). No further comparisons were possible because the normal values reported in Nunan et al. [40] did not report on all the estimated HRV metrics in this study.

4.2. The Association within HRV Indices

The most credible estimate of correlation value found in this study was first between SDNN (ms) (which reflects all factors contributing to HRV including SNS and PNS activities [7,8,10]) and LF ms^2 band (*rho* = 0.9; 95% HDI = 0.568–0.982; Table 5). This relationship is in line with most of the reported studies [6–8,10]. However, HRV can be analyzed using the HF band (0.15–0.4 Hz) and the LF band (0.04–0.15 Hz). The LF band has been shown to reflect mainly the SNS activities in several studies [2,3,6,7,10,16,40,55,56]; however, due to the fact the this study measured HRV in resting condition, the relationship between SDNN (ms) and LF ms^2 could be explained by baroreflex activity affecting the LF band compared to cardiac sympathetic innervation [2,3,6,7,10,16,40,55,56]. Hence, the fact that the PNS affects heart rhythms down to 0.05 Hz compared to the SNS, which has been reported to produce up to 0.1 Hz [6,16], explains the oscillations in the heart rhythms that can occur during resting vagal activities which cross over into the LF band [2,3,6,7,10,16,40,55,56], thus explaining the observed association in the present study. This explanation can be further confirmed by the strong association observed between the RMSSD and HF band compared to the LF band (Table 5) as RMSSD was suggested to be mainly influenced by PNS [6,10,57]. Similar results can be observed between SDNN and SD2 which represent the short- and long-term HRV [6,7] with the most credible correlation value of *rho* = 0.918 (95% HDI = 0.654–0.987; Table 5). Since SD2 reflects both SNS and PNS activities contributing to HRV (similar to LF), this association was expected and in line with what has been reported in the literature [6,7]. The similarity between SD2 and LF can be further demonstrated by the most credible relationship values found between the two in this study (*rho* = 0.893; 95% HDI = 0.575–0.98; Table 5).

Considering that the LF band does not cross the HF band [6,16], researchers concluded that the HF band reflects PSN/vagal activities [2,3,6,7,10,13,16,40,56], which is why it was later named the respiratory band as it relates to HRV indices related to breathing [6]. Therefore, it was expected that HF ms^2 would have a strong relationship with RMSSD, as the RMSSD was classified as the primary time domain measure that reflects changes related to vagal activities affecting HRV [7,16,57]. This relationship was confirmed in the current study, and the results showed that the most credible correlation value between the two was *rho* = 0.9 (95% HDI = 0.567–0.982; Table 5). Furthermore, since pNN50 and RMSSD were reported to reflect short-term HRV changes and both reflect the PNS activities [6,57], it was expected that the pNN50 would add further affirmation to the results in this study when compared to the other studies. Indeed, the relationship found between pNN50 (%) and HF ms^2 in this study confirms the association between RMSSD and HF ms^2 (Table 5; *rho* = 0.896; 95% HDI = 0.574–0.984). Moreover, the SD1, which represents the fast beat to beat variability in IBI [7], has been reported to be the nonlinear domain metric that is identical to the time domain metric RMSSD [6]; the similarity between SD1 and HF, which correlates with baroreflex sensitivity [6,7], dictated the expectation that SD1 would correlate with RMSSD (*rho* = 0.92; 95% HDI = 0.665–0.987) and HF (*rho* = 0.895; 95% HDI = 0.582–0.982) which further confirms the relationship between the HF and RMSSD (Table 5).

It should be noted that no further confirmed probable associations were observed between time, frequency and nonlinear-domain variables in comparison to those reported by the task force [3] (Table 5). However, this might be due to the short-term measurement (5 min) used in this study compared to the 24 h measurements reported in the task force report, where the lack of association was caused by "both mathematical and physiological relationships [3]". Furthermore, the used statistical analysis in this study, which is based on the Bayesian estimation of correlation [49], indicates that the highest probability (95% HDI) of the correlation values overlapped zero or near zero; therefore, those relationships were regarded as unclear. Finally, the reported short-term estimated relationships between time, frequency and nonlinear-domain variables reported in the literature [2,3,6,7,10,13,16,56] are comparable to the associations observed in this study.

4.3. The Relationship between Measures of HRV Indices and Both Measures of Blood Pressure Indices and Aerobic Capacity Parameters

The Bayesian estimation of correlation relocates credibility across possibilities [49–51]. Thus, the possibilities are reflected by the 95% HDI, and the probability of the estimated Bayesian correlation falling at any point within the 95% HDI is equal. Based on the Bayes' rule, an estimated coefficient (*rho* = median) would not be enough evidence of association if the 95% HDI overlapped zero [48,49]. Therefore, the findings from this study did not provide enough evidence of the association between the measures of HRV indices and the parameters from the aerobic capacity test (i.e., $VO2_{Peak}$, BPM, HR_{max} and Time to exhaustion; Table 6). Nevertheless, the results (Table 6 and Figure 2) indicate a possible association (regardless of the strength) between pNN50% and MAP, MeanRR (ms) and RPP, SDNN (ms) and RPP, LF (ms^2) and RPP and SD2 and RPP (Figure 2).

Several studies have investigated changes in HRV indices as a result of performance adaptations in response to different exercise protocols. The results of these studies indeed confirm that changes in $VO2_{max}$ are accompanied by changes in HRV indices [21,23,26–28,31]. The changes observed differed based on age and measuring condition (i.e., supine, standing) [28], duration of intervention [27,28,38], participants' background [23,26] and measurement of time of day [39]. Nevertheless, the fact that research shows that the measures of resting HRV were not affected by exercise in the middle-aged group (50–59 years old) compared to the young group [26,28], that changes in HRV indices appear to flatten after 12 weeks of exercise [27] and that the maintenance of those changes could be achieved by exercising regularly [26], could in part explain *i)* the lack of evidence of association between measures of HRV indices and variables from the aerobic capacity test in this study and ii) the conflicting results reported in the literature. Another possible explanation is the newly reported results by Phoemsapthawee et al. [38], showing that changes in vagal-related HRV are related to individual ability to adapt to exercise. This was further confirmed by the multiple stepwise regression, which did not show a meaningful relationship between measures of HRV indices and changes in $VO2_{peak}$ [38].

Studies investigated the relationship between measures of HRV indices and aerobic capacity directly and/or indirectly through establishing a prediction model to estimate aerobic capacity using the frequentist approach to data analysis [21,27,29,30,32,33,36,37,58]. Interestingly and regardless of whether the association was observed [30,33,36,37] or not [27,32], all the correlations reported in these studies falls within the 95% HDI reported in this study (Table 6). Several authors proposed explanations for the disparity in the results across those studies, which can be summarized by 3 major reasons: The first reason is the differences in the participants' background, type of sport and age [26,29,32,33,35,58]. The results from these reports confirm that associations were detected in soccer players, distance runners, patients with chronic obstructive pulmonary disease and young people [26,29,32,33,58], but were not confirmed in middle-aged participants, untrained subjects, sprinters and throwers [26,29,32,36]. The variation related to the participants' background was explained by the fact that the participants with already high values of vagal-related HRV indices in resting conditions tend to reach their anaerobic threshold at a higher exercise intensity compared to those who have lower values of vagal-related HRV indices [33]. The second reason is measurement position (i.e., supine, standing etc.). Studies have reported notably higher PNS activities in the seated rest compared to the standing position [21]. It was further investigated and reported that out of 30 possible correlations between HRV indices and aerobic capacity, only two from the supine position were associated with aerobic capacity compared to 15 from a standing position [32]. The third reason was the measuring time of day and condition (i.e., sleeping, early morning, evening); reported results showed that HRV indices measured in a resting supine position early in the morning (at wake up) did not differ between young and older participants. Nevertheless, the results indicate that there were differences in vagal-related HRV between age groups when measured during sleep, with the young group having higher values [28]. Furthermore, a review conducted by Vitale et al. [39] concluded that higher vagal-related HRV indices in the morning, compared to the evening, were observed and that they differed between individuals, which the authors used further to advise coaches and trainers to consider when planning the timing of exercise. Among all the studies above, no association was reported in a similar age group to the one in this study.

In this study, a possible inverse relationship was detected between MeanRR and RPP (Table 6, Figure 2). This was expected and was confirmed in the majority of published studies: simply stated, when the human body is exposed to a stressful demand (such as standing, performing daily activities and exercise), the SNS activities trigger the heart, and an increase in HR can be observed to meet the demands imposed on the body. This increase in HR is coupled with a decrease in time between the beat to beat interval [22]. This process is a good example of the combined actions of PNS and SNS in opposite directions, where the HR speeds up in response to a stimulus from the SNS and slows down in response to a stimulus from the PNS [59]. This can be further extended to explain the possible positive association observed between HRV indices reflecting mainly SNS activities (LF ms2 and SD2) and RPP (Table 6), indicating that an increase in SNS activities would cause higher RPP [10,16,59]. It is important to be reminded, as described earlier in this article, that the relationship between PNS and SNS is dynamic and that PNS activity could be associated with low, high or no SNS activities [6]. Therefore, the trivial (lower band of the 95% HDI at zero but not overlapping; Table 6) possible association between SDNN and RPP could be explained by the fact that measurements were carried out at resting condition, causing the PNS to be the dominant system. However, since RPP is the product of HR and systolic arterial pressure, and the systolic arterial pressure is only affected by the SNS [59], which has been reported to produce up to 0.1 Hz and crosses over to the LF band, it is expected that this trivial possibility will vanish with increased activity (see Section 4.2.). Finally, the relationship between HRV indices and MAP showed a potential but trivial (since the 95% HDI was almost at zero but not overlapping) possibility for association between pNN50 (a parameter primarily reflecting PNS activity) and MAP (Table 6). Nevertheless, while it was not expected to find a relationship at rest, it was expected that measures of PNS correlate positively with MAP [18]. This association could also be explained by the dynamic relationship between PNS and SNS explained earlier [6]. Furthermore, MAP involves both systolic and diastolic blood pressure [19,24], and the possible association could further be explained by the fact that the autonomic nervous system's role in regulating MAP is to maintain it at the homeostasis level [18]. Hence, an elevation in MAP has been reported to cause a decrease in SNS activities and an increase in PSN activities [6,18,59].

In line with other studies, this study is not without limitations. Due to the difficulties involved in conducting such studies, the sample size was small, but still in line with the recommendation from the task force [3] to be able to establish norms through meta-analysis studies. The small sample size was compensated for by using the within-subjects experimental design as advised [4,5,9], the simulation of data using MCMC producing a simulated sample [49], the retrospective power analysis based on PPC and the assessment of representativeness and accuracy by examining the convergence of the MCMC algorithm. Furthermore, the number of participants in this study is in line with the majority of studies examining HRV in the field [12,15,28,31,35,60]. Participants' in this study were tested during resting supine position only, which can also be viewed as a limitation; however, due to the measurement equipment used in this study, the measurements under other conditions (reactivation (during training) and rest (post-activation)) would have produced unreliable results. For those reasons, and due to the fact that this is the first study within sport sciences that uses the Bayesian estimation of correlation on MCMC simulated data using the 95% HDI, the author has attached all the necessary information for replicability (supplementary materials) in order to contribute to future advancements in the field.

5. Conclusions

The normal values reported in the literature were based on several studies which can be seen as a stable reference to evaluate HRV values. The relationships within the HRV indices can also be seen as stable relationships that are hard to change due to the dynamics between PNS and SNS activities. Hence, the Bayesian estimation of correlation using MCMC simulated data produced similar HRV values to the norms reported in the literature, and the associations found within HRV indices (time, frequency and nonlinear) were also in line with what has been reported in the literature. Nevertheless, while the measures in this study fell within the reported norms, the values were lower, which may have been caused by the Bayesian hierarchical model having a higher precision in calculating the most credible values of the Mean compared to the frequentist Mean value. However, this argument is not completely valid unless more studies are carried out. Therefore, it would be helpful if the reported studies could publish their data sources for other researchers to able to assess the data using the Bayesian hierarchical model and compare the results with what has been reported. Alternatively, the lower values could also have been caused by different recording conditions (supine, reactivation, rest), recording systems, time of day (morning, evening, sleep etc.) and age of participants, which would clearly give different results. Hence, it is advised to use the same condition and recording system when the repeated measure is intended. Furthermore, it could be noted that PNS and SNS activities are dynamic and depend on the individual's baseline physiological and psychologically abilities and the ability to adapt to stressors, suggesting that the disparity in the association between the measures of HRV indices and aerobic capacity could be caused by a different dynamic between the two systems among individuals. Hence, it is expected that two individuals with the same aerobic capacity would have different PNS and SNS activities dynamics. Furthermore, the fact that PNS activity could be associated with low, high or no SNS activities and that it is individually based could explain the disparity in the results reported in the literature. Therefore, further investigation of the dynamics between PNS and SNS in different participants who share the same physiological abilities is strongly advised. Hence, the results from this investigation are valid only for the participants in this study and at the time of participation. Finally, the use of the Bayesian estimation of correlation with 95% HDI on MCMC simulated data is a new technique for data analysis in sport science and seems to provide a more robust approach to allocating credibility through a meaningful mathematical model. However, the 95% HDI found in this study, accompanied by the theoretical explanations regarding the dynamics between PNS and SNS in relation to different recording conditions (supine, reactivation, rest), recording systems, time of day (morning, evening, sleep etc.) and age of participants, suggests that the association between measures of HRV indices and aerobic performance parameters has yet to be explicated.

Supplementary Materials: The following are available online at http://www.mdpi.com/1660-4601/17/18/6750/s1; S1: Methodological details; S1: Source data and all calculations of HRV; S1: The R code; S1: The complete correlation figures.

Funding: This research received no external funding.

Acknowledgments: The author would like to acknowledge Mia Alvestad Bay assistant in administrating, coordinating and testing.

Conflicts of Interest: The author declares no conflict of interest.

References

1. Berntson, G.G.; Bigger, J.T., Jr.; Eckberg, D.L.; Grossman, P.; Kaufmann, P.G.; Malik, M.; Nagaraja, H.N.; Porges, S.W.; Saul, J.P.; Stone, P.H.; et al. Heart rate variability: Origins, methods, and interpretive caveats. *Psychophysiology* **1997**, *34*, 623–648. [CrossRef] [PubMed]
2. Sessa, F.; Anna, V.; Messina, G.; Cibelli, G.; Monda, V.; Marsala, G.; Ruberto, M.; Biondi, A.; Cascio, O.; Bertozzi, G.; et al. Heart rate variability as predictive factor for sudden cardiac death. *Aging* **2018**, *10*, 166–177. [CrossRef] [PubMed]
3. Task_Force. Heart rate variability: Standards of measurement, physiological interpretation and clinical use. Task Force of the European Society of Cardiology and the North American Society of Pacing and Electrophysiology. *Circulation* **1996**, *93*, 1043–1065. [CrossRef]
4. Laborde, S.; Mosley, E.; Thayer, J.F. Heart Rate Variability and Cardiac Vagal Tone in Psychophysiological Research—Recommendations for Experiment Planning, Data Analysis, and Data Reporting. *Front. Psychol.* **2017**, *8*. [CrossRef] [PubMed]
5. Quintana, D.S.; Heathers, J.A.J. Considerations in the assessment of heart rate variability in biobehavioral research. *Front. Psychol* **2014**, *5*, 805. [CrossRef] [PubMed]
6. Shaffer, F.; Ginsberg, J.P. An overview of heart rate variability metrics and norms. *Front. Public Health* **2017**, *5*, 258. [CrossRef]
7. Dong, J.G. The role of heart rate variability in sports physiology (Review). *Exp. Ther. Med.* **2016**, *11*, 1531–1536. [CrossRef]
8. Bradley, M.A.; Luecken, L.J. Heart rate variability as an index of regulated emotional responding. *Rev. Gen. Psychol.* **2006**, *10*, 229–240. [CrossRef]
9. Quintana, D.S.; Alvares, G.A.; Heathers, J.A. Guidelines for Reporting Articles on Psychiatry and Heart rate variability (GRAPH): Recommendations to advance research communication. *Transl. Psychiatry* **2016**, *6*, e803. [CrossRef]
10. Shaffer, F.; McCraty, R.; Zerr, C.L. A healthy heart is not a metronome: An integrative review of the heart's anatomy and heart rate variability. *Front. Psychol.* **2014**, *5*, 1040. [CrossRef]
11. Castaneda, D.; Esparza, A.; Ghamari, M.; Soltanpur, C.; Nazeran, H. A review on wearable photoplethysmography sensors and their potential future applications in health care. *Int. J. Biosens. Bioelectron.* **2018**, *4*, 195–202. [CrossRef] [PubMed]
12. Kingsley, M.; Lewis, M.J.; Marson, R.E. Comparison of Polar 810s and an ambulatory ECG system for RR interval measurement during progressive exercise. *Int. J. Sports Med.* **2005**, *26*, 39–44. [CrossRef] [PubMed]
13. Nunan, D.; Donovan, G.; Jakovljevic, D.G.; Hodges, L.D.; Sandercock, G.R.; Brodie, D.A. Validity and reliability of short-term heart-rate variability from the Polar S810. *Med. Sci. Sports Exerc.* **2009**, *41*, 243–250. [CrossRef] [PubMed]
14. Hernando, D.; Garatachea, N.; Almeida, R.; Casajus, J.A.; Bailon, R. Validation of Heart Rate Monitor Polar RS800 for Heart Rate Variability Analysis During Exercise. *J. Strength Cond. Res.* **2016**, *32*, 716–725. [CrossRef] [PubMed]

15. Cassirame, J.; Vanhaesebrouck, R.; Chevrolat, S.; Mourot, L. Accuracy of the Garmin 920 XT HRM to perform HRV analysis. *Australas. Phys. Eng. Sci. Med.* **2017**, *40*, 831–839. [CrossRef] [PubMed]
16. Fatisson, J.; Oswald, V.; Lalonde, F. Influence diagram of physiological and environmental factors affecting heart rate variability: An extended literature overview. *Heart Int.* **2016**, *11*, e32–e40. [CrossRef]
17. Triplett, N.T. Structure and function of body systems. In *Essentials of Strength Training and Conditioning*, 4th ed.; Haff, G.G., Triplett, N.T., Eds.; Human Kinetics: Champaign, IL, USA, 2016; pp. 1–18.
18. DeMers, D.; Wachs, D. *Physiology, Mean Arterial Pressure*; StatPearls Publishing: Treasure Island, FL, USA, 2019.
19. Ansari, M.; Javadi, H.; Pourbehi, M.; Mogharrabi, M.; Rayzan, M.; Semnani, S.; Jallalat, S.; Amini, A.; Abbaszadeh, M.; Barekat, M.; et al. The association of rate pressure product (RPP) and myocardial perfusion imaging (MPI) findings: A preliminary study. *Perfusion* **2012**, *27*, 207–213. [CrossRef]
20. Chapleau, M.W. Baroreceptor Reflexes. In *Primer on the Autonomic Nervous System*; Low, P.A., Polinsky, R.J., Robertson, D., Robertson, D., Paton, J.F.R., Low, P.A., Eds.; Elsevier Science & Technology: San Diego, CA, USA, 2011; pp. 161–165.
21. Figueroa, M.A.; Demeersman, R.E.; Manning, J. The autonomic and rate pressure product responses of tai chi practitioners. *N. Am. J. Med. Sci.* **2012**, *4*, 270–275. [CrossRef]
22. Kazmi, S.Z.H.; Zhang, H.; Aziz, W.; Monfredi, O.; Abbas, S.A.; Shah, S.A.; Kazmi, S.S.H.; Butt, W.H. Inverse Correlation between Heart Rate Variability and Heart Rate Demonstrated by Linear and Nonlinear Analysis. *PLoS ONE* **2016**, *11*, e0157557. [CrossRef]
23. Papp, M.E.; Lindfors, P.; Storck, N.; Wändell, P.E. Increased heart rate variability but no effect on blood pressure from 8 weeks of hatha yoga—A pilot study. *BMC Res. Notes* **2013**, *6*, 59. [CrossRef]
24. Swank, A.; Sharp, C. Adaptations to aerobic endurance training programs. In *Essentials of Strength Training and Conditioning*, 4th ed.; Haff, G.G., Triplett, N.T., Eds.; Human Kinetics: Champaign, IL, USA, 2016; pp. 115–134.
25. Herda, T.J.; Cramer, J.T. Bioenergetics of Exercise and Training. In *Essentials of Strength Training and Conditioning*, 4th ed.; Haff, G.G., Triplett, N.T., Eds.; Human Kinetics: Champaign, IL, USA, 2016; pp. 43–64.
26. De Meersman, R.E. Heart rate variability and aerobic fitness. *Am. Heart J.* **1993**, *125*, 726–731. [CrossRef]
27. Melanson, E.L.; Freedson, P.S. The effect of endurance training on resting heart rate variability in sedentary adult males. *Eur. J. Appl. Physiol.* **2001**, *85*, 442–449. [CrossRef] [PubMed]
28. Catai, A.M.; Chacon-Mikahil, M.P.; Martinelli, F.S.; Forti, V.A.; Silva, E.; Golfetti, R.; Martins, L.E.; Szrajer, J.S.; Wanderley, J.S.; Lima-Filho, E.C.; et al. Effects of aerobic exercise training on heart rate variability during wakefulness and sleep and cardiorespiratory responses of young and middle-aged healthy men. *Braz. J. Med. Biol. Res.* **2002**, *35*, 741–752. [CrossRef] [PubMed]
29. Kouidi, E.; Haritonidis, K.; Koutlianos, N.; Deligiannis, A. Effects of athletic training on heart rate variability triangular index. *Clin. Physiol. Funct. Imaging* **2002**, *22*, 279–284. [CrossRef] [PubMed]
30. Marocolo, M.; Nadal, J.; Benchimol Barbosa, P.R. The effect of an aerobic training program on the electrical remodeling of heart high-frequency components of the signal-averaged electrocardiogram is a predictor of the maximal aerobic power. *Braz. J. Med. Biol. Res.* **2007**, *40*, 199–208. [CrossRef]
31. Schmitt, L.; Fouillot, J.P.; Millet, G.P.; Robach, P.; Nicolet, G.; Brugniaux, J.; Richalet, J.P. Altitude, heart rate variability and aerobic capacities. *Int. J. Sports Med.* **2008**, *29*, 300–306. [CrossRef]
32. Grant, C.C.; Clark, J.R.; Janse van Rensburg, D.C.; Viljoen, M. Relationship between exercise capacity and heart rate variability: Supine and in response to an orthostatic stressor. *Auton Neurosci.* **2009**, *151*, 186–188. [CrossRef]
33. Leite, M.R.; Ramos, E.M.; Kalva-Filho, C.A.; Rodrigues, F.M.; Freire, A.P.; Tacao, G.Y.; de Toledo, A.C.; Cecílio, M.J.; Vanderlei, L.C.; Ramos, D. Correlation between heart rate variability indexes and aerobic physiological variables in patients with COPD. *Respirology* **2015**, *20*, 273–278. [CrossRef]
34. Flatt, A.A.; Esco, M.R. Evaluating individual training adaptation with smartphone-derived heart rate variability in a collegiate female soccer team. *J. Strength Cond. Res.* **2016**, *30*, 378–385. [CrossRef]
35. Flatt, A.A.; Esco, M.R.; Nakamura, F.Y. Individual Heart Rate Variability Responses to Preseason Training in High Level Female Soccer Players. *J. Strength Cond. Res.* **2017**, *31*, 531–538. [CrossRef]
36. Materko, W. Stratification of the level of aerobic fitness based on heart rate variability parameters in adult males at rest. *Motricidade* **2018**, *14*, 51–57. [CrossRef]

37. Materko, W.; Bartels, R.; Peçanha, T.; Perrout de Lima, J.R.; Carvalho, A.R.S.; Nadal, J. Maximum oxygen uptake prediction model based on heart rate variability parameters for young healthy adult males at rest. *Open Access Biostat. Bioinform.* **2018**, *2*, 1–7. [CrossRef]
38. Phoemsapthawee, J.; Prasertsri, P.; Leelayuwat, N. Heart rate variability responses to a combined exercise training program: Correlation with adiposity and cardiorespiratory fitness changes in obese young men. *J. Exerc. Rehabil.* **2019**, *15*, 114–122. [CrossRef] [PubMed]
39. Vitale, J.A.; Bonato, M.; La Torre, A.; Banfi, G. Heart rate variability in sport performance: Do time of day and chronotype play a role? *J. Clin. Med.* **2019**, *8*, 723. [CrossRef] [PubMed]
40. Nunan, D.; Sandercock, G.R.; Brodie, D.A. A quantitative systematic review of normal values for short-term heart rate variability in healthy adults. *Pacing Clin. Electrophysiol.* **2010**, *33*, 1407–1417. [CrossRef]
41. Society, B.A.I.H. Validated BP Monitors for For Specialist Use. Available online: https://bihsoc.org/bp-monitors/for-specialist-use/ (accessed on 26 February 2020).
42. Kallioinen, N.; Hill, A.; Horswill, M.S.; Ward, H.E.; Watson, M.O. Sources of inaccuracy in the measurement of adult patients' resting blood pressure in clinical settings: A systematic review. *J. Hypertens.* **2017**, *35*, 421–441. [CrossRef]
43. Berntson, G.G.; Quigley, K.S.; Jang, J.F.; Boysen, S.T. An approach to artifact identification: Application to heart period data. *Psychophysiology* **1990**, *27*, 586–598. [CrossRef]
44. Vyaire, m. Vyntus CPX Powered by SentrySuite. Available online: https://www.vyaire.com/Documents/international/brochures/respiratory-care/cardiopulmonary/RC_Vyntus-CPX_BR_EN.pdf (accessed on 10 December 2018).
45. Gibson, A.L.; Wagner, D.R.; Heyward, V.H. *Advanced Fitness Assessment and Exercise Prescription*; Human Kinetics: Champaign, IL, USA, 2019.
46. Nevill, A.M.; Ramsbottom, R.; Williams, C. Scaling physiological measurements for individuals of different body size. *Eur. J. Appl. Physiol. Occup. Physiol.* **1992**, *65*, 110–117. [CrossRef]
47. Kaufmann, T.; Sutterlin, S.; Schulz, S.M.; Vogele, C. ARTiiFACT: A tool for heart rate artifact processing and heart rate variability analysis. *Behav. Res. Methods* **2011**, *43*, 1161–1170. [CrossRef]
48. Hooten, M.B.; Hefley, T.J. *Bringing Bayesian Models to Life*; CRC Press, Taylor & Francis Group: Boca Raton, FL, USA, 2019.
49. Kruschke, J.K. *Doing Bayesian Data Analysis. A Tutorial with R, JAGS, and Stan*, 2nd ed.; Elsevier: Oxford, UK, 2015.
50. Kruschke, J.K.; Liddell, T.M. Bayesian data analysis for newcomers. *Psychon. Bull. Rev.* **2018**, *25*, 155–177. [CrossRef]
51. Kruschke, J.K.; Liddell, T.M. The Bayesian New Statistics: Hypothesis testing, estimation, meta-analysis, and power analysis from a Bayesian perspective. *Psychon. Bull. Rev.* **2018**, *25*, 178–206. [CrossRef]
52. DeCarlo, L.T. On the meaning and use of kurtosis. *Psychol. Methods* **1997**, *2*, 292–307. [CrossRef]
53. Cohen, J. *Statistical Power Analysis for the Behavioral Sciences*; Routledge: New York, NY, USA, 1988.
54. Kruschke, J.K. Posterior predictive checks can and should be Bayesian: Comment on Gelman and Shalizi, 'Philosophy and the practice of Bayesian statistics'. *Br. J. Math. Stat. Psychol.* **2013**, *66*, 45–56. [CrossRef]
55. Jarrin, D.C.; McGrath, J.J.; Giovanniello, S.; Poirier, P.; Lambert, M. Measurement fidelity of heart rate variability signal processing: The devil is in the details. *Int. J. Psychophysiol.* **2012**, *86*, 88–97. [CrossRef]
56. Rajendra Acharya, U.; Paul Joseph, K.; Kannathal, N.; Lim, C.M.; Suri, J.S. Heart rate variability: A review. *Med. Biol. Eng. Comput.* **2006**, *44*, 1031–1051. [CrossRef]
57. Stein, P.K. Assessing heart rate variability from real-world Holter reports. *Card. Electrophysiol. Rev.* **2002**, *6*, 239–244. [CrossRef]
58. Sendelides, T.; Metaxas, T.; Koutlianos, N.; Kouidi, E.; Deligiannis, A. Heart rate variability changes in soccer players. *OÉsterr. J. Sportmed.* **2003**, *33*, 10–13.
59. Sherldine, T. The Usefulness of the Rate Pressure Product (RPP) for cardiac rehabilitation exercise prescription. *Intern. Med. Res. Open J.* **2017**, *2*, 1–3.
60. Nasario-Junior, O.; Benchimol-Barbosa, P.R.; Pedrosa, R.C.; Nadal, J. Beat-to-beat ventricular repolarization duration variability assessed by cardiac acceleration and deceleration phases in athletes. *EC Cardiol.* **2015**, *1*, 33–42.

International Journal of
Environmental Research and Public Health

MDPI

Article

Can Post-Activation Performance Enhancement (PAPE) Improve Resistance Training Volume during the Bench Press Exercise?

Michal Krzysztofik [1], Michal Wilk [1,*], Aleksandra Filip [1], Piotr Zmijewski [2], Adam Zajac [1] and James J. Tufano [3]

1 Institute of Sport Sciences, Jerzy Kukuczka Academy of Physical Education in Katowice, 40-065 Katowice, Poland; m.krzysztofik@awf.katowice.pl (M.K.); a.filip@awf.katowice.pl (A.F.); a.zajac@awf.katowice.pl (A.Z.)
2 Jozef Pilsudski University of Physical Education in Warsaw, 00-809 Warsaw, Poland; piotr.zmijewski@insp.waw.pl
3 Faculty of Physical Education and Sport, Charles University, 16000 Prague, Czech Republic; tufano@ftvs.cuni.cz
* Correspondence: m.wilk@awf.katowice.pl

Received: 24 March 2020; Accepted: 7 April 2020; Published: 8 April 2020

Abstract: *Background*: The aim of the present study was to evaluate the effects of post-activation performance enhancement (PAPE) on resistance training volume during the bench press exercise (BP). The study included 12 healthy strength-trained males (age 25.2 ± 2.1 years, body mass 92.1 ± 8.7 kg, BP one-repetition maximum (1RM) 28.8 ± 10.5 kg, training experience 6.3 ± 2.1 years). *Methods*: The experiment was performed following a randomized crossover design, where each participant performed two different exercise protocols with a conditioning activity (CA) consisting of the BP with three sets of three repetitions at 85% 1RM (PAPE), and a control without the CA (CONT). To assess the differences between PAPE and CONT, the participants performed three sets of the BP to volitional failure at 60% 1RM. The differences in the number of performed repetitions (REP), time under tension (TUT), peak power output (PP), mean of peak power output (PP_{MEAN}), mean power output (MP), peak bar velocity (PV), mean of peak bar velocity (PV_{MEAN}), and mean bar velocity (MV) between the CONT and PAPE conditions were examined using repeated measures ANOVA. *Results*: The post-hoc analysis for the main condition effect indicated significant increases in TUT ($p < 0.01$) for the BP following PAPE, compared to the CONT condition. Furthermore, there was a significant increase in TUT ($p < 0.01$) in the third set for PAPE compared to the CONT condition. No statistically significant main effect was revealed for REP, PP, PV, PP_{MEAN}, PV_{MEAN}, MP, and MV. *Conclusion*: The main finding of the study was that the PAPE protocol increased training volume based on TUT, without changes in the number of preformed REP.

Keywords: strength-endurance; repetition; time under tension; power output; bar velocity

1. Introduction

Athletic performance requires a high level of various training components that can be developed through a sports conditioning program. Recently, much attention has been given to acute increases in exercise performance through methods that induce a post-activation performance enhancement (PAPE) evoked by prior muscle activity [1]. PAPE has been defined as a physiological phenomenon which acutely improves voluntary muscular performance (e.g., jumps and throws) following a conditioning activity (CA) which includes a single heavy loaded resistance exercise [2–4] or consecutive sets of a single resistance exercise [5,6]. In training practice, PAPE can be achieved by the use of a CA with a wide range of external loads, ranging from 70% of one-repetition maximum (1RM) [6] to even supramaximal loads of 110–130% 1RM [7]. Furthermore, training experience [8], individual strength level [3], as well as muscle groups involved in the activity may affect the magnitude of subsequent performance enhancement.

To date, studies have focused on the acute changes in power output and velocity of movement during explosive activities (e.g., jumps and throws) directly after various types of CA [4,7]. However, little attention has been given to the potential impact of PAPE on training volume. To achieve a desired training volume, performing a certain number of repetitions (REP) per set, per exercise, and per session significantly affects the adaptive changes to resistance training [9,10]. However, the duration of a single REP is not always the same (it depends on the tempo of movement used), which is why, in addition to the number of performed REP in a set or a whole session, the time under tension (TUT) is considered as a variable describing training volume [11,12]. Furthermore, according to Wilk et al. [12,13], TUT during resistance exercise is a more accurate and credible indicator of the training volume performed compared to the number of performed REP. To date, only two studies have examined the effect of PAPE on resistance training volume of the upper body, yet only one of them considered TUT. Sevilmiş and Atalağ [14] indicated a significantly increased number of performed REP and TUT during a single set of the bench press exercise (BP) performed to volitional failure at 65% 1RM after a CA performed with eccentric only contractions at 120% 1RM, compared to control conditions. Furthermore, Alves et al. [15] also reported improved training volume evaluated by the total lifted load (REP x load) and the maximum number of performed REP after a CA.

However, it should be noted that most studies considering the acute effects of PAPE were assessed on the basis of only a single set of a post-activation exercise [7,16,17], while most resistance training guidelines recommend multiple sets of each exercise to achieve the desired adaptation [10]. To the best of our knowledge, only Alves et al. [15] evaluated the PAPE effect on resistance training volume during an upper-body exercise consisting of several sets. Alves et al. [15] showed that the PAPE effect increases total lifted load and the number of performed REP during three sets of the BP to volitional failure at 75% 1RM after a CA of three REP at 90% 1RM. However, there are no more studies confirming this effect, especially when using other training variables (external load, time rest, number of sets, tempo of movement), both during the CA and in the post-activation exercise.

Furthermore, the effectiveness of PAPE during resistance exercise preformed to volitional failure is not only related to the volume of work, but also to the ability to maintain a high level of movement velocity and power output. Decreases in bar velocity during particular sets of an exercise have been accepted as a valid indicator of neuromuscular fatigue [18]. However, currently there is no research available on the impact of PAPE on exercise volume, with a simultaneous analysis of power output and bar velocity changes. Another factor in the optimal utilization of PAPE includes the determination of individual intra-complex rest intervals (IRT) between the CA and the post-activation exercise. According to Golas et al. [4], the IRT should be customized individually for each study participant. Recovery duration shows a large inter-individual variability that is associated with numerous factors such as strength level, training experience, and myotypology [4,19–21]. Therefore, the estimation of the individual IRT for each participant should be optimized, most likely using the trial and error method, experimenting with a rest interval from 2 to 10–12 min.

Since, numerous studies have confirmed the PAPE effect during intensive, short-duration activities, it would be interesting to investigate whether this phenomenon affects training volume during resistance exercise carried on to volitional failure. Furthermore, it would be interesting to investigate how PAPE protocols may attenuate the decrease in movement velocity and power output commonly observed during sets performed to volitional failure. Thus, the aim of the present study was to evaluate the effects of PAPE on training volume assessed by the number of performed REP and TUT during the BP exercise among strength trained participants. An additional aim of the study was to assess the impact of PAPE on power output and bar velocity during the BP exercise performed to concentric volitional failure.

2. Materials and Methods

The experiment was performed following a randomized crossover design, where each participant performed the following test protocols: one with a CA consisting of 3 sets of 3 repetitions at 85% 1RM (PAPE) and a control without the CA (CONT). Before the main experiment each participant performed two familiarization sessions, one with the 1RM test and the second with an individual intra-complex rest interval (IRT). The entire research procedure lasted 4 weeks with a one-week interval between each trial. During the experimental sessions, the participants performed 3 sets of the BP exercise to establish the maximum number of preformed REP to volitional failure with a load of 60% 1RM. The repetitions were performed with maximal velocity in the eccentric and concentric phases of movement. The following variables were registered: number of performed repetitions (REP), time under tension (TUT), peak power output (PP), mean of peak power output (PP_{MEAN}), mean power output (MP), peak bar velocity (PV), mean of peak bar velocity (PV_{MEAN}), and mean bar velocity (MV). All testing was performed in the Strength and Power Laboratory at the Academy of Physical Education in Katowice.

2.1. Participants

Twelve healthy strength-trained men participated in this study (age = 25.2 ± 2.1 years, body mass = 92.1 ± 8.7 kg, BP 1RM = 128.8 ± 10.5 kg), with a minimum 3 years of resistance training experience (6.3 ± 2.1 years). The inclusion criteria was a BP personal record of at least 120% of body mass. Participants were allowed to withdraw from the experiment at any moment and were free from any musculoskeletal disorders. The participants were instructed to maintain their normal dietary habits over the course of the study and not to use any supplements or stimulants for the duration of the experiment. They were informed about the benefits and potential risks of the study before providing their written informed consent for participation. The study protocol was approved by the Bioethics Committee for Scientific Research at the Academy of Physical Education in Katowice, Poland (10/2018), and performed according to the ethical standards of the Declaration of Helsinki, 1983.

2.2. Procedures

Familiarization Session

Two weeks before the main experiment, the participants performed 2 familiarization sessions, once per week. The first familiarization session included the 1RM test. During the second familiarization session, one week before the main experiment, IRT testing was performed [4]. The participants arrived at the laboratory at the same time of day as the upcoming experimental sessions and performed a standardized general and specific warm-up before each of the familiarization and main sessions. The warm-up protocol included 5 min cycling on a stationary ergometer (heart rate of around 130 bpm), followed by a general upper-body warm-up of 10 trunk rotations and trunk side-bends on each side, 10 internal and external rotary movements of the shoulders, and 10 push-ups. Next, the participants performed 15, 10, and 5 BP repetitions using 20%, 40%, and 60% of their estimated 1RM. The first test load was set to an estimated 80% 1RM and was increased by 2.5 to 10 kg for each subsequent attempt. This process was repeated until failure. During the 1RM test, 5 min rest intervals were given between each attempt and the 1RM was attained within 5 attempts. According to Wilk et al. [22], all trials during the 1RM test were performed with a constant duration in the eccentric phase (2 s). Hand placement on the barbell was set at 150% of the individual bi-acromial distance. The positioning of the hands was recorded to ensure consistent hand placement during all experimental sessions.

During the second familiarization session the IRT test was performed. The participants performed 2 repetitions of an explosive BP (60% 1RM) at baseline. After a 5 min rest interval they performed a CA consisting of 3 sets of 3 repetitions at 85% 1RM with 4 min rest intervals between each set. After 4, 8, 12 and 16 min of recovery, the participant performed a test similar to baseline (2 repetitions at 60% 1RM) to establish an optimal rest interval for each participant. An optimal individual IRT was selected as the best single repetition in peak power output in comparison to baseline [4].

2.3. Experimental Sessions

The general and specific warm-up for the experimental sessions was identical to the one used during familiarization. After the warm-up, the participants started the evaluations. In a randomized, cross-over fashion, the participants performed 3 sets of the BP exercise to volitional failure at a load of 60% 1RM with maximal possible velocity in the concentric and eccentric phases of movement, either preceded by a CA (PAPE) or without activation (CONT). During the CA the participants performed 3 sets of 3 repetitions with a constant duration of 2 s for the eccentric movement and maximal velocity for the concentric phase at a load of 85% 1RM. The rest interval between successive sets equaled 4 min. The time between the CA and post-activation exercise was determined in accordance with the IRT. Every repetition was performed without bouncing the barbell off the chest and without intentionally pausing at the transition between the eccentric and concentric phases. A linear position transducer system (Tendo Power Analyzer, Tendo Sport Machines, Trencin, Slovakia) was used for the evaluation of bar mechanics. The Tendo Power Analyzer is a reliable system for measuring movement velocity and power output [23,24]. The measurement was made independently for each repetition and automatically converted into the values of power output and bar velocity.

The peak power output (PP) and peak bar velocity (PV) were obtained from the best repetition performed in a particular set. The mean of peak power output (PP_{MEAN}) and mean of peak bar velocity (PV_{MEAN}) were obtained from the peak of all repetitions performed in a particular set. The mean power output (MP) as well as mean bar velocity (MV) were obtained as the mean of all repetitions performed in particular sets. All participants completed the described testing protocol, which was carefully replicated in subsequent experimental sessions.

2.4. Statistical Analysis

Data were presented as the mean ± SD. All variables presented a normal distribution according to the Shapiro-Wilk test. Verification of differences between CONT and PAPE in REP, TUT, PP, PP_{MEAN}, MP, PV, PV_{MEAN}, and MV was performed using a two-way 2 X 3 (condition x set) analysis of variance (ANOVA) with repeated measures. In cases of a significant main effect, post-hoc comparisons were conducted using Tukey's test. Percent changes and 95% confidence intervals were also calculated. Effect sizes (Cohen's d) were reported where appropriate and interpreted as large ($d \geq 0.80$), moderate (d between 0.79 and 0.50), small (d between 0.49 and 0.20), and trivial ($d < 0.20$) [25]. All statistical analyses were performed using Statistica 9.1 (Hillview Avenue, Palo Alto, CA, USA). The statistical significance was set at $p < 0.05$.

3. Results

The two-way repeated measures ANOVA indicated a significant conditions x set main interaction effect for TUT ($p < 0.01$). There was also a significant main effect for the condition in TUT ($p < 0.01$). No statistically significant main effect was revealed for REP, PP, PP_{MEAN}, MP, PV, PV_{MEAN}, and MV (Table 1). The post-hoc analysis for the main effect indicated significant increases in TUT ($p < 0.01$) for the BP following PAPE, compared to the CONT condition. Finally, there was a significant increase in TUT ($p < 0.01$) in the third set for PAPE compared to the CONT condition (Table 2). The results of the IRT test showed that 4 min was an optimal rest interval for 7 participants, 8 min for 3 participants and 12 min for 2 of them (Figure 1).

Table 1. Performance variables during 3 sets of the bench press exercise.

Variables	Conditions (3 Sets)		p
	CONTROL	PAPE	
REP [n]	17.4 ± 7.0	17.8 ± 6.8	0.38
TUT [s]	25.1 ± 9.6	26.78 ± 8.3	0.01 *
MP [W]	379 ± 74	385 ± 82	0.13
PP [W]	774 ± 160	727 ± 164	0.18
PP_{MEAN} [W]	570 ± 129	570 ± 127	0.71
MV [m/s]	0.53 ± 0.07	0.52 ± 0.08	0.15
PV [m/s]	0.92 ± 0.14	0.90 ± 0.14	0.14
PV_{MEAN} [m/s]	0.68 ± 0.10	0.68 ± 0.11	0.75

These data present the mean values of the 3 sets. All data are presented as mean ± standard deviation; REP—the number of performed repetitions, TUT—time under tension, MP—mean power output, PP—peak power output, PP_{MEAN}—mean of peak power output, MV—mean bar velocity output, PV—peak bar velocity, PV_{MEAN}—mean of peak bar velocity; * statistically significant difference $p < 0.05$.

Table 2. Performance variables for particular sets of the bench press exercise.

Performance	Conditions	Set 1 (95% CI)	Set 2 (95% CI)	Set 3 (95% CI)
			REP [n]	
REP [n]	CONTROL	25.8 ± 2.5 (24.3 to 27.4)	16.3 ± 2.1 (14.9 to 17.6)	10.0 ± 2.3 (8.5 to 11.5)
	PAPE	25.8 ± 3.3 (23.6 to 27.9)	16.7 ± 2.5 (15.1 to 18.3)	10.9 ± 2.5 (9.3 to 12.5)
	ES	0	0.17	0.37
TUT [s]	CONTROL	35.3 ± 4.9 (32.2 to 38.3)	25.9 ± 3.4 (23.7 to 28.1)	14.1 ± 3.8 * (11.7 to 16.5)
	PAPE	35.4 ± 5.6 (31.9 to 38.9)	25.8 ± 4.2 (23.1 to 28.4)	19.2 ± 4.8 * (16.1 to 22.2)
	ES	0.02	0.03	1.18
MP [W]	CONTROL	423 ± 68 (380 to 466)	373 ± 68 (330 to 416)	340 ± 68 (297 to 383)
	PAPE	431 ± 71 (386 to 476)	376 ± 75 (328 to 423)	349 ± 84 (296 to 403)
	ES	0.12	0.04	0.12
PP [W]	CONTROL	843 ± 112 (771 to 914)	734 ± 139 (645 to 823)	656 ± 175 (544 to 767)
	PAPE	832 ± 112 (761 to 903)	702 ± 150 (607 to 798)	647 ± 176 (535 to 759)
	ES	0.10	0.22	0.05
PP_{MEAN} [W]	CONTROL	639 ± 99 (576 to 702)	565 ± 115 (492 to 638)	513 ± 145 (421 to 605)
	PAPE	637 ± 108 (569 to 706)	553 ± 128 (472 to 635)	521 ± 125 (441 to 600)
	ES	0.02	0.10	0.06

Table 2. *Cont.*

Performance	Conditions	Set 1 (95% CI)	Set 2 (95% CI)	Set 3 (95% CI)
MV [m/s]	CONTROL	0.59 ± 0.03 (0.57 to 0.62)	0.52 ± 0.05 (0.49 to 0.56)	0.46 ± 0.03 (0.45 to 0.48)
	PAPE	0.60 ± 0.05 (0.56 to 0.63)	0.50 ± 0.04 (0.47 to 0.53)	0.45 ± 0.05 (0.42 to 0.49)
	ES	0.24	0.44	0.24
PV [m/s]	CONTROL	1.05 ± 0.10 (0.99 to 1.11	0.91 ± 0.09 (0.85 to 0.97)	0.81 ± 0.11 (0.74 to 0.88)
	PAPE	1.04 ± 0.09 (0.98 to 1.10)	0.87 ± 0.11 (0.80 to 0.94)	0.80 ± 0.11 (0.73 to 0.87)
	ES	0.11	0.40	0.10
PV_{MEAN} [m/s]	CONTROL	0.79 ± 0.06 (0.75 to 0.83)	0.67 ± 0.08 (0.62 to 0.71)	0.60 ± 0.07 (0.56 to 0.64)
	PAPE	0.78 ± 0.07 (0.74 to 0.83)	0.65 ± 0.08 (0.60 to 0.71)	0.61 ± 0.08 (0.56 to 0.66)
	ES	0.15	0.25	0.13

Data are presented as mean ± standard deviation and 95% confidence interval (95% CI). Effect size (ES) was assessed using Cohen's *d*. These data present the mean values of the 3 sets. All data are presented as mean ± standard deviation; REP—the number of performed repetitions, TUT—time under tension, MP—mean power output, PP—peak power output, PP_{MEAN}—mean of peak power output, MV—mean bar velocity, PV—peak bar velocity, PV_{MEAN}—mean of peak bar velocity * statistically significant difference $p < 0.05$.

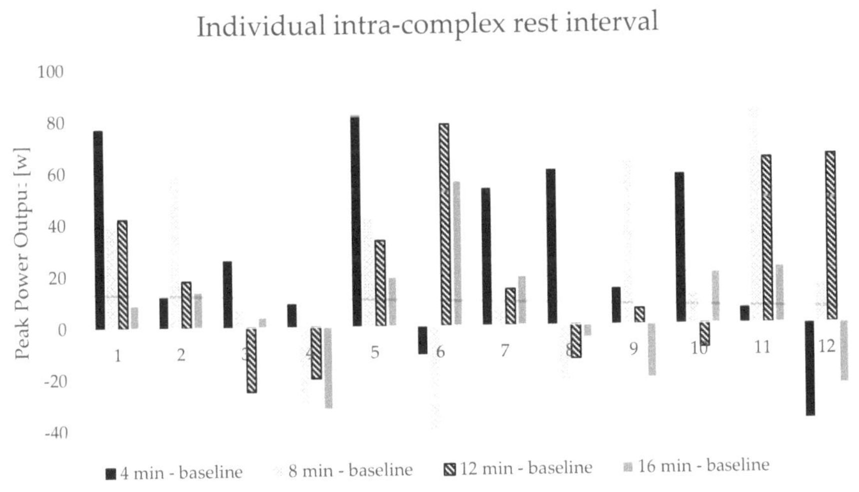

Figure 1. Individual differences in peak power output between baseline and rest interval for each individual during the intra-complex rest interval test. The y-axis represents the difference in peak power output between the baseline and rest interval for each individual.

4. Discussion

The main finding of the study was that the PAPE protocol increased training volume based on TUT in the BP performed to volitional failure compared to CONT conditions. Despite the fact that there was an increase in TUT for the PAPE conditions, the study did not show significant changes in the number of performed REP. Greater TUT, when volume load (REP × load) was equated, may result in greater neuromuscular fatigue, but in our study, we did not observe effects of fatigue reflected by decreasing power output or bar velocity between the PAPE and CONT conditions during the BP exercise performed to volitional failure. Therefore, these results suggest that the PAPE effect can be used to acutely increase the time of effort during resistance exercise, without affecting the concentric bar velocity and power output of each set.

To the best of the authors knowledge, the presented study is the first to analyze both the changes in training volume as well as in power output and bar velocity following PAPE effects in trained men. Despite the large body of evidence investigating the effect of PAPE on the performance of explosive activities, only two studies have examined the impact of PAPE on resistance training volume [14,15]. However, neither of them analyzed training volume as well as power output and bar velocity simultaneously during sets performed to volitional failure. In terms of the impact of PAPE on training volume based on the number of performed REP, the results obtained in our study contradict those of Sevilmiş and Atalağ [14] and Alves et al. [15], which showed an increase in the number of preformed REP following CA. However, it should be noted that Sevilmiş and Atalağ [14] analyzed only one set of an exercise (compared to three sets in our study), which is not habitual practice during sports training, where several sets of each exercise are used in order to obtain significant adaptive changes. The impact of the PAPE effect on the number of performed REP during more than one set was analyzed only in the study of Alves et al. [15], who showed that the number of performed REP in the first and second sets were greater under PAPE, compared to the control conditions. However, no significant difference was found in the third set. This result is contrary to the presented results, where no significant changes in the number of preformed REP were observed in any of the three sets. Furthermore, the result of effect size showed higher differences between PAPE and CONT conditions in the third set (10.9 ± 2.5 vs. 10.0 ± 2.3 respectively; ES = 0.37) compared to the first (25.8 ± 3.3 vs. 25.8 ± 2.5 respectively; ES = 0) and second set (16.7 ± 2.5 vs. 16.3 ± 2.1 respectively; ES = 0.17), which is opposite to the results obtained by Alves et al. [15].

The differences in impact of PAPE on the maximal number of performed REP during sets performed to volitional failure between the presented results and the study of Sevilmiş and Atalağ [14] and Alves et al. [15] may be related to the level of experience in resistance training [8,26], as well as to the movement tempo used during exercise [6,13]. Compared to the presented research, where the participants had a minimum of three years of resistance training experience (6.3 ± 2.1 years), in the study of Sevilmiş and Atalağ [14] and Alves et al. [15], the participants had a minimum of 1 year of resistance training experience. Furthermore, in the study by Sevilmiş and Atalağ [14], as well as that by Alves et al. [15], the movement tempo of each performed REP was controlled and amounted to 2 s in the eccentric phase and 1 s in the concentric phase, while in the present study the participants used maximal tempo of movement. According to Wilk et al. [13], movement tempo has a significant effect on the maximal number of performed REP in a particular set, as well as on the PAPE effect during successive sets of a resistance exercise [6].

Moreover, according to Wilk et al. [13,27] not only the number of performed REP, but also TUT is an important variable to consider when evaluating training volume. However, only one previous study analyzed the impact of PAPE on TUT [14]. Sevilmiş and Atalağ [14] showed a significant increase in TUT for the PAPE condition compared to the control, during the BP exercise performed to volitional failure, which is consistent with the presented study. Furthermore, the presented study showed not only a significant increase of total training TUT, but also a significant increase of TUT in the third set of the BP exercise for the PAPE condition, compared to the CONT. Regardless of the mechanisms underpinning PAPE performance improvement, it can be speculated that the increase in time of the resistance effort could have been obtained as a result of increased muscle temperature and blood flow as well as water content following the CA. Thus, the PAPE protocol may contribute to enhancing the general effects of the warm-up [1]. Furthermore, the increase of TUT during the PAPE condition compared to the CONT (especially in third set) can also be attributed to increased phosphorylation of myosin light chains rendering the actin and myosin molecules more sensitive to Ca^{2+} availability [5], which would allow the participants to maintain a certain amount of force even in the presence of biochemical changes within the working muscle that lead to fatigue. However, an assessment of power output and bar velocity did not show differences between PAPE and CONT conditions, which indicates that the increase in TUT was not related to the changes in concentric bar velocity and power output. Therefore, the increase in TUT with the simultaneous lack of significant differences in the number of performed REP as well as the lack of significant differences in concentric bar velocity and power output indicate that a longer TUT for the PAPE condition was related to the extension of the eccentric phase of movement only.

The present study has several limitations which should be addressed. Although the results showed a significantly greater value of TUT, following the CA, the direct causes of these changes cannot be determined and explained. There was no analysis of direct physiological changes, as well as no electromyography recordings that would be the basis for explaining the obtained results. Since there is no evidence regarding the possible cause for the increased TUT in the PAPE condition, further research is needed to assess the physiological and mechanical variables responsible for these changes.

Practical Implications

The impact of a CA can been used effectively to extend the duration of effort during resistance exercise performed to volitional failure; therefore, it can be useful in increasing the efficiency of strength-endurance performance. Furthermore, combining several sets of high-load exercises before sets performed to volitional failure can be an effective way to develop both maximal strength and strength-endurance in a single session, without losing the effectiveness of sets whose goal is strength-endurance performance. In addition, such a complex training system can be particularly useful in sports disciplines that, due to a high number of competitions, do not leave adequate time to perform separate training sessions for maximal strength and strength-endurance.

5. Conclusions

In summary, the presented study showed that compared to CONT conditions, PAPE did not significantly affect the number of performed REP during the BP exercise performed to volitional failure. However, an increase in TUT was observed. Even if the applied CA did not increase the training volume (based on REP), it did not adversely affect the level of training volume. Therefore, a training program that combines both a high-load exercise prior to several sets performed to volitional failure could be a valuable alternative, especially for athletes whose sports discipline requires both a high level of muscular power and appropriate strength endurance.

Author Contributions: Data curation, M.K., A.F., P.Z.; formal analysis, MK. and M.W.; investigation, M.W., A.F., and P.Z.; methodology, M.W.; software, M.K., M.W., and A.F.; supervision, M.W., A.Z., and J.J.T.; writing—original draft, M.K., M.W., and J.J.T.; writing—review and editing, M.W., A.Z., and J.J.T. All authors have read and agreed to the published version of the manuscript.

Funding: This study would not have been possible without our participants' commitment, time, and effort. The study was supported and funded by the statutory research of the Jerzy Kukuczka Academy of Physical Education in Katowice, Poland.

Conflicts of Interest: The authors declare no conflict of interest.

References

1. Blazevich, A.J.; Babault, N. Post-activation Potentiation Versus Post-Activation Performance Enhancement in Humans: Historical Perspective, Underlying Mechanisms, and Current Issues. *Front. Physiol.* **2019**, *10*, 1359. [CrossRef]
2. Sale, D.G. Postactivation potentiation: Role in human performance. *Exerc. Sport Sci. Rev.* **2002**, *30*, 138–143. [CrossRef]

3. Seitz, L.B.; Haff, G.G. Factors Modulating Post-Activation Potentiation of Jump, Sprint, Throw, and Upper-Body Ballistic Performances: A Systematic Review with Meta-Analysis. *Sports Med.* **2016**, *46*, 231–240. [CrossRef]
4. Golas, A.; Maszczyk, A.; Zajac, A.; Mikolajec, K.; Stastny, P. Optimizing post activation potentiation for explosive activities in competitive sports. *J. Hum. Kinet.* **2016**, *52*, 95–106. [CrossRef] [PubMed]
5. Tillin, N.A.; Bishop, D. Factors Modulating Post-Activation Potentiation and its Effect on Performance of Subsequent Explosive Activities. *Sports Med.* **2009**, *39*, 147–166. [CrossRef] [PubMed]
6. Wilk, M.; Krzysztofik, M.; Drozd, M.; Zajac, A. Changes of Power Output and Velocity During Successive Sets of the Bench Press with Different Duration of Eccentric Movement. *Int. J. Sports Physiol. Perform.* **2020**, *15*, 1–6. [CrossRef] [PubMed]
7. Krzysztofik, M.; Wilk, M.; Golas, A.; Lockie, R.G.; Maszczyk, A.; Zajac, A. Does Eccentric-only and Concentric-only Activation Increase Power Output? *Med. Sci. Sports Exerc.* **2020**, *52*, 484–489. [CrossRef] [PubMed]
8. Wilson, J.M.; Duncan, N.M.; Marin, P.J.; Brown, L.E.; Loenneke, J.P.; Wilson, S.M.C.; Jo, E.; Lowery, R.P.; Ugrinowitsch, C. Meta-Analysis of Postactivation Potentiation and Power: Effects of Conditioning Activity, Volume, Gender, Rest Periods, and Training Status. *J. Strength Cond. Res.* **2013**, *27*, 854–859. [CrossRef] [PubMed]
9. Krzysztofik, M.; Wilk, M.; Wojdala, G.; Golas, A. Maximizing Muscle Hypertrophy: A Systematic Review of Advanced Resistance Training Techniques and Methods. *Int. J. Environ. Res. Public Health* **2019**, *16*, 4897. [CrossRef]
10. American College of Sports Medicine. American College of Sports Medicine position stand: Progression models in resistance training for healthy adults. *Med. Sci. Sports Exerc.* **2002**, *34*, 364–380. [CrossRef]
11. Tran, Q.T.; Docherty, D. Dynamic training volume: A construct of both time under tension and volume load. *J. Sports Sci. Med.* **2006**, *5*, 707–713.
12. Wilk, M.; Krzysztofik, M.; Maszczyk, A.; Chycki, J.; Zajac, A. The acute effects of caffeine intake on time under tension and power generated during the bench press movement. *J. Int. Soc. Sports Nutr.* **2019**, *16*, 8. [CrossRef]
13. Wilk, M.; Golas, A.; Stastny, P.; Nawrocka, M.; Krzysztofik, M.; Zajac, A. Does Tempo of Resistance Exercise Impact Training Volume? *J. Hum. Kinet.* **2018**, *62*, 241–250. [CrossRef]
14. Sevilmiş, E.; Atalağ, O. Effects of post activation potentiation on eccentric loading: Is it possible to do more repetitions after supra-maximal loading? *J. Hum. Sport Exerc.* **2019**, *14*, 584–590. [CrossRef]
15. Alves, R.R.; Viana, R.B.; Silva, M.H.; Guimarães, T.C.; Vieira, C.A.; de Santos, D.A.T.; Gentil, P.R.V. Postactivation Potentiation Improves Performance in a Resistance Training Session in Trained Men. *J. Strength Cond. Res.* **2019**. [CrossRef]
16. Esformes, J.I.; Keenan, M.; Moody, J.; Bampouras, T.M. Effect of Different Types of Conditioning Contraction on Upper Body Postactivation Potentiation. *J. Strength Cond. Res.* **2011**, *25*, 143–148. [CrossRef]
17. Suchomel, T.J.; Sato, K.; DeWeese, B.H.; Ebben, W.P.; Stone, M.H. Potentiation Effects of Half-Squats Performed in a Ballistic or Nonballistic Manner. *J. Strength Cond. Res.* **2016**, *30*, 1652–1660. [CrossRef]
18. Sánchez-Medina, L.; González-Badillo, J.J. Velocity Loss as an Indicator of Neuromuscular Fatigue during Resistance Training. *Med. Sci. Sports Exerc.* **2011**, *43*, 1725–1734. [CrossRef]
19. Hamada, T.; Sale, D.G.; Macdougall, J.D.; Tarnopolsky, M.A. Interaction of fiber type, potentiation and fatigue in human knee extensor muscles. *Acta Physiol. Scand.* **2003**, *178*, 165–173. [CrossRef]
20. Chen, Z.R.; Lo, S.L.; Wang, M.H.; Yu, C.F.; Peng, H.T. Can different complex training improve the individual phenomenon of post- activation potentiation? *J. Hum. Kinet.* **2017**, *56*, 167–175. [CrossRef]
21. Naclerio, F.; Chapman, M.; Larumbe-Zabala, E.; Massey, B.; Neil, A.; Triplett, T.N. Effects of three different conditioning activity volumes on the optimal recovery time for potentiation in college athletes. *J. Strength Cond. Res.* **2015**, *29*, 2579–2585. [CrossRef]
22. Wilk, M.; Golas, A.; Zmijewski, P.; Krzysztofik, M.; Filip, A.; Del Coso, J.; Tufano, J.J. The Effects of the Movement Tempo on the One-Repetition Maximum Bench Press Results. *J. Hum. Kinet* **2020**, *72*, 151–159.
23. García-Ramos, A.; Pestaña-Melero, F.L.; Pérez-Castilla, A.; Rojas, F.J.; Haff, G.G. Differences in the Load–Velocity Profile Between 4 Bench-Press Variants. *Int. J. Sports Physiol. Perform.* **2018**, *13*, 326–331. [CrossRef]

24. Goldsmith, J.A.; Trepeck, C.; Halle, J.L.; Mendez, K.M.; Klemp, A.; Cooke, D.M.; Haischer, M.H.; Byrnes, R.K.; Zoeller, R.F.; Whitehurst, M.; et al. Validity of the Open Barbell and Tendo Weightlifting Analyzer Systems Versus the Optotrak Certus 3D Motion-Capture System for Barbell Velocity. *Int. J. Sports Physiol. Perform.* **2019**, *14*, 540–543. [CrossRef]
25. Cohen, J. *Statistical Power Analysis for the Behavioral Sciences*; Elsevier Science: Burlington, NJ, USA, 2013; ISBN 978-1-4832-7648-9.
26. Maszczyk, A.; Wilk, M.; Krzysztofik, M.; Gepfert, M.; Zajac, A.; Petr, M.; Stastny, P. The effects of resistance training experience on movement characteristics in the bench press exercise. *Biol. Sport* **2020**, *37*, 79–83. [CrossRef]
27. Wilk, M.; Tufano, J.J.; Zajac, A. The influence of movement tempo on acute neuromuscular, hormonal, and mechanical responses to resistance exercise–a mini-review. *J. Strength Cond. Res* **2020**, in press.

International Journal of
Environmental Research and Public Health

MDPI

Article

Influence of Interval Training Frequency on Time-Trial Performance in Elite Endurance Athletes

Espen Tønnessen [1,*], Jonny Hisdal [2] and Bent R. Ronnestad [3]

1 School of Health Sciences, Kristiana University College, 0153 Oslo, Norway
2 Department of Vascular Investigations, Oslo University Hospital—Aker, 0586 Oslo, Norway; jonny.hisdal@medisin.uio.no
3 Section for Health and Exercise Physiology, Inland Norway University, 2624 Lillehammer, Norway; bent.ronnestad@inn.no
* Correspondence: espen.tonnessen@kristiania.no; Tel.: +47-990-98-767

Received: 9 April 2020; Accepted: 29 April 2020; Published: 4 May 2020

Abstract: Purpose: To determine the impact of interval training frequency in elite endurance athletes. It was hypothesized that two longer sessions would elicit greater performance improvements and physiological adaptation than four shorter sessions at the same intensity. Methods: Elite cross-country skiers and biathletes were randomly assigned to either a high-frequency group (HF group) (5 M, 1 F, age 22 (19–26), VO_{2max} 67.8 (65.5–70.2) mL/kg/min) doing four short interval sessions per week or a low-frequency group (LF group) (8 M, 1 F, age 22 (18–23), VO_{2max} 70.7 (67.0–73.9) mL/kg/min) doing two longer interval sessions. All interval sessions were performed at ~85% of maximum heart rate, and groups were matched for total weekly training volume. Pre- and post-intervention, athletes completed an 8 km rollerski time-trial, maximal oxygen uptake (VO_{2max}) test, and an incremental, submaximal exercise test. Results: The LF group had a statistically significant improved time-trial performance following the intervention ($p = 0.04$), with no statistically significant changes in the HF group. Similarly, percentage utilization of VO_{2max} at anaerobic threshold ($p = 0.04$) and exercise economy ($p = 0.01$) were statistically significantly improved following the intervention in the LF group only. No statistically significant changes in VO_{2max} were observed in either group. Conclusions: Two longer interval sessions appear superior to four shorter sessions per week in promoting endurance adaptations and performance improvements in elite endurance athletes. Despite matched training volume and exercise intensity, the larger, more concentrated exercise stimulus in the LF group appears to induce more favorable adaptations. The longer time between training sessions in the LF group may also have allowed athletes to recover more effectively and better "absorb" the training. These findings are in line with the "best practice" observed by many of the world's best endurance athletes.

Keywords: cross-country skiers; exercise economy; VO_{2max}

1. Introduction

At a senior level, endurance athletes frequently train up to 1000 h per year, of which 80%–90% is typically conducted at low intensity [1–3]. The remaining 10%–20% is composed of high-intensity training in the form of competition, high-intensity continuous training, and interval training.

The principle of interval training was first described by Reindell & Roskamm in 1959 [4] and is a method of training which alternates between exercise periods with high and low intensity. Compared to continuous exercise, interval training allows the athlete to maintain a higher intensity and work for longer time at high intensities (>85% maximal heart rate (HRmax)) [5–8]. Increased training time at high intensity creates better conditions to optimally stimulate the development of performance capacity, maximal oxygen uptake (VO_{2max}), percentage utilization of maximal oxygen uptake (% VO_{2max}) and exercise economy [9,10].

Six factors determine total workload: duration per interval, exercise intensity, recovery duration, recovery intensity, movement patterns, and total training time [11,12]. Depending on the purpose of the training session, these variables can be manipulated to give countless different combinations. Studies of well-trained endurance athletes indicate that the best training effect, i.e., increased stroke volume and oxygen delivery, is achieved at intensities between 85%–95% of HRmax [13–15], although studies have also demonstrated positive effects of training at higher intensities [12,16].

The optimal interval duration for well-trained endurance athletes appears to be 4–10 min [13–15], with a beneficial effect observed at a total effective duration of approximately 15 min [5,13]. However, durations of 30–45 min appear to elicit the best effect [14,15].

The optimal number of high-intensity interval training sessions per week in order to maximally stimulate the development of performance has not yet been elucidated. In a retrospective study it was found that world-class endurance athletes performed 2–3 high-intensity training sessions per week (100–140 sessions per year) [17]. Half of these sessions were completed as interval training, with 30%–50% of these performed at an intensity around 85% HR_{max}, with a total effective duration of 30–75 min per session [17].

The aim of the present study was therefore to determine the effect of frequency of high-intensity interval training in elite cross-country skiers. Based on the "best practice" observed in world-class endurance athletes, our hypothesis was that two longer interval sessions at an intensity of ~85% HR_{max} would elicit greater improvements in time-trial performance, VO_{2max}, %VO_{2max} at anaerobic threshold (AT), and work economy than four shorter sessions at the same intensity.

2. Materials and Methods

2.1. Subjects

Twenty elite cross-country skiers and biathletes volunteered their written, informed consent to take part in the study, which was approved by the institution's ethics committee, in accordance with the Declaration of Helsinki; the study was further approved by the Norwegian center for research data (number: 26732). All participants had competed in cross-country skiing or a biathlon at a national level for a minimum of three years. Athletes were randomly assigned to either a high-frequency group (HF group, n = 10) doing four interval sessions per week or a low-frequency group (LF group, n = 10) doing two longer interval sessions. There was one drop-out in the LF group due to illness. There were four drop-outs in the HF group, three due to illness and one to an accident not related to the project. The athletes' physiological and anthropometric characteristics and initial training status are shown in Table 1.

Table 1. Baseline characteristics of test subjects in the high-frequency group (HF group) performing four interval sessions per week, and in the low-frequency group (LF group) that performed two interval sessions per week. Values are presented as the median and inter quartile range (IQR). There were no significant differences between the groups.

Characteristics of the Subjects	HF Group	LF Group
Gender	♂= 5, ♀= 1	♂= 8, ♀= 1
Age (years)	22.0 (18.8–26.0)	22.0 (18.0–22.5)
Height (m)	1.81 (1.75–1.86)	1.82 (1.80–1.84)
Body mass (kg)	72.3 (64.6–78.0)	76.9 (72.1–79.9)
VO_{2max} (mL/min/kg)	67.8 (65.5–70.2)	70.7 (67.0–73.9)
Training volume last 12 months (hours)	565 (431–638)	650 (520–755)
Training volume last 2 months (hours)	65 (58–81)	75 (63–80)

2.2. Procedures

During the 12-week intervention period, the LF group performed two interval sessions per week, whilst the HF group performed four sessions per week, at the same intensity and matched for weekly training volume (Figure 1). Oxygen consumption (VO_2), heart rate (HR), and blood lactate were measured, and exercise economy was calculated pre- and post-intervention. In addition, a performance test (8 km roller-skiing time trial) was conducted before and after the intervention period.

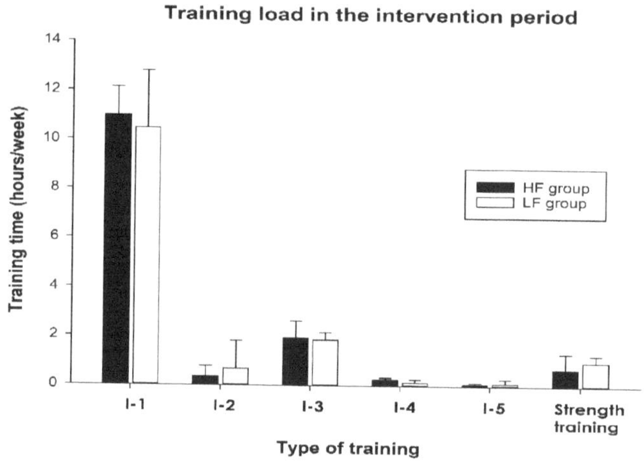

Figure 1. Weekly training load in the 12-week intervention period. The figure shows the distribution of endurance training in the different intensity zones (I-1 to I-5) and duration of strength training in the high- and low-frequency group (HF- and LF group). Values are presented as the median and IQR. There were no statistically significant differences between the groups.

2.2.1. Interval Training

The intervention was performed as dry land training during the summer period from May to August. The exercise intensity scale developed by the Norwegian Olympic Centre (NOC) was used for classification of training intensity (Table 2). Interval durations and work intensity for both interventions were selected to correspond with what the literature suggests to be an effective model to elicit performance adaptations in endurance athletes.

Outside of the planned intervention sessions, athletes were instructed to train normally, with low-intensity training (<82% HR_{max} I-zones 1–2) and a maximum of one additional session per week of high-intensity interval training (>87% HR_{max}, I-zones 4–5). To ensure that the training load during the intervention period outside of prescribed training did not differ between groups, subjects were provided with an electronic training diary with both written and verbal instructions on how to record their training. Data recorded in these diaries were used to calculate the training volume and intensity distribution.

During the intervention period, the LF group completed one session per week of 8 × 8 min intervals in I-zone 3 with 2 min recoveries (total time 64 min) and one session of 6 × 12 min intervals in I-zone 3 with 3 min recoveries (total time 72 min). The HF group performed twice-weekly sessions of 4 × 8 min in I-zone 3 separated by 2 min recoveries (total time 32 min) and two sessions of 3 × 12 min in I-zone 3 with 3 min recoveries (total time 36 min). All interval sessions were performed as rollerski skating. For both groups, the total prescribed weekly training time in I-zone 3 was 136 min. The LF group had a minimum of one day, and typically two days, between each session in I-zone 3. The HF group performed two I-zone 3 sessions on two consecutive days, while there was one day off before the remaining I-zone 3 session.

Each interval session included a self-selected warm-up and warm-down. During the first four weeks of the intervention period, 1–2 interval sessions per week were organized as group training sessions, during which blood lactate and HR were monitored and controlled to ensure that athletes were training at the planned intensity. During the remaining weeks of the intervention, once participants had become accustomed to maintaining the correct intensity during training sessions, only a selection of sessions were monitored.

Table 2. The exercise intensity scale developed by the Norwegian Olympic Centre (NOC) used for classification of training intensity (I-zones).

Intensity Zone	% of HR_{max}	Blood Lactate (mmol/L) *	Examples of Training Models
I-zone 5	92–100	6.0–10.0	Interval training with maximal or near maximal exertion. Recovery period equivalent to 70%–90% of the work interval time.
I-zone 4	87–92	4.0–6.0	High-intensity continuous training or intervals with a high level of exertion. Recovery periods equivalent to approximately 50% of the work time.
I-zone 3	82–87	2.5–4.0	Natural interval training, intensive continuous training, or long intervals. Recovery periods equivalent to 20%–30% of the work time.
I-zone 2	72–82	1.5–2.5	Moderate intensity continuous work.
I-zone 1	55–72	<1.5	Recovery sessions and low-intensity continuous work.

* Values determined via a hand-held or portable lactate analyzer using red cell lysed blood.

2.2.2. Test Day 1: Submaximal Exercise Test and VO_{2max}

Pre- and post-intervention, subjects performed a submaximal incremental rollerskiing (skating) test on a motorized treadmill (Lode Valiant Special, Lode B.V. Groningen, Netherlands) in a laboratory maintained at 17–21 °C and 25%–40% relative humidity. Participants completed a ~15-min standardized warm-up. The test started at 5% incline and 10.8 km/h for men and 9 km/h for women. Each stage lasted 5 min, followed by a one-minute recovery. The treadmill incline was increased by 2% between each stage. The test was terminated when blood lactate concentration exceeded 4.0 mmol/L (Lactate Pro LT-1710t, ArkRay Inc., Kyoto, Japan). Expired air was analyzed continuously with VO_2 determined at 30 s intervals throughout the test (Oxycon Pro, Erich Jaeger, Hoechberg, Germany). HR was measured continuously using short-range telemetry (Polar S620i, Kempele, Finland). For both HR and VO_2, the average values recorded during the final three minutes of each stage were used for analyses. A finger-prick blood sample was taken during the recovery between each stage for blood lactate determination. Exercise economy was calculated from body mass-adjusted oxygen consumption, and HR and lactate recorded for the lowest test workload (5% incline 10.8 km/h for men and 9 km/h for women). This workload was chosen to ensure aerobic metabolism, indicated by a lactate level < 2.5 mmol/L.

VO_2 at an estimated lactate concentration of 4.0 mmol/L was calculated by a forecast algorithm. We used a built-in algorithm in Excel 2016, using the measured values beyond and above an intensity corresponding to 4.0 mmol/L to predict a given y-value (VO_2) at a given x-value (4.0 mmol/L), based on the measured values in the data set, using the algorithm $a + bx$:

$$a = \overline{y} - b\overline{x} \quad \text{and} \quad b = \frac{\sum(x-\overline{x})(y-\overline{y})}{\sum(x-\overline{x})^2} \tag{1}$$

Here, x and y are the sample means average (x = lactate, y = VO_2).

Following ~10 min recovery, VO_{2max} was measured via a continuous, incremental rollerskiing (skating) test to volitional exhaustion. The test started at a 5% incline and 10.8 km/h for men and

9 km/h for women. Every minute, the treadmill incline was increased by 2%. When an incline of 15% was reached, treadmill speed was then increased by 0.5 km/h every minute. VO_2 was measured continuously, and the average of the two highest consecutive 30 s measurements was defined as VO_{2max}. Respiratory exchange ratio ≥ 1.05, a plateau in VO_2 with increasing workload, and blood lactate concentration ≥ 8 mmol/L were used as criteria to evaluate if VO_{2max} was obtained [18]. HR was measured continuously, with the highest value during the test defined as HRpeak.

2.2.3. Test Day 2: Rollerski Time Trial Performance

Pre- and post-intervention, each athlete completed an 8 km rollerski (skating) uphill time-trial outdoors. This had a typical duration of 30–35 min and was preceded by a 30 min standardized warm-up. Athletes started in a random order at 30 s intervals pre-intervention, and again in this same order post-intervention to prevent any possible motivational effects. Performance times were recorded by two synchronized stopwatches (Regnly RT3, Emit AS, Oslo, Norway). The weather conditions pre- and post-intervention were stable, with ambient temperature between 17–20 °C, no wind and dry asphalt. All athletes were familiar with the 8 km course.

Subjects used identical rollerskis (Swenor Skate, Sport Import AS. Sarpsborg, Norway), with each athlete using the same pair of skis pre- and post-intervention. These were not used between pre- and post-testing to avoid changes in rolling resistance. Participants also used the same skating poles (SWIX CT3, Swix Sport AS. Lillehammer, Norway) of self-selected length. The two test days were separated by a minimum of 48 h and a maximum of 6 days. Prior to testing, participants underwent a standardized 2 day tapering period. Tests were performed at the same time of day (± 1 h) and following a 1 h fast. Participants were required to abstain from strenuous exercise, alcohol, and caffeine during the 24 h leading up to each test. Athletes not able to participate in whole intervention period were excluded from the study ($n = 1$ in the LF group and $n = 4$ in the HF group).

2.3. *Statistical Analyses*

Since not all variables passed the normality test, all results are presented as median values with the corresponding inter-quartile range (IQR). A Wilcoxon matched-pairs signed rank test was used to test for differences between each parameter before and after the 12-week intervention period. In all comparisons, two-tailed tests were used. Differences were considered significant at $p < 0.05$. Due to the small sample size and expectations of small changes in these already well-trained athletes, the data were further analyzed with mean effects size (ES). ES was calculated as Cohen's d to compare the practical significance of the performance improvements among the two groups. The criteria to interpret the magnitude of the ES were 0.0–0.2 trivial, 0.2–0.6 small, 0.6–1.2 moderate, 1.2–2.0 large, and >2.0 very large. The calculations were performed in Microsoft Excel 2010 (Microsoft Corporation), and the statistical analyses were conducted in SigmaPlot for Windows, version 12.2 (Systat Software GmbH, Erkrath, Germany).

3. Results

All included test subjects completed > 80% of the interval sessions and no statistically significant differences were observed in training compliance between the groups. When prescribed interval sessions were skipped, that was mainly due to the athletes requesting a rest due to a feeling of tiredness.

3.1. *Baseline*

At baseline, no statistically significant differences were observed between the LF- and HF group with respect to age, height, weight, VO_{2max} or training volume (Table 1). Further, there were no statistically significant differences in exercise economy, $\%VO_{2max}$, $\%VO_{2max}$ at 4 mmol/L lactate or time-trial performance.

3.2. Training Load in the Intervention Period

There was no difference in the weekly training load between groups in terms of training volume, intensity distribution, or resistance training during the intervention period (Figure 1). Despite a higher median training load in both the last 12 and last 2 months, the statistical analysis revealed that there was no systematic differences between the groups. In our opinion, it is therefore unlikely that difference in training volume had a significant impact on the results.

3.3. Time-Trial Performance

In the LF group, seven out of nine subjects showed an improvement in rollerski time-trial performance following the intervention, with median time-trial time that was statistically significantly lower at post-intervention (30.6 (30.1–34.1) min vs. 31.8 (30.3–35.0) min, $p = 0.04$). In the HF group, no statistically significant improvement between pre- and post-test was observed ($p = 0.16$). ES of the changes revealed only a trivial effect of LF training vs. HF training (ES = 0.17). Individual results from the time-trial performance test are shown in Figure 2.

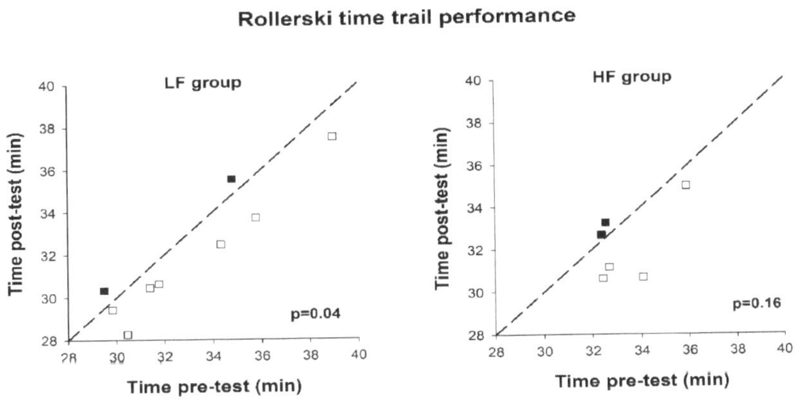

Figure 2. Time taken to complete the 8 km rollerski time-trial, pre-test and post-test, in the low-frequency group (LF group) and high-frequency group (HF group). Reference lines indicate identical values pre- and post-test. Each box represents a test subject. Open boxes indicate an improvement, and filled boxes indicate a decline, compared to the pre-test.

3.4. VO_{2max} and % VO_{2max} at AT

No statistically significant changes in VO_{2max} were observed between pre- and post-intervention in either group. Individual values for all subjects are shown in Figure 3. There was no statistically significant change in body mass in either group. % VO_{2max} at anaerobic threshold (lactate 4.0 mmol/L) was statistically significantly increased after the intervention period in the LF group (85.4 (79.9–88.2)% vs. 80.7 (79.7–84.9)%, $p = 0.04$) but not in the HF group ($p = 1.00$). Individual results are shown in Figure 4. The mean ES revealed a small practical effect of the LF training vs. HF training (ES = 0.52).

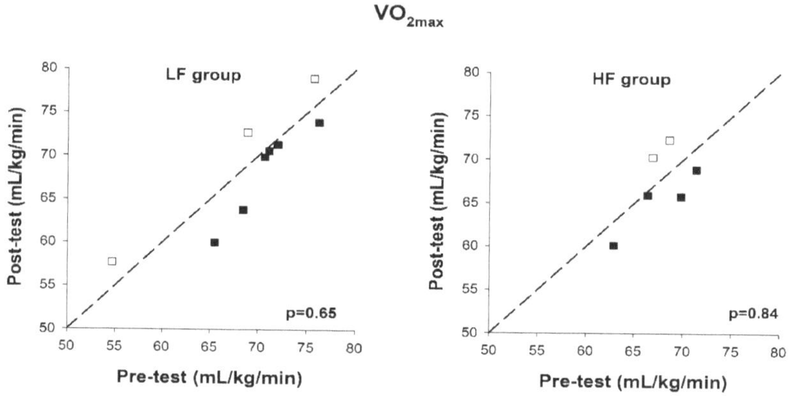

Figure 3. VO_{2max} at pre-test and post-test, in the low-frequency group (LF group) and high-frequency group (HF group). Reference lines indicate identical values pre- and post-test. Each box represents a test subject. Open boxes indicate an improvement and filled boxes indicate a decline, compared to the pre-test.

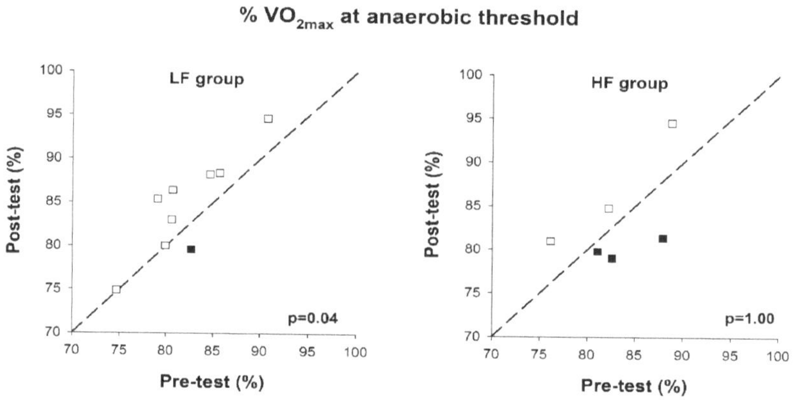

Figure 4. % of VO_{2max} at anaerobic threshold at pre-test and post-test, in the low-frequency group (LF group) and high-frequency group (HF group). Reference lines indicate identical values at pre- and post-test. Each box represents a test subject. Open boxes indicate an improvement and filled boxes indicate a decline, compared to the pre-test.

3.5. Exercise Economy

A statistically significant reduction in submaximal oxygen consumption at 10.9 km/h and 5% incline was observed in the LF group (39.6 (39.3–41.2) mL/kg/min vs. 41.0 (40.3–42.8) mL/kg/min, $p = 0.01$), but not in the HF group at post-test. Individual values are shown in Figure 5. The ES showed a moderate practical effect of the LF training vs. HF training on improvements in exercise economy (ES = 1.14).

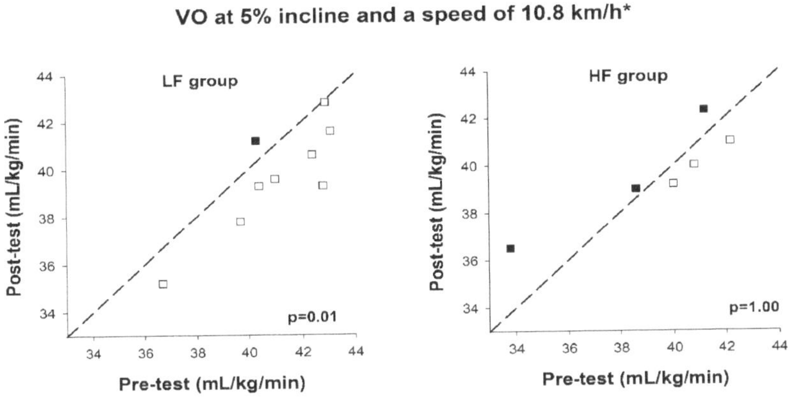

Figure 5. VO_2 at 5% incline and a speed of 10.8 km/h at pre-test and post-test, in the low-frequency group (LF group) and high-frequency group (HF group). Reference lines indicate identical values at pre- and post-test. Each box represents a test subject. Open boxes indicate an improvement and filled boxes indicate a decline, compared to the pre-test. * = 9.0 km/h for women.

There was a statistically significant reduction in submaximal HR for the LF group (134 (124–144) vs. 144 (137–152) bpm, p = 0.01) but not for the HF group. Individual results are demonstrated in Figure 6. Mean ES of the improvement in submaximal HR revealed a moderate practical effect of performing LF training vs. HF training (ES = 0.95).

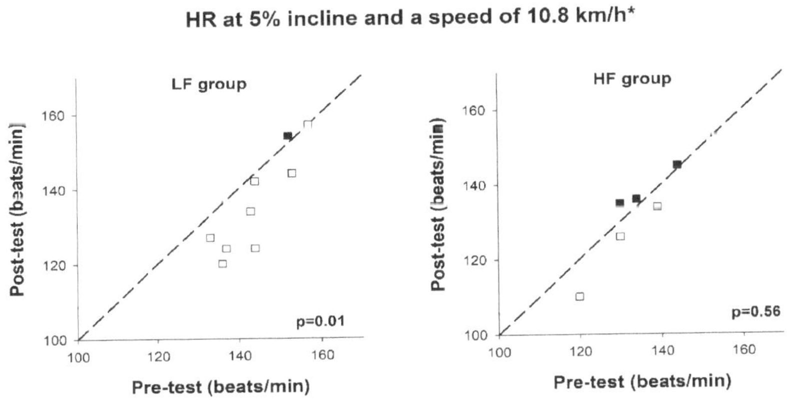

Figure 6. Heart rate at a speed of 10.8 km/h at pre- and post-test, in the low-frequency group (LF group) and high-frequency group (HF group). Reference lines indicate identical values at pre- and post-test. Each box represents a test subject. Open boxes indicate an improvement and filled boxes indicate a decline, compared to the pre-test. * = 9.0 km/h for women.

At the lowest workload, blood lactate for all subjects was <2.5 mmol/L both pre- and post-intervention. There were no statistically significant differences observed for either group.

4. Discussion

The main finding in the present study is that highly trained cross-country skiers and biathletes performing two longer high-intensity interval sessions per week (LF group) for a period of 12 weeks, showed a statistically significant improvement in 8 km rollerski time-trial performance. These improvements can likely be explained by a concurrent improvement in % VO_{2max} at AT and exercise economy. There were no statistically significant improvements in rollerski time-trial performance, % VO_{2max} at AT or exercise economy in the HF group, who performed the same weekly volume of high-intensity training as the LF group but distributed among four shorter sessions.

4.1. Rollerski Time-Trial Performance

The improvement in the time-trial performance in the LF group is in line with that presented by Seiler et al. [15], showing that training around the anaerobic threshold is effective in improving long-duration endurance exercise performance. It is possible to speculate that significant improvements in performance may not have been seen if a shorter time-trial had been used, whereas improvements may have been even more pronounced with a longer duration test.

The external conditions such as asphalt, weather conditions, and competitive element of the task and roller ski equipment were similar pre-and post-intervention and should therefore not have impacted the time-trial results.

4.2. VO_{2max} Test

The present findings of no statistically significant change in VO_{2max} in either group is in accordance with findings from previous studies with well-trained cross-country skiers following a similar length training intervention [19,20]. The most likely explanation for this is probably that all the athletes had a long training history, with many years of training at a high level. With prolonged training, improvements in VO_{2max} eventually plateau and there is some evidence for a genetic "ceiling", making it difficult to further increase VO_{2max} in already highly-trained endurance athletes [21,22]. Another possible explanation is that the interval training sessions used in the current study were not of a sufficiently high exercise intensity to stimulate improvements in VO_{2max}. Previous studies have shown that training at an intensity above the anaerobic threshold is necessary in order to stimulate an increase in VO_{2max} in trained athletes [13,15].

4.3. Submaximal Rollerskiing

The increase in %VO_{2max} at AT in the LF group is in line with our hypothesis. However, other studies finding improved aerobic endurance performance reported no changes or minor improvements in %VO_{2max} at AT in endurance trained athletes [13,23]. A possible explanation for this may be differences in the length of the intervention period, interval duration or effective training time in I-zone 3.

Despite equivalent total training volume and intensity, the longer duration per session in the LF group may better stimulate peripheral adaptations such as capillarization, increased size and number of mitochondria, and increased activity of enzymes involved in aerobic respiration [24]. The main stimulus for exercise-induced capillarization in skeletal muscle is increased shear stress due to reactive hyperemia and high strain (e.g., muscle stretch; reviewed by Egginton [25]). It has therefore been suggested that in well-trained endurance athletes, a larger and more concentrated exercise stimulus leads to a higher level of capillarization [26]. As the effective duration in I-zone 3 in the LF group was 64–72 min per session compared to 32–36 min in the HF group, athletes in the LF group were exposed to a larger and more concentrated exercise stimulus. Hence, improved capillarization may partly explain the finding of improved exercise economy in the LF group only. It has been suggested that gross efficiency is improved with high intensity training [27]. Furthermore, it has recently been observed that a higher rate of glycogen utilization during exercise is associated with increased activation of intracellular signaling cascades central in mitochondrial biogenesis [28]. Despite these speculations, the latter may suggest a potential superiority of an exercise session with large glycogen utilization, and theoretically, there was a larger glycogen consumption in the LF training compared to the HF training [29]. It has previously been reported that training in a state of low muscle glycogen to a greater degree stimulates adaptation to endurance exercise [30].

Improved exercise economy in the LF group likely explains the concurrent reduction in submaximal HR. The observed improvement in exercise economy should, in theory, have been coupled with reduced submaximal blood lactate concentration in the LF group. However, this was not the case at the specific workload at which exercise economy was measured in the current study. This is likely related to the aerobic nature of this workload and low blood lactate values at pre-intervention making it difficult to detect changes.

At inclusion, group sizes were matched. However, due to greater drop-out in the HF group, the statistical power of the study was slightly reduced. The present study is too small and it was not decided to elucidate potential differences in adherence to LF- vs. HF-interventions. Recruiting a sufficient number of participants becomes challenging when conducting research with elite athletes. However, we considered as a strength of the study that highly trained athletes were included, rather than sedentary or recreationally active participants. It should be noted that even though there were no differences between groups in weekly training duration in I-zone 3, the difference in the number of work intervals during each session probably induced differences between groups in the session rate of perceived exertion. Unfortunately, the rate of perceived exertion during the sessions was not recorded in the present study.

4.4. Practical Applications and Limitation of the Study

The results of the current study indicate that in order to stimulate improvements in rollerski time-trial performance, $\%VO_{2max}$ at AT, and exercise economy in elite endurance athletes, an interval training model with lower training frequency but longer duration per session appears to be more effective. Interval sessions in I-zone 3 appear to elicit the best effect when the total effective duration is $\geq$60 min. Regardless of whether the total training load remains the same, more frequent sessions of a shorter duration appear less effective in stimulating peripheral adaptations and performance improvements. These findings may be particularly applicable to endurance athletes competing in sports with a long competition time, as previous literature indicates that training at this intensity is particularly beneficial to prolonged exercise performance. One of the limitations of the present study was the number of participants ($n = 20$). However, it is very difficult to achieve high number of participants from individual sports and therefore we believe that this study could contribute to future meta-analysis studies in the field.

5. Conclusions

In a group of elite endurance athletes, two long interval sessions appeared to be more effective than four shorter sessions per week in promoting endurance adaptations and performance improvements. Despite both groups performing the same training volume at the same exercise intensity, it appears that the larger and more concentrated exercise stimulus in the LF group induced more favorable endurance adaptations. The longer time between training sessions in the LF group may have allowed the athletes to recover better and more effectively "absorb" the training. These findings are in line with the current endurance training philosophy in Norwegian elite sport and with the "best practice" observed by many of the world's best endurance athletes [2,3].

Author Contributions: Conceptualization, E.T. and B.R.R.; methodology, E.T., J.H., and B.R.R.; validation, E.T., J.H., and B.R.R.; formal analysis, E.T., J.H., and B.R.R.; investigation, E.T., J.H. and B.R.R.; resources, E.T.; data curation, E.T. and B.R.R.; writing—original draft preparation, E.T.; writing—review and editing, E.T., J.H. and B.R.R.; supervision, E.T., J.H., and B.R.R.; project administration, B.R.R.; funding acquisition, E.T. All authors have read and agreed to the published version of the manuscript.

Funding: This research was funded by the Norwegian Olympic Federation. The APC was funded by School of Health Sciences, Kristiana University College, Oslo, Norway.

Conflicts of Interest: The authors declare no conflict of interest.

References

1. Billat, V.L.; Demarle, A.; Slawinski, J.; Paiva, M.; Koralsztein, J.P. Physical and training characteristics of top-class marathon runners. *Med. Sci. Sports Exerc.* **2001**, *33*, 2089–2097. [CrossRef] [PubMed]
2. Seiler, S.; Tønnessen, E. Intervals, thresholds and long slow distance: The role of intensity and duration in endurance training. *Sport Sci.* **2009**, *13*, 32–53.
3. Tønnessen, E. *Hvorfor ble de Beste Best? En Casestudie av tre Kvinnelige Verdensenere i Orientering, Langrenn og Langdistanseløp*; Norwegian School of Sport Sciences: Oslo, Norway, 2009.
4. Reindell, H.; Roskamm, H. Ein Beitrag zu den physiologischen Grundlagen des Intervalltrainings unter besonderer Berücksichtigung des Kreislaufes. *Schweiz. Z. Sportmed.* **1959**, *7*, 1–8.
5. Billat, V.L.; Slawinski, J.; Bocquet, V.; Demarle, A.; Lafitte, L.; Chassaing, P.; Koralsztein, J.P. Intermittent runs at the velocity associated with maximal oxygen uptake enables subjects to remain at maximal oxygen uptake for a longer time than intense but submaximal runs. *Eur. J. Appl. Physiol.* **2000**, *81*, 188–196. [CrossRef] [PubMed]
6. Hurley, B.F.; Hagberg, J.M.; Allen, W.K.; Seals, D.R.; Young, J.C.; Cuddihee, R.W.; Holloszy, J.O. Effect of training on blood lactate levels during submaximal exercise. *J. Appl. Physiol. Respir. Environ. Exerc. Physiol.* **1984**, *56*, 1260–1264. [CrossRef]
7. MacDougall, D.; Sale, D. Continuous vs. interval training: A review for the athlete and the coach. *Can. J. Appl. Sport Sci.* **1981**, *6*, 93–97. [PubMed]
8. Smith, D.J.; Wenger, H.A. The 10 day aerobic mini-cycle: The effects of interval or continuous training at two different intensities. *J. Sports Med. Phys. Fit.* **1981**, *21*, 390–394.
9. Daniels, J.; Scardina, N. Interval training and performance. *Sports Med.* **1984**, *1*, 327–334. [CrossRef]
10. Daussin, F.N.; Ponsot, E.; Dufour, S.P.; Lonsdorfer-Wolf, E.; Doutreleau, S.; Geny, B.; Piquard, F.; Richard, R. Improvement of VO_{2max} by cardiac output and oxygen extraction adaptation during intermittent versus continuous endurance training. *Eur. J. Appl. Physiol.* **2007**, *101*, 377–383. [CrossRef]
11. Laursen, P.B.; Jenkins, D.G. The scientific basis for high-intensity interval training: Optimising training programmes and maximising performance in highly trained endurance athletes. *Sports Med.* **2002**, *32*, 53–73. [CrossRef]
12. Rozenek, R.; Funato, K.; Kubo, J.; Hoshikawa, M.; Matsuo, A. Physiological responses to interval training sessions at velocities associated with VO_{2max}. *J. Strength Cond. Res.* **2007**, *21*, 188–192.
13. Helgerud, J.; Hoydal, K.; Wang, E.; Karlsen, T.; Berg, P.; Bjerkaas, M.; Simonsen, T.; Helgesen, C.; Hjorth, N.; Bach, R.; et al. Aerobic high-intensity intervals improve VO_{2max} more than moderate training. *Med. Sci. Sports Exerc.* **2007**, *39*, 665–671. [CrossRef]
14. Sandbakk, O.; Sandbakk, S.B.; Ettema, G.; Welde, B. Effects of intensity and duration in aerobic high-intensity interval training in highly trained junior cross-country skiers. *J. Strength Cond. Res.* **2013**, *27*, 1974–1980. [CrossRef]
15. Seiler, S.; Joranson, K.; Olesen, B.V.; Hetlelid, K.J. Adaptations to aerobic interval training: Interactive effects of exercise intensity and total work duration. *Scand. J. Med. Sci. Sports* **2013**, *23*, 74–83. [CrossRef]
16. Wenger, H.A.; Bell, G.J. The interactions of intensity, frequency and duration of exercise training in altering cardiorespiratory fitness. *Sports Med.* **1986**, *3*, 346–356. [CrossRef]
17. Wakefield, B.R.; Glaister, M. Influence of work-interval intensity and duration on time spent at a high percentage of VO_{2max} during intermittent supramaximal exercise. *J. Strength Cond. Res.* **2009**, *23*, 2548–2554. [CrossRef]
18. Howley, E.T.; Bassett, D.R., Jr.; Welch, H.G. Criteria for maximal oxygen uptake: Review and commentary. *Med. Sci. Sports Exerc.* **1995**, *27*, 1292–1301. [CrossRef]
19. Losnegard, T.; Mikkelsen, K.; Ronnestad, B.R.; Hallen, J.; Rud, B.; Raastad, T. The effect of heavy strength training on muscle mass and physical performance in elite cross country skiers. *Scand. J. Med. Sci. Sports* **2011**, *21*, 389–401. [CrossRef]
20. Ronnestad, B.R.; Kojedal, O.; Losnegard, T.; Kvamme, B.; Raastad, T. Effect of heavy strength training on muscle thickness, strength, jump performance, and endurance performance in well-trained Nordic Combined athletes. *Eur. J. Appl. Physiol.* **2012**, *112*, 2341–2352. [CrossRef]
21. Jones, A.M. A five year physiological case study of an Olympic runner. *Br. J. Sports Med.* **1998**, *32*, 39–43. [CrossRef]

22. Rusko, H.K. Development of aerobic power in relation to age and training in cross-country skiers. *Med. Sci. Sports Exerc.* **1992**, *24*, 1040–1047. [CrossRef]
23. Bangsbo, J. Estimation of lactate release from contracting muscles in man. *Acta Physiol. Scand* **1994**, *150*, 349–350. [CrossRef] [PubMed]
24. Holloszy, J.O.; Coyle, E.F. Adaptations of skeletal muscle to endurance exercise and their metabolic consequences. *J. Appl. Physiol. Respir. Environ. Exerc. Physiol.* **1984**, *56*, 831–838. [CrossRef]
25. Egginton, S. Physiological factors influencing capillary growth. *Acta Physiol.* **2011**, *202*, 225–239. [CrossRef]
26. Ronnestad, B.R.; Ellefsen, S.; Nygaard, H.; Zacharoff, E.E.; Vikmoen, O.; Hansen, J.; Hallen, J. Effects of 12 weeks of block periodization on performance and performance indices in well-trained cyclists. *Scand. J. Med. Sci. Sports* **2014**, *24*, 327–335. [CrossRef]
27. Hopker, J.; Coleman, D.; Passfield, L. Changes in cycling efficiency during a competitive season. *Med. Sci. Sports Exerc.* **2009**, *41*, 912–919. [CrossRef]
28. Tokmakidis, S.P.; Leger, L.A.; Pilianidis, T.C. Failure to obtain a unique threshold on the blood lactate concentration curve during exercise. *Eur. J. Appl. Physiol. Occup. Physiol.* **1998**, *77*, 333–342. [CrossRef]
29. Sahlin, K. Metabolic factors in fatigue. *Sports Med.* **1992**, *13*, 99–107. [CrossRef]
30. Hansen, A.K.; Fischer, C.P.; Plomgaard, P.; Andersen, J.L.; Saltin, B.; Pedersen, B.K. Skeletal muscle adaptation: Training twice every second day vs. training once daily. *J. Appl. Physiol.* **2005**, *98*, 93–99. [CrossRef]

International Journal of
Environmental Research and Public Health

MDPI

Article

Sprint Interval Running and Continuous Running Produce Training Specific Adaptations, Despite a Similar Improvement of Aerobic Endurance Capacity—A Randomized Trial of Healthy Adults

Sigbjørn Litleskare [1,2], Eystein Enoksen [1], Marit Sandvei [1], Line Støen [1], Trine Stensrud [1], Egil Johansen [1] and Jørgen Jensen [1,*]

1 Department of Physical Performance, Norwegian School of Sport Sciences, 0863 Oslo, Norway; sigbjorn.litleskare@inn.no (S.L.); eystein.enoksen@nih.no (E.E.); maritsandvei@hotmail.com (M.S.); linemor@gmail.com (L.S.); trine.stensrud@nih.no (T.S.); e.i.johansen@nih.no (E.J.)

2 Department of Sports and Physical Education, Inland Norway University of Applied Sciences, 2406 Elverum, Norway

* Correspondence: jorgen.jensen@nih.no

Received: 9 April 2020; Accepted: 26 May 2020; Published: 29 May 2020

Abstract: The purpose of the present study was to investigate training-specific adaptations to eight weeks of moderate intensity continuous training (CT) and sprint interval training (SIT). Young healthy subjects (n = 25; 9 males and 16 females) performed either continuous training (30–60 min, 70–80% peak heart rate) or sprint interval training (5–10 near maximal 30 s sprints, 3 min recovery) three times per week for eight weeks. Maximal oxygen consumption, 20 m shuttle run test and 5·60 m sprint test were performed before and after the intervention. Furthermore, heart rate, oxygen pulse, respiratory exchange ratio, lactate and running economy were assessed at five submaximal intensities, before and after the training interventions. Maximal oxygen uptake increased after CT (before: 47.9 ± 1.5; after: 49.7 ± 1.5 mL·kg^{-1}·min^{-1}, $p < 0.05$) and SIT (before: 50.5 ± 1.6; after: 53.3 ± 1.5 mL·kg^{-1}·min^{-1}, $p < 0.01$), with no statistically significant differences between groups. Both groups increased 20 m shuttle run performance and 60 m sprint performance, but SIT performed better than CT at the 4th and 5th 60 m sprint after the intervention ($p < 0.05$). At submaximal intensities, CT, but not SIT, reduced heart rate ($p < 0.05$), whereas lactate decreased in both groups. In conclusion, both groups demonstrated similar improvements of several performance measures including VO_{2max}, but sprint performance was better after SIT, and CT caused training-specific adaptations at submaximal intensities.

Keywords: maximal oxygen consumption; heart rate; oxygen pulse; shuttle run; repeated sprint ability

1. Introduction

Manipulation of duration and intensity of exercise bouts change the demands of metabolic pathways within muscle cells, as well as oxygen delivery to exercising muscles [1]. The training adaptations that occur after repeated bouts of exercise are to some degree specific to that particular exercise [1,2], but both high intensity interval training and continuous training bouts increase VO_{2max} and oxidative capacity in skeletal muscles [1–3]. Within this context, it is of interest to clarify the specific adaptations of different training protocols to optimize endurance training, health and performance.

There has recently been a lot of interest in a type of high intensity interval training known as sprint interval training (SIT). SIT is (often) performed as 30 s of "all out" sprints with 2.5–4.5 min of rest between sprints [4–6]. Several cycling studies have reported that this type of training improves maximal oxygen consumption (VO_{2max}), endurance performance and the oxidative capacity of skeletal muscle [3–12]. Previous studies have also demonstrated that the magnitude of improvement in endurance performance and VO_{2max} after SIT is comparable to continuous cycling at moderate intensity [3,4]. Furthermore, research also suggest that SIT is an efficient approach to improve several important health parameters in addition to VO_{2max}, such as insulin sensitivity, blood pressure, cardiovascular function, and body composition [13].

Because most previous studies on SIT adaptations have used a cycling protocol, there is limited knowledge about sprint interval running [14]. This is unfortunate, as running is a basic and popular type of exercise. More importantly, there are several fundamental differences between cycling and running exercise. Power output during sprint exercise is substantially higher in cycling than in running [15]. There are also several physiological differences, such as higher heart rate (HR), higher fat oxidation and higher muscle mass activation in running than in cycling [16,17]. Thus, results from sprint interval cycling may not be directly applicable to sprint interval running [18].

Only a few previous studies have investigated the effects of sprint interval running. In most of these studies, SIT is added to the training program of trained endurance athletes [19–21]. However, one previous study has compared the effect of sprint interval and traditional endurance running in healthy untrained subjects [22]. Macpherson et al. [22] reported similar improvements of VO_{2max} and endurance performance after SIT and continuous running at moderate intensity. Interestingly, VO_{2max} improved in the SIT group without affecting cardiac output, whereas continuous running increased cardiac output, as expected. The study by Macpherson et al. [22] revealed that sprint interval running and continuous running produced similar improvements of aerobic performance, but still caused training-specific physiological adaptations. Because there is limited data available on this topic, it is of great interest to investigate training-specific adaptations of sprint interval running and continuous running.

The purpose of this study was therefore to compare performance and health related adaptations of continuous training (CT) and SIT, performed as running, on VO_{2max}, 20 m shuttle run performance, repeated sprint ability (RSA) and the physiological response to submaximal exercise. We hypothesized that both types of training would improve VO_{2max} and 20 m shuttle run similarly, and that training-specific adaptations would occur at submaximal exercise in favor of CT and during RSA in favor of SIT.

2. Materials and Methods

2.1. Participants

Participants were recruited through the official webpage of the Norwegian School of Sport Sciences, and printed and electronic flyers posted in various places in the local area of northern Oslo and in social media, respectively. Forty-eight subjects volunteered and were screened for participation. The inclusion criteria for participation were: (1) non-smokers; (2) body mass index (BMI) < 30 kg·m^{-2}; (3) no cardiovascular or metabolic disease; (4) no systematic endurance training during the last two years (≤2 sessions per week). Twenty-nine subjects met these criteria and were invited to participate. Subjects were matched based on gender and VO_{2max}, and then randomly assigned by coin toss to either CT or SIT. Four subjects dropped out during the training intervention; One dropped out during week 1 due to receiving a job offer (CT, male 21 years), one, during week 2, after realizing that participation in the intervention was not compatible with his life situation (SIT, male, 21 years), one during week 5, due to unspecified reasons (CT, male, 22 years), and one during week 8, due to moving to a different region (SIT, female, 22 years). Thus, 25 subjects (9 males and 16 females) completed the training intervention.

2.2. Training Protocol

Both groups completed eight weeks of training. Each week consisted of three training sessions, separated by at least one resting day. Training sessions were organized and supervised by qualified instructors. Subjects were occasionally allowed to perform sessions at home if participation in organized sessions was problematic. The training intensity was controlled during all sessions by heart rate monitors (Polar Sport Tester RS800CX, Polar Electro, OY, Kempele, Finland). An adherence of >85% (19 of 24 training sessions, including sessions performed at home) was required. Subjects were instructed to maintain their normal diet and lifestyle throughout the intervention.

The CT group was instructed to maintain an intensity corresponding to 70–80% HR_{peak} at all training sessions. Organized training sessions were performed on slightly undulating terrain. During the first week, the CT group performed 30 min of running. The time then increased by five minutes per week, up to a total of 60 min. The SIT group consisted of 30 s sprints at near maximal effort, with three minutes of rest between each sprint. The training intensity of SIT sessions was evaluated subjectively during sessions, while the HR data was used to verify that the individual participant did not have a session or interval that deviated from their usual level of effort. During the first week, the SIT group performed five sprints per session. The number of sprints then increased gradually, until a total of 10 sprints per session in weeks 7 and 8. When the number of sprints reached seven, subjects were given six minutes of rest midway through the training session. All sprints were performed on slightly uphill terrain. Prior to all training sessions, the CT group performed a ten-minute warm-up at an intensity corresponding to 60–75% of HR_{peak}. The SIT group performed a ten-minute warm-up at an intensity corresponding to 60–85% of HR_{peak}, followed by three incremental strides of about 80 m. After each training session, all subjects performed five minutes of walking or running at intensities below 70% of HR_{peak}. The training volume in CT and SIT was not matched.

2.3. Measures

Incremental treadmill test to exhaustion. The test was performed on a motorized treadmill (Woodway pps55 sport, Woodway Gmbh, Weil an Rhein, Germany). Oxygen consumption (VO_2) was measured through a 2-way mouthpiece (Hans Rudolph Instr., Shawnee, KS, USA) and a sling, which was connected to an O_2 and CO_2 analyzer (Oxycon Champion, Jaeger Instruments, Hoechberg, Germany). Samples of O_2 and CO_2 were collected continuously from a mixing chamber, with average values obtained over 30-s intervals. The gas analyzer was calibrated before each test with ventilated indoor air and standardized gas concentrations, to span the concentration range observed during exercise. The expired volume was measured with a turbine (Triple V volume transducer, Leipzig, Germany), and volume calibration was performed regularly with a 3-L syringe.

The incremental test to exhaustion followed current recommendations for test duration [23], and was performed according to the standard protocol of the Norwegian Olympic Sports Centre (see e.g., [24]). Prior to the pre-test, subjects performed two familiarization tests to reduce the learning effect, following the recommendations of Edgett et al. [25]. Identical procedures were conducted for familiarization, pre- and post-test. All subjects performed a 15-min warm-up of gradually increasing intensity. The last five minutes of the warm-up were performed with an inclination of 5.3%, as was the incremental test. The starting speed was chosen in order to exhaust the subjects after ~5 min. Running speed was initially increased by 1 $km \cdot h^{-1}$ every minute. At the end of the test, running speed was either maintained or increased by 0.5 $km \cdot h^{-1}$, to allow at least one minute running at the final speed. VO_{2max} was determined as the average of the highest values achieved over two subsequent 30-s measurements. Verbal encouragement was given throughout the test. Two minutes after completion, a capillary blood sample was obtained and 20 μl of blood was injected into a lactate analyzer (1500 SPORT, YSI Inc., Yellow Springs Instr., Yellow spring, OH, USA), with the help of a standard injector. The lactate analyzer was calibrated before each test with a 5.0 mM lactate standard. The main criterion for evaluating whether VO_{2max} was achieved was a plateau in oxygen consumption. A levelling-off of the VO_2 curve was used in conjunction with a lactate value ≥ 6 $mmol \cdot l^{-1}$ and respiratory exchange ratio (RER) > 1.10 as secondary criteria. HR was monitored throughout the test (Polar Sport Tester RS800CX, Polar Electro, OY, Kempele, Finland) and the highest value achieved was defined as HR_{peak}.

Submaximal treadmill test. The submaximal treadmill test was conducted with the same equipment as described above and consisted of four stages of five minutes on a motorized treadmill. The running speed at each stage was individualized based on each subject's VO_{2max} and a general relationship between running speed and VO_2. This relationship was estimated based on data from a pilot study. The purpose of the procedure was to establish four individualized stages of gradually increasing running velocities at approximate intensities of 50%, 60%, 70% and 80% of VO_{2max}. The same velocity (absolute intensity) was used for both the pre- and post-test. Measurements of VO_2 and RER were made between the third and fourth minute. After the fourth minute, the mouthpiece was removed and HR was monitored until the end of the stage. Between each stage, the subjects were given one minute rest for measurement of lactate, as described above. The post-test was conducted at the same running velocities as the pre-test. Running economy (RE; $mL \cdot kg^{-1} \cdot km^{-1}$) was defined as VO_2 divided by body mass and running speed. O_2 pulse ($mL \cdot beat^{-1}$) was calculated by dividing VO_2 ($mL \cdot min^{-1}$) by HR ($beat \cdot min^{-1}$).

Training adaptations at the same relative intensity were evaluated by examining the running speed that elicited the VO_2 value closest to 70% of the individual subject's VO_{2max}. This intensity was chosen because it produced the least variation in VO_2 values.

Repeated sprint test. After completing the submaximal treadmill test, all subjects performed a 5·60 m repeated sprint test in an indoor sports hall. The test was considered appropriate to induce the performance decrement associated with repeated sprint exercise [26]. All subjects performed a test-specific warm-up prior to the sprint test consisting of 3·60 m incremental runs. The sprints were performed with a 1 m flying start and each sprint was separated by 30 s of rest. Time was measured by photoelectric detectors (Brower Speed Trap II Timing system, Brower Timing system, Salt Lake USA). Verbal encouragement was given throughout the test.

20 m shuttle run test. The 20 m shuttle run test procedure was the same as previously described [27]. In short, subjects ran repeatedly between two lines, 20 m apart. The test started at a running speed of 8.5 $km \cdot h^{-1}$, which then increased by 0.5 $km \cdot h^{-1}$ per minute. The test was terminated when subjects failed to reach the 20 m line before the signal on two successive occasions. To stimulate competition, the subjects ran in groups.

2.4. Procedures

All tests were performed before and after the training interventions. The submaximal treadmill test and the repeated sprint test were performed on the same day, and only separated by the time to relocate from the laboratory to the sports hall. All other tests were separated by at least one resting day. Subjects were familiarized with testing procedures to minimize any potential learning effect.

The data for this study were collected in relation to a larger study [28]. The study was approved by the Regional Ethics Committee of Oslo, Norway (ref. number 2010/1567-1) and was performed according to the Declaration of Helsinki. All subjects were informed about the purpose of the study and associated risks before they gave their written informed consent to participate.

A few subjects did not obtain valid results for all tests due to sickness, injury and unspecified withdrawal from the study. These subjects were excluded from both pre and post analysis for these particular tests. The number of participants for each test is stated in the captions of tables and figures.

2.5. Analysis

Data are presented as group means ± SEM. All statistical analyses were performed in SPSS version 18 (SPSS inc., Chicago, IL, USA). The assumption of normality was evaluated by a Shapiro–Wilk test. Student's paired t-test was used to investigate within-group differences, and a Student's unpaired t-test was used to investigate between-group differences. A repeated measures ANOVA with a Greenhouse–Geisser correction was used to evaluate a potential increase in VO_{2max} as a function of the number of tests performed before the intervention. In cases where data was not normally distributed, a Wilcoxon signed-rank test was used to verify within-group differences, and a Mann–Whitney test was used to verify between-group differences. Statistical significance was accepted at the $p < 0.05$ level.

3. Results

The number of females in each group was eight, while the number of males was four in CT and five in SIT. The mean age, height, weight and BMI was 25 ± 1 years, 175 ± 2 cm, 72.6 ± 3.8 kg and 23.6 ± 0.9 $kg \cdot m^{-2}$ in CT at the start of the intervention. In SIT, the mean age, height, weight and BMI was 25 ± 1 years, 173 ± 3 cm, 71.2 ± 4.1 kg and 24.0 ± 0.8 $kg \cdot m^{-2}$. There was no statistical difference between groups and these characteristics did not change during the intervention. Heart rate registrations at all training sessions confirmed that the subjects performed the training as recommended, including the sessions performed at home (19% of sessions). Three participants experienced minor injuries during the training intervention, including one injury unrelated to the intervention. All three were in the SIT group, and all managed to complete > 85% of training sessions.

Maximal oxygen consumption and 20 m shuttle run performance. Maximal oxygen uptake was measured three times prior to the intervention, and VO_{2max} increased from test to test. The repeated measures ANOVA revealed that VO_{2max} increased from 48.2 ± 1.1 at the first familiarization test to 49.3 ± 1.3 in the second, and eventually to 49.9 ± 1.3 $mL \cdot kg^{-1} \cdot min^{-1}$ at the third test when combining both groups ($F(1.434, 28.683) = 10.320$, $p < 0.01$). VO_{2max} was improved in both CT ($p < 0.05$) and SIT ($p < 0.01$) after training (Table 1). The improvement of VO_{2max} corresponded to a 3.8% increase in CT and 5.5% in SIT. The increase in VO_{2max} varied between subjects and five subjects did not increase VO_{2max} (Figure 1). In accordance with the improved VO_{2max}, both groups also increased maximal O_2 pulse ($p < 0.05$) and the number of laps performed on the 20 m shuttle run test (CT $p < 0.05$; SIT $p < 0.01$).

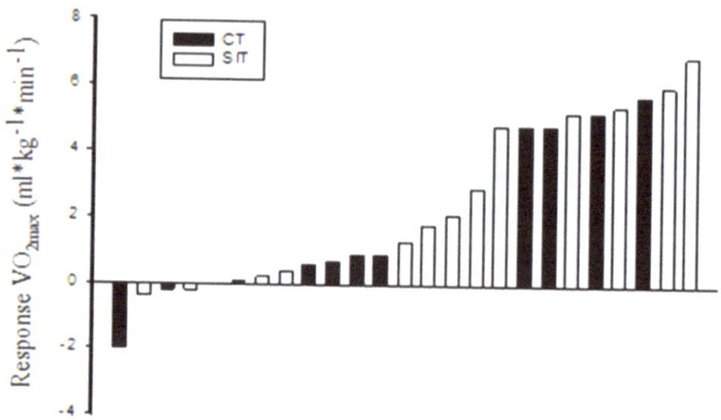

Figure 1. Individual change in maximal oxygen consumption (VO_{2max}) after eight weeks of either continuous training (CT) or sprint interval training (SIT) (one subject in CT did not experience any change).

Repeated sprint test. Both the CT and SIT groups improved sprint performance for the first sprint (Table 2) and thereby improved maximal 60 m sprint performance. Both groups also improved performance on all successive sprints. However, the SIT group performed better than the CT group on sprints number four ($p < 0.05$) and five ($p < 0.05$) after the intervention (Table 2).

Table 1. Parameters of maximal endurance performance before and after eight weeks of continuous training (CT) and sprint interval training (SIT).

	CT		SIT	
	Pre	Post	Pre	Post
VO_{2max} ($mL{\cdot}kg^{-1}{\cdot}min^{-1}$)	47.9 ± 1.5	49.7 ± 1.5 *	50.5 ± 1.6	53.3 ± 1.5 *
Maximal O_2 pulse	17.4 ± 1.0	18.1 ± 1.0 *	18.0 ± 1.0	19.2 ± 1.0 *
Laps	71.5 ± 6.1	79.4 ± 5.2 *	69.5 ± 3.8	81.7 ± 4.0 *

Values are mean ± SEM. CT, n = 12 (4 males, 8 females). SIT, n = 13 (5 males, 8 females). VO_{2max}, maximal oxygen consumption; O_2 pulse, oxygen pulse; Laps, number of laps completed during the 20 m shuttle run test. * Statistically significant difference from pre (student's t-test), $p < 0.05$. There were no statistically significant differences between groups.

Table 2. Performance on the repeated sprint test before and after eight weeks of continuous training (CT) and sprint interval training (SIT).

	CT				SIT			
	Pre		Post		Pre		Post	
	Time (s)	%dec.	Time (s)	%dec	Time (s)	%dec	Time (s)	%dec
1. 60 m	9.92 ± 0.25		9.69 ± 0.26 *		9.64 ± 0.26		9.20 ± 0.21 *	
2. 60 m	10.44 ± 0.33	5.2	10.06 ± 0.27 *	3.8	9.98 ± 0.23	3.5	9.48 ± 0.18 *	3.0
3. 60 m	10.76 ± 0.29	8.5	10.31 ± 0.23 *	6.4	10.27 ± 0.22	6.5	9.89 ± 0.20 *	7.5
4. 60 m	10.87 ± 0.30	9.6	10.54 ± 0.23 *	8.8	10.37 ± 0.25	7.6	9.91 ± 0.19 *,†	7.7
5. 60 m	10.93 ± 0.21	10.2	10.70 ± 0.22 *	10.4	10.53 ± 0.25	9.2	9.96 ± 0.20 *,†	8.3

Values are mean ± SEM. CT, n = 10. SIT, n = 11. %dec = percent performance decrement compared to the fastest sprint time * Statistically significant difference from pre.† Statistically significant difference from CT (student's t-test), $p < 0.05$.

Physiological response to submaximal exercise at the same absolute intensity. The submaximal treadmill test was performed at the same velocity, before and after the intervention. Both groups ran at a lower percentage of VO_{2max} after eight weeks of training (Table 3). The CT group decreased VO_2 at all stages (i.e., running economy), while the SIT group decreased VO_2 at stage 4 and RE at stages 2 and 4 (Table 3). HR was lower after CT at all stages ($p < 0.01$), but remained unchanged after SIT (Table 3). O_2 pulse at submaximal intensities did not change in any group (Table 3).

Physiological response to submaximal exercise at the same relative intensity. Adaptations to running, performed at the same relative intensity before and after the intervention, were evaluated at the velocity closest to 70% VO_{2max}. At this intensity, HR remained unchanged after CT, while O_2 pulse increased by 0.6 $mL{\cdot}beat^{-1}$ ($p < 0.05$; Table 4). In contrast, HR increased ($p < 0.05$) and O_2 pulse remained unchanged after SIT (Table 4). RER was reduced at 70% VO_{2max} after CT ($p < 0.05$), but not statistically significant after SIT ($p = 0.07$; Table 4). Lactate was reduced at 70% of VO_{2max} in both groups after the intervention.

Table 3. Physiological responses at submaximal velocities, before (pre) and after (post) eight weeks of either continuous training (CT) or sprint interval training (SIT).

		1		2		3		4	
		Pre	**Post**	**Pre**	**Post**	**Pre**	**Post**	**Pre**	**Post**
CT	VO_2 (mL·min^{-1})	1553 ± 139	1381 ± 159 *,#	2307 ± 177	1876 ± 157 *	2414 ± 175	2275 ± 174 *	2754 ± 186	2620 ± 172 *
	% VO_{2max}	45.1 ± 3.4	37.8 ± 2.1 *	58.4 ± 3.1	52.4 ± 2.8 *	71.1 ± 2.3	64.6 ± 2.4 *	79.4 ± 2.0	73.3 ± 1.8 *
	RE (mL·kg^{-1}·km^{-1})	213 ± 16	186 ± 10 *,#	229 ± 12	213 ± 10 *	238 ± 8	224 ± 8 *	232 ± 6	223 ± 6 *
	% HR_{peak}	66.9 ± 2.1	59.6 ± 2.3 *	76.8 ± 2.2	70.8 ± 2.5 *	85.3 ± 1.5	80.2 ± 2.1 *	90.0 ± 1.0	86.3 ± 1.4 *
	O_2pulse (mL·beat^{-1})	11.5 ± 0.7	11.5 ± 1.0	13.1 ± 0.8	13.3 ± 0.9	14.2 ± 0.8	14.1 ± 0.9	15.3 ± 0.9	15.2 ± 0.9
	RER (VCO_2·$VO_2$$^{-1}$)	0.89 ± 0.01	0.84 ± 0.01 *	0.93 ± 0.01	0.88 ± 0.01 *	0.94 ± 0.01	0.90 ± 0.01 *	0.97 ± 0.01	0.93 ± 0.01 *
	Lactate (mmol·l^{-1})	1.22 ± 0.13	0.77 ± 0.06 *	1.76 ± 0.26	1.16 ± 0.13 *	2.39 ± 0.25	1.75 ± 0.17 *	3.84 ± 0.30	2.66 ± 0.24 *
SIT	VO_2 (mL·min^{-1})	1544 ± 152	1523 ± 150	2221 ± 168	2076 ± 158	2574 ± 181	2500 ± 165	2909 ± 204	2832 ± 196 *,#
	% VO_{2max}	42.6 ± 2.2	40.1 ± 2.5 *	61.9 ± 1.6	55.3 ± 2.0 *	71.8 ± 1.2	66.5 ± 1.5 *	81.2 ± 0.9	75.2 ± 1.2 *
	RE (mL·kg^{-1}·km^{-1})	201 ± 10	199 ± 10	243 ± 8	228 ± 8 *	240 ± 5	234 ± 4	237 ± 4	231 ± 4 *
	% HR_{peak}	61.6 ± 2.4	61.6 ± 2.5	75.0 ± 1.6	72.0 ± 2.0	82.6 ± 1.2	81.1 ± 1.5	88.6 ± 0.9	87.2 ± 1.2
	O_2pulse (mL·beat^{-1})	12.8 ± 1.0	12.6 ± 1.0	14.9 ± 1.0	14.5 ± 1.1	15.8 ± 1.0	15.6 ± 0.9	16.6 ± 1.0	16.4 ± 1.0
	RER (VCO_2·$VO_2$$^{-1}$)	0.86 ± 0.02	0.83 ± 0.02	0.91 ± 0.01	0.87 ± 0.02 *,#	0.92 ± 0.01	0.89 ± 0.01 *	0.96 ± 0.01	0.92 ± 0.01 *
	Lactate (mmol·l^{-1})	1.12 ± 0.08	0.89 ± 0.06 *	1.79 ± 0.15	1.20 ± 0.07 *,#	2.38 ± 0.17	1.68 ± 0.12 *	3.45 ± 0.24	2.66 ± 0.19 *,#

Values are mean ± SEM. VO_2, oxygen consumption; % VO_{2max}, percent of maximal oxygen consumption; RE, running economy; % HF_{peak}, percent of peak heart rate; O_2 pulse, oxygen pulse; RER, respiratory exchange ratio. Velocities at stage 1, 2, 3 and 4 equaled 6.2 ± 0.2, 7.5 ± 0.2, 8.8 ± 0.3 and 10.1 ± 0.3 km·h^{-1} in CT, and 6.4 ± 0.2, 7.7 ± 0.2, 9.1 ± 0.3 and 10.4 ± 0.3 km·h^{-1} in SIT. CT, n = 11. SIT, n = 13. Values for % HF_{peak} and O_2 pulse represents only 12 subjects in SIT. * Statistically significant difference from pre (student's t-test), $p < 0.05$. # Statistically significant difference from pre (verified by Wilcoxon signed rank test), $p < 0.05$. There were no statistically significant differences between groups.

Table 4. Physiological responses to running at the velocity closest to 70 percent of maximal oxygen consumption, before (pre) and after (post) eight weeks of either continuous training (CT) or sprint interval training (SIT).

	CT		SIT	
	Pre	**Post**	**Pre**	**Post**
Velocity ($km \cdot h^{-1}$)	8.7 ± 0.4	9.7 ± 0.3 *	8.8 ± 0.4	9.6 ± 0.3 *
% VO_{2max}	70.5 ± 0.9	71.4 ± 0.7	70.3 ± 0.7	70.2 ± 0.6
% HR_{peak}	84.3 ± 1.0	85.1 ± 0.9	81.9 ± 1.6	84.9 ± 1.4 *
O_2 pulse ($mL \cdot beat^{-1}$)	14.5 ± 0.9	15.1 ± 0.9 *	15.7 ± 1.0	16.0 ± 0.9
RER ($VCO_2 \cdot VO_2^{-1}$)	0.94 ± 0.01	0.91 ± 0.01 *	0.93 ± 0.01	0.91 ± 0.01
Lactate ($mmol \cdot l^{-1}$)	2.62 ± 0.16	2.18 ± 0.19 *,#	2.33 ± 0.12	2.03 ± 0.15 *,#

Values are mean ± SEM. % VO_{2max}, percent of maximal oxygen consumption; % HF_{peak}, percent of peak heart rate; O_2 pulse, oxygen pulse; RER, respiratory exchange ratio. CT, $n = 11$. SIT, $n = 13$. Values for % HF_{peak} and O_2 pulse represents only 12 subjects in SIT. * Statistically significant difference from pre (student's t-test), $p < 0.05$. # Statistically significant difference from pre (verified by Wilcoxon signed rank test), $p < 0.05$. There were no statistically significant differences between groups.

4. Discussion

The main findings of the present study were that both training protocols increased VO_{2max} and shuttle run performance, but also produced training-specific adaptations. The SIT group performed better than the CT group on the last two 60 m sprints, while only CT improved HR and O_2 pulse adaptations at submaximal intensities.

The higher VO_{2max} in both groups after eight weeks of training holds implications for both performance and health, and is supported by previous research, showing a comparable improvement of VO_{2max} after sprint interval running and cycling [4,22]. Interestingly, previous research suggests that the adaptations that lead to the comparable improvement of VO_{2max} are different in the two types of training interventions. Macpherson et al. [22] showed that continuous endurance running improved maximal cardiac output, while sprint interval running did not. These reports suggest that the improvement of VO_{2max} in the present study was due to peripheral adaptations [5,6]. Importantly, the increase in VO_{2max} varied substantially between participants whether they performed CT or SIT, and five subjects did not increase their VO_{2max}, even though the training was supervised by qualified instructors, and heart rate recordings confirmed that the training was performed with the recommended HR. These data agree with previous studies showing large variation in the increase in VO_{2max} after endurance training [29,30]. Genetic variation has been suggested to explain differences in the increase of VO_{2max}, but research also suggests that a large number of genetic variations collectively determine increases in VO_{2max} [31]. No genetic variation predicting has so far been validated.

The increase of VO_{2max} observed after endurance exercise is caused by an improvement of cardiac output and/or arteriovenous oxygen difference [32], which results in higher VO_2 per heartbeat (i.e., O_2 pulse). At submaximal intensities, an increased O_2 pulse results in lower HR [32]. In the present study, HR was reduced after CT at all submaximal velocities, while it remained unchanged after SIT. However, the participants improved running economy, which precludes the comparison of cardio-respiratory adaptations at the same absolute intensities. Therefore, to investigate the submaximal training adaptations independent of running economy, we examined HR and O_2 pulse at the same relative intensity (~70% VO_{2max}), pre and post training. At ~70% VO_{2max}, O_2 pulse increases after CT as expected (please see Table 4). In contrast, SIT did not change O_2 pulse at ~70% VO_{2max} and HR was higher after the training intervention, supporting Macpherson et al. [22], who reported unchanged cardiac output after sprint interval running. Increased cardiac output leads to higher O_2 pulse and decreased HR at submaximal intensities [31]. The limited cardiac adaptations after SIT in the present study suggest that CT is a superior option for cardiac adaptations, which holds implications for the health benefits of SIT, as improved cardiac function is an important part of the health benefits of exercise [33].

Several studies have shown that SIT increases the expression of oxidative enzymes in skeletal muscle [3,5,6]. In the present study, blood lactate and RER were reduced after both CT and SIT (although $p = 0.07$ for RER in SIT at 70% VO_{2max}). It is well known that lactate production and RER are influenced by the oxidative capacity of skeletal muscle [34] and, thus, our results suggest that both CT and SIT improved the oxidative capacity of skeletal muscle. Results from the 20 m shuttle run test also revealed that both groups improved endurance performance and that the improvement was similar in both groups. These results are in accordance with previous investigations of both sprint interval cycling and running [3,22]. Endurance performance is a complex characteristic that is dependent on several factors, which makes it difficult to identify any single factor responsible for improved performance. Several adaptions could potentially contribute to the improved endurance performance observed in this study, but the correlation between the change of VO_{2max} and the change of 20 m shuttle run performance ($r = 0.56$, $p = 0.01$) suggest that VO_{2max} is central.

Results from the test of repeated sprints showed that both CT and SIT improved the performance of the first sprint and thereby improved maximal sprint performance. Improved maximal 60 m sprint performance after CT may be surprising based on the "slow paced" nature of the training intervention. However, previous research has reported similar results for untrained people, including two studies of endurance cycling reporting improved sprint performance after continuous training [34,35]. The mechanisms behind these improvements are uncertain, but mechanical efficiency has been suggested as the most important factor [35]. In the present study, CT improved RE, which is a common measure of mechanical efficiency [36]. Improved RE could therefore offer an explanation for improved maximal sprint performance after CT. Improvements of mechanical efficiency is often associated with increased stiffness of muscles and tendons, but improved running technique by wasting less energy on braking forces and excessive vertical oscillation may be a likely cause for the improvement in CT [36], since the participants were inexperienced runners with a high potential for improving running technique. Improved maximal running velocity after SIT has previously been reported [22], and is supported by findings of improved peak power after sprint interval cycling [4,8,9,19].

Both groups also improved repeated sprint ability. These results are in accordance with previous studies that have investigated RSA after continuous training and high intensity interval training [34,35,37]. Interestingly, the SIT group performed better than the CT group on sprints number four and five after the intervention, thus demonstrating a superior ability to resist fatigue. The reason for the improved performance on the last two sprints could be related to the ability of SIT to increase muscle buffer capacity and levels of anaerobic enzymes [3,6], and to prevent metabolic and ionic perturbation during high-intensity exercise [8]. All of these adaptations can potentially improve performance during repeated sprint exercise [26]. The benefit of improved buffer capacity and ability to prevent ionic and metabolic perturbations would be progressively more beneficial during repeated sprint exercise, which may explain why SIT performed better at sprint number 4 and 5, and not 1, 2 and 3.

Some limitations in the present study need to be recognized. The number of participants included in this study was based on an a priori power analysis for the between group comparison of VO_{2max}. However, the statistical power may still be limited for the other comparisons in this study, in particular for tests with missing data. The results at the 70% intensity should be considered carefully. As explained in the methods, running speed was not adjusted to exactly 70% VO_{2max} and there was some individual variation in running intensity from pre- to post-test. However, these variations were small, and mean relative intensity varied by less than one percentage-point between pre- and post-test (Table 4). The majority of participants were female, and although training groups were gender matched, we did not control for oral contraceptive use and menstrual cycle phase. Furthermore, high intensity exercise is commonly associated with increased risk of injury [38], and in the present study, we were unable to prevent the occurrence of injuries in the SIT group, despite a standardized warm-up and supervision of highly qualified personnel. Strengths of this study include the fact that heart rate was recorded at all training sessions, and that both females and males were included. Furthermore, a substantial effort was made during familiarization, to reduce the potential impact of a learning effect on VO_{2max} from pre- to post-test. VO_{2max} did increase during the familiarization process, but levelled off from the last familiarization test to the pre-test, which indicates that the efforts was successful at minimizing the learning effect in this study. However, the inclusion of the familiarization tests in addition to an already high number of pre-tests may have resulted in some minor training adaptations before the onset of the training interventions.

5. Conclusions

In conclusion, both types of training produced similar improvements of VO_{2max}, endurance capacity and sprint performance. Despite these similarities, O_2 pulse and HR during submaximal exercise was improved after CT only, which suggests superior adaptations of cardiac health after CT compared to SIT. In addition, SIT improved RSA significantly more compared to CT. The present study therefore suggest that training-specific adaptations occur after sprint interval running and continuous running with moderate intensity. The presumption of training-specific adaptations should be taken into consideration when composing an optimal endurance training program.

Author Contributions: Conceptualization, S.L., E.E., M.S., L.S., E.J., T.S. and J.J.; methodology, S.L., E.E., M.S., L.S., E.J., and J.J.; formal analysis, S.L.; investigation, S.L., E.E., M.S., L.S., E.J. and J.J.; writing—original draft preparation, S.L.; writing—review and editing, E.E., M.S., L.S., E.J., T.S. and J.J.; supervision, E.E. and J.J.; project administration, S.L., M.S. and L.S. All authors have read and agreed to the published version of the manuscript.

Funding: This research received no external funding.

Acknowledgments: The authors thank Puma, Norway, for supplying subjects with training equipment. We also thank Line Hårklau for technical assistance and Kristoffer Jensen Kolnes for help as training instructor.

Conflicts of Interest: The authors declare no conflict of interest.

References

1. Laursen, P.B.; Jenkins, D.G. The scientific basis for high-intensity interval training: Optimising training programmes and maximising performance in highly trained endurance athletes. *Sports Med.* **2002**, *32*, 53–73. [CrossRef] [PubMed]
2. Seiler, S.; Tønnessen, E. Intervals, Thresholds, and Long Slow Distance: The Role of Intensity and Duration in Endurance Training. *Sport Sci.* **2009**, *13*, 32–53.
3. Gibala, M.J.; Little, J.P.; Van Essen, M.; Wilkin, G.P.; Burgomaster, K.A.; Safdar, A., Raha, S.; Tarnopolsky, M.A. Short-term sprint interval versus traditional endurance training: Similar initial adaptations in human skeletal muscle and exercise performance. *J. Physiol.* **2006**, *575 Pt 3*, 901–911. [CrossRef]
4. Burgomaster, K.A.; Howarth, K.R.; Phillips, S.M.; Rakobowchuk, M.; MacDonald, M.J.; McGee, S.L.; Gibala, M.J. Similar metabolic adaptations during exercise after low volume sprint interval and traditional endurance training in humans. *J. Physiol.* **2008**, *586*, 151–160. [CrossRef] [PubMed]
5. Burgomaster, K.A.; Hughes, S.C.; Heigenhauser, G.J.; Bradwell, S.N.; Gibala, M.J. Six sessions of sprint interval training increases muscle oxidative potential and cycle endurance capacity in humans. *J. Appl. Physiol.* **2005**, *98*, 1985–1990. [CrossRef]
6. MacDougall, J.D.; Hicks, A.L.; MacDonald, J.R.; McKelvie, R.S.; Green, H.J.; Smith, K.M. Muscle performance and enzymatic adaptations to sprint interval training. *J. Appl. Physiol.* **1998**, *84*, 2138–2142. [CrossRef]
7. Burgomaster, K.A.; Heigenhauser, G.J.; Gibala, M.J. Effect of short-term sprint interval training on human skeletal muscle carbohydrate metabolism during exercise and time-trial performance. *J. Appl. Physiol.* **2006**, *100*, 2041–2047.
8. Harmer, A.R.; McKenna, M.J.; Sutton, J.R.; Snow, R.J.; Ruell, P.A.; Booth, J.; Thompson, M.W.; Mackay, N.A.; Stathis, C.G.; Crameri, R.M.; et al. Skeletal muscle metabolic and ionic adaptations during intense exercise following sprint training in humans. *J. Appl. Physiol.* **2000**, *89*, 1793–1803. [CrossRef]
9. Hazell, T.J.; MacPherson, R.E.; Gravelle, B.M.; Lemon, P.W. 10 or 30-s sprint interval training bouts enhance both aerobic and anaerobic performance. *Eur. J. Appl. Physiol.* **2010**, *110*, 153–160.

10. Macpherson, T.W.; Weston, M. The effect of low-volume sprint interval training on the development and subsequent maintenance of aerobic fitness in soccer players. *Int. J. Sports Physiol. Perform.* **2015**, *10*, 332–338.
11. Naves, J.P.A.; Viana, R.B.; Rebelo, A.C.S.; de Lira, C.A.B.; Pimentel, G.D.; Lobo, P.C.B.; de Oliveira, J.C.; Ramirez-Campillo, R.; Gentil, P. Effects of High-Intensity Interval Training vs. Sprint Interval Training on Anthropometric Measures and Cardiorespiratory Fitness in Healthy Young Women. *Front. Physiol.* **2018**, *9*, 1738. [CrossRef] [PubMed]
12. Yamagishi, T.; Babraj, J. Effects of reduced-volume of sprint interval training and the time course of physiological and performance adaptations. *Scand. J. Med. Sci. Sports* **2017**, *27*, 1662–1672. [CrossRef] [PubMed]
13. Vollaard, N.B.J.; Metcalfe, R.S. Research into the Health Benefits of Sprint Interval Training Should Focus on Protocols with Fewer and Shorter Sprints. *Sports Med.* **2017**, *47*, 2443–2451. [CrossRef] [PubMed]
14. Sloth, M.; Sloth, D.; Overgaard, K.; Dalgas, U. Effects of sprint interval training on VO2max and aerobic exercise performance: A systematic review and meta-analysis. *Scand. J. Med. Sci. Sports* **2013**, *23*, e341–e352. [CrossRef]
15. Ratel, S.; Williams, C.A.; Oliver, J.; Armstrong, N. Effects of age and mode of exercise on power output profiles during repeated sprints. *Eur. J. Appl. Physiol.* **2004**, *92*, 204–210. [CrossRef]
16. Achten, J.; Venables, M.C.; Jeukendrup, A.E. Fat oxidation rates are higher during running compared with cycling over a wide range of intensities. *Metabolism* **2003**, *52*, 747–752. [CrossRef]
17. Millet, G.P.; Vleck, V.E.; Bentley, D.J. Physiological differences between cycling and running: Lessons from triathletes. *Sports Med.* **2009**, *39*, 179–206. [CrossRef]
18. Kavaliauskas, M.; Jakeman, J.; Babraj, J. Early Adaptations to a Two-Week Uphill Run Sprint Interval Training and Cycle Sprint Interval Training. *Sports* **2018**, *6*, 72. [CrossRef]
19. Bangsbo, J.; Gunnarsson, T.P.; Wendell, J.; Nybo, L.; Thomassen, M. Reduced volume and increased training intensity elevate muscle Na^+-K^+ pump alpha2-subunit expression as well as short- and long-term work capacity in humans. *J. Appl. Physiol.* **2009**, *107*, 1771–1780. [CrossRef]
20. Iaia, F.M.; Hellsten, Y.; Nielsen, J.J.; Fernström, M.; Sahlin, K.; Bangsbo, J. Four weeks of speed endurance training reduces energy expenditure during exercise and maintains muscle oxidative capacity despite a reduction in training volume. *J. Appl. Physiol.* **2009**, *106*, 73–80. [CrossRef]
21. Iaia, F.M.; Thomassen, M.; Kolding, H.; Gunnarsson, T.; Wendell, J.; Rostgaard, T.; Nordsborg, N.; Krustrup, P.; Nybo, L.; Hellsten, Y.; et al. Reduced volume but increased training intensity elevates muscle Na+-K+ pump alpha1-subunit and NHE1 expression as well as short-term work capacity in humans. *Am. J. Physiol. Regul. Integr. Comp. Physiol.* **2008**, *294*, R966–R974. [CrossRef] [PubMed]
22. Macpherson, R.E.; Hazell, T.J.; Olver, T.D.; Paterson, D.H.; Lemon, P.W. Run sprint interval training improves aerobic performance but not maximal cardiac output. *Med. Sci. Sports Exerc.* **2011**, *43*, 115–122.
23. Midgley, A.W.; Bentley, D.J.; Luttikholt, H.; McNaughton, L.R.; Millet, G.P. Challenging a dogma of exercise physiology: Does an incremental exercise test for valid VO 2 max determination really need to last between 8 and 12 minutes? *Sports Med.* **2008**, *38*, 441–447.
24. Grendstad, H.; Nilsen, A.K.; Rygh, C.B.; Hafstad, A.; Kristoffersen, M.; Iversen, V.V.; Nybakken, T.; Vestbøstad, M.; Algrøy, E.A.; Sandbakk, Ø.; et al. Physical capacity, not skeletal maturity, distinguishes competitive levels in male Norwegian U14 soccer players. *Scand. J. Med. Sci. Sports* **2020**, *30*, 254–263. [CrossRef] [PubMed]
25. Edgett, B.A.; Bonafiglia, J.T.; Raleigh, J.P.; Rotundo, M.P.; Giles, M.D.; Whittall, J.P.; Gurd, B.J. Reproducibility of peak oxygen consumption and the impact of test variability on classification of individual training responses in young recreationally active adults. *Clin. Physiol. Funct. Imaging* **2018**, *38*, 630–638. [CrossRef] [PubMed]
26. Girard, O.L.; Mendez-Villanueva, A.; Bishop, D. Repeated-sprint ability—Part I: Factors contributing to fatigue. *Sports Med.* **2011**, *41*, 673–694. [CrossRef] [PubMed]
27. Liu, N.Y.; Plowman, S.A.; Looney, M.A. The reliability and validity of the 20-meter shuttle test in American students 12 to 15 years old. *Res. Q. Exerc. Sport* **1992**, *63*, 360–365.
28. Sandvei, M.; Jeppesen, P.B.; Stoen, L.; Litleskare, S.; Johansen, E.; Stensrud, T.; Enoksen, E.; Hautala, A.; Martinmäki, K.; Kinnunen, H.; et al. Sprint interval running increases insulin sensitivity in young healthy subjects. *Arch. Physiol. Biochem.* **2012**, *118*, 139–147. [CrossRef]

29. Bouchard, C.; Rankinen, T. Individual differences in response to regular physical activity. *Med. Sci. Sports Exerc.* **2001**, *33* (Suppl. 6), S446–S451, discussion S452–S453. [CrossRef]
30. Hautala, A.J.; Kiviniemi, A.M.; Mäkikallio, T.H.; Kinnunen, H.; Nissilä, S.; Huikuri, H.V.; Tulppo, M.P. Individual differences in the responses to endurance and resistance training. *Eur. J. Appl. Physiol.* **2006**, *96*, 535–542.
31. Bouchard, C.; Sarzynski, M.A.; Rice, T.K.; Kraus, W.E.; Church, T.S.; Sung, Y.J.; Rao, D.C.; Rankinen, T. Genomic predictors of the maximal O_2 uptake response to standardized exercise training programs. *J. Appl. Physiol.* **2011**, *110*, 1160–1170. [CrossRef] [PubMed]
32. Jones, A.M.; Carter, H. The effect of endurance training on parameters of aerobic fitness. *Sports Med.* **2000**, *29*, 373–386. [CrossRef] [PubMed]
33. Seo, D.Y.; Kwak, H.B.; Kim, A.H.; Park, S.H.; Heo, J.W.; Kim, H.K.; Ko, J.R.; Lee, S.J.; Bang, H.S.; Sim, J.W.; et al. Cardiac adaptation to exercise training in health and disease. *Pflug. Arch.* **2020**, *472*, 155–168. [CrossRef] [PubMed]
34. Edge, J.; Bishop, D.; Goodman, C.; Dawson, B. Effects of high- and moderate-intensity training on metabolism and repeated sprints. *Med. Sci. Sports Exerc.* **2005**, *37*, 1975–1982. [CrossRef]
35. Glaister, M.; Stone, M.H.; Stewart, A.M.; Hughes, M.G.; Moir, G.L. The influence of endurance training on multiple sprint cycling performance. *J. Strength Cond. Res.* **2007**, *21*, 606–612.
36. Saunders, P.U.; Pyne, D.B.; Telford, R.D.; Hawley, J.A. Factors affecting running economy in trained distance runners. *Sports Med.* **2004**, *34*, 465–485.
37. Iaia, F.M.; Bangsbo, J. Speed endurance training is a powerful stimulus for physiological adaptations and performance improvements of athletes. *Scand. J. Med. Sci. Sports* **2010**, *20* (Suppl. 2), 11–23.
38. Rynecki, N.D.; Siracuse, B.L.; Ippolito, J.A.; Beebe, K.S. Injuries sustained during high intensity interval training: Are modern fitness trends contributing to increased injury rates? *J. Sports Med. Phys. Fit.* **2019**, *59*, 1206–1212.

International Journal of
Environmental Research and Public Health

MDPI

Article

Acute Effects of Open Kinetic Chain Exercise Versus Those of Closed Kinetic Chain Exercise on Quadriceps Muscle Thickness in Healthy Adults

Soul Cheon [1,2], Joo-Hyun Lee [1], Hyung-Pil Jun [3], Yong Woo An [4] and Eunwook Chang [1,2,*]

1 Department of Kinesiology, Inha University, Incheon 22212, Korea; soul9879@gmail.com (S.C.); joohyun09@gmail.com (J.-H.L.)
2 Institute of Sports & Arts Convergence (ISAC), Inha University, Incheon 22212, Korea
3 Department of Physical Education, Dong-A University, Busan 49236, Korea; hjun@dau.ac.kr
4 Department of Health and Human Sciences, Loyola Marymount University, Los Angeles, CA 90045, USA; anyong0047@gmail.com
* Correspondence: change@inha.ac.kr; Tel.: +82-32-860-8185; Fax: +82-32-860-8188

Received: 9 June 2020; Accepted: 28 June 2020; Published: 29 June 2020

Abstract: This study aimed to compare immediate changes in the thickness of the rectus femoris (RF), vastus intermedius (VI), vastus lateralis (VL), vastus medialis (VM), and vastus medialis oblique (VMO) muscles after open kinetic chain exercise (OKCE) and closed kinetic chain exercise (CKCE) and identify the effect of both exercise types on each quadricep muscle for early rehabilitation to prevent knee joint injury. Twenty-six healthy participants (13 males and 13 females) were randomly divided into the OKCE (n = 13) and CKCE (n = 13) groups. The thickness of their quadriceps muscles was measured using a portable ultrasonic imaging device before and after exercise in the sequence RF, VI, VL, VM, and VMO. A two-way repeated measures analysis of variance was used to compare the thickness of each component of the quadriceps muscles between the two groups. The thickness of the RF, VL, VM, and VMO muscles increased after OKCE, and the thickness of the VI muscle showed the greatest increase with a medium–large effect size (F = 8.52, p = 0.01, and d = 0.53). The thickness of the VI, VL, VM, and VMO muscles increased after CKCE, and the VMO muscle had the largest effect size (F = 11.71, p = 0.00, and d = 1.02). These results indicate that the thickness of the quadriceps muscles can be selectively improved depending on the type of exercise.

Keywords: quadriceps atrophy; vastus intermedius; vastus medialis; vastus medialis oblique; muscle hypertrophy; resistance exercise; type of exercise

1. Introduction

The quadriceps femoris muscle belongs to the primary muscle group that is involved in the function of the knee joint. Various sports injuries could result in altered quadriceps characteristics, such as muscle strength, activation, mass, and size of the quadriceps [1–4]. Previous studies have reported weakness and atrophy of quadriceps muscles after knee joint injuries [2,5]. Recovery of these muscles to their pre-injury state is needed to restore the function of the knee joint [6–8]. The quadriceps femoris muscle is made up of five specific muscles—the rectus femoris (RF), vastus intermedius (VI), vastus lateralis (VL), vastus medialis (VM), and vastus medialis oblique (VMO). Although this group of muscles normally functions as a knee extensor, previous studies have reported a specific function of each muscle component. The RF is a biarticular muscle that connects the hip joint to the knee joint and acts as a primary knee muscle extensor; 33% force is exerted while bending the hip joint [9]. The VM is a primary knee extensor muscle, and the VMO muscle acts as a medial stabilizer of the patella [10]. Although the VMO muscle is weaker than the VL muscle, it controls the lateral deviation of the patella [11,12]. The imbalance of forces between the VM and VL muscles results in patellar instability, causing movement dysfunction and inducing patella femoral pain syndrome (PFPS) [13]. Each quadriceps muscle has a specific role in movement; hence, it is necessary to investigate the characteristic of each quadricep muscle for functional improvement.

Open kinetic chain exercise (OKCE) and closed kinetic chain exercise (CKCE) are the types of exercise based on the fixed point of the extremity during movements. Although they have been used in the clinical field, each exercise has a specific purpose and characteristics. OKCE is considered less functional than CKCE, but it plays an important role in improving muscle strength during rehabilitation in patients with a limited range of motion [14]. Additionally, it improves the muscle strength of each quadricep muscle or the entire muscle without compensating the movement [15]. CKCE can be performed by applying varying ranges of motion with a functional speed. This type of exercise requires action of the antagonistic muscles to eccentrically control the movements by providing stability to the damaged joints [16]. Therefore, CKCE has been recommended in the early stages of rehabilitation after the anterior cruciate ligament reconstruction (ACLR) [14].

In previous studies evaluating the effects of OKCE and CKCE on the quadriceps femoris muscle [14,17,18], the activity of the RF muscle increased by 45% after OKCE compared to that after CKCE [14]. In another study, OKCE was effective for the activation of the quadriceps muscles during the first two weeks of rehabilitation [17] and restoring the ratio of the VM muscle to the VL muscle after knee joint surgery [18]. In a recent study, muscle thickness was considered a significant factor for identifying muscle strength and knee extension torque, and joint functions were predicted by the thickness of the VI and VMO muscles after ACLR [19]. While these previous investigations revealed the different effects on quadriceps activity by exercise type and the importance of muscle thickness, the acute effect on the thickness of each quadricep muscle after OKCE and CKCE was not investigated. Therefore, this study aimed to compare the acute effect of OKCE and CKCE on the thickness of each quadricep muscle. We hypothesized that there is a significant difference in the thickness of the quadricep femoris muscles before and after OKCE and CKCE.

2. Materials and Methods

2.1. Participants

Twenty-six healthy adults (13 males and 13 females; age: 24.3 ± 3.8 years; height: 169.3 ± 7.2 cm; weight: 66.4 ± 12.9 kg; and body mass index (BMI) [17]: 23 ± 3.6 kg/m^2) who participated in this study were randomly divided into the OKCE (n = 13; male: 8, female: 5) and CKCE (n = 13; male: 7, female: 6) groups. Participants having current knee joint pain and those who had undergone surgeries of the lower back and extremities in the past 6 months were excluded from the study. The general characteristics of the study participants are shown in Table 1. All participants signed an informed consent form after understanding the purpose of the study. All procedures were approved by the University's Institutional Review Board (Study ID: 190404).

Table 1. General characteristics of the study participants.

Characteristics	OKCE (n = 13)	CKCE (n = 13)	p-Value
Age (years)	23.5 ± 1.7	25.1 ± 5.1	0.30
Height (cm)	170.2 ± 6.5	168.4 ± 8.0	0.53
Mass (kg)	67.8 ± 15.6	65.1 ± 9.8	0.61
BMI (kg/m^2)	23.2 ± 4.6	22.9 ± 2.5	0.82

Values are presented as the mean ± standard deviation (SD). OKCE: open kinetic chain exercise; CKCE: closed kinetic chain exercise; BMI: body mass index.

2.2. Study Design

The study design is presented in Figure 1. All participants visited the laboratory for a day during the period of the study. Before the exercises, the thickness of the quadriceps muscles was measured using a portable B-mode ultrasound device (Healcerion, Seoul, Korea) with a linear-array transducer (7.5 MHz). The ultrasound device was set for gain (dB), depth (5 cm), and frequency (12 MHz) for all images. Each participant in the OKCE and CKCE groups performed three exercises and the thickness of their quadriceps muscles was measured in the same position immediately after the exercises.

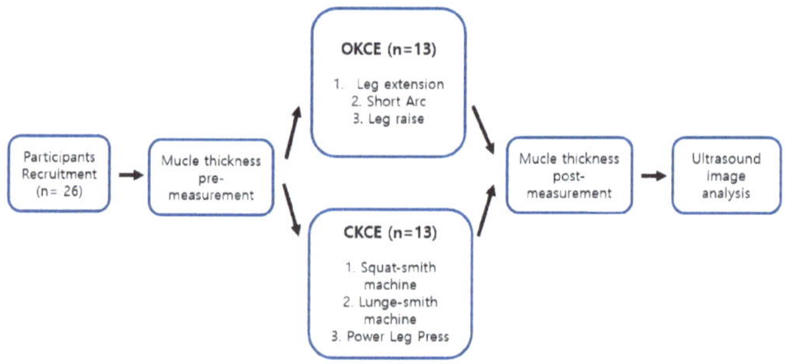

Figure 1. Overview of the study design, demonstrating the muscle thickness pre- and post-measurement.

2.3. Experimental Methods

2.3.1. Muscular Thickness Measurement

Ultrasound images were obtained using a portable ultrasonic imaging device and a portable tablet personal computer (IPad, Foxconn, Taipei, Taiwan). All muscle thickness measurements were performed by one investigator. Previous investigations reported excellent intra-rater (Intraclass Correlation Coefficients (ICCs) 0.95–0.97) and acceptably good inter-rater (ICCs 0.62–0.90) reliability of the quadriceps thickness measurements using ultrasound [20,21]. To measure the thickness of each quadricep muscle, the participants were made to lie in a supine position to prevent external hip rotation. The leg of the participants that was farthest away from the ball was considered the dominant leg [22]. The dominant leg of the participants was assessed after the participants were made to lie in a supine position with both legs fully extended for 10 min to stabilize the fluid shifts [23]. A water-soluble gel that was applied between the transducer and skin enhanced the acoustic contact and reduced the risk of image misinterpretation [24]. The transversal images of the quadriceps muscles were acquired in the sequence RF, VI, VL, VM, and VMO. To obtain the images, a virtual line was marked along the length of the thigh from the superior pole of the patella to the anterior superior iliac spine (ASIS). The RF and VI were measured on and at 50% of the virtual line. In order to measure VL, thigh circumference at 50% of the virtual line was measured, and then VL was measured as 10% of the measured circumference distance laterally from the virtual line. The VM muscle was measured at 20% distance of the virtual line, and then the circumference was measured on the same point. Once the measurement of the circumference was completed, VM was measured at 12.5% of the measured circumference distance medially from the virtual line [25]. The VMO muscle was measured 4 cm superior and 3 cm medial of the superior pole of the patella (Figure 2) [26]. The gain was adjusted until the femur was in the center of the screen such that the boundary of the muscle was visible, and then the depth of the image was measured. Images of each muscle were recorded three times. The ultrasound images were saved for further analysis after the muscle thickness was measured.

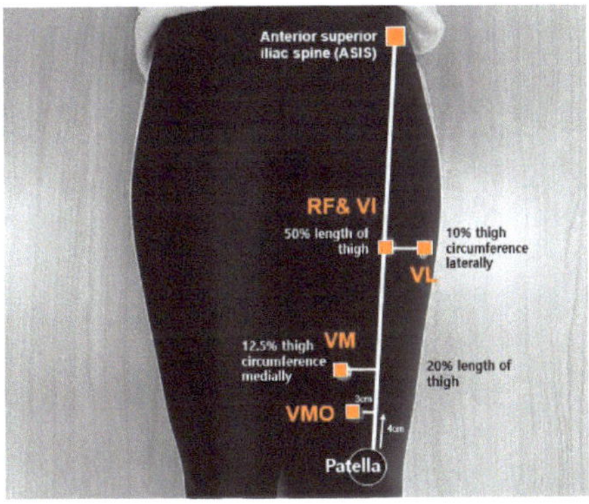

Figure 2. Location of quadriceps thickness measurement. RF: rectus femoris; VI: vastus intermedius; VL: vastus lateralis; VM: vastus medialis; VMO: vastus medialis oblique.

2.3.2. Exercise

The National Strength and Conditioning Association standard states that 3–6 sets of an exercise at 6–12 repeated maximums (RM: 67–75% of 1 RM) is effective for muscle hypertrophy [27]. Therefore, the intensity of the exercises was set at 10 RM. The participants performed three sets of exercises with 10 repetitions each, with a 60-s rest between sets [28].

2.3.3. Open Kinetic Chain Exercise

OKCE consisted of leg extension, short-arc, and straight leg raise exercises. Leg extension and short-arc exercises were performed using an exercise machine and straight leg raise exercise was performed as a free-weight exercise (Figure 3).

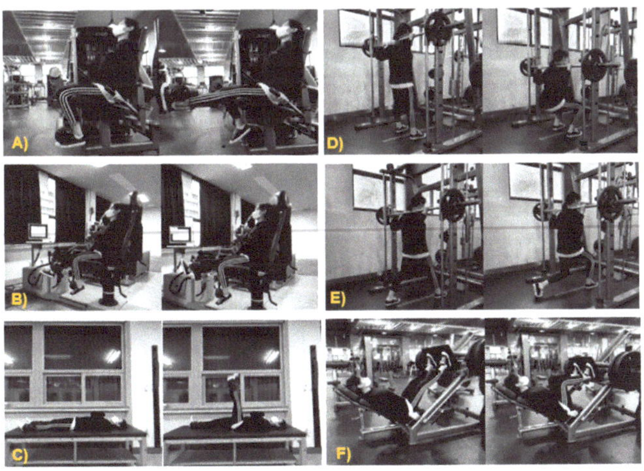

Figure 3. OKCE and CKCE exercise. OKCE: (**A**) leg extension; (**B**) short-arc; (**C**) leg raise. CKCE: (**D**) squat—Smith machine; (**E**) lunge—Smith machine; (**F**) leg press.

1. Leg extension exercise

   - Participants were positioned on the center of the back of a machine such that their thighs, backs, and heads were not tilted on one side. Their knees were aligned in a straight line along the axis of the machine and their hips and thighs were positioned such that the back of their knees touched the edge of the chair. The starting position was set at a flexion of 90°. The knees of the participants were not in hyperextension or hyperflexion during the exercise and their upper body was stationary [27].

2. Short-arc exercise

- The short-arc exercise was performed using a knee extension exercise machine. Although the participant was positioned in the same way as that of the leg extension exercise, the starting position of the knee was at a flexion of 20°. Participants performed knee extensions and a hold of 2–3 s in the fully extended position.

3. Leg Raises Exercise

- Sandbags with a predetermined weight of 10 RM were attached to ankle of each of the participant. They initiated a straight leg raise while lying on the table with both hands on their chest and one leg extended. The other leg was stabilized at the knee flexed with 90°.

2.3.4. Closed Kinetic Chain Exercise

The participants in the CKCE group performed three exercises—squat, lunge, and leg press. Squat and lunge exercises were performed using a Smith machine and the leg press exercise was performed on a linear 45° leg press machine (Figure 3).

1. Squat—Smith machine

- Participants were made to stand while they held a bar in pronation grip across their shoulders. Their feet were positioned at a slightly wider distance than the shoulders and toes were pointed slightly outside. The participants initiated the exercise in the squat position while slowly flexing their hips and knees and keeping the body angle constant [27].

2. Lunge—Smith machine

- Participants were made to stand and a bar was placed above the posterior deltoid and upper trapezius in pronation grip that was wider than their shoulder. They maintained a straight posture and one foot was placed forward and the other was placed behind. Their front leg was horizontal to the floor and their rear leg was vertical to the floor, while the knees and hips of their front legs were bent gradually. They were instructed not to bend the front knee past the front foot and not to bend the trunk forward. The trial was repeated if this requirement was not met [27].

3. Leg press machine

- Participants were positioned on the center of the back of a machine such that their thigh, back, and head were not tilted on one side and they held the handle on both sides. Their knees were extended and their feet were positioned above the footpad within shoulder width. Participants were seated at an angle of approximately 120°. The knee of each participant extended and protracted back to the starting position. The heels of the participants remained on the footpads and the knees were not in hyperextension or hyperflexion. The upper body of the participants remained stationary [27].

2.3.5. Ultrasound Image Analysis

The recorded ultrasound images were analyzed using Image J software (National Institute for Health, Bethesda, MD, USA). Each image was scaled individually for converting an area in pixels to centimeters using the straight-line function to analyze the muscle thickness [29]. According to previous studies, the region of interest within each muscle was selected, excluding the surrounding bone and fascia [30–32]. Muscle thickness was defined as the widest distance between the adipose muscle upper interface and the lower interface for all quadriceps muscles, excluding the VI muscle [33]. The VI muscle was measured as the widest distance between the adipose muscle upper interface and the femur (Figure 4) [33]. One middle line and two lines were placed at regular intervals on both sides around middle line and the average values of the three lines were obtained [34]. The images were analyzed by an investigator who was unable to see the participants' identity. The average values of the three images per muscle were statistically analyzed.

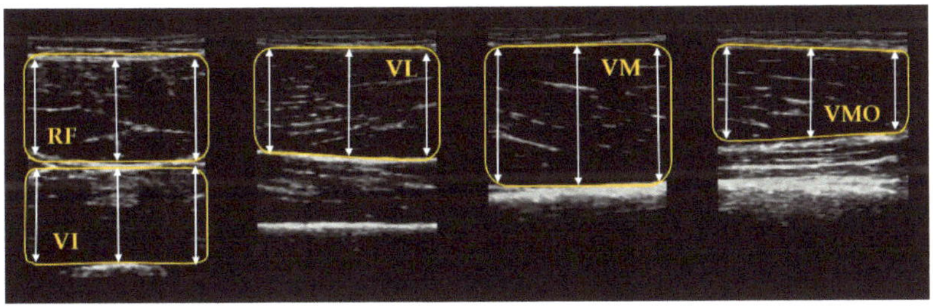

Figure 4. Image of the thickness of the quadriceps muscles. RF: rectus femoris; VI: vastus intermedius; VL: vastus lateralis; VM: vastus medialis; VMO: vastus medialis oblique.

2.4. Statistical Analysis

Demographic characteristics of the participants were compared between the two groups using an independent t-test. Continuous variables, such as age, height, mass, and BMI, are presented as the mean ± SD. A two-way repeated measures analysis of variance (ANOVA) (group: OKCE and CKCE; by time: pre-exercise and post-exercise) compared the thickness of each quadricep muscle before and after the exercise. A post hoc analysis was performed using the Tuckey method for a group-by-time interaction effect. Cohen's d effect size was calculated to determine the magnitude of change in muscle thickness before and after exercise (small = 0.2–0.49, medium = 0.5–0.79, and large > 0.8) [35]. All data are expressed as the mean and SD. Statistical analyses were performed using SPSS 25.0 software (SPSS Inc., Chicago, IL, USA). A p-value < 0.05 was considered statistically significant.

3. Results

For the general characteristics, a significant statistical difference was not observed ($p > 0.05$) between the groups (Table 1).

The thickness of the VI muscle increased in both groups (OKCE pre: 13.92 ± 4.08 mm, post: 15.86 ± 3.13 mm; CKCE pre: 15.3 ± 2.46 mm, post: 16.47 ± 3.66 mm). For the VI muscle, there was a significant time effect in the thickness ($F = 8.52$, $p = 0.01$) and its effect size was greater for OKCE ($d = 0.53$) than CKCE ($d = 0.38$) (Table 2) (Figure 4). The thickness of the VMO muscle was increased in both groups (OKCE pre: 14.37 ± 3.50 mm, post: 15.42 ± 3.70 mm; CKCE pre: 12.59 ± 2.96 mm, post: 15.72 ± 3.19 mm). For VMO muscle, there was a significant time effect in the thickness only ($F = 11.71$, $p = 0.00$). While CKCE exhibited a large effect size ($d = 1.02$), OKCE showed a small effect size ($d = 0.29$) (Table 2) (Figure 5). Finally, there was no significant time-by-group interaction, group, and time main effect on RF, VL, and VM ($p > 0.05$) (Table 2 and Figure 5).

Table 2. Comparison of the quadriceps muscle thickness between the groups pre- and post-intervention.

Muscles	OKCE			CKCE			*p*-Value
	Pre	Post	ES	Pre	Post	ES	
RF(mm)	19.72 ± 2.98	20.70 ± 3.70	0.29	18.71 ± 2.47	18.45 ± 3.68	−0.08	0.59
VI(mm)	13.92 ± 4.08	15.86 ± 3.13	0.53	15.30 ± 2.46	16.47 ± 3.66	0.38	* 0.01
VL(mm)	20.39 ± 2.77	20.87 ± 3.46	0.15	18.68 ± 3.00	19.77 ± 3.36	0.34	0.20
VM(mm)	25.61 ± 3.92	24.58 ± 3.95	−0.26	23.71 ± 4.51	24.83 ± 4.20	0.26	0.98
VMO(mm)	14.37 ± 3.50	15.42 ± 3.70	0.29	12.59 ± 2.96	15.72 ± 3.19	1.02	* 0.00

Values are presented as the mean ± SD. ES: Cohen's d effect size; OKCE: open kinetic chain exercise; CKCE: closed kinetic chain exercise; RF: rectus femoris; VI: vastus intermedius; VL: vastus lateralis; VM: vastus medialis; VMO: vastus medialis oblique. * $p < 0.05$ indicates a significant difference between pre- and post-intervention within the group.

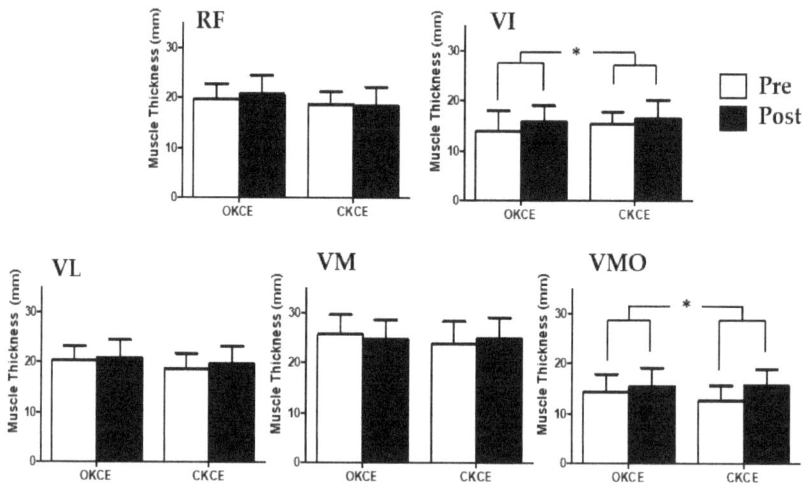

Figure 5. Comparison of the changes in quadricep muscle thickness. OKCE: open kinetic chain exercise, CKCE: closed kinetic chain exercise, RF: rectus femoris; VI: vastus intermedius; VL: vastus lateralis; VM: vastus medialis; VMO: vastus medialis oblique. * $p < 0.05$ indicates a significant difference between pre- and post-intervention within the group.

4. Discussion

This study aimed to compare the effects of OKCE and CKCE on the thickness of each quadricep muscle. Previous studies have reported that many patients with lower extremity injuries developed quadriceps atrophy after surgery or injury [36,37]. Since each quadricep muscle has different functions, the patterns of atrophy are different [19,38,39]. Therefore, it is important to identify an appropriate method of exercise for each quadricep muscle. In this study, the thickness of the VI muscle increased significantly after OKCE, and the thickness of the VMO muscle increased significantly after CKCE, resulting in the medium–large effect size. These findings suggest that the effects of OKCE and CKCE in improving the overall thickness of the quadriceps muscles, especially in early rehabilitation training, is appropriate for patients with ACLR or PFPS who need selective strengthening of the VI and VMO muscles.

According to a previous study, the VMO and VL are the principle muscles that stabilize the patella during dynamic knee extension [11]. Although the ideal ratio of the EMG activity of the VMO-to-VL for healthy people is 1:1 [12], patients with PFPS in a previous study had a ratio of 0.54:1, resulting in a weakening of the VMO muscle [40]. In another previous study, the ultrasonographic measurements of the VMO muscle were smaller in individuals with PFPS knees than in healthy people [41]; this imbalance between the two muscles resulted in an abnormal tracking of the patella, causing joint pain [42]. Therefore, rehabilitation exercises are important to strengthen the VMO muscles in such patients. In the present study, a large effect size was observed in the thickness of the VMO muscle after CKCE.

In the current study, three CKCEs were performed, including squat, lunge, and leg press; previous investigations reported that these exercises were naturally accompanied by hip adduction with knee joint movement [11,43]. These findings support the results of a prior study, in which CKCE with isometric hip adduction significantly improved the ratio of VMO muscle to VL muscle compared to OKCE, where only knee joints were involved independently [11]. An anatomic cadaver study has suggested the origin of the VMO muscle from the distal part of the adductor magnus and has revealed that the VMO muscle exerts a greater force after CKCE than OKCE [44]. Therefore, CKCE could be useful during the initial stage of rehabilitation of patients with PFPS.

The VI muscle acts on knee extension torque and is essential for athletes who need explosive movements [19]. A previous study has found a reduction in the thickness of the VI muscle in patients with ACLR and has suggested that increasing this thickness during the early phases of rehabilitation is a key factor for restoring the knee function [45]. In a prior study, the range of motion of the knee joint was limited in the early stages of the knee rehabilitation program; hence, it suggests that partial muscle strengthening exercises should be performed along with OKCE [18]. In the present study, the thickness of the VI muscles showed medium–large effect sizes after OKCE compared to that after CKCE. OKCE can be a more effective rehabilitation exercise than CKCE to restore the thickness of the VI muscle after ACLR.

It could be interesting that OKCE showed the greatest influence in increasing VI thickness compared to the other quadricep muscle components. VI is the quadriceps component that originate from the femur and it functions in knee extension only, whereas another component helps for hip flexion [46]. Therefore, it could be speculated that the independent movement of the knee joint, such as knee extension during OKCE, requires the greatest efforts on VI. Additionally, VI exhibited the highest estimated torque contribution during isometric knee extension among the quadriceps components [47], which supports the results of the current study.

Both exercises were able to improve the thickness of the quadriceps muscles. Further, proper methods can be used to effectively exercise the individual muscles for improvement. Hooper et al. (2001) [48] and Perry et al. (2005) [49] have reported that although CKCE is more effective in improving functional movements than OKCE, there is no significant difference when they were measured by actual clinical evaluation indicators in patients with ACLR. However, sophisticated research is needed because the results vary depending on the subjects or methods for evaluating the functions and errors. The study has some limitations. First, it was not possible to ascertain whether each participant performed the exercise effectively. Secondly, although both men and women participated in this study, sex-related hormones were not checked. Thirdly, the sample size was small and the adults were healthy. Therefore, further studies enrolling participants of different age groups and patients with various lower-limb injuries are needed to generalize the current study results. Fourthly, exercise selection was decided based on the feasibility of the clinical setting and it was not controlled. Finally, we obtained an acute effect, not a long-term effect, after the intervention. Further studies are needed to compare the muscle reactions before and after exercise as well as between acute and chronic exercise.

5. Conclusions

This study was conducted to investigate the acute effects of OKCE and CKCE on the thickness of the five individual quadriceps muscles. The thickness of the VI muscle improved after OKCE and the thickness of the VMO muscle increased significantly after CKCE. The findings of this study can help athletes and patients with knee joint injuries choose the most appropriate exercise during the early stages of rehabilitation. OKCE and CKCE should be properly used for selective strengthening of the quadriceps muscles.

Author Contributions: Conceptualization, S.C. and E.C.; methodology, S.C., J.-H.L. and E.C.; software, S.C., and J.-H.L.; validation, S.C., J.-H.L., Y.W.A., and E.C.; formal analysis, S.C., H.-P.J. and E.C.; investigation, S.C., H.-P.J. and Y.W.A.; resources, S.C., H.-P.J., Y.W.A. and E.C.; data curation, S.C. and E.C.; writing—original draft preparation, S.C. and J.-H.L.; writing—review and editing, S.C., J.-H.L., H.-P.J., Y.W.A. and E.C.; visualization, S.C. and J.-H.L.; supervision, E.C.; project administration, E.C.; funding acquisition, E.C. All authors have read and agreed to the published version of the manuscript.

Funding: This research was funded by the National Research Foundation of South Korea (NRF-2017R1C1B5076644) and the Ministry of Education of the Republic of Korea (NRF-2019S1A5C2A03082727).

Conflicts of Interest: The authors declare no conflict of interest.

References

1. Callaghan, M.; Oldham, J. Quadriceps atrophy: To what extent does it exist in patellofemoral pain syndrome? *Br. J. Sports Med.* **2004**, *38*, 295–299. [CrossRef] [PubMed]
2. Lynch, A.D.; Logerstedt, D.S.; Axe, M.J.; Snyder-Mackler, L. Quadriceps activation failure after anterior cruciate ligament rupture is not mediated by knee joint effusion. *J. Orthop. Sports Phys. Ther.* **2012**, *42*, 502–510. [CrossRef] [PubMed]
3. Suter, E.; Herzog, W.; De Souza, K.; Bray, R. Inhibition of the quadriceps muscles in patients with anterior knee pain. *J. Appl. Biomech.* **1998**, *14*, 360–373. [CrossRef]
4. Werner, S. An evaluation of knee extensor and knee flexor torques and EMGs in patients with patellofemoral pain syndrome in comparison with matched controls. *Knee Surg. Sports Traumatol. Arthrosc.* **1995**, *3*, 89–94. [CrossRef]
5. Chmielewski, T.L.; Stackhouse, S.; Axe, M.J.; Snyder-Mackler, L. A prospective analysis of incidence and severity of quadriceps inhibition in a consecutive sample of 100 patients with complete acute anterior cruciate ligament rupture. *J. Orthop. Res.* **2004**, *22*, 925–930. [CrossRef]
6. Eitzen, I.; Moksnes, H.; Snyder-Mackler, L.; Risberg, M.A. A progressive 5-week exercise therapy program leads to significant improvement in knee function early after anterior cruciate ligament injury. *J. Orthop. Sports Phys. Ther.* **2010**, *40*, 705–721. [CrossRef]
7. Liu-Ambrose, T.; Taunton, J.; MacIntyre, D.; McConkey, P.; Khan, K. The effects of proprioceptive or strength training on the neuromuscular function of the ACL reconstructed knee: A randomized clinical trial. *Scand. J. Med. Sci. Sports* **2003**, *13*, 115–123. [CrossRef]
8. Wilk, K.E.; Romaniello, W.T.; Soscia, S.M.; Arrigo, C.A.; Andrews, J.R. The relationship between subjective knee scores, isokinetic testing, and functional testing in the ACL-reconstructed knee. *J. Orthop. Sports Phys. Ther.* **1994**, *20*, 60–73. [CrossRef]
9. Hyoungsu, K.; Eunyoung, K.; Jiwon, H. The effects of quadriceps femoris muscle activation by closed and open kinetic chain exercise. *J. Korean Soc. Integr. Med.* **2015**, *3*, 71–80.
10. Hubbard, J.K.; Sampson, H.W.; Elledge, J.R. Prevalence and morphology of the vastus medialis oblique muscle in human cadavers. *Anat. Rec.* **1997**, *249*, 135–142. [CrossRef]
11. Irish, S.E.; Millward, A.J.; Wride, J.; Haas, B.M.; Shum, G.L. The effect of closed-kinetic chain exercises and open-kinetic chain exercise on the muscle activity of vastus medialis oblique and vastus lateralis. *J. Strength Cond. Res.* **2010**, *24*, 1256–1262. [CrossRef] [PubMed]
12. Souza, D.R.; Gross, M.T. Comparison of vastus medialis obliquus: Vastus lateralis muscle integrated electromyographic ratios between healthy subjects and patients with patellofemoral pain. *Phys. Ther.* **1991**, *71*, 310–316. [CrossRef] [PubMed]
13. Wong, Y.-M. Recording the vastii muscle onset timing as a diagnostic parameter for patellofemoral pain syndrome: Fact or fad? *Phys. Ther. Sport* **2009**, *10*, 71–74. [CrossRef] [PubMed]
14. Escamilla, R.F.; Fleisig, G.S.; Zheng, N.; Barrentine, S.W.; Wilk, K.E.; Andrews, J.R. Biomechanics of the knee during closed kinetic chain and open kinetic chain exercises. *Med. Sci. Sports Exer.* **1998**, *30*, 556–569. [CrossRef] [PubMed]
15. Kisner, C.; Colby, L. *Therapeutic Exercise: Foundations and Techniques*; FA Davis Co: Philadelphia, PA, USA, 2007.
16. Iwasaki, T.; Shiba, N.; Matsuse, H.; Nago, T.; Umezu, Y.; Tagawa, Y.; Nagata, K.; Basford, J.R. Improvement in knee extension strength through training by means of combined electrical stimulation and voluntary muscle contraction. *Tohoku J. Exp. Med.* **2006**, *209*, 33–40. [CrossRef]

17. Kwon, Y.J.; Bae, S.S.; Park, S.J. The Effect of Static Balance Recovery by Open Kinetic Chain and Closed Kinetic Chain Exercises. *J. Korean Soc. Phys. Ther.* **2009**, *4*, 23–30.
18. Han, S.W. A SEMG analysis of knee joint angle during close kinetic chain exercise and open kinetic chain exercises in quadriceps muscle. *J. Korean Soc. Phys. Ther.* **2004**, *16*, 192–204.
19. Ando, R.; Saito, A.; Umemura, Y.; Akima, H. Local architecture of the vastus intermedius is a better predictor of knee extension force than that of the other quadriceps femoris muscle heads. *Clin. Physiol. Funct. Imaging* **2015**, *35*, 376–382. [CrossRef]
20. Cheon, S.; Chang, E. Inter-rater Reliability of a Portable Ultrasound for the Quadriceps and Hamstrings Thickness Measurement in Healthy Adults. *Exerc. Sci.* **2020**, *29*, 71–76. [CrossRef]
21. Ruas, C.V.; Pinto, R.S.; Lima, C.D.; Costa, P.B.; Brown, L.E. Test-retest reliability of muscle thickness, echo-intensity and cross sectional area of quadriceps and hamstrings muscle groups using B-mode ultrasound. *Int. J. Kinesiol. Sports Sci.* **2017**, *5*, 35–41. [CrossRef]
22. van Melick, N.; Meddeler, B.M.; Hoogeboom, T.J.; Nijhuis-van der Sanden, M.W.; van Cingel, R.E. How to determine leg dominance: The agreement between self-reported and observed performance in healthy adults. *PLoS ONE* **2017**, *12*, e0189876. [CrossRef] [PubMed]
23. Berg, H.; Tedner, B.; Tesch, P. Changes in lower limb muscle cross-sectional area and tissue fluid volume after transition from standing to supine. *Acta Physiol. Scand.* **1993**, *148*, 379–385. [CrossRef] [PubMed]
24. Pinto, R.S.; Correa, C.S.; Radaelli, R.; Cadore, E.L.; Brown, L.E.; Bottaro, M. Short-term strength training improves muscle quality and functional capacity of elderly women. *AGE* **2014**, *36*, 365–372. [CrossRef] [PubMed]
25. Giles, L.; Webster, K.; McClelland, J.; Cook, J. Can ultrasound measurements of muscle thickness be used to measure the size of individual quadriceps muscles in people with patellofemoral pain? *Phys. Ther. Sport* **2015**, *16*, 45–52. [CrossRef]
26. Miao, P.; Xu, Y.; Pan, C.; Liu, H.; Wang, C. Vastus medialis oblique and vastus lateralis activity during a double-leg semisquat with or without hip adduction in patients with patellofemoral pain syndrome. *BMC Musculoskelet. Disord.* **2015**, *16*, 289. [CrossRef]
27. Coburn, J.W.; Malek, M.H. *NSCA's Essentials of Personal Training*, 2nd ed.; Human Kinetics: Champaign, IL, USA, 2012.
28. Ouellette, M.M.; LeBrasseur, N.K.; Bean, J.F.; Phillips, E.; Stein, J.; Frontera, W.R.; Fielding, R.A. High-intensity resistance training improves muscle strength, self-reported function, and disability in long-term stroke survivors. *Stroke* **2004**, *35*, 1404–1409. [CrossRef]
29. Scanlon, T.C.; Fragala, M.S.; Stout, J.R.; Emerson, N.S.; Beyer, K.S.; Oliveira, L.P.; Hoffman, J.R. Muscle architecture and strength: Adaptations to short-term resistance training in older adults. *Muscle Nerve* **2014**, *49*, 584–592. [CrossRef]
30. Cadore, E.L.; Izquierdo, M.; Conceição, M.; Radaelli, R.; Pinto, R.S.; Baroni, B.M.; Vaz, M.A.; Alberton, C.L.; Pinto, S.S.; Cunha, G. Echo intensity is associated with skeletal muscle power and cardiovascular performance in elderly men. *Exp. Gerontol.* **2012**, *47*, 473–478. [CrossRef]
31. Rosenberg, J.G.; Ryan, E.D.; Sobolewski, E.J.; Scharville, M.J.; Thompson, B.J.; King, G.E. Reliability of panoramic ultrasound imaging to simultaneously examine muscle size and quality of the medial gastrocnemius. *Muscle Nerve* **2014**, *49*, 736–740. [CrossRef]
32. Palmer, T.B.; Akehi, K.; Thiele, R.M.; Smith, D.B.; Thompson, B.J. Reliability of panoramic ultrasound imaging in simultaneously examining muscle size and quality of the hamstring muscles in young, healthy males and females. *Ultrasound Med. Biol.* **2015**, *41*, 675–684. [CrossRef]
33. Rech, A.; Radaelli, R.; Goltz, F.R.; da Rosa, L.H.T.; Schneider, C.D.; Pinto, R.S. Echo intensity is negatively associated with functional capacity in older women. *Age* **2014**, *36*, 9708. [CrossRef] [PubMed]
34. Fujisawa, C.; Tamaki, A.; Yamada, E.; Matsuoka, H. Influence of gender on muscle fatigue during dynamic knee contractions. *Phys. Ther. Res.* **2017**, *20*, E9889. [CrossRef] [PubMed]
35. Cohen, J. Statistical power analysis. *Curr. Direct. Psychol. Sci.* **1992**, *1*, 98–101. [CrossRef]
36. Thomas, A.C.; Wojtys, E.M.; Brandon, C.; Palmieri-Smith, R.M. Muscle atrophy contributes to quadriceps weakness after anterior cruciate ligament reconstruction. *J. Sci. Med. Sport* **2016**, *19*, 7–11. [CrossRef]
37. Wurtzel, C.N.; Gumucio, J.P.; Grekin, J.A.; Khouri, R.K., Jr.; Russell, A.J.; Bedi, A.; Mendias, C.L. Pharmacological inhibition of myostatin protects against skeletal muscle atrophy and weakness after anterior cruciate ligament tear. *J. Orthop. Res.* **2017**, *35*, 2499–2505. [CrossRef]

38. Panagiotopoulos, E.; Strzelczyk, P.; Herrmann, M.; Scuderi, G. Cadaveric study on static medial patellar stabilizers: The dynamizing role of the vastus medialis obliquus on medial patellofemoral ligament. *Knee Surg. Sports Traumatol. Arthrosc.* **2006**, *14*, 7–12. [CrossRef]
39. Yang, J.-H.; Eun, S.-P.; Park, D.-H.; Kwak, H.-B.; Chang, E. The Effects of Anterior Cruciate Ligament Reconstruction on Individual Quadriceps Muscle Thickness and Circulating Biomarkers. *Int. J. Environ. Res. Public Health* **2019**, *16*, 4895. [CrossRef]
40. Powers, C.M. Patellar kinematics, part I: The influence of vastus muscle activity in subjects with and without patellofemoral pain. *Phys. Ther.* **2000**, *80*, 956–964. [CrossRef]
41. Jan, M.-H.; Lin, D.-H.; Lin, J.-J.; Lin, C.-H.J.; Cheng, C.-K.; Lin, Y.-F. Differences in sonographic characteristics of the vastus medialis obliquus between patients with patellofemoral pain syndrome and healthy adults. *Am. J. Sports Med.* **2009**, *37*, 1743–1749. [CrossRef]
42. Fulkerson, J.P. Diagnosis and treatment of patients with patellofemoral pain. *Am. J. Sports Med.* **2002**, *30*, 447–456. [CrossRef]
43. Koh, E.-K.; Lee, K.-H.; Jung, D.-Y. The effect of isometric hip adduction and abduction on the muscle activities of vastus medialis oblique and vastus lateralis during leg squat exercises. *Korean J. Sport Biomech.* **2011**, *21*, 361–368. [CrossRef]
44. Hanten, W.P.; Schulthies, S.S. Exercise effect on electromyographic activity of the vastus medialis oblique and vastus lateralis muscles. *Phys. Ther.* **1990**, *70*, 561–565. [CrossRef]
45. van Melick, N.; van Cingel, R.E.; Brooijmans, F.; Neeter, C.; van Tienen, T.; Hullegie, W.; Nijhuis-van der Sanden, M.W. Evidence-based clinical practice update: Practice guidelines for anterior cruciate ligament rehabilitation based on a systematic review and multidisciplinary consensus. *Br. J. Sports Med.* **2016**, *50*, 1506–1515. [CrossRef]
46. RL, D.; Vogl, A. *Gray's Anatomy for Students*; Churchill Livingstone/Elsevier: Philadelphia, PA, USA, 2015; pp. 592–594.
47. Zhang, L.Q.; Wang, G.; Nuber, G.W.; Press, J.M.; Koh, J.L. In vivo load sharing among the quadriceps components. *J. Orthop. Res.* **2003**, *21*, 565–571. [CrossRef]
48. Hooper, D.M.; Morrissey, M.C.; Drechsler, W.; Morrissey, D.; King, J. Open and closed kinetic chain exercises in the early period after anterior cruciate ligament reconstruction: Improvements in level walking, stair ascent, and stair descent. *Am. J. Sports Med.* **2001**, *29*, 167–174. [CrossRef] [PubMed]
49. Perry, M.C.; Morrissey, M.C.; King, J.B.; Morrissey, D.; Earnshaw, P. Effects of closed versus open kinetic chain knee extensor resistance training on knee laxity and leg function in patients during the 8-to 14-week post-operative period after anterior cruciate ligament reconstruction. *Knee Surg. Sports Traumatol. Arthrosc.* **2005**, *13*, 357–369. [CrossRef] [PubMed]

International Journal of
Environmental Research and Public Health

MDPI

Article

Efficacy of a Six-Week Dispersed Wingate-Cycle Training Protocol on Peak Aerobic Power, Leg Strength, Insulin Sensitivity, Blood Lipids and Quality of Life in Healthy Adults

Chun Hou Wun [1,†], Mandy Jiajia Zhang [2,†], Boon Hor Ho [2], Kenneth McGeough [3], Frankie Tan [1,4] and Abdul Rashid Aziz [4,*]

1. Department of Physiology, Yong Loo Lin School of Medicine, National University of Singapore, Singapore 117597, Singapore; chunhou.wun@gmail.com (C.H.W.); frankie_tan@sport.gov.sg (F.T.)
2. Changi Sports Medicine Centre, Changi General Hospital, Singapore 529889, Singapore; Mandy_Zhang@cgh.com.sg (M.J.Z.); Boon_Hor_ho@cgh.com.sg (B.H.H.)
3. ActiveSG, Active Health Division, Sport Singapore, Singapore 397630, Singapore; kenneth_mcGeough@sport.gov.sg
4. Sport Science and Sport Medicine, Singapore Sport Institute, Sport Singapore, Singapore 397630, Singapore

* Correspondence: abdul_rashid_aziz@sport.gov.sg

† These authors contributed equally to the study.

Received: 25 May 2020; Accepted: 30 June 2020; Published: 6 July 2020

Abstract: *Background*: The aim of this study was to evaluate the efficacy of a six-week dispersed Wingate Anaerobic test (WAnT) cycle exercise training protocol on peak aerobic power (VO_{2peak}), isokinetic leg strength, insulin sensitivity, lipid profile and quality of life, in healthy adults. *Methods*: We conducted a match-controlled cohort trial and participants were assigned to either the training (intervention, INT, $N = 16$) or non-training (control, CON, $N = 17$) group. INT performed 30-s WAnT bouts three times a day in the morning, afternoon and evening with each bout separated by ~4 h of rest, performed for 3 days a week for 6 weeks. Criterion measures of peak oxygen uptake (VO_{2peak}), leg strength, insulin markers such as homeostatic model assessment (HOMA) and quantitative insulin-sensitivity check index (QUICKI), blood lipids profile and health-related quality of life (HRQL) survey were assessed before and after 6 weeks in both groups. *Results*: Absolute VO_{2peak} increased by 8.3 ± 7.0% ($p < 0.001$) after INT vs. 0.9 ± 6.1% in CON ($p = 0.41$) group. Maximal voluntary contraction at $30°{\cdot}s^{-1}$ of the dominant lower-limb flexors in INT increased significantly post-training ($p = 0.03$). There were no changes in the INT individuals' other cardiorespiratory markers, HOMA, QUICKI, blood lipids, and HRQL measures (all $p > 0.05$) between pre- and post-training; but importantly, no differences were observed between INT and CON groups (all $p > 0.05$). *Conclusions*: The results indicate that 6 weeks of dispersed sprint cycle training increased cardiorespiratory fitness and dynamic leg strength but had minimal impact on insulin sensitivity, blood lipids and quality of life in the exercising individuals.

Keywords: aerobic; anaerobic; high-intensity interval training; sprint interval training; cardiometabolic markers

1. Introduction

Exercise and a well-balanced diet are the cornerstone of good health. Engaging in regular aerobic-type of exercise has proven to elicit several beneficial adaptations including increased cardiorespiratory fitness, and enhanced glycemic control [1]. In line with these benefits, the World Health Organization (WHO) recommends that adults engage in a minimum 150 min per week of moderate-intensity or 75 min per week of vigorous-intensity continuous aerobic physical activity to achieve meaningful improvements in cardiorespiratory fitness and metabolic health [2]. Unfortunately, less than 50% of the population cohort studied have met these physical activity recommendations, often citing 'lack of time' as a common barrier to exercise [3,4]. In this regard, high-intensity interval training (HIIT) has been proposed as a time-efficient intervention that can bring about similar benefits as compared to the typically much longer duration of moderate-intensity continuous training (MICT) [5,6].

HIIT is described as an intermittent period of short intense exercise interspersed by recovery period [6]. Two main forms of HIIT exist, known as 'high-intensity training' (HIT) and 'sprint interval training' (SIT), respectively. HIT incorporates bouts of close to maximum intensity exercise performed between one to several minutes at between >80% peak oxygen uptake (or VO_{2peak}) to <100% VO_{2peak}, with several minutes of low-intensity recovery between bouts. SIT on the other hand, consists of bouts of supramaximal, i.e., 'all-out' effort at >100% VO_{2peak} with passive rest or light active recovery between each sprint bout [6].

The scientific literature has shown the effectiveness of SIT in enhancing cardiorespiratory fitness [7]. The mechanisms underlying skeletal muscle metabolic adaptations to SIT however, have not fully been elucidated [8,9]. Studies have shown that SIT increases mitochondrial capacity through activation of peroxisome-proliferator activated receptor coactivator (PGC)-1α. PGC-1α is also known as the 'master switch' of mitochondrial biogenesis in muscle cells which participates in the regulation of carbohydrate and glucose uptake, oxidative capacity, anti-oxidant defense and anti-inflammatory pathways [6,9]. The SIT protocol of low-volume 'all-out' sprint bouts has the potential to increase PGC-1α messenger-ribonucleic acid (mRNA) by multiple folds when measured post exercise [8], which is comparable to the effects observed after a bout of continuous moderate-intensity endurance-type exercise [10,11]. Indeed, as little as six exercise sessions of 4 to 7 bouts of 30-s 'all-out' sprints with 4 min recovery performed over two weeks, positively impacted the muscle's maximal capacity to use oxygen, or otherwise known as skeletal muscle oxidative capacity [12].

A typical example of the traditional SIT exercise protocol employs the Wingate anaerobic cycle test (WAnT) which consists of two to four 30-s bouts of 'all-out' or supramaximal efforts (>100% VO_{2peak}) performed consecutively and interspersed with only between ~2 to 4 min of active or passive recovery periods [12,13]. The traditional SIT exercise protocol is likened to a 'clustered' protocol. This 'clustered' WAnT protocol is known to be physically strenuous and requires high levels of self-motivation to complete successfully [14–16]. Thus, for clustered WAnT training protocol to be more appealing, we proposed to increase the rest periods between each of the sprint bout, in what we termed as the 'dispersed' WAnT protocol. In this dispersed protocol, a single 30-s WAnT bout is performed three times a day, but with ~4 h of rest between each bout. Using this exercise protocol, for the same volume and/or number of sprint bouts per day (e.g., 3 × 30-s cycle bouts), the dispersed protocol requires less than half the amount of time to complete as compared to the clustered protocol due to the elimination of recovery between the bouts (see Table 1). Thus, the dispersed protocol is deemed to be more time-efficient. Previous research has indicated that individuals can accrue similar health benefits from exercising in a single bout or accumulating activity from shorter bouts throughout the day [17]. With the concept of 'accumulated' benefits of exercise, the dispersed WAnT protocol may be a potential exercise strategy for individuals who are unwilling or unable to spent time in prolonged physical activity. Indeed, two recent training studies that employed the dispersed WAnT protocol observed improvements in VO_{2peak}. The first was a pilot study conducted by our research group on sedentary females, consisting of 3 × 30-s WAnT sprint bouts with 4 h of rest between bouts, 3 days per week for 8 weeks. We showed an average of ~14% improvement in VO_{2peak} [18]. Another study that employed a similar protocol also reported that 3 × 20-s WAnT sprint bouts with 1 to 4 h rest duration performed for 3 days per week for a total of 6 weeks, led to ~4% improvement in VO_{2peak}, among inactive but moderately fit college-aged individuals [19]. These two studies showed that WAnT bouts performed in a dispersed fashioned could result in modest improvements in cardiorespiratory fitness in trained and untrained individuals. However, several limitations were noted in these two studies. These include the lack of non-training control group to quantify the magnitude of training-induced improvements, and the effects of the dispersed WAnT protocol on other important health markers such as insulin sensitivity, lipid profile, functional strength, and perceived quality of life were not assessed.

Table 1. Comparison of time commitment to perform a clustered vs. dispersed Wingate Anaerobic test (WAnT) cycle exercise training protocol.

Exercise Component Variables	Clustered WAnT Bouts Protocol	Dispersed WAnT Bouts Protocol
Warm-up duration	1 × 60-s = 1.0 min	3 × 60-s = 3.0 min
Bouts duration	3 × 30-s = 1.5 min	3 × 30-s = 1.5 min
Recovery duration between bouts	2 × 4 min = 8 min	~4 h (but this duration is part of individual's official work time and is hence excluded from the exercise time)
Total exercise time per day or per session	10.5 min	4.5 min
Total exercise time per week (based on 3 training days per week)	31.5 min	13.5 min (~60% less time commitment vs. clustered protocol)

Therefore, our aim in the present study was to address these limitations and provide additional evidence of the efficacy of a dispersed WAnT cycle training protocol. Based on the findings of previous studies [18,19], the working hypothesis of the present study was that a dispersed WAnT exercise training protocol is effective in improving cardiovascular fitness, leg strength, insulin sensitivity and lipid profile of healthy individuals.

2. Methods

2.1. Participants

A total of thirty-four healthy male and female participants, aged 21–45 y, were recruited from ~320 staff working for an organization whom had convenient access to the laboratory facilities where all testing and training sessions were conducted. A validated pre-screening physical activity tool was administered to all volunteers, followed by a screening process performed by a sport physician. This is to ensure that participants were free from risk factors associated with metabolic, cardiovascular or pulmonary disease, and have had no pre-existing musculoskeletal conditions that would limit their physical function. Participants were also informed that lifestyle changes may potentially affect the outcome of the study, and hence, were instructed to maintain their routine diet and daily activities. The experimental procedures and potential risks were fully explained to all participants prior to obtaining their written-informed consent. The study was approved by the institutional review board and conformed to the Declaration of Helsinki.

A match-controlled cohort trial was carried out and volunteers were assigned to either the training/intervention (INT) or non-training/control (CON) group. Several blocks of recruitment exercise took place over a 16-week period. Approximately 4 to 8 participants were recruited during each block, and they were tested for their pre-training or baseline VO_{2peak} before being assigned to either the INT or CON groups based on their VO_{2peak}, age and body mass index (BMI), to ensure similar baseline characteristics for both groups.

2.2. Pre- and Post-Experimental Procedures

All participants arrived in the laboratory in the morning after at least 8 h of overnight fasting. They were advised to consume 500 mL of water in the morning of the test. They were instructed to abstain from strenuous exercise 2–3 days before the test and avoid alcohol and smoking the evening before the test. Baseline measurements for all participants consisted of the assessment of basic anthropometric measures, resting blood pressure (BP), resting heart rate (HR), body fat, VO_{2peak}, blood lipids, fasting blood glucose and fasting insulin, as well as a survey on their quality of life. After the completion of 6 weeks of training, post-training tests similar to baseline measures were obtained to determine the efficacy of the training intervention. The post-training measures were conducted between 3 to 7 d after the final training session.

Anthropometric measures, resting heart rate and resting blood pressure: Stature was measured in centimeters without shoes. Body mass and body fat percentage were determined using bioimpedance technique (Inbody770, Chungcheong, Korea) following the manufacturer's standard procedures. Resting BP and HR were assessed in a seated position, with the individuals seated upright on a chair with a back support and arm positioned at chest level for a minimum of 3 min before any measurement was taken. BP and HR measures were manually taken by the same trained physician throughout the study. Two blood pressure measurements were taken at each time point, with a 2-min rest between measures, and these were averaged to reduce variability.

2.3. Peak Oxygen Uptake

All participants performed a progressive exercise ramp test on a cycle ergometer (Lode BV, Excalibur Sport, Groningen, The Netherlands) to determine their peak oxygen uptake or VO_{2peak}. Participants completed a standardized 3 min warm-up between 40 to 60 W. For the VO_{2peak} test, the cycle resistance was increased by 1 W every 3 s until volitional exhaustion. Volitional exhaustion is determined as the physical limit beyond which the participant was no longer able to continue the prescribed pedal rate, i.e., between 50 revolutions per min (rpm) for women and 60 rpm for men. Subsequently, after a passive rest of ~8 min, a verification test of the initial VO_{2peak} value was undertaken. Based on the peak power attained in the initial test, the individual cycled at 50%, 70%, 105% for 60-s, followed by cycle to volitional exhaustion at 120%. The expired respiratory gases during initial and verification tests were measured using a calibrated metabolic cart (TrueOne 2400MMS, Parvomedics, East Sandy, UT, USA), and VO_{2peak} was recorded as the highest value over a 30-s period during the initial and verification tests. The coefficient of variation for VO_{2peak} measurement in our laboratory is 2% (unpublished data).

2.4. Leg Strength

As the criterion measure of dynamic leg strength, maximal voluntary contraction (MVC) was assessed via the maximal knee extension and flexion of the dominant leg on a isokinetic dynamometer (Biodex System 3 PRO dynamometer, Biodex Medical Systems, Shirley, NY, USA). Participants warmed-up by cycling for 8 min followed by 3 min of dynamic stretching of the hip, knee and ankle joints. Participants were then securely strapped across the upper body and the hips while seated on the dynamometer chair with the arms folded across the chest. The dynamometer lever arm was secured 2–4 cm above the ankle malleolus of the dominant leg and the participant's knee joint was then adjusted to align with the axis of rotation of the dynamometer lever arm. The range of motion of the tested leg was then set accordingly for the knee extension/flexion movement. As part of familiarization, each participant was asked to perform 5 repetitions (rep) at $300°\cdot s^{-1}$, followed by 3 rep at $30°\cdot s^{-1}$ at their perceived 50–60% submaximal effort. Subsequently, the participant was then instructed to forcefully extend and flex the lower leg as fast as possible, at the tested speed of $30°\cdot s^{-1}$ and $300°\cdot s^{-1}$, respectively. Each individual had to perform three reps of flexion and extension interspersed with ~15-s of passive rest between each rep. MVC was defined and recorded as the highest peak torque (in Newton-meters, N·m) of the 3 rep. The dynamometer was calibrated prior to each testing session and was corrected for gravity.

2.5. Lipid Profile

Following at least 8 h of overnight fasting, venous blood sample (~5 mL) was obtained using BD vacutainer blood collection system. The blood was kept in the refrigerator at 4 °C and transported to an accredited commercial biochemistry laboratory (Quest Laboratories, Singapore) within 2 h of the blood draw. Analyses for fasting glucose, fasting insulin, plasma triglyceride, low-density lipoprotein (LDL)-cholesterol and high-density lipoprotein (HDL)-cholesterol were performed using standardized procedures. The intra-assay coefficients of variation of these markers are within 3% (Quest Laboratories, Singapore).

2.6. Insulin Resistance Markers

Fasting insulin and fasting glucose were obtained from venous blood sample (~3 mL) after an overnight fast for at least 8 h. Two indirect indices, the Homeostatic model assessment (HOMA) and Quantitative insulin-sensitivity check index (QUICKI), were used to estimate insulin resistance as these measures are identified as reliable and simple indirect methods for detection of insulin sensitivity [19]. HOMA index uses the formula previously described [20]: Insulin (UM^{-1}) × [Glucose ($mmol{\cdot}L^{-1}/22.5$]. The QUICKI is based on the logarithmic transformation: 1/(log insulin log glycaemia in $mg{\cdot}dL^{-1}$) [21]. The blood measures of glucose and insulin were performed under standardized procedures in an accredited biochemistry laboratory (Quest Laboratories, Singapore). The intra-assay coefficient of variation for fasting glucose and fasting insulin measures are within 3% (Quest Laboratories, Singapore).

2.7. Psychological Measures

Health-related quality of life (HRQL) was assessed using the validated Short Form-36 (SF-36) RAND questionnaire [22]. This self-evaluated questionnaire assesses the individual's perceived health over the training period that includes eight sub-scales grouped into the physical component summary (PCS) and mental component summary (MCS). An algorithm generates the total score using the Orthotool kit SF-36 calculator. Each subcomponent was scored using a scale ranging between 0 and 100 (arbitrary units, au). The description of the scores are: 0–20 = 'very bad', 20–40 = 'bad', 40–60 = 'moderate', 60–80 = 'good' and 'optimal' = 80–100 HRQL [23], whereby a score closer to 100 indicates a higher quality of life.

2.8. Exercise Training Intervention

Participants allocated to INT group performed the dispersed WAnT exercise training protocol on a cycle ergometer (Wattbike Pro, Nottingham, UK). They were required to perform a single 30-s 'all-out' sprint bout three times a day, for 3 days per week over 6 weeks, for a total of 54 bouts during the study period. Due to the challenging nature of the SIT, the duration of each cycle sprint bout commenced with 15-s for training week 1, then increased to 20-s per bout for week 2 and finally to 30-s from week 3 to week 6. On each training day, the participant performed a total of 3 sprint bouts. Every sprint bout was preceded with a 60-s warm-up at ~40 W or 50 W resistance, followed by a single 'all-out' sprint effort. All exercise sessions were conducted in the laboratory situated within the participants' working environment; the estimated walking distance from the participants' workstations to the laboratory was between 2 to 5 min. In addition, participants were strongly encouraged to perform the cycle sprint exercise in comfortable work attire, without the need to change into sports gear (Figure 1). About 398 of the exercise sessions (~70% of total of 568 sessions of the study) were performed in the individuals' working attire.

It was purposefully designed that each cycle sprint bout was interspersed with at least 4 h of rest that corresponded to their work schedule. Individuals in the INT group were encouraged to perform their first WAnT cycle (i.e., the morning bout) before work (08:30 to 10:30), the second bout around lunch time (afternoon bout; 12:30 to 14:30), and the last bout before leaving the office (evening bout; 16:30 to 18:30). This schedule was to mimic the work pattern of a regular office worker. In the present study, because of work exigencies however, the duration of the rest periods varies between and within individuals. We recorded the actual rest duration between the morning and afternoon bouts, and between the afternoon and evening bouts, in the INT group throughout the study (see Table 2).

Ratings of perceived exertion (RPE, Borg's 0–10 scale) [24] and their affect ("how enjoyable is this exercise", using Likert scale from 1 = 'not enjoyable at all', 4 = 'moderately enjoyable', to 7 = 'extremely enjoyable'), were administered to participants at the end of each exercise session and prior to leaving the laboratory. The value of RPE and enjoyability post-training were summed every week across the entire training period. Participants used the same cycle ergometer throughout the 6 weeks of training. All training sessions were closely supervised by the two primary researchers. Participants set their preferred cycle resistance with the assistance of the researchers during the familiarization phase with the objective of exerting maximal power output during each cycle sprint. In the instance that a participant missed a training session, a make-up session was organized on the next available date, with the aim of completing all 54 training sessions within 6 ± 1 week. Participants in the CON group were instructed to maintain their usual lifestyle habits and behavior patterns throughout the study duration. A weekly reminder was made through telephone or text message to remind them to not to engage in any unaccustomed exercise and to keep to their normal diet.

(A) (B)

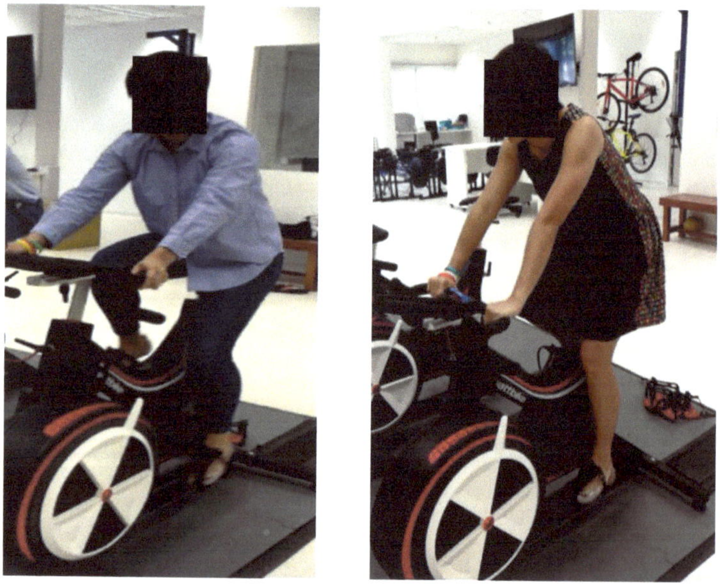

Figure 1. Participating individuals performing the dispersed protocol of the 30 s Wingate Anaerobic cycle Test (WAnT) bouts in two of the most common non-sporting attires; in (**A**) jeans with shirt or t-shirt, and (**B**) long-skirt.

Table 2. Frequencies of the rest periods between the morning and afternoon exercise bouts, and between the afternoon and evening exercise bouts.

Duration of the Rest Periods	Frequencies (%)
Between 0–1 h	0
Between 1–2 h	0.88
Between 2–3 h	17.61
Between 3–4 h	31.16
Between 4–4.5 h	50.35

3. Statistical Analysis

The sample size of 16 individuals in each group was adequate to estimate the mean of VO_{2peak} scale between two groups in healthy individuals with effect size: (5 points difference with standard deviation 6.5) using a one-way analysis of variance (ANOVA) test (two-tailed, alpha = 0.05 with statistical power 0.80) including 10% attrition rate. All numeric data were presented as mean ± SD. All statistical data were completed using SPSS version 22 (IBM Corp., Armonk, NY, USA). Data were assessed by a Shapiro-Wilk test for normality, and by a Levene test for the homogeneity of variance assumption. The Greenhouse-Geisser correction was used to account for the sphericity assumption of unequal variances across groups. Baseline values of each variable were compared between INT and CON groups by a *t*-test. Changes in the dependent variables from the baseline to post 6 weeks training were compared between the groups by a mixed-design two-way ANOVA for raw data, and their normalized changes were compared between groups by a *t*-test. Two-way mixed model ANOVAs (group [INT, CON] × time [pre, post]) were performed to test the effects of training on VO_{2peak}, total cholesterol, HDL, LDL, triglycerides, fasting insulin, fasting glucose, HOMA, QUICKI and SF-36. A significant training X group interaction was used to identify training-induced changes in these variables. When ANOVA showed a significant interaction (group × time) effect, Tukey's post-hoc test was used to detect differences between means. Time course data (i.e., peak power, mean power, weekly level of enjoyability and RPE) were compared via repeated measures of ANOVA. The effect size for the difference in the magnitude of the change from pre-training to post-training between the INT and CON groups was calculated for each outcome measure using Cohen's *d*, and 0.2, 0.5, and 0.8 were considered as a small, medium, and large effect, respectively. Statistical significance was set at $p < 0.05$.

4. Results

Of the 34 participants enrolled in the study, one participant in the INT group withdrew due to prolonged febrile illness. Thus, 33 participants (INT, $N = 16$; CON, $N = 17$) completed the study.

INT participants completed 861 of 864 WAnT bouts in total, i.e., training adherence of 99.6%, with no injuries or clinical complications sustained over the period of the study. At baseline, both INT and CON groups had similar physical and physiological characteristics, strength and metabolic-health markers (Table 3). We have also included the pre- and post- 6 weeks of intervention results of both groups as Table S1.

There were significant interaction effects in absolute and relative VO_{2peak} ($F_{1,31}$ ratio = 8.77, $p = 0.006$ and $F_{1,31}$ ratio = 8.85, $p = 0.004$, respectively). Comparison between pre- to post-training indicates that there was significant improvement in both the absolute and relative VO_{2peak} in the INT group ($p = 0.004$ and $p < 0.001$, respectively) but not in the CON group ($p = 0.42$ and 0.64, respectively) (Figure 2).

Table 3. Baseline characteristics and measures between the two groups in the study.

Measured Variables	CON Group (N = 17; 8 M + 9 F)	INT Group (N =16; 8 M + 9 F)	p Value between Groups
Age (y)	35.1 ± 6.9	34.1 ± 6.3	0.68
Stature (cm)	167 ± 8	168 ± 11	0.82
Body mass (kg)	69.0 ± 14.7	69.3 ± 14.2	0.86
Body fat (%)	26.3 ± 9.8	24.9 ± 7.2	0.63
Resting Systolic BP (mmHg)	120 ± 14	117 ± 13	0.53
Resting Diastolic BP (mmHg)	79 ± 11	76 ± 8	0.33
Resting HR (b·min^{-1})	65 ± 10	63 ± 10	0.84
VO_{2peak} (L·min^{-1})	2.50 ± 0.68	2.58 ± 0.86	0.75
VO_{2peak} (mL·kg^{-1}·min^{-1})	36.9 ± 9.6	36.7 ± 6.7	0.97
MVC flexion 30°·s^{-1} (Nm)	158 ± 42	168 ± 59	0.59
MVC extension 30°·s^{-1} (Nm)	91 ± 31	86 ± 25	0.66
MVC flexion 300°·s^{-1} (Nm)	80 ± 27	87 ± 31	0.46
MVC extension 300°·s^{-1} (Nm)	55 ± 23	48 ± 16	0.36
Total cholesterol (mmol·L^{-1})	4.97 ± 0.75	4.74 ± 0.93	0.45
Triglycerides (mmol·L^{-1})	2.00 ± 1.06	1.79 ± 0.99	0.56
HDL (mmol·L^{-1})	1.68 ± 0.46	1.60 ± 0.37	0.58
LDL (mmol·L^{-1})	2.87 ± 0.71	2.77 ± 0.75	0.71
Fasting Glucose (mmol·L^{-1})	4.79 ± 0.57	4.56 ± 0.42	0.21
Fasting Insulin (mmol·L^{-1})	5.96 ± 3.70	4.68 ± 3.16	0.29
Insulin resistance–HOMA (au)	1.32 ± 0.89	0.96 ± 0.71	0.22
Insulin sensitivity–QUICKI (au)	0.39 ± 0.07	0.39 ± 0.06	0.99

Key: M = males; F = females; CON = control or non-training; INT = Intervention or training; BP = blood pressure; HR = heart rate; VO_{2peak} = peak oxygen uptake; MVC = maximal voluntary contraction; HDL = High-density lipoprotein; LDL = low-density lipoprotein; HOMA = Homeostatic model assessment; QUICKI = Quantitative insulin-sensitivity check index; au = arbitrary unit.

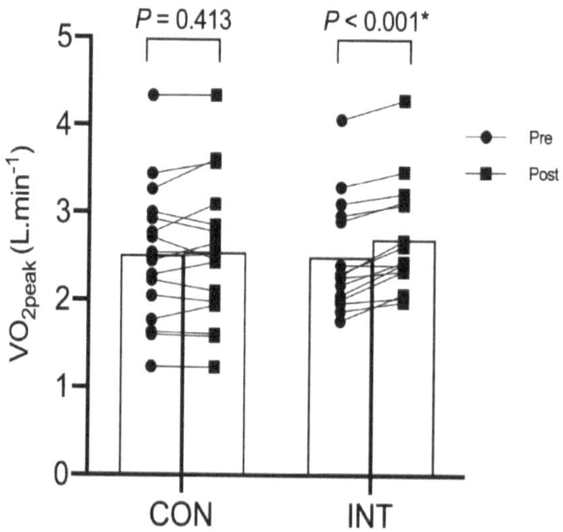

Figure 2. Peak oxygen uptake (or VO_{2peak}) at pre- and post-6 weeks of training in the non-training or control (CON, N = 17) and intervention training (INT; N = 16) group. * Significance difference from pre-training in INT group only.

The magnitude of increase in VO_{2peak} was 2.7 ± 2.1 mL·kg^{-1}·min^{-1} ($p < 0.001$) in the INT group and 0.32 ± 2.51 mL·kg^{-1}·min^{-1} ($p = 0.62$) in the CON group; with a large effect size difference between the two groups (Figure 3).

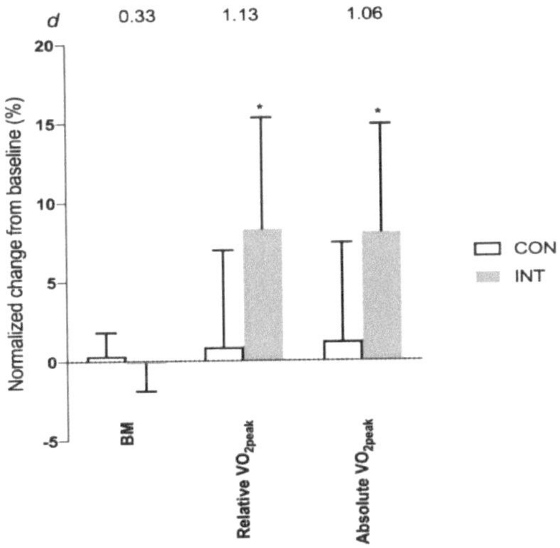

Figure 3. Normalized changes (mean ± SD) in body mass (BM) and VO_{2peak} from baseline (0%) to post-6 weeks training for non-training or control (CON, $N = 17$) group and intervention training (INT; $N = 16$) group. * Significance ($p < 0.01$) difference from CON group. Effect size (d) for the difference between CON and INT groups is shown on the top of the graph.

There were no significant time and interaction effects in body fat %, resting BP and resting HR, within and between the two groups (all F ratio values with $p > 0.05$; Figure 4).

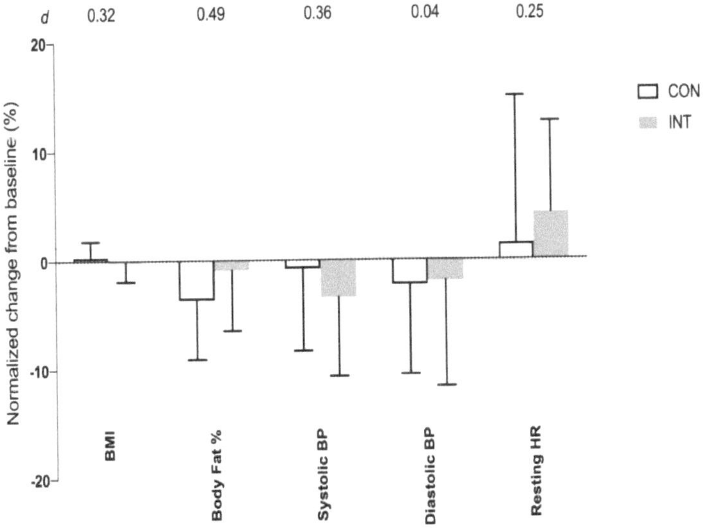

Figure 4. Normalized changes (mean ± SD) in body mass index (BMI), body fat percentage (%), systolic blood pressure (BP), diastolic BP and resting heart rate (HR) from baseline (0%) to post-6 weeks training for non-training or control (CON, $N = 17$) group and intervention training (INT; $N = 16$) group. Effect size (d) for the difference between CON and INT groups is shown on the top of the graph.

For leg strength measures, there were interaction effects for MVC at $30°·s^{-1}$ for flexion and extension ($F_{1,31}$ ratio = 4.36, $p = 0.045$ and $F_{1,31}$ ratio = 4.42, $p = 0.04$, respectively), and for MVC at

300°·s^{-1} for flexion ($F_{1,31}$ ratio = 5.00, p = 0.03). However, post-hoc analysis indicates only MVC at 30°·s^{-1} for flexion was statistically significantly different between INT and CON groups (p = 0.03, with a moderate effect size; Figure 5).

Fasting insulin, fasting glucose, insulin sensitivity markers of HOMA, QUICKI and blood lipids did not show any time nor interaction effects between the two groups (all F ratio values with p > 0.05; Figure 6).

There was also no significant difference in cycle sprints peak ($F_{1,285}$ ratio = 0.12, p = 0.89) and mean power ($F_{1,285}$ ratio = 0.01, p = 0.99) between the morning, afternoon and evening WAnT bouts, throughout the 6 weeks (Table 4).

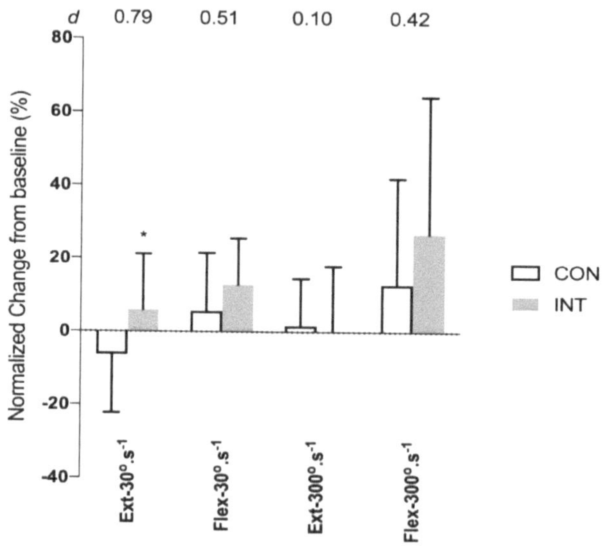

Figure 5. Normalized changes (mean ± SD) in maximum voluntary contraction (MVC) of the dominant lower limb on isokinetic dynamometer at knee extension at velocity of 30°·s^{-1} and 300°·s^{-1}, and knee flexion at velocity of 30°·s^{-1} and 300°·s^{-1}, from baseline (0%) to post-6 weeks training for non-training or control (CON, N = 17) group and intervention training (INT; N = 16) group. * Significance (p < 0.05) difference from CON group. Effect size (d) for the difference between CON and INT groups is shown on the top of the graph.

Table 4. The average peak and mean power of the morning, afternoon and evening 30-s Wingate Anaerobic cycle test (WAnT) bouts performed throughout the six-weeks training period.

WAnT Bouts of the Day	Peak Power (W)	Mean Power (W)
Morning Bout	838 ± 312	555 ± 189
Afternoon Bout	839 ± 318	552 ± 191
Evening Bout	850 ± 317	555 ± 194

In relation to the quality-of-life survey, no significant group x time interactions were detected between INT and CON, at pre- and post-training. During training week 1 and week 2 when sprint bouts were shorter (15-s and 20-s, respectively), participants generally indicated a higher level of enjoyment to the exercise compared to training week 3 to 6; although they were not statistically different across the training weeks, $F_{1,94}$ ratio = 0.66, p = 0.65 (Figure 7). RPE showed a significant time effect ($F_{1,94}$ ratio = 3.04, p = 0.014), but post-hoc analysis showed no statistically significant differences between any of the training weeks, all p > 0.05 (Figure 7).

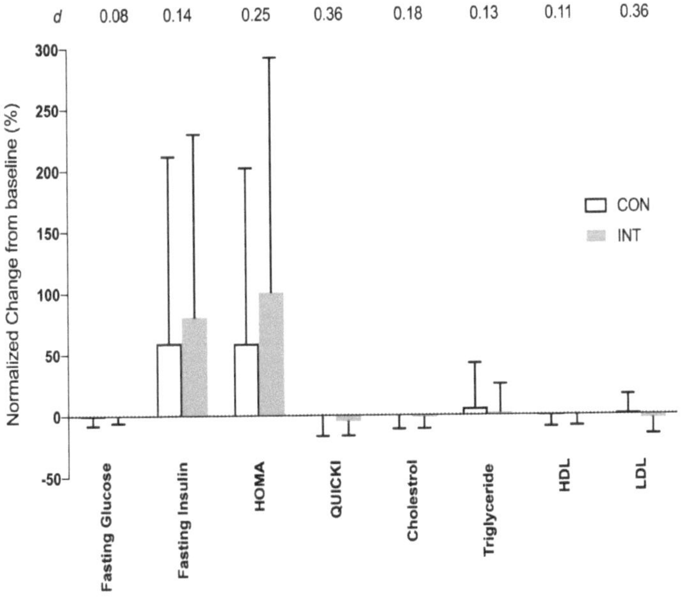

Figure 6. Normalized changes (mean ± SD) in fasting glucose, fasting insulin, Homeostatic model assessment (HOMA), Quantitative insulin-sensitivity check index (QUICKI), total cholesterol, triglyceride, high-density lipoprotein (HDL), low-density lipoprotein (LDL) from baseline (0%) to post-6 weeks training for non-training or control (CON, $N = 17$) group and intervention training (INT; $N = 16$) group. Effect size (d) for the difference between CON and INT groups is shown on the top of the graph.

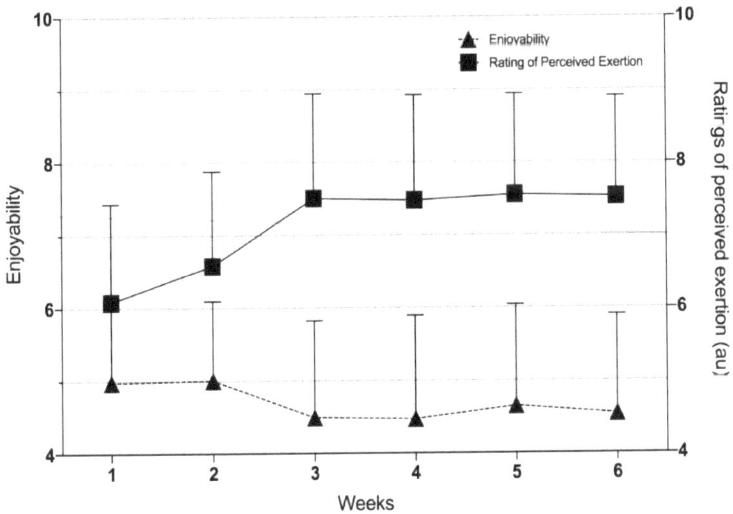

Figure 7. Weekly training levels of enjoyability and ratings of perceived exertion or RPE at the end of the exercise sessions across the 6 weeks of training of participants in the intervention or training group (INT, $N = 16$). The mean data is the average of all sessions performed over that week.

5. Discussion

The key findings of this study were that a dispersed WAnT exercise training protocol on cycle ergometer for 6 weeks enhanced cardiovascular fitness and dynamic lower-limb muscular strength in healthy adults. In the present study, 6 weeks of 30-s sprints, 3 bouts per day, separated by ~4 h rest, 3 days per week was effective in improving aerobic fitness by ~8% compared to a non-training group.

The present study's findings corroborated the results of earlier studies. Using a similar dispersed WAnT exercise protocol, Little and colleagues reported a ~4% increase in VO_{2peak} following 6 weeks of 20-s sprints, 3 bouts per day, separated by 1–4 h rest for 3 days a week [19]. And our own pilot study of 8 weeks of 30-s sprints, 3 bouts per day, separated by ~4 h rest, 3 days per week, reported ~14% improvement in VO_{2peak} [18]. Collectively, these three studies contribute to the growing evidence that very short duration of 'all-out' supramaximal sprint cycle bouts performed multiple times throughout the day, with extended rest duration between the bouts can result in modest improvements in cardiorespiratory fitness within a wide range of healthy individuals. Interestingly, despite the brief duration of exercise commitment (exercise duration ~1.0–1.5 min), the magnitude of training induced improvements in cardiovascular fitness improvement is comparable to longer, traditional SIT using a clustered protocol (exercise duration ~10.0–15.0 min) [7]. Rapid improvements in physiological adaptation with a clustered WAnT protocol have been attributed to increased cardiac output and peripheral oxygen extraction in response to increased muscle oxidative potential [25]. In a clustered WAnT exercise protocol, it has clearly been shown that individuals were not able to sustain their maximum power output throughout all of the three 30-s bouts [26]. In contrast, in the present dispersed WAnT exercise training protocol, there were no significant differences in the average peak and mean power obtained during the morning, afternoon and evening bouts across the 6 weeks (Table 4), which indicates that individuals were able to sustain their maximal power output exertion for all of the three 30-s bouts performed throughout the day, i.e., the overall exercise intensity across the entire training programme would theoretically, be higher in the dispersed compared to the clustered protocol. Perhaps, the consistency of being able to maximize the level of exercise intensity for every single WAnT bout performed throughout the 6 weeks of training is the key stimulus that allows the dispersed protocol to be as, if not more, potent than the same number of WAnT bouts performed in a clustered fashioned [27]. However, to our knowledge, no direct study has been undertaken to determine the underlying physiological mechanism(s) of the training-induced adaptations to a dispersed WAnT exercise training protocol, which implies a fertile area for future research.

The present study's low volume, maximal-intensity WAnT training bouts dispersed throughout the day significantly improved leg strength as indicated by the increased in MVC at $30°{\cdot}s^{-1}$ for flexion. The findings are in sharp contrast with two previous studies that examined the impact of a clustered WAnT training protocol on leg strength. Astorino and colleagues [28] had males and females performed a clustered WAnT protocol 6–8 times over a three-week period and their results showed no significant changes in their subjects' MVC of the knee flexor and extensor muscle torque. Similarly, Bagley et al. [29] found that 12 weeks of clustered WAnT training did not increase the knee muscular torque in their participants, although the same subjects showed increase in their lower-limb muscle mass. We were unable to provide any mechanism(s) nor reasons for the contrasting observations between these studies, but it is likely that the same reason of the ability to elicit the greatest peak power and mean power possible during each of the three daily WAnT bouts and thus an overall higher resistance throughout the entire training programme relative to the previous studies is a key difference to the stark improvement observed in the lower limb strength in the present study. Nonetheless, our results showed a modest increased in the INT group's knee flexor strength, which may suggest that a dispersed WAnT exercise training protocol may enhance the functional working capability and physical function of an individual's lower-limbs. This positive impact on lower-limb strength may have important implications in exercise programming for the elderly, which requires further investigation.

WAnT bouts training performed in the clustered fashioned has been shown to accrue many positive benefits such as greater glucose uptake by skeletal muscle, increased intramuscular expression of glucose transporter type 4 (GLUT-4), and greater depletion of intramuscular glycogen that may explain the observed improvements in insulin sensitivity in some studies [6,30,31]. In the present study however, six weeks of dispersed WAnT training was not sufficient to improve insulin resistance nor various metabolic health markers when measured 3 to 7 days after the final exercise training session. It should be noted that improvement in aerobic fitness is not obligatory for training-induced improvements to cardiovascular risk factors [32] and that factor such as heterogeneity (as the case in the present study due to the use of both males and female as subjects) caused by genetic variability such as the expression of RNA, may contribute to training susceptibility [33]. Nonetheless, the current study's findings did corroborate with those of earlier studies conducted on healthy asymptomatic adolescents. For example, Buchan and colleagues [34] reported no change in fasting glucose or insulin following 7 weeks of 4 to 6 × 30-s maximal sprints 3 times per week. Further, a published meta-regression analyses suggest that to achieve a reduction of HOMA-IR of 0.5 units, the baseline HOMA needs to be at least 3.18, indicating that insulin sensitivity can only be improved in those who are already insulin resistant [35,36]. It is possible that the minimum threshold of insulin resistant was not sufficiently met in the present study's healthy participants. Indeed, when exercise volume was increased and sprint bouts were performed in a clustered fashioned of 3–4 times × 30-s or 7–12 times × 60-s, [37–39], improvements in insulin sensitivity, albeit small in magnitude, were observed. We speculate that the differing energy fluxes and substrate utilization during the clustered and dispersed WAnT exercise protocol may be the reason for the contrasting results. During the first 30-s sprint bout of the clustered WAnT exercise protocol, adenosine triphosphate (ATP) demand is primarily met via phosphocreatine breakdown and glycolysis, with oxidative metabolism contributing to about 30% of overall energy requirements [40]. In subsequent bouts, the proportional contribution from oxidative phosphorylation is progressively increased. With the partial recovery between bouts, aerobic energy contribution progressively increases in the subsequent 30-s bouts, even though the exercise is of maximal physical effort. For the dispersed protocol, each of the 30-s morning, afternoon and evening bout of WAnT exercise would predominantly be fueled via ATP and glycolysis processes, which meant a greater anaerobic contribution in total relative to that of the clustered WAnT protocol. As such, it is assumed that there would be a greater energy flux through the oxidative mitochondrial generated substrate pathways during a clustered WAnT compared to a dispersed WAnT exercise training protocol, and correspondingly, greater insulin sensitizing effect in the clustered WAnT protocol [41].

Research focused on blood lipid changes after exercise of maximal and supramaximal efforts have shown contrasting outcomes [42]. Some studies reported significant positive changes [43–45], while others [46,47] did not observe any improvement in blood lipid profile following chronic HIT. Racil and colleagues observed an improvement in blood lipids, cardiometabolic markers and blood leptin in obese adolescent females after 12 weeks of 12 × 30-s running sprints at 50% maximal aerobic speed, three times a week [44]. Similarly, Koubaa et al. noted significant improvement in blood lipids in obese children following 2 min run at 80% VO_{2peak}, performed three times a week over 12 weeks [43]. On the other hand, Crouse and colleagues did not show any influence of exercise intensity on lipid profile following a progressive exercise of 15 to 60 min three times per week for 24 weeks of cycle ergometer training at intensity of either 50% and 80% VO_{2max} [46]. Ouerghi and colleagues reported an improvement in lipid profile in sedentary obese but not in the normal weight individuals following three times a week for 8 weeks of 2 × 30-s running sprint at 100–110% maximal aerobic velocity [48]. It remains plausible that lipid lowering effects following HIIT-type of exercise is more pronounced in metabolically challenged individuals than in normal weight individuals. It may also be that there is a relationship between body fat and cholesterol levels, insofar a relatively higher volume of training relative to the present study's SIT programme, is required to elicit changes in fat mass [47]. In short, the volume of training completed as opposed to the intensity of exercise training may be the key factor to improving lipid profile, and as such, the low volume albeit supramaximal-intensity exercise protocol in the present study may not have significant impact on blood lipids.

The design of the current study's exercise protocol provides a practical prescription that can be easily incorporated into an office worker's daily routine, to form an integral component between work and active lifestyle. Thus, instead of having individuals to set aside time for exercise, an exercise program built into their daily routine can help to eliminate the common excuse of 'lack of time' barrier to exercise [15]. Participants were further encouraged to exercise in their work attire without the need to change into specific exercise or sportswear, which saved even more time and improved efficiency. This dispersed WAnT exercise training protocol reduced training time by 60% compared to a traditional clustered protocol; to a mere 4.5 min per day or 13.5 min per week (Table 1). The side effects of 'faints, respiratory events, nausea, light-headedness, and vomiting' that have been associated with a clustered WAnT protocol is well-known [49]. We thus were able to circumvent these negative responses by introducing a prolonged rest periods between each cycle sprint bout. It is heartening to note that the present dispersed WAnT exercise training protocol achieved >99% compliance or attendance rate and was rated as 'fairly' enjoyable in the study. In addition, there were no adverse clinical events over the six weeks of training. These suggest that a dispersed WAnT exercise training protocol can be well adopted and prescribed safely to healthy adults, and possibly for special population cohorts such as the diseased and elderly, albeit more studies are required to confirm the latter.

6. Strengths and Limitations of the Study

The present dispersed WAnT exercise training protocol is specifically designed around a typical office worker's schedule and helped eliminate the barrier of lack of time for exercise. The major strength of the study was that it was conducted within a 'real-life' office-workplace scenario and therefore the findings have much practical applications. It is envisaged that cycle ergometers can be conveniently placed around the office workstations to allow individuals to perform the current proposed short-bouts of exercise throughout the work-day. The benefits of the present dispersed WAnT exercise protocol may also entice sedentary individuals who are in a state of 'exercise resistance' to start exercising because of the low time commitment required [50]. There are several limitations in the present study. Firstly, the study was conducted on healthy rather than metabolically challenged individuals, such as the obese or those with pre-diabetic conditions. Secondly, it was not possible to fully control for physical activities outside of the prescribed training program and dietary intake, although participants were instructed to maintain their normal habits. Also, the study did not control for the amount and type of foods ingested in the evening prior to the overnight fast which could have influenced the morning-after blood drawn serum lipid values. Thirdly, measures of insulin resistance were not determined using the hyperinsulinemia euglycemic clamp technique, which is considered to be the gold-standard measurement of insulin sensitivity, due to its invasive procedures. Finally, the inclusion of both sexes may potentially compound the results (e.g., insulin sensitivity) as there was no control for menstrual cycle variations when testing the female participants at pre- and post-training time points [51].

7. Conclusions

The results of the present study confirmed that a dispersed WAnT exercise training protocol, with rest periods of ~4 h between bouts is a practical and effective exercise strategy to improve cardiovascular fitness and lower-limb muscular strength. However, it had no significant impact on blood lipids or insulin sensitivity. It is suggested that this training regime may have important positive implications on functional work capacity, especially to the time-constrained office-workers. Finally, considering the high compliance rate observed, further research using a dispersed WAnT exercise training protocol to try to improve cardiorespiratory fitness and metabolic health in the diseased and challenging population cohort should be explored.

Supplementary Materials: The following are available online at http://www.mdpi.com/1660-4601/17/13/4860/s1, Table S1: Mean pre and post-intervention results in the Control ($n = 17$) and Intervention ($n = 16$) groups.

Author Contributions: C.H.W., M.J.Z., B.H.H. and A.R.A. conceived the study's aims and designed the study's experiment and training protocols. C.H.W., M.J.Z., K.M. and F.T. contributed to recruitment of participants, access to facilities and experiment equipping. C.H.W., M.J.Z., and A.R.A. conducted the experiments and data collection. C.H.W. and M.J.Z., helped to tabulate and collate the raw data. C.H.W., M.J.Z., and A.R.A. analyzed and interpreted the data. C.H.W., M.J.Z., and A.R.A. prepared the initial draft of the manuscript. B.H.H., K.M., and F.T. provided constructive feedback to the progress of the written manuscript. All authors read and approved the final version of the manuscript.

Funding: This research received no external funding.

Acknowledgments: The authors would like to thank the participating individuals for showing their all-round enthusiasm and highest-level of discipline and motivation in completing this study's demanding requirements.

Conflicts of Interest: All authors declare no conflict of interest to the outcome of the study.

References

1. Centers for Disease Control and Prevention. Fastats: Exercise or Physical Activity. Available online: http://www.cdc.gov/nchs/fastats/exercise.htm (accessed on 26 March 2019).
2. World Health Organization. Global Recommendations on Physical Activity for Health. Available online: http://www.who.int/dietphysicalactivity/publications/9789241599979/en/ (accessed on 26 March 2019).
3. Chua, L.; Soh, I.; Health Status and Health Related Behaviors in Adults with Self-Reported Diabetes. Statistics Singapore Newsletter. 2016. Available online: https://www.singstat.gov.sg/-/media/files/publications/society/ssnsep16-pg5-9.pdf (accessed on 26 March 2019).
4. Roth, M. Self-reported physical activity in adults. In *Health Survey for England*; Craig, R., Mindell, J., Hirani, V., Eds.; National Centre for Social Research: London, UK, 2008; pp. 21–42.
5. Gibala, M.J.; Little, J.P.; Essen, M.V.; Wilkin, G.P.; Burgomaster, K.A.; Safdar, A.; Raha, S.; Tarnopolsky, M.A. Short-term sprint interval versus traditional endurance training: Similar initial adaptations in human skeletal muscle and exercise performance. *J. Physiol.* **2006**, *575*, 901–911. [CrossRef] [PubMed]
6. Gibala, M.J.; Little, J.P.; MacDonald, M.J.; Hawley, J.A. Physiological adaptations to low volume high intensity interval training in health and disease. *J. Physiol.* **2012**, *590*, 1077–1084. [CrossRef]
7. Gist, N.H.; Fedewa, M.V.; Dishman, R.K.; Cureton, K.J. Sprint interval training effects on aerobic capacity: A systematic review and meta-analysis. *Sports Med.* **2014**, *44*, 269–279. [CrossRef] [PubMed]
8. Gibala, M.J.; McGee, S.L. Metabolic adaptations to short term high intensity interval training. *Exerc. Sport Sci. Rev.* **2008**, *36*, 58–63. [CrossRef] [PubMed]
9. Wu, Z.; Puigserver, P.; Andersson, U.; Zhang, C.; Adelmant, C.; Mootha, V.; Troy, C.; Cinti, S.; Lowell, B.; Scarpulla, R.C.; et al. Mechanisms controlling mitochondrial biogenesis and respiration through the thermogenic coactivator PGC-1. *Cell* **1999**, *98*, 115–124. [CrossRef]
10. Egan, B.; Carson, B.P.; Garcia-Roves, P.M.; Chibalin, A.V.; Sarsfield, F.M.; Barron, N.; McCaffrey, N.; Moyna, N.M.; Zierath, J.R.; O'Gorman, D.J. Exercise intensity-dependent regulation of PGC-1a mRNA abundance is associated with differential activation of upstream signalling kinases in human skeletal muscle. *J. Physiol.* **2010**, *588*, 1779–1790. [CrossRef]
11. Norrbom, J.; Sundberg, C.J.; Ameln, H.; Kraus, W.E.; Jansson, E.; Gustafsson, T. PGC-1a mRNA expression is influenced by metabolic perturbation in exercising human skeletal muscle. *J. Appl. Physiol.* **2004**, *96*, 189–194. [CrossRef]
12. Burgomaster, K.A.; Hughes, S.C.; Heigenhauser, G.J.; Bradwell, S.N.; Gibala, M.J. Six sessions of sprint interval training increases muscle oxidative potential and cycle endurance capacity in human. *J. Appl. Physiol.* **2005**, *98*, 1985–1990. [CrossRef]
13. Burgomaster, K.A.; Heigenhauser, G.J.; Gibala, M.J. Effect of short-term sprint interval training on human skeletal muscle carbohydrate metabolism during exercise and time-trial performance. *J. Appl. Physiol.* **2006**, *100*, 2041–2047. [CrossRef]
14. Gillen, J.B.; Percival, M.E.; Skelly, L.E.; Martin, B.J.; Tan, R.B.; Tarnopolsky, M.A.; Gibala, M.J. Three minutes of all-out intermittent exercise per week increases skeletal muscle oxidative capacity and improves cardiometabolic health. *PLoS ONE* **2014**, *9*, e111489. [CrossRef]
15. Herazo-Beltrán, Y.; Pinillos, Y.; Vidarte, J.; Crissien, E.; Suarez, D.; Garcia, R. Predictors of perceived barriers to physical activity in the general adult population: A cross-sectional study. *Braz. J. Phys. Ther.* **2017**, *21*, 44–50. [CrossRef]

16. Vollaard, N.B.; Metcalfe, R.; Williams, S. Effect of number of sprints in a SIT session on change in VO_{2max}: A meta-analysis. *Med. Sci. Sports Exerc.* **2017**, *49*, 1147–1156. [CrossRef] [PubMed]
17. Mitranun, W.; Deerochanawong, C.; Tanaka, H.; Suksom, D. Continuous vs interval training on glycemic control and macro-and microvascular reactivity in type 2 diabetic patients. *Scand. J. Med. Sci. Sports* **2014**, *24*, 69–76. [CrossRef] [PubMed]
18. Ho, B.H.; Lim, I.; Tian, R.; Tan, F.; Aziz, A.R. Effects of novel exercise training protocol of Wingate-based sprint bouts dispersed over a day on selected cardiometabolic health markers in sedentary females: A pilot study. *BMJ. Open Sport Exerc. Med.* **2018**, *4*. [CrossRef] [PubMed]
19. Little, J.P.; Langley, J.; Lee, M.; Myette-Côté, E.; Jackson, G.; Durrer, C.; Gibala, M.J.; Jung, M.E. Sprint exercise snacks: A novel approach to increase aerobic fitness. *Eur. J. Appl. Physiol.* **2019**, *119*, 1203–1212. [CrossRef]
20. Matthews, D.R.; Hosker, J.P.; Rudenski, A.S.; Naylor, B.A.; Treacher, D.F.; Turner, R.C. Homeostasis model assessment: Insulin resistance and b cell function from fasting plasma glucose and insulin concentration in man. *Diabetologia* **1985**, *28*, 412–419. [CrossRef]
21. Kaz, A.; Nambi, S.S.; Mather, K.; Baron, A.D.; Follmann, D.A.; Sulivan, G.; Quon, M.J. Quantitative insulin sensitivity check index: A simple, accurate method for assessing insulin sensitivity in humans. *J. Clin. Endocrinol. Metab.* **2000**, *85*, 2402–2410.
22. Knowles, A.M.; Herbert, P.; Easton, C.; Sculthorpe, N.; Grace, F.M. Impact of low volume, high intensity interval training on maximal aerobic capacity, health-related quality of life and motivation to exercise in ageing man. *Aging* **2015**, *37*. [CrossRef]
23. Campolina, A.G.; Ciconelli, R.M. SF 36 and the development of new assessment tools for quality of life. *Acta Reumatol. Port.* **2008**, *33*, 127–133.
24. Borg, G. *Perceived Exertion and Pain Scales*; Human Kinetics: Champaign, IL, USA, 1998.
25. Laursen, P.B.; Jenkins, D.G. The scientific basis for high-intensity interval training: Optimizing training programmes and maximizing performance in highly trained endurance athletes. *Sports Med.* **2002**, *32*, 53–73. [CrossRef]
26. McCartney, N.; Spriet, L.L.; Heigenhauser, G.J.F.; Kowalchuk, J.M.; Sutton, R.; Jones, N.L. Muscle power and metabolism in maximal intermittent exercise. *J. Appl. Physiol.* **1986**, *60*, 1164–1169. [CrossRef] [PubMed]
27. MacInnis, M.J.; Skelly, L.E.; Gibala, M.J. CrossTalk proposal: Exercise training intensity is more important than volume to promote increases in human skeletal muscle mitochondrial content. *J. Physiol.* **2019**, *597*, 4111–4113. [CrossRef]
28. Astorino, T.A.; Allen, R.P.; Roberson, D.W.; Jurancich, M. Effect of high intensity interval training on cardiovascular function, VO_{2max} and muscular force. *J. Strength Cond. Res.* **2012**, *26*, 138–145. [CrossRef]
29. Bagley, L.; Al-Shanti, N.; Bradburn, S.; Baig, O.; Slevin, M.; McPhee, J.S. Sex comparison of knee extensor size, strength and fatigue adaptation to sprint interval training. *J. Strength Cond. Res.* **2018**. [CrossRef] [PubMed]
30. Jellyman, C.; Yates, T.; O'Donovan, G.; Gray, L.J.; King, J.A.; Khunti, K.; Davies, M.J. The effects of high intensity interval training on glucose regulation and insulin resistance: A meta-analysis. *Obes. Rev.* **2015**, *16*, 942–961. [CrossRef] [PubMed]
31. Little, J.P.; Gillen, J.B.; Percival, M.E.; Safdar, A.; Tarnopolsky, M.A.; Punthakee, Z.; June, M.E.; Gibala, M.J. Low volume high intensity interval training reduces hyperglycaemia and increases muscle mitochondrial capacity in patients with type 2 diabetes. *J. Appl. Physiol.* **2011**, *111*, 1554–1560. [CrossRef] [PubMed]
32. Hartman, Y.A.; Hopman, M.T.; Schreuder, T.H.; Verheggen, R.J.; Scholten, R.R.; Oudegeest-Sander, M.H.; Poelkens, F.; Maiorana, A.J.; Naylor, L.H.; Willems, P.H.; et al. Improvements in fitness are not obligatory for exercise training-induced improvements in CV risk factors. *Physiol. Rep.* **2018**, *6*. [CrossRef] [PubMed]
33. Timmons, J.A.; Knudsen, S.; Rankinen, T.; Koch, L.G.; Sarzynski, M.; Jensen, T.; Keller, P.; Scheele, C.; Vollaard, N.B.; Nielsen, S.; et al. Using molecular classification to predict gains in maximal aerobic capacity following endurance exercise training in humans. *J. Appl. Physiol.* **1985**, *108*, 1487–1496. [CrossRef] [PubMed]
34. Buchan, D.S.; Ollis, S.; Young, J.D.; Cooper, S.M.; Shield, J.P.; Baker, J.S. High intensity interval running enhances measures of physical fitness but not metabolic measures of cardiovascular disease risk in healthy adolescents. *BMC Public Health* **2013**, *13*. [CrossRef]
35. Hanley, A.J.G.; Williams, K.; Stern, M.P.; Haffner, S.M. Homeostasis model assessment of insulin resistance in relation to the incidence of cardiovascular disease: The San Antonio heart study. *Diabetes Care.* **2002**, *25*, 1177–1184. [CrossRef]

36. Bonora, E.; Formentini, G.; Calcaterra, F.; Lombardi, S.; Marini, F.; Zenari, L.; Saggiani, F.; Poli, M.; Perbellini, S.; Raffaelli, A.; et al. HOMA-estimated insulin resistance is an independent predictor of cardiovascular disease in type 2 diabetic subjects- prospective data from the Verona Diabetes Complicated Study. *Diabetes Care* **2002**, *25*, 1135–1141. [CrossRef] [PubMed]
37. Fox, E.L.; Bartels, R.L.; Billings, C.E.; Mathews, D.K.; Bason, R.; Webb, W.M. Intensity and distance of interval training programs and changes in aerobic power. *Med. Sci. Sports* **1973**, *5*, 18–22.
38. Little, J.P.; Safdar, A.; Wilkin, G.P.; Tarnopolsky, M.A.; Gibala, M.J. A practical model of low-volume high-intensity interval training induces mitochondrial biogenesis in human skeletal muscle: Potential mechanisms. *J. Physiol.* **2010**, *588*, 1011–1022. [CrossRef] [PubMed]
39. Babraj, J.A.; Vollard, N.B.; Keast, C.; Guppy, F.M.; Cottrell, G.; Timmons, J.A. Extremely short duration high intensity interval training substantially improves insulin action in young healthy males. *BMC Endocr. Disord.* **2009**, *9*. [CrossRef] [PubMed]
40. Withers, R.T.; Sherman, W.M.; Clark, D.G.; Esselbach, P.C.; Nolan, S.R.; Mackay, M.H.; Brinkman, M. Muscle metabolism during 30, 60 and 90s of maximal cycling on an air-braked ergometer. *Eur. J. Appl. Physiol.* **1991**, *63*, 354–362. [CrossRef] [PubMed]
41. Thyfault, J.P. Setting the stage: Possible mechanism by which acute contraction restores insulin sensitivity in muscle. *Am. J. Physiol. Regul. Integr. Comp. Physiol.* **2008**, *294*, 1103–1110. [CrossRef]
42. Mann, S.; Beedie, C.; Jimenez, A. Differential effects of aerobic exercise, resistance training and combined exercise modalities on cholesterol and the lipid profile: Review, synthesis and recommendations. *Sports Med.* **2014**, *44*, 211–221. [CrossRef]
43. Koubaa, A.; Trabelsi, H.; Masmoudi, L.; Elloumi, M.; Sahnoun, Z.; Zeghal, K.M.; Hakim, A. The effects of intermittent and continuous training on body composition, cardiorespiratory fitness and lipid profile in obese adolescents. *J Pharm.* **2013**, *3*, 31–37. [CrossRef]
44. Racil, G.; Ben Ounis, O.; Hammouda, O.; Kallel, A.; Zouhal, H.; Chamari, K.; Amri, M. Effects of high vs. moderate exercise intensity during interval training on lipids and adiponectin levels in obese young females. *Eur. J. Appl. Physiol.* **2013**, *113*, 2531–2540. [CrossRef]
45. Racil, G.; Coquart, J.B.; Elmontassar, W.; Haddad, M.; Goebel, R.; Chaouachi, A.; Amri, M.; Chamari, K. Greater effects of high- compared with moderate-intensity interval training on cardio-metabolic variables, blood leptin concentration and ratings of perceived exertion in obese adolescent females. *Biol. Sport.* **2016**, *33*, 145–152. [CrossRef]
46. Crouse, S.F.; O'Brien, B.C.; Grandjean, P.W.; Lowe, R.C.; Rohack, J.J.; Green, J.S.; Tolson, H. Training intensity, blood lipids and apolipoproteins in men with high cholesterol. *J. Appl. Physiol.* **1997**, *82*, 270–277. [CrossRef] [PubMed]
47. Nybo, L.; Sundstrup, E.; Jakobsen, M.D.; Mohr, M.; Hornstrup, T.; Simonsen, L.; Bülow, J.; Randers, M.B.; Nielsen, J.J.; Aagaard, P.; et al. High intensity training versus traditional exercise interventions for promoting health. *Med. Sci. Sports Exerc.* **2010**, *42*, 1951–1958. [CrossRef] [PubMed]
48. Ouergil, N.; Fradj, M.K.; Bezrati, I.; Khammassi, M.; Feki, M.; Kaabachi, N.; Bouassida, A. Effects of high intensity interval training on body composition, aerobic and anaerobic performance in plasma lipids in overweight/obese and normal weight young men. *Biol. Sport* **2017**, *34*, 385–392.
49. Verney, J.; Duclos, M.; Thivel, D. Sprint interval training: What are the clinical implications and precautions? *Med. Sci. Sports Exerc.* **2017**, *49*, 2361–2362. [CrossRef]
50. Akins, J.D.; Crawford, C.K.; Burton, H.M.; Wolfe, A.S.; Vardarli, E.; Coyle, E.F. Inactivity induces resistance to the metabolic benefits following acute exercise. *J. Appl. Physiol.* **2019**, *126*, 1088–1094. [CrossRef]
51. Masharani, U.; Goldfine, I.D.; Youngren, J.F. Influence of gender on the relationship between insulin sensitivity, adiposity and plasma lipids in lean non-diabetic subjects. *Metabolism* **2009**, *58*, 1602–1608. [CrossRef] [PubMed]

International Journal of
Environmental Research and Public Health

MDPI

Article

Assessing the Anthropometric Profile of Spanish Elite Reserve Soccer Players by Playing Position over a Decade

Jon Manuel Vega [1], Asier Gonzalez-Artetxe [1,*], Jon Ander Aguinaco [1] and Asier Los Arcos [2,*]

1 Department of Physical Education and Sport, University of the Basque Country UPV/EHU, 01007 Vitoria-Gasteiz, Spain; jonmanuel10@gmail.com (J.M.V.); j.aguinaco96@gmail.com (J.A.A.)

2 Society, Sports and Physical Exercise Research Group (GIKAFIT), Department of Physical Education and Sport, University of the Basque Country UPV/EHU, 01007 Vitoria-Gasteiz, Spain

* Correspondence: asierjfkz@gmail.com (A.G.-A.); asier.losarcos@ehu.eus (A.L.A.); Tel.: +34-945-013-519 (A.G.-A.)

Received: 3 July 2020; Accepted: 26 July 2020; Published: 28 July 2020

Abstract: The aims of this study were to describe the evolution of the anthropometric profile of soccer players over a decade and to compare the anthropometric profiles of players promoted from an elite reserve team to high-level soccer with those players who were not promoted. We examined the body mass, height, body-mass index, and body fat of 98 players enrolled in the reserve team from 2008 to 2018. The players were classified in terms of (a) the highest competitive level they achieved up to the 2019/2020 season (i.e., Spanish 1st–2nd divisions or semi-professional); (b) the period in which they played their last season on the team; and (c) their playing position. Over time, the height of goalkeepers, lateral midfielders, and attackers has increased (effect size = 0.66 ± 1.13) but has decreased in central midfielders (effect size = 0.83). The body fat of defenders has also fallen (effect size = 0.55 ± 0.95). Spanish high-level goalkeepers, lateral midfielders, and attackers were taller than their semi-professional player counterparts (effect size = 1.20 ± 1.98). Body fat did not determine promotion from a reserve team to high-level soccer, but height may be an advantage for several playing positions. The assessment of the anthropometric profile and the application of interventions should be designed according to the playing position.

Keywords: team sport; talent; body composition; weight; body fat

---

1. Introduction

Because the financial resources of elite soccer clubs are not evenly distributed and the transfer of qualified players is a very high economic expense, less wealthy clubs must adopt different strategies in order to survive in this competitive industry [1]. One such strategy is to invest in soccer academies [2]. Such academies identify potential youth soccer players and incorporate them into their club's youth teams with the aim of developing them into top-class soccer players [3].

Evaluating the anthropometric profile of players is common practice in soccer academies in order to optimize physical fitness performance and reduce injuries. Body fat levels correlate negatively with aerobic fitness [4] and with the sprint decrement score (observed during a repeated-sprint ability test in soccer players [5]). Similarly, an increased body-mass index and a low fat percentage have been identified as anthropometric injury risk factors in elite-standard young soccer players (under-11s to under-19s) [6]. In addition, anthropometric characteristics could determine the selection of players and their progression to the professional level [7]. Many studies have assessed the relevance of anthropometric profiles in the selection process of young soccer players [8,9]. It appears that the most talented young players (from the under-9s to under-19s) tend to be heavier and taller, as well as having more advanced skeletal maturation [8]. Elite soccer players have also been found to have a lower percentage of body fat compared with players at the lower competition levels [10]. However, despite the transition from reserve team to high-level soccer being seen as a pivotal [2] and critical [11] stage, little is known about the relevance of anthropometric factors in the final step to high-level soccer [12]. To our knowledge, only one other study has compared the anthropometric profile of players promoted from an elite reserve team to Spanish elite professional soccer (LFP players) with those not promoted (non-LFP players) [12]. The authors of that paper found differences in the height and weight values between the LFP and non-LFP players in several playing positions [12]. However, the study was carried out exclusively in a high-level club. Moreover, relevant anthropometric characteristics in soccer, such as body fat and the body-mass index [4–6], were not considered. Thus, further research into body fat and the body-mass index is necessary to assess the impact of anthropometric profiles on promotion from an elite reserve team to the professional level.

The physical demands in elite soccer matches have increased in recent years [13], while the physical fitness performance of the professional and reserve team soccer players has varied little over different periods [12,14,15]. Similarly, several studies have found that the anthropometric profile of youth soccer players in elite soccer academies has also barely changed [16,17]. For example, one investigation found no significant differences in the anthropometric profile (i.e., body mass, height, and body-mass index) of senior and junior Norwegian soccer players over time [14]. However, to our knowledge no study has examined the evolution of the anthropometric profile in elite reserve soccer players over a long period of time. Doing so may allow for a link to be drawn between the evolution of the anthropometric profile and the characteristics of those players who are promoted to high-level soccer.

Several studies have compared the anthropometric profile of senior soccer players according to their competition level [18–20]. However, none of these compared profiles in terms of the playing position of the players [18–20]. Given that the anthropometric profile varies substantially between playing positions [10,19,21,22], and given that the physical, physiological, and perceived demands in matches [23–25] (and changes over recent years [23]) have also been found to differ substantially according to playing position, comparison of anthropometric profiles in accordance with this factor should be carried out.

Therefore, the aims of this study were to evaluate whether there were any changes in the players' anthropometric profile over a decade (i.e., 2008/2009–2017/2018), and to compare the anthropometric profile of Spanish elite reserve soccer players according to the competitive level they subsequently achieved.

2. Materials and Methods

2.1. Participants

We took anthropometric measurements for a reserve soccer team of a first-division Spanish club between the 2008/2009 and 2017/2018 seasons. Ninety-eight (age = 21.3 years ± 1.8) young professional players took part in the study, being evaluated at least twice during their last season with the team. The averages of all the assessments for each anthropometric measure (i.e., body mass, height, body-mass index, and body fat) were computed for each player (3 ± 1 pieces of data per player). After studying their sporting careers up to the beginning of the 2019/2020 season, we classified the players according to the highest competitive level they had achieved [12,15]: (i) Spanish LFP (LFP), comprising players who had signed a contract with a Spanish first- or second-division team and who had played at least one match as a full-time professional; or (ii) semi-professional (non-LFP), comprising players who had never competed in the Spanish first or second division. Thirty-nine of the forty-one players promoted to the 1st team of the club (i.e., 95%) came directly from the reserve team. The 10-year period examined was divided into two five-year terms: Period 1 (Period-1): 2008/2009–2012/2013; and Period 2 (Period-2): 2013/2014–2017/2018. Each player was assigned to the period in which he had played his last season in the reserve team. In addition, players were classified according to their playing position [12,15,26]: (a) goalkeepers; (b) defenders—lateral defenders and central defenders; (c) midfielders—lateral midfielders and central midfielders); and (d) attackers. The allocation of the playing positions was carried out by the team's technical staff. To decide on the few controversial cases, the playing position in which the player competed more times was considered. This study was performed in accordance with the Declaration of Helsinki and approved by the Ethics Committee of the University of the Basque Country (UPV/EHU), reference number M10_2018_181.

2.2. Measures

According to the protocols established by the club over the last 10 years, anthropometric measurements (i.e., body mass, height, and body fat) were taken four times during each season: (i) one month before the competition period (i.e., July/August); (ii) one month after the start of the competition period (i.e., October/November); (iii) in the middle of the season (i.e., January/February); and (iv) at the end of the season (i.e., April/May). In addition, the body-mass index was calculated.

All measurements were taken by the same club's medical staff, in accordance with guidelines outlined by the ISAK (International Society for the Advancement of Kinanthropometry). Body mass was recorded to the nearest 0.1 kg (Seca 719, Medical Measuring Systems and Scales, Germany) and height was measured with a stadiometer (Seca 213, Medical Measuring Systems and Scales, Germany) to the nearest 0.1 cm. The body-mass index was calculated by dividing body mass by squared height (kilograms per square meter) and used to assess the weight relative to height. Six skinfold thicknesses (triceps, subscapular, supraspinale, abdominal, thigh, and calf) were measured using a skinfold caliper (Harpenden, Holtain Ltd., Crymych, UK). Each measurement was taken three times, in accordance with the recommendations of the Spanish International Group of Kinanthropometry and International Standards for Anthropometric Assessment (ISAK), and the average value for each skinfold calculated. The sum of these six measurements was then calculated (sum of skinfolds). The body fat percentage was estimated using the equation proposed by Yuhasz [27]: body fat (%) = $\sum$skinfolds · 0.1051 + 2.585.

2.3. Statistical Analysis

Descriptive statistics were computed for each anthropometrical measurement (mean ± SD). Practical differences, Cohen's d effect size [28], were used to compare the anthropometric profile of the players according to period (Period-1 (2008/2009–2012/2013) vs. Period-2 (2013/2014–2017/2018)) and promotion level (non-LFP vs. LFP), as well as separately by playing position. Effect sizes (d) above 0.8, between 0.8 and 0.5, between 0.5 and 0.2, and lower than 0.2 were considered large, moderate, small, and trivial, respectively. We considered effect size values greater than small as worthy of discussion in the results section.

3. Results

LFP goalkeepers were largely heavier and taller (effect size = 1.27–1.35) than non-LFP goalkeepers and had moderately greater body fat (effect size = 0.77) than the latter did (Table 1). The goalkeepers in Period-2 were moderately heavier (effect size = 0.52) and largely taller (effect size = 1.13) than the goalkeepers in Period-1 (Table 1).

Table 1. Comparison of the anthropometric profile of goalkeepers in Period-1 (2008/2009–2012/2013) with that of goalkeepers in Period-2 (2013/2014–2017/2018) and of Spanish non-LFP players with that of Spanish LFP players (2008/2009–2017/2018).

Variable	Period-1	Period-2	Effect Size	Non-LFP	LFP	Effect Size
	n = 5 *	*n* = 7 **		*n* = 9	*n* = 3	
Body mass (kg)	79.38 ± 4.09	81.64 ± 4.59	0.52 (*moderate*)	79.59 ± 4.49	84.03 ± 1.20	1.35 (*large*)
Height (m)	1.85 ± 0.03	1.89 ± 0.04	1.13 (*large*)	1.86 ± 0.04	1.90 ± 0.02	1.27 (*large*)
Body-mass index	23.22 ± 0.50	23.00 ± 1.25	0.21 (*small*)	23.05 ± 1.25	23.22 ± 0.67	0.17 (*trivial*)
Body fat (%)	7.51 ± 1.23	7.22 ± 1.00	0.26 (*small*)	7.16 ± 1.10	7.91 ± 0.83	0.77 (*moderate*)

Non-LFP: players who had never competed in the Spanish first or second division; LFP: players who had signed a contract with a Spanish first- or second-division team and who had played at least one match as a full-time professional. * Non-LFP players: 3, LFP players: 2; ** Non-LFP players: 6, LFP players: 1.

The body-mass index of the LFP lateral defenders was moderately lower (effect size = 0.53) than that of non-LFP lateral defenders (Table 2). The body-mass index of the LFP central defenders was moderately greater (effect size = 0.54) than that of the non-LFP central defenders (Table 2). The body fat of defenders, lateral defenders, and central defenders in Period-2 was moderately/largely lower (effect size = 0.55–0.95) than that of the same players in Period-1 (Table 2). The lateral defenders in Period-1 were moderately slimmer (effect size = 0.62) and their body-mass index moderately lower (effect size = 0.51) than that of lateral defenders in Period-2 (Table 2).

Table 2. Comparison of the anthropometric profile of defenders in Period-1 (2008/2009–2012/2013) with that of defenders in Period-2 (2013/2014–2017/2018) and of Spanish non-LFP players with that of Spanish LFP players (2008/2009–2017/2018).

Variable	Period-1	Period-2	Effect Size	Non-LFP	LFP	Effect Size
Defenders	*n* = 16 *	*n* = 19 **		*n* = 20	*n* = 15	
Body mass (kg)	75.59 ± 5.26	73.76 ± 5.29	0.35 (*small*)	74.87 ± 5.48	74.24 ± 5.17	0.12 (*trivial*)
Height (m)	1.79 ± 0.07	1.78 ± 0.06	0.15 (*trivial*)	1.78 ± 0.07	1.79 ± 0.05	0.16 (*trivial*)
Body-mass index	23.69 ± 1.46	23.17 ± 0.83	0.44 (*small*)	23.53 ± 1.32	23.24 ± 0.96	0.25 (*small*)
Body fat (%)	7.42 ± 0.95	6.79 ± 0.76	0.73(*moderate*)	6.99 ± 0.86	7.19 ± 0.97	0.22 (*small*)
Lateral defenders	*n* = 9 ^	*n* = 12 ^^		*n* = 11	*n* = 10	
Body-mass (kg)	73.24 ± 4.39	70.85 ± 3.31	0.62 (*moderate*)	72.10 ± 4.05	71.63 ± 3.92	0.12 (*trivial*)
Height (m)	1.75 ± 0.06	1.75 ± 0.03	0.00 (*trivial*)	1.74 ± 0.04	1.76 ± 0.04	0.50 (*small*)
Body-mass index	23.97 ± 1.90	23.22 ± 0.89	0.51 (*moderate*)	23.89 ± 1.61	23.15 ± 1.14	0.53 (*moderate*)
Body fat (%)	7.24 ± 0.88	6.76 ± 0.88	0.55 (*moderate*)	6.83 ± 0.88	7.11 ± 0.94	0.31 (*small*)
Central defenders	*n* = 7 #	*n* = 7 ##		*n* = 9	*n* = 5	
Body-mass (kg)	78.62 ± 4.95	78.74 ± 4.24	0.03 (*trivial*)	78.24 ± 5.23	79.46 ± 2.79	0.30 (*small*)
Height (m)	1.84 ± 0.04	1.85 ± 0.03	0.28 (*small*)	1.84 ± 0.04	1.84 ± 0.03	0.00 (*trivial*)
Body-mass index	23.32 ± 0.51	23.09 ± 0.78	0.35 (*small*)	23.09 ± 0.71	23.42 ± 0.50	0.54 (*moderate*)
Body fat (%)	7.65 ± 1.06	6.84 ± 0.57	0.95 (*large*)	7.19 ± 0.84	7.34 ± 1.13	0.15 (*trivial*)

Non-LFP: players who had never competed in the Spanish first or second division; LFP: players who had signed a contract with a Spanish first- or second-division team and who had played at least one match as a full-time professional. * Non-LFP players: 10, LFP players: 6; ** Non-LFP players: 10, LFP players: 9; ^ Non-LFP players: 5, LFP players: 4; ^^ Non-LFP players: 6 LFP players: 6; # Non-LFP players: 5, LFP players: 2; ## Non-LFP players, 4; LFP players: 3.

The weight of the LFP midfielders was moderately greater (effect size = 0.56) than that of non-LFP midfielders; and LFP lateral midfielders were largely heavier and taller (effect size = 1.38–1.98) than non-LFP lateral midfielders (Table 3). The body-mass index of the LFP central midfielders was moderately greater (effect size = 0.51) than that of the non-LFP central midfielders (Table 3). Lateral midfielders in Period-1 were largely taller (effect size = 1.05) than those in Period-2 (Table 3); in turn, central midfielders in Period-2 were moderately slimmer (effect size = 0.63) and mainly shorter (effect size = 0.83) than central midfielders in Period-1 (Table 3).

Table 3. Comparison of the anthropometric profile of midfielders in Period-1 (2008/2009–2012/2013) with that of midfielders in Period-2 (2013/2014–2017/2018) and of Spanish non-LFP players with that of Spanish LFP players (2008/2009–2017/2018).

Variable	Period-1	Period-2	Effect Size	Non-LFP	LFP	Effect Size
Midfielders	*n* = 13 *	*n* = 23 **		*n* = 20	*n* = 16	
Body mass (kg)	72.65 ± 6.88	70.58 ± 6.01	0.32 (*small*)	69.82 ± 6.71	73.21 ± 5.42	0.56 (*moderate*)
Height (m)	1.78 ± 0.07	1.77 ± 0.06	0.15 (*trivial*)	1.76 ± 0.07	1.78 ± 0.05	0.33 (*small*)
Body-mass index	22.88 ± 1.21	22.65 ± 1.73	0.15 (*trivial*)	22.46 ± 0.92	23.08 ± 2.08	0.39 (*small*)
Body fat (%)	6.98 ± 0.50	7.04 ± 0.80	0.09 (*trivial*)	7.01 ± 0.75	7.02 ± 0.64	0.01 (*trivial*)
Lateral midfielders	*n* = 5 ^	*n* = 10 ^^		*n* = 10	*n* = 5	
Body mass (kg)	67.42 ± 3.43	69.00 ± 5.22	0.36 (*small*)	66.73 ± 4.32	71.97 ± 3.19	1.38 (*large*)
Height (m)	1.72 ± 0.02	1.76 ± 0.05	1.05 (*large*)	1.72 ± 0.03	1.79 ± 0.04	1.98 (*large*)
Body-mass index	22.78 ± 0.75	22.34 ± 1.13	0.46 (*small*)	22.48 ± 1.03	22.49 ± 1.09	0.01 (*trivial*)
Body fat (%)	6.96 ± 0.56	7.02 ± 0.86	0.08 (*trivial*)	6.97 ± 0.81	7.07 ± 0.70	0.13 (*trivial*)
Central midfielders	*n* = 8 #	*n* = 13 ##		*n* = 10	*n* = 11	
Body mass (kg)	75.91 ± 6.54	71.80 ± 6.49	0.63 (*moderate*)	72.92 ± 7.42	73.77 ± 6.24	0.12 (*trivial*)
Height (m)	1.82 ± 0.06	1.77 ± 0.06	0.83 (*large*)	1.80 ± 0.08	1.78 ± 0.05	0.30 (*small*)
Body-mass index	22.95 ± 1.47	22.90 ± 2.10	0.03 (*trivial*)	22.44 ± 0.84	23.35 ± 2.39	0.51 (*moderate*)
Body fat (%)	7.00 ± 0.49	7.05 ± 0.79	0.08 (*trivial*)	7.06 ± 0.74	7.01 ± 0.65	0.07 (*trivial*)

Non-LFP: players who had never competed in the Spanish first or second division; LFP: players who had signed a contract with a Spanish first- or second-division team and who had played at least one match as a full-time professional.* Non-LFP players: 7, LFP players: 6; ** Non-LFP players: 13, LFP players: 10; ^ Non-LFP players: 3, LFP players: 2; ^^ Non-LFP players: 7, LFP players: 3; # Non-LFP players: 4, LFP players: 4; ## Non-LFP players: 6; LFP players: 7.

The LFP attackers were largely heavier (effect size = 0.88) and taller (effect size = 1.20) than the non-LFP attackers (Table 4). The attackers in Period-1 were moderately taller (effect size = 0.66) than the attackers in Period-2 (Table 4).

Table 4. Comparison of the anthropometric profile of attackers in Period-1 (2008/2009–2012/2013) with that of attackers in Period-2 (2013/2014–2017/2018) and of Spanish non-LFP players with that of Spanish LFP players (2008/2009–2017/2018).

Variable	Period-1	Period-2	Effect Size	Non-LFP	LFP	Effect Size
	n = 8 *	*n* = 7 **		*n* = 8	*n* = 7	
Body mass (kg)	75.32 ± 5.46	77.23 ± 6.62	0.32 (*small*)	73.93 ± 4.57	78.82 ± 6.44	0.88 (*large*)
Height (m)	1.80 ± 0.05	1.84 ± 0.07	0.66 (*moderate*)	1.79 ± 0.05	1.85 ± 0.05	1.20 (*large*)
Body-mass index	23.16 ± 1.08	22.90 ± 1.21	0.23 (*small*)	23.10 ± 1.24	22.97 ± 1.04	0.11 (*trivial*)
Body fat (%)	7.31 ± 1.47	7.34 ± 0.97	0.02 (*trivial*)	7.41 ± 1.20	7.23 ± 1.32	0.14 (*trivial*)

Non-LFP: players who had never competed in the Spanish first or second division; LFP: players who had signed a contract with a Spanish first- or second-division team and who had played at least one match as a full-time professional. * Non-LFP players: 4, LFP players 4; ** Non-LFP players: 4, LFP players: 3.

4. Discussion

The aims of this study were to evaluate whether the anthropometric profile of soccer players changed over a decade (i.e., 2008/2009–2017/2018), and to compare the anthropometric profile of the Spanish elite reserve soccer players according to the competitive level they subsequently achieved. We found that changes in the anthropometric profile over time differed by playing position. In the same vein, the relevance of each anthropometric characteristic to promotion to Spanish high-level soccer varied according to playing position. The height of the goalkeepers, lateral midfielders, and attackers increased substantially over time. At the academy level, it appears that being taller is an advantage for goalkeepers, lateral midfielders, and attackers when it comes to being promoted to high-level soccer. Despite the body fat of defenders declining over time, this factor did not determine the competition level attained for any playing position.

We found a substantial decrease (effect size = 0.55–0.95, moderate–large) in body-fat values over time in the defenders, lateral defenders, and central defenders (Table 2). This reduction should be viewed positively, given that body fat levels correlate negatively with aerobic fitness [4] and the physical demands on defenders in matches at high-level have increased substantially [23]. Despite the fact that the physical demands of matches on players have been found to vary substantially between lateral defenders and central defenders [23], it appears that after a continuum selection process in elite soccer academies [29] the body fat of elite reserve defenders is optimal and its decrease is not an advantage for promotion to the Spanish LFP (Table 2). On the other hand, while the body-mass index of the LFP lateral defenders was lower than that of the non-LFP lateral defenders, the body-mass index of the LFP central defenders was greater compared with that of the non-LFP central defenders (Table 2). This suggests that greater weight per height is an advantage for central defenders. Martínez-Santos et al. [12] found that elite Spanish reserve LFP central defenders were moderately smaller than non-LFP central defenders (1.82 ± 0.04 vs. 1.85 ± 0.04; effect size = 0.62) in a similar high-level Spanish reserve team. In contrast, we found trivial differences between both groups (LFP: 1.84 ± 0.03 m vs. non-LPF: 1.84 ± 0.04 m) (Table 2). The moderate differences (1.82 ± 0.04 vs. 1.84 ± 0.03; effect size = 0.50) between the LFP central defenders in both academies suggest that each club assesses the height of their central defenders in different ways.

Taking all midfielders together as a whole, there has been barely any change in anthropometric profile over time. However, when we differentiated between lateral midfielders and central midfielders, several considerable differences could be seen. Furthermore, the evolution of the height of the lateral midfielders and central midfielders over time showed contrasting trends (Table 3). Thus, the generic classification of "midfielders" may be insufficient when it comes to assessing the anthropometric profile of elite reserve players. At the academy level, the increase in height of the lateral midfielders appears to be coherent with the selection of lateral midfielders to Spanish high-level soccer; that is, the LFP lateral midfielders were largely taller (effect size = 1.98) than the non-LFP lateral midfielders (Table 3), suggesting that a greater height is an advantage for lateral midfielders in this regard. In contrast, Martínez-Santos et al. [12] found no substantial differences between LFP and non-LFP lateral midfielders in a very similar soccer academy. Unfortunately, they did not provide the height values so we cannot compare both groups of lateral midfielders [12]. On the other hand, our central midfielders in Period-2 were moderately slimmer (effect size = 0.63) and largely shorter (effect size = 0.83) than the central midfielders in Period-1. However, it seems that being slimmer and shorter than other central midfielders in the elite reserve team is not an advantage when it comes to promotion to Spanish elite soccer, although a higher body-mass index can be. Linking this with the results for the LFP central defenders, we suggest that a greater weight per height can be an advantage for those who play in a central position in the team. In contrast, Martínez-Santos et al. [12] found that the LFP central midfielders in their elite reserve team were moderately taller than their non-LFP central midfielders (effect size = 0.67). The moderate differences (1.82 ± 0.05 vs. 1.78 ± 0.05 m; effect size = 0.67) between the LFP central midfielders in both academies suggest that, as mentioned for central defenders, each club views height in different way (1.82 ± 0.05 vs. 1.78 ± 0.05 m; effect size = 0.67).

The LFP attackers were largely heavier (effect size = 0.88) and taller (effect size = 1.20) than the non-LFP attackers. At the academy level, the moderate increase (effect size = 0.66) in the height of attackers over time suggests a consistent selection process in the reserve team. In their study, Martínez-Santos et al. [12] also found that the LFP attackers (1.81 ± 0.05 vs. 1.77 + 0.06 m; effect size = moderate) were taller than the non-LFP attackers (although the LFP attackers in our study were moderately taller than the LFP attackers in their high-level reserve team; 1.85 ± 0.05 vs. 1.81 ± 0.05; effect size = moderate). It would appear that here, too, the two soccer academies view the height of those that play in central playing positions (i.e., central defenders, central midfielders, and attackers) in a different way.

A previous study showed that height and body mass in goalkeepers differentiated elite from non-elite junior players (under-19s) (effect size > 0.6) [30]. In addition, Martínez-Santos et al. [12] found that LFP goalkeepers were largely taller (effect size = 1.12) and moderately heavier (effect size = 0.71) than non-LFP goalkeepers [12]. Similarly, we found the LFP goalkeepers to be largely heavier (effect size = 1.35) and taller (effect size = 1.27) than the non-LFP goalkeepers (Table 1). These results suggest that despite being heavier and having more body fat (Table 1), the tallest goalkeepers in high-level reserve teams have an advantage over their teammates (1.90 ± 0.02 vs. 1.86 ± 0.04 m) when it comes to promotion to the Spanish 1st and 2nd divisions. At the academy level, the moderate increase (effect size = 1.13) in the height of goalkeepers over time suggests a consistent selection process in the elite reserve team.

The main limitation of this study was that no other factors were considered, such as the physical fitness performance and socioeconomic status of the players. Despite this, the assessment of the anthropometric profile during a decade in an elite Spanish reserve team could be very interesting for physical coaches and club medical staff.

5. Conclusions

The changes in anthropometric profile over time differed by playing position. Similarly, the relevance of each anthropometric characteristic for promotion to Spanish high-level soccer varied according to playing position. The height of goalkeepers, lateral midfielders, and attackers has increased substantially over time. At the academy level, it appears that being taller is an advantage for goalkeepers, lateral midfielders, and attackers in terms of promotion to high-level soccer. Despite the finding that the body fat of defenders has fallen over time, body fat did not determine the competition level attained for any playing position.

The study shows the reference values of the anthropometric profile of elite reserve soccer players in a Spanish first-division club. In addition to other characteristics, it would be interesting to consider the height of players in the selection process of young goalkeepers, lateral midfielders, and attackers. The assessment of the anthropometric profile and the application of interventions by medical staff should be designed according to the playing position of the players.

Author Contributions: Conceptualization, J.M.V. and A.L.A.; methodology, A.L.A.; formal analysis, A.G.-A. and J.A.A.; investigation, J.M.V.; data curation, A.G.-A. and J.A.A.; writing—original draft preparation, J.M.V., A.G.-A., J.A.A. and A.L.A.; writing—review and editing, J.M.V., A.G.-A., J.A.A. and A.L.A.; funding acquisition, A.L.A. All authors have read and agreed to the published version of the manuscript.

Funding: The authors gratefully acknowledge the support of the Spanish government's subproject Integration paths between qualitative and quantitative data, multiple case development, and synthesis review as the main axis for an innovative future in physical activity and sports research [PGC2018-098742-B-C31] (Ministerio de Ciencia, Innovación y Universidades, Programa Estatal de Generación de Conocimiento y Fortalecimiento Científico y Tecnológico del Sistema I+D+i), which is part of the coordinated project's new approach towards research in physical activity and sport from a mixed-methods perspective (NARPAS_MM) [SPGC201800X098742CV0].

Conflicts of Interest: The authors declare no conflict of interest. The funders had no role in the design of the study; in the collection, analyses, or interpretation of data; in the writing of the manuscript, or in the decision to publish the results.

References

1. Liu, X.F.; Liu, Y.-L.; Lu, X.-H.; Wang, Q.-X.; Wang, T.-X. The anatomy of the global football player transfer network: Club functionalities versus network properties. *PLoS ONE* **2016**, *11*, e0156504. [CrossRef]
2. Mills, A.; Butt, J.; Maynard, I.; Harwood, C. Identifying factors perceived to influence the development of elite youth football academy players. *J. Sports Sci.* **2012**, *30*, 1593–1604. [CrossRef] [PubMed]
3. Dodd, K.D.; Newans, T.J. Talent identification for soccer: Physiological aspects. *J. Sci. Med. Sport* **2018**, *21*, 1073–1078. [CrossRef]
4. Reilly, T.; Williams, A.M.; Nevill, A.; Franks, A. A multidisciplinary approach to talent identification in soccer. *J. Sports Sci.* **2000**, *18*, 695–702. [CrossRef]
5. Brocherie, F.; Girard, O.; Forchino, F.; Al Haddad, H.; Dos Santos, G.A.; Millet, G.P. Relationships between anthropometric measures and athletic performance, with special reference to repeated-sprint ability, in the Qatar national soccer team. *J. Sports Sci.* **2014**, *32*, 1243–1254. [CrossRef] [PubMed]
6. Kemper, G.L.J.; van der Sluis, A.; Brink, M.S.; Visscher, C.; Frencken, W.G.P.; Elferink-Gemser, M.T. Anthropometric injury risk factors in elite-standard youth soccer. *Int. J. Sports Med.* **2015**, *36*, 1112–1117. [CrossRef] [PubMed]

7. Milsom, J.; Naughton, R.; O'Boyle, A.; Iqbal, Z.; Morgans, R.; Drust, B.; Morton, J.P. Body composition assessment of English Premier League soccer players: A comparative DXA analysis of first team, U21 and U18 squads. *J. Sports Sci.* **2015**, *33*, 1799–1806. [CrossRef] [PubMed]
8. Sarmento, H.; Anguera, M.T.; Pereira, A.; Araújo, D. Talent identification and development in male football: A systematic review. *Sports Med.* **2018**, *48*, 907–931. [CrossRef] [PubMed]
9. Bergkamp, T.L.G.; Niessen, A.S.M.; den Hartigh, R.J.R.; Frencken, W.G.P.; Meijer, R.R. Methodological issues in soccer talent identification research. *Sports Med.* **2019**, *49*, 1317–1335. [CrossRef]
10. Slimani, M.; Nikolaidis, P.T. Anthropometric and physiological characteristics of male soccer players according to their competitive level, playing position and age group: A systematic review. *J. Sports Med. Phys. Fit.* **2019**, *59*, 141–163. [CrossRef]
11. Vaeyens, R.; Coutts, A.; Philippaerts, R.M. Evaluation of the "under-21 rule": Do young adult soccer players benefit? *J. Sports Sci.* **2005**, *23*, 1003–1012. [CrossRef] [PubMed]
12. Martinez-Santos, R.; Castillo, D.; Los Arcos, A. Sprint and jump performances do not determine the promotion to professional elite soccer in Spain, 1994–2012. *J. Sports Sci.* **2016**, *34*, 2279–2285. [CrossRef] [PubMed]
13. Barnes, C.; Archer, D.T.; Hogg, B.; Bush, M.; Bradley, P.S. The evolution of physical and technical performance parameters in the English Premier League. *Int. J. Sports Med.* **2014**, *35*, 1095–1100. [CrossRef] [PubMed]
14. Haugen, T.A.; Tønnessen, E.; Seiler, S. Anaerobic performance testing of professional soccer players 1995–2010. *Int. J. Sports Physiol. Perform.* **2013**, *8*, 148–156. [CrossRef]
15. Castillo, D.; Los Arcos, A.; Martínez-Santos, R. Aerobic endurance performance does not determine the professional career of elite youth soccer players. *J. Sports Med. Phys. Fit.* **2018**, *58*, 392–398. [CrossRef]
16. Carling, C.; Le Gall, F.; Malina, R.M. Body size, skeletal maturity, and functional characteristics of elite academy soccer players on entry between 1992 and 2003. *J. Sports Sci.* **2012**, *30*, 1683–1693. [CrossRef]
17. Gonaus, C.; Birklbauer, J.; Lindinger, S.J.; Stöggl, T.L.; Müller, E. Changes over a decade in anthropometry and fitness of elite Austrian youth soccer players. *Front. Physiol.* **2019**, *10*, 333. [CrossRef]
18. Arnason, A.; Sigurdsson, S.B.; Gudmundsson, A.; Holme, I.; Engebretsen, L.; Bahr, R. Physical fitness, injuries, and team performance in soccer. *Med. Sci. Sports Exerc.* **2004**, *36*, 278–285. [CrossRef]
19. Sutton, L.; Scott, M.; Wallace, J.; Reilly, T. Body composition of English Premier League soccer players: Influence of playing position, international status, and ethnicity. *J. Sports Sci.* **2009**, *27*, 1019–1026. [CrossRef]
20. Tønnessen, E.; Hem, E.; Leirstein, S.; Haugen, T.; Seiler, S. Maximal aerobic power characteristics of male professional soccer players, 1989–2012. *Int. J. Sports Physiol. Perform.* **2013**, *8*, 323–329. [CrossRef]
21. Carling, C.; Orhant, E. Variation in body composition in professional soccer players: Interseasonal and intraseasonal changes and the effects of exposure time and player position. *J. Strength Cond. Res.* **2010**, *24*, 1332–1339. [CrossRef] [PubMed]
22. Sporis, G.; Jukic, I.; Ostojic, S.M.; Milanovic, D. Fitness profiling in soccer: Physical and physiologic characteristics of elite players. *J. Strength Cond. Res.* **2009**, *23*, 1947–1953. [CrossRef]
23. Bush, M.; Barnes, C.; Archer, D.T.; Hogg, B.; Bradley, P.S. Evolution of match performance parameters for various playing positions in the English Premier League. *Hum. Mov. Sci.* **2015**, *39*, 1–11. [CrossRef] [PubMed]
24. White, A.; Hills, S.P.; Cooke, C.B.; Batten, T.; Kilduff, L.P.; Cook, C.J.; Roberts, C.; Russell, M. Match-play and performance test responses of soccer goalkeepers: A review of current literature. *Sports Med.* **2018**, *48*, 2497–2516. [CrossRef] [PubMed]
25. Bush, M.D.; Archer, D.T.; Hogg, R.; Bradley, P.S. Factors influencing physical and technical variability in the English Premier League. *Int. J. Sports Physiol. Perform.* **2015**, *10*, 865–872. [CrossRef] [PubMed]
26. Los Arcos, A.; Martins, J. Physical fitness performance of young professional soccer players does not change during several training seasons in a Spanish elite reserve team: Club study, 1996–2013. *J. Strength Cond. Res.* **2018**, *32*, 2577–2583. [CrossRef]
27. Yuhasz, M. *Physical Fitness Manual*; University of Western Canada: London, ON, Canada, 1974.
28. Cohen, J. *Statistical Power Analysis for the Behavioral Sciences*, 2nd ed.; Lawrence Erlbaum Associates: Mahwah, NJ, USA, 1988.

29. Bidaurrazaga-Letona, I.; Lekue, J.A.; Amado, M.; Gil, S.M. Progression in youth soccer: Selection and identification in youth soccer players aged 13–15 years. *J. Strength Cond. Res.* **2019**, *33*, 2548–2558. [CrossRef]
30. Rebelo, A.; Brito, J.; Maia, J.; Coelho-e-Silva, M.J.; Figueiredo, A.J.; Bangsbo, J.; Malina, R.M.; Seabra, A. Anthropometric characteristics, physical fitness and technical performance of under-19 soccer players by competitive level and field position. *Int. J. Sports Med.* **2013**, *34*, 312–317. [CrossRef]

International Journal of
Environmental Research
and Public Health

MDPI

Article

Influence of a Six-Week Swimming Training with Added Respiratory Dead Space on Respiratory Muscle Strength and Pulmonary Function in Recreational Swimmers

Stefan Szczepan [1,*], Natalia Danek [2], Kamil Michalik [2], Zofia Wróblewska [3] and Krystyna Zatoń [1]

1 Department of Swimming, Faculty of Physical Education, University School of Physical Education in Wroclaw, Ignacego Jana Paderewskiego 35, Swimming Pool, 51-612 Wroclaw, Poland; krystyna.zaton@awf.wroc.pl

2 Department of Physiology and Biochemistry, Faculty of Physical Education, University School of Physical Education in Wroclaw, Ignacego Jana Paderewskiego 35, P-3 Building, 51-612 Wroclaw, Poland; natalia.danek@awf.wroc.pl (N.D.); kamil.michalik@awf.wroc.pl (K.M.)

3 Faculty of Pure and Applied Mathematics, Wroclaw University of Science and Technology, Zygmunta Janiszewskiego 14a, C-11 Building, 50-372 Wroclaw, Poland; zofia.wroblewska12@gmail.com

* Correspondence: stefan.szczepan@awf.wroc.pl; Tel.: +48-713-473-404

Received: 5 July 2020; Accepted: 6 August 2020; Published: 8 August 2020

Abstract: The avoidance of respiratory muscle fatigue and its repercussions may play an important role in swimmers' health and physical performance. Thus, the aim of this study was to investigate whether a six-week moderate-intensity swimming intervention with added respiratory dead space (ARDS) resulted in any differences in respiratory muscle variables and pulmonary function in recreational swimmers. A sample of 22 individuals (recreational swimmers) were divided into an experimental (E) and a control (C) group, observed for maximal oxygen uptake (VO_2max). The intervention involved 50 min of front crawl swimming performed at 60% VO_2max twice weekly for six weeks. Added respiratory dead space was induced via tube breathing (1000 mL) in group E during each intervention session. Respiratory muscle strength variables and pulmonary and respiratory variables were measured before and after the intervention. The training did not increase the inspiratory or expiratory muscle strength or improve spirometric parameters in any group. Only in group E, maximal tidal volume increased by 6.3% ($p = 0.01$). The ARDS volume of 1000 mL with the diameter of 2.5 cm applied in moderate-intensity swimming training constituted too weak a stimulus to develop respiratory muscles and lung function measured in the spirometry test.

Keywords: swimming; added respiratory dead space; respiratory muscle strength; pulmonary function; respiratory variables

1. Introduction

Increased work of respiratory muscles can lead to their fatigue and a sense of dyspnoea, which, in turn, can impair the ability to perform physical exercise [1]. Respiratory muscle fatigue is defined as a loss in the capacity for developing force and/or velocity resulting from muscle activity under load, which reverses by rest [2]. It has been shown that the emerging respiratory muscle fatigue may be caused by the accumulation of metabolites in these muscles and sympathetic vasoconstriction in locomotor muscles as a result of the metabolic reflex of respiratory muscles [3]. This metaboreflex involves reduced blood flow in the extremities and thus decreased supply of oxygen (O_2) to the respiratory muscles [4]. It is believed that the need for increased blood flow to the diaphragm is a potential reason for working muscle vasoconstriction, which can stimulate the development of locomotor muscle fatigue, reducing exercise tolerance [3,5].

The efficiency of the respiratory system depends not only on the amount of oxygen supplied by the cardiovascular system but also on the efficiency of removing the excess carbon dioxide (CO_2) [6,7]. Increased minute ventilation (VE) during exercise allows for the adjustment of the partial pressure of CO_2 in arterial blood ($PaCO_2$), which can be measured noninvasively by establishing the end-tidal gas composition and its CO_2 pressure ($PetCO_2$) [8]. A high $PaCO_2$ level implies an insufficient increase in VE during exercise and a limited ability to maximize exercise. This may be due to mechanical respiratory restrictions when reaching the upper limit of peak expiratory flow, such as insufficient respiratory muscle strength or reduced chemoreceptor reactivity. On the other hand, lower ventilation is also associated with reduced respiratory muscle work and can decrease blood flow in respiratory muscles, with a simultaneous increase (by ca. 10%) of extremity muscle blood flow. This mechanism can delay the appearance of fatigue [8]. This seems particularly important with reference to exercises in which VE pattern regulation, i.e., the adjustment of tidal volume (VT) and respiratory frequency (Rf), is associated with the rhythm of locomotor activities, e.g., swimming [9]. As respiratory muscle capacity is considered to be one of the many important factors determining exercise efficiency, it seems right to look for effective ways to increase it.

Respiratory muscle training (RMT) under normocapnic hyperpnoea conditions is applied to develop respiratory muscle strength and improve lung function [1,10]. Positive effects of this approach are based on several physiological adaptations, which include diaphragm hypertrophy, elevated nitric oxide concentration in the airways, change in the efficiency of muscle fibre contractions, improvement of the nervous control and economy of respiratory muscle work, delayed metabolic fatigue, reduced dyspnoea, and improved lung function [11–13]. These adaptations lead to decreases in the rating of perceived breathlessness or rating of perceived exertion. Moreover, the above mentioned attenuation of the metaboreflex phenomenon may result in the redirection of blood flow from locomotor muscles to respiratory muscles [1]. Studies lasting several weeks and using various types of devices to stimulate inspiratory resistance have already been conducted among trained swimmers [14,15]. However, similar research in recreational swimmers is still lacking. Knowledge of the training responses among this population should contribute to more effective training planning in order to counteract limiting the effort capacity of the respiratory system.

Other RMT methods that have been suggested involve breathing through a special mask [16] or tube breathing to increase the volume of the respiratory dead space [17]. As for the latter, the authors concluded that tube breathing was well tolerated by healthy individuals, did not cause desaturation or adverse events, and led to hypercapnia in most participants. In addition, it was speculated that a slight increase in $PaCO_2$ during tube breathing might even provide a more intense training stimulus [17]. Previous research on exercise interventions including added respiratory dead space (ARDS) focused primarily on circulatory and respiratory responses to a single exercise session on a cycle ergometer [18] or on long-term training adaptations in physical performance during moderate-intensity continuous training in elite cyclists [19–21], high-intensity swim training in well-trained cohorts [22], or high-intensity interval training in amateur triathletes [23]. Our latest research examined the effects of swimming with ARDS on cardiorespiratory fitness and lipid metabolism among recreational swimmers [24]. While the cardiorespiratory response to ARDS is better understood, no studies to date have investigated the effects of a long-term intervention (six weeks) with ARDS on respiratory muscle variables and pulmonary function in recreational swimmers; this is therefore the subject of our present considerations. Increasing the distance that the air has to cover to reach the lungs raises airway resistance. The higher the gas flow rate, the higher the friction forces [25]. The compensatory mechanism (as in the case of raised respiratory minute ventilation) consists in increasing the tidal volume and decreasing the respiratory frequency. Poon [26] explains this in terms of so-called mechanical and respiratory optimization, as the body determines the value of ventilation that allows to bear the lowest possible cost of the respiratory muscles work in response to chemoreceptor pulsation. In this context, the aims of this study were to investigate whether there appeared any differences in respiratory muscle variables and pulmonary function after a six-week moderate-intensity swimming intervention with ARDS in recreational swimmers, as well as to determine if there were any performance advantages of applying a low-cost method that could safely induce ARDS. This information may be used by recreational swimmers to improve their pulmonary function, by coaches to support making decisions on enhancing the performance of developmental level and trained swimmers during the workout process and by untrained individuals to increase their pulmonary function and health. It was hypothesized that the ARDS intervention would bring about large improvements in respiratory muscle strength and beneficial changes in pulmonary variables. To our knowledge, this theory has not been empirically addressed yet. The rationale behind these postulates comes from the research on ARDS which has shown positive effects on selected cardiorespiratory variables.

2. Materials and Methods

2.1. Participants

The research involved 22 healthy and physically active people, including women (n = 11) and men (n = 11). Their physical activity was limited to swimming the average distance of 2 km twice a week with an intensity of 65–75% of maximum heart rate (HRmax). The participants were divided into 2 groups, the control group (C: 7 men, 4 women) and the experimental group (E: 4 men, 7 women) (Table 1). During the first visit, all participants' body mass (kg) and height (m) were measured by using WPT 200 medical scales (RADWAG, Radom, Poland). The groups were compared in terms of the somatic parameters, i.e., age (p = 0.72), body height (p = 0.50), body mass (p = 0.65), and maximal oxygen uptake (VO_2max) (p = 0.65), and the Wilcoxon nonparametric test was applied in the assessment (alpha error: 0.05). This generated comparable groups with an objective baseline level of somatic build.

Table 1. Participants' characteristics (mean ± standard deviation).

Variables	E	C
Age (years)	24.3 ± 2.7	24.0 ± 3.3
Body height (m)	1.7 ± 0.1	1.7 ± 0.1
Body mass (kg)	70.0 ± 13.1	72.3 ± 10.1
VO_2max (mL kg^{-1} min^{-1})	45.6 ± 7.5	47.1 ± 8.9

VO_2max—maximal oxygen uptake.

The individuals' assignment to the study groups was based on VO_2max values measured during a progressive test performed in accordance with the protocol by Michalik et al. [27] on an Excalibur Sport cycle ergometer (Lode BV, Groningen, the Netherlands) 3 days prior to the ARDS intervention. The VO_2max values were arranged from highest to lowest. The study participants were ascribed sequential numbers in accordance with their VO_2max results. The individuals with odd numbers were assigned to group E and those with even numbers to group C. Before entering the experiment, all swimmers provided their written consent to participate in the study; they could withdraw at any time. The experiment was approved by the University Research Ethics Committee (#14/2017) and carried out in accordance with the standards of the Declaration of Helsinki.

2.2. Design and Procedures

Added respiratory dead space intervention protocol.

A week before the start of the tests, a familiarization session was held to adapt the participants to the study protocol with ARDS, as none of them had previously used this method. The familiarization session involved a 1000-mL low-intensity front crawl swimming in a 25-m indoor swimming pool, with breathing through an ARDS device.

The participants in group E took part in a 6-week ARDS training. During the 6 weeks, they completed a total of 12 swimming sessions with ARDS. The ARDS intervention was limited to 2 swimming sessions per week. During each 50-min session, the individuals were front crawling. The interval between sessions was 72 h. During each swimming session, the participants undertook constant, moderate-intensity physical effort of aerobic character. The effort intensity was individually determined on the basis of the heart rate (HR) achieved at 60% VO_2max in the progressive test, corresponding to individual HR values in the range of 125–140 beats min^{-1}. While swimming, the participants monitored their HR with an RS400 sports watch (Polar Electro, Kempele, Finland). Intensity below the lactate threshold was chosen because it was suitable for long-term effort of untrained individuals involved in the experiment.

Group E swam with a custom ARDS apparatus consisting of a polypropylene centre-mount swimming snorkel with a mouthpiece (Speedo International Ltd., Nottingham, UK) integrated with 2.5-cm diameter ribbed tubing to provide ARDS of 1000 mL (Figure 1). Dead space volume (1000 mL) was identical for each participant and measured by filling the snorkel with water and then transferring the volume to a graduated cylinder, as described by Szczepan et al. [24]. The snorkel was sufficiently rigid to maintain a constant volume when swimming.

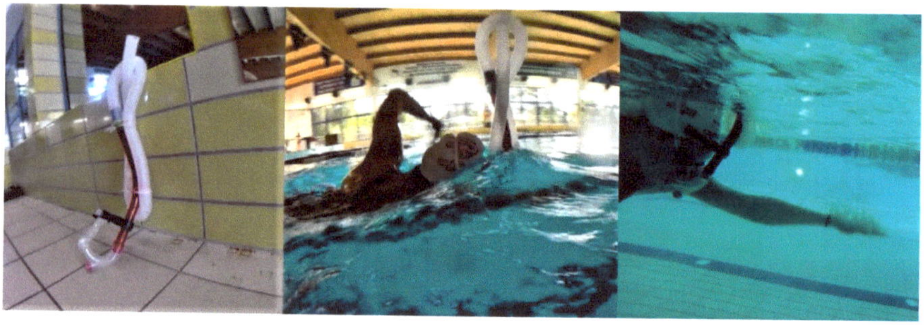

Figure 1. An instrument increasing added respiratory dead space: a custom added respiratory dead space (ARDS) apparatus consisting of a polypropylene centre-mount swimming snorkel with a mouthpiece (Speedo International Ltd., Nottingham, UK) integrated with 2.5-cm diameter ribbed tubing to provide 1000 mL of dead space.

The swimmers in group C took part in the same training but without ARDS intervention. In group C, no additional respiratory changes were introduced; the group applied a standard breathing pattern for the front crawl technique.

All sessions took place in a 25-m swimming pool, under uniform conditions (water temperature: 27 °C, air temperature: 28 °C, relative humidity: 60%, lighting: 600 lx). Throughout the experimental period, the individuals from both groups led a lifestyle and maintained a diet normal for people of that age and did not participate in any additional training. The participants' diet was not controlled.

2.3. *Independent Variable Measurements*

Respiratory muscle, pulmonary function, and cardiorespiratory tests were administered 3 days before and after the intervention with ARDS to assess changes in respiratory muscle strength and pulmonary function between the pre- and postintervention status. Both testing series were performed in the same controlled conditions (temperature: 24 °C, relative humidity: 50%) in a climate-controlled exercise laboratory (PN-EN ISO 9001:2009 certified). The measurements were taken by a laboratory worker with a device calibrated before each trial.

2.3.1. Respiratory Muscle Strength Variable Measurements

Inspiratory muscle strength (maximal inspiratory pressure [PImax] [cm H_2O]) and expiratory muscle strength (maximal expiratory pressure [PEmax] [cm H_2O]) were measured in a test using a

Micro RPM respiratory pressure meter (CareFusion, San Diego, CA, USA). To assess PImax, the tested person, in a standing position, performed a maximum inspiration from the level of a maximum expiration. Then, to evaluate PEmax, the individual exhaled starting from the maximum inspiration level. In both cases, a special stopper was fitted. The PImax and PEmax tests were conducted at rest [28]. Each participant took 2 trials for maximum inspiration and maximum expiration each, and the higher values were selected for further analysis.

2.3.2. Pulmonary Variable Measurements

Pulmonary function was measured by spirometry as a functional examination of the respiratory system. Spirometry was performed by using a Quark b^2 ergospirometer (Cosmed, Milan, Italy). It involved an inspiration with a maximum volume preceded by 2–3 quiet breaths and ended with an intense exhalation with a maximum airflow, resulting in a minimum volume of residual air. In the course of the respiratory test, the following parameters were recorded: forced vital capacity (FVC) [L], forced expiratory volume in 1 s (FEV_1) [L], peak expiratory flow (PEF) [L s^{-1}], and peak inspiratory flow (PIF) [L s^{-1}]. Each participant took 2 trials, and the one with higher FEV_1 value was selected for further analysis.

2.3.3. Respiratory Variable Measurements

An incremental exercise test on a cycle ergometer was applied to assess VO_2max [mL kg^{-1} min^{-1}], VE [L min^{-1}], Rf [breaths min^{-1}], VT [L $breath^{-1}$] and other respiratory parameters: Total duration of the inspiratory cycle (Ti) [s], total duration of the expiratory cycle (Te) [s], total duration of the respiratory cycle (Ttot) [s], ratio of mean inspiratory time to the total time of the respiratory cycle (Ti/Ttot) [%], $PetCO_2$ [mm Hg]. Heart rate [beats min^{-1}] was also continuously measured with a noninvasive HR monitor (S810, Polar Electro, Kempele, Finland).

The incremental exercise test was administered 3 days before the training intervention. Gas exchange was evaluated breath-by-breath by using a metabolic cart (Quark b^2, Cosmed, Italy). The device was calibrated with a reference gas mixture of CO_2 (5%), O_2 (16%), and N_2 (79%). Pulmonary function assessment began 2 min prior to the test start and continued 5 min after the test conclusion, with data averaged over 30-s intervals. VO_2 was measured and VO_2max was automatically indicated. VO_2max was defined as the highest 30-s average at which relative VO_2 values plateaued (<1.35 mL kg^{-1} min^{-1}) despite an increase in workload or 2 of the following criteria: (a) respiratory exchange ratio > 1.10; (b) attainment of HRmax (within 10 beats min^{-1} of age-predicted maximum [220-age]); (c) voluntary exhaustion. Primary cardiorespiratory outcome measures of Rf [breaths·min^{-1}], VT [L $breath^{-1}$], VE [L min^{-1}] were determined at 4 workloads (50, 100, 150, 200 W) and at maximal power (max). The outcome measures of Ti [s], Te [s], Ttot [s], Ti/Ttot [%], $PetCO_2$ [mm Hg] were determined at 4 workloads (50, 100, 150, 200 W).

2.4. Statistical Analysis

The quantitative investigation planning involved a 4-dimensional approach (alpha, power, sample size, and effect size) and followed the accepted methodology [29].

Data are presented as means ± standard deviations, the difference (Δ) between pre- and postintervention values, and the standard deviation for the difference. In addition, parameter changes (increase or decrease) are expressed as a dimensionless ratio of two quantities (%). Significance was set at an alpha level of 0.05 for all statistical procedures, with p values provided for all results.

The distribution of the data set was screened for normality by using the Kolmogorov–Smirnov test. The homogeneity of variances was checked with the Levene's test. Respiratory muscle strength variables (PImax, PEmax), pulmonary variables (FVC, FEV_1, PEF, PIF), and respiratory variables (Rf, VT) for each workload (50, 100, 150, 200 W, max), and Ti, Te, Ttot, Ti/Ttot, $PetCO_2$ were compared with the use of one-way ANOVA with repeated measures (measurement × group) and Tukey's honest significant difference (HSD) test for pairwise posthoc comparisons. The VE and VO_2max variables values derived from Szczepan et al. [25].

Furthermore, effect sizes for ANOVA were calculated by using partial eta squared (η_p^2). Effect sizes were interpreted as small (0.02), moderate (0.13), or large (≥0.26) [30,31].

The sample size was estimated with a stand-alone power analysis program for statistical tests (G*Power 3.1.9.2, Kiel University, Kiel, Germany) [32] with a small effect size of f2 = 0.29. With the assumption of an alpha error of 0.05 and power of (1-β) 0.80, the required total sample size was estimated to be 26 participants in total. However, owing to the length and commitment of the intervention, we were able to include only 22 individuals in the final analysis.

All calculations of the analysed variables were performed with the IBM SPSS Statistics version 26 software package (IBM, Inc., Chicago, IL, USA).

3. Results

Pre- and postintervention respiratory muscle strength, pulmonary function, and respiratory outcomes for within-group comparisons are presented in Tables 1–3. Between-group comparisons are provided in the text only.

Table 2. Pre- and postintervention within-group comparisons (PImax, PEmax, FVC, FEV_1, PEF, PIF).

Variables	Pre-Intervention	Post-Intervention	Δ (Post-Pre)	± of Δ (Post-Pre)	% Difference	p Value	η_p^2
Control Group							
PImax [cm H_2O]	127.6 ± 38.1	124.1 ± 36.2	−3.5	52.6	−2.7	0.47	0.05
PEmax [cm H_2O]	162.6 ± 33.0	166.5 ± 32.5	3.8	46.3	2.3	0.46	0.06
FVC [L]	6.6 ± 1.6	6.5 ± 1.6	−0.1	2.2	−1.8	0.68	0.02
FEV_1 [L]	4.8 ± 0.9	4.9 ± 1.0	0.1	1.4	1.9	0.74	0.01
PEF [L s^{-1}]	8.9 ± 2.2	8.9 ± 1.9	0.0	2.9	0.3	0.89	0.01
PIF [L s^{-1}]	2.6 ± 0.9	2.2 ± 1.0	−0.5	1.4	−18.3	0.10	0.24
Experimental Group							
PImax [cm H_2O]	122.9 ± 40.7	131.2 ± 26.4	8.3	48.5	6.7	0.47	0.05
PEmax [cm H_2O]	136.1 ± 52.8	156.6 ± 49.0	20.4	72.0	15.0	0.21	0.01
FVC [L]	6.0 ± 1.2	6.1 ± 1.6	0.1	2.0	1.5	0.80	≥0.00
FEV_1 [L]	4.9 ± 0.9	4.6 ± 0.9	−0.3	1.2	−5.4	0.22	0.15
PEF [L s^{-1}]	8.2 ± 2.2	7.9 ± 2.2	−0.3	3.1	−3.6	0.58	0.03
PIF [L s^{-1}]	1.9 ± 1.0	2.6 ± 1.8	0.7	2.1	34.7	0.26	0.13

Data presented as mean ± standard deviation. Δ and % difference with respect to preintervention status. Positive Δ indicates an increase in variables. Positive % indicates an increase in variables. ± of Δ (post-pre)—standard deviation for the difference. PImax—maximal inspiratory pressure, PEmax—maximal expiratory pressure, FVC—forced vital capacity; FEV_1—forced expiratory volume in 1 s; PEF—peak expiratory flow, PIF—peak inspiratory flow.

Table 3. Pre- and postintervention within-group comparisons (Rf, VT, VE, VO_2max).

Variables	Power [W]	Pre-Intervention	Post-Intervention	Δ (Post-Pre)	± of Δ (Post-Pre)	% Difference	p Value	η_p^2
Control Group								
Rf [breaths min^{-1}]	50	20.4 ± 2.8	20.4 ± 5.5	0.0	6.2	−0.1	0.99	≥0.00
	100	23.1 ± 4.7	22.6 ± 4.0	−0.5	6.1	−2.0	0.68	0.02
	150	25.3 ± 4.1	25.9 ± 4.5	0.6	6.1	2.4	0.61	0.03
	200	29.5 ± 7.9	31.3 ± 6.6	1.8	10.2	6.0	0.22	0.15
	Max	47.8 ± 10.3	47.1 ± 7.6	−0.7	12.8	−1.4	0.72	0.01
VT [L $breath^{-1}$]	50	1.4 ± 0.2	1.4 ± 0.3	0.1	0.4	3.6	0.65	0.02
	100	1.7 ± 2.0	1.7 ± 0.2	0.0	2.0	−1.8	0.65	0.02
	150	2.0 ± 0.3	2.1 ± 0.3	0.1	0.4	4.0	0.32	0.01
	200	2.4 ± 0.4	2.4 ± 0.3	0.0	0.5	−0.8	0.85	0.01
	Max	2.6 ± 0.6	2.6 ± 0.5	0.0	0.8	−0.8	0.82	≥0.00

Table 3. *Cont.*

Control Group								
Variables	Power [W]	Pre-Intervention	Post-Intervention	Δ (Post-Pre)	± of Δ (Post-Pre)	% Difference	p Value	η_p^2
VE [L min^{-1}]	50	28.8 ± 4.8	28.2 ± 4.2	−0.6	6.4	−2.1	0.99	0.01
	100	39.0 ± 4.1	37.4 ± 2.6	−1.6	4.9	−4.1	0.80	0.11
	150	51.9 ± 5.3	53.4 ± 4.3	1.5	6.8	2.9	0.89	0.07
	200	71.5 ± 12.3	72.4 ± 7.0	0.9	14.2	1.3	0.99	0.01
	Max	132.3 ± 35.1	135.8 ± 39.8	3.5	53.1	2.6	0.93	0.03
VO_2max [mL kg^{-1} min^{-1}]	Max	47.1 ± 8.9	47.6 ± 10.2	0.5	13.5	1.1	0.97	0.05
Experimental Group								
Variables	Power [W]	Pre-Intervention	Post-Intervention	Δ (Post-Pre)	± of Δ (Post-Pre)	% Difference	p Value	η_p^2
Rf [breaths min^{-1}]	50	18.2 ± 5.1	18.5 ± 5.9	0.3	7.8	1.4	0.87	≥0.00
	100	19.5 ± 6.3	20.9 ± 4.8	1.4	8.0	7.1	0.36	0.09
	150	22.1 ± 7.0	23.3 ± 5.3	1.2	8.7	5.5	0.52	0.04
	200	28.8 ± 8.7	27.9 ± 8.0	−0.9	11.8	−3.2	0.58	0.03
	Max	41.8 ± 6.2	40.5 ± 7.9	−1.2	10.1	−2.9	0.60	0.03
VT [L breath^{-1}]	50	1.6 ± 0.5	1.4 ± 0.5	−0.1	0.7	−8.3	0.15	0.2
	100	2.1 ± 0.7	1.8 ± 0.4	−0.3	0.8	−13.7	0.03 *	0.39
	150	2.3 ± 0.6	2.2 ± 0.4	−0.1	0.7	−5.7	0.34	0.09
	200	2.4 ± 0.5	2.5 ± 0.5	0.1	0.7	4.6	0.40	0.07
	Max	2.5 ± 0.6	2.7 ± 0.6	0.2	0.8	6.3	0.01 *	0.52
VE [L min^{-1}]	50	26.9 ± 6.0	24.6 ± 3.3	−2.3	6.8	−8.6	0.63	0.11
	100	36.9 ± 5.0	35.6 ± 2.1	−1.3	5.4	−3.5	0.84	0.05
	150	47.6 ± 6.2	48.7 ± 3.8	1.1	7.3	2.3	0.95	0.02
	200	66.4 ± 12.0	66.8 ± 7.4	0.4	14.1	0.6	1.00	0.01
	Max	121.5 ± 39.5	124.8 ± 37.1	3.3	54.2	2.7	0.94	0.04
VO_2max [mL kg^{-1} min^{-1}]	Max	45.6 ± 7.5	46.7 ± 8.3	1.1	11.2	2.4	0.80	0.15

Data presented as mean ± standard deviation. * Significant difference at $p < 0.05$ vs. preintervention value. Δ and % difference with respect to preintervention status. Positive Δ indicates an increase in variables. Positive % indicates an increase in variables. ± of Δ (post-pre)—standard deviation for the difference. Rf—respiratory frequency, VT—tidal volume, VE—respiratory minute ventilation, VO_2max—maximal oxygen uptake. The VE and VO_2max variables values derived from Szczepan et al. [25]

No between- or within-group differences were observed after the intervention for respiratory muscle strength variables (PImax, PEmax) or pulmonary/spirometry variables (FVC, FEV_1, PEF, PIF) (Table 2).

Among respiratory variables (Rf, VT, VE), the difference analysis revealed changes only within the experimental group for the VT variable at 100 W workload (decrease by 13.7%; $p = 0.03$; $\eta_p^2 = 0.39$) and at maximum workload (increase by 6.3%; $p = 0.01$; $\eta_p^2 = 0.52$) (Table 3). Pre- and postintervention between-group comparisons (control group vs. experimental group) did not indicate any changes.

For the other respiratory variables (Ti, Te, Ttot, Ti/Ttot, $PetCO_2$), the difference analysis showed changes within the control group for the Ti/Ttot variable at 150 W workload (decrease by 2.1%; $p = 0.01$; $\eta_p^2 = 0.46$) and at 200 W workload (decrease by 2.0%; $p = 0.04$; $\eta_p^2 = 0.36$). Differences were also observed within the control group for $PetCO_2$ at 200 W workload (decrease by 2.7%; $p = 0.02$; $\eta_p^2 = 0.44$). Changes were recorded within the experimental group for the Ti variable at 100 W workload (decrease by 16.7%; $p = 0.01$; $\eta_p^2 = 0.52$), Ttot at 100 W workload (decrease by 11.5%; $p = 0.02$; $\eta_p^2 = 0.45$), Ti/Ttot at 100 W workload (decrease by 4.4%; $p = 0.04$; $\eta_p^2 = 0.35$), and $PetCO_2$ at 100 W workload (decrease by 2.6%; $p = 0.01$; $\eta_p^2 = 0.47$) and at 150 W workload (decrease by 5.6%; $p = 0.04$; η_p^2= 0.35) (Table 4).

Table 4. Pre- and postintervention within-group comparisons (Ti, Te, Ttot, Ti/Ttot, $PetCO_2$).

Control Group								
Variables	Power [W]	Pre-Intervention	Post-Intervention	Δ (Post-Pre)	± of Δ (Post-Pre)	% Difference	p Value	η_p^2
Ti [s]	50	1.4 ± 0.2	1.4 ± 0.4	0.1	0.4	4.4	0.62	0.03
	100	1.3 ± 0.3	1.3 ± 0.2	0.0	0.4	−0.8	0.92	≥0.00
	150	1.2 ± 0.2	1.1 ± 0.2	−0.1	0.3	−6.0	0.20	0.18
	200	1.1 ± 0.3	1.0 ± 0.2	−0.1	0.4	−12.0	0.11	0.24
Te [s]	50	1.6 ± 0.3	1.7 ± 0.4	0.1	0.5	4.9	0.52	0.04
	100	1.4 ± 0.3	1.5 ± 0.2	0.0	0.4	2.1	0.68	0.02
	150	1.3 ± 0.2	1.3 ± 0.2	0.0	0.3	0.8	0.79	0.01
	200	1.1 ± 0.3	1.0 ± 0.2	−0.1	0.3	−4.6	0.32	0.01
Ttot [s]	50	3.0 ± 0.4	3.1 ± 0.8	0.1	0.8	4.7	0.56	0.04
	100	2.7 ± 0.6	2.7 ± 0.4	0.0	0.7	1.1	0.87	≥0.00
	150	2.4 ± 0.4	2.4 ± 0.4	−0.1	0.6	−2.5	0.56	0.03
	200	2.2 ± 0.6	2.0 ± 0.4	−0.2	0.7	−8.3	0.16	0.17
Ti/Ttot [%]	50	45.0 ± 3.0	44.0 ± 3.0	−1.0	4.2	−2.2	0.51	0.05
	100	46.0 ± 3.0	46.0 ± 2.0	0.0	3.6	0.0	0.36	0.08
	150	47.0 ± 2.0	46.0 ± 2.0	−1.0	2.8	−2.1	0.01 *	0.46
	200	49.0 ± 2.0	48.0 ± 2.0	−1.0	2.8	−2.0	0.04 *	0.36
$PetCO_2$ [mm Hg]	50	38.0 ± 1.8	37.6 ± 3.2	−0.4	3.6	−1.0	0.63	0.02
	100	39.5 ± 2.4	40.4 ± 3.0	0.9	3.8	2.3	0.15	0.20
	150	40.9 ± 2.7	39.9 ± 2.8	−1.0	3.9	−2.4	0.18	0.17
	200	40.3 ± 2.8	39.2 ± 2.7	−1.1	3.9	−2.7	0.02 *	0.44
Experimental Group								
Variables	Power [W]	Pre-Intervention	Post-Intervention	Δ (Post-Pre)	± of Δ (Post-Pre)	% Difference	p Value	η_p^2
Ti [s]	50	1.5 ± 0.4	1.5 ± 0.5	0.0	0.6	−0.7	0.94	≥0.00
	100	1.6 ± 0.5	1.3 ± 0.3	−0.3	0.6	−16.7	0.01 *	0.52
	150	1.3 ± 0.4	1.2 ± 0.3	−0.1	0.5	−8.2	0.36	0.08
	200	1.0 ± 0.2	1.1 ± 0.2	0.0	0.3	2.9	0.51	0.04
Te [s]	50	2.0 ± 0.6	2.1 ± 0.7	0.0	0.9	1.5	0.81	≥0.00
	100	1.8 ± 0.5	1.7 ± 0.4	−0.1	0.7	−7.6	0.12	0.23
	150	1.6 ± 0.4	1.4 ± 1.4	−0.2	1.5	−10.0	0.21	0.16
	200	1.2 ± 0.3	1.2 ± 0.4	0.0	0.5	0.8	0.84	≥0.00
Ttot [s]	50	3.5 ± 1.0	3.6 ± 1.1	0.0	1.5	0.6	0.93	≥0.00
	100	3.4 ± 1.0	3.0 ± 0.7	−0.4	1.2	−11.5	0.02 *	0.45
	150	2.9 ± 0.8	2.7 ± 0.6	−0.3	1.0	−8.8	0.27	0.12
	200	2.3 ± 0.5	2.3 ± 0.6	0.0	0.7	1.8	0.71	0.02
Ti/Ttot [%]	50	42.0 ± 3.0	42.0 ± 2.0	0.0	3.6	0.0	0.43	0.06
	100	45.0 ± 2.0	43.0 ± 2.0	−2.0	2.8	−4.4	0.04 *	0.35
	150	45.0 ± 1.0	45.0 ± 2.0	0.0	2.2	0.0	0.38	0.08
	200	46.0 ± 2.0	46.0 ± 2.0	0.0	2.8	0.0	0.45	0.06
$PetCO_2$ [mm Hg]	50	39.6 ± 3.1	38.7 ± 2.8	−0.9	4.2	−2.3	0.09	0.27
	100	41.5 ± 2.8	40.5 ± 2.5	−1.1	3.8	−2.6	0.01 *	0.47
	150	43.5 ± 4.1	41.0 ± 2.6	−2.5	4.9	−5.6	0.04 *	0.35
	200	41.1 ± 3.7	40.1 ± 3.6	−1.0	5.2	−2.4	0.22	0.15

Data presented as mean ± standard deviation. * Significant difference at $p < 0.05$ vs. preintervention value. Δ and % difference with respect to preintervention status. Positive Δ indicates an increase in variables. Positive % indicates an increase in variables. ± of Δ (post-pre)—standard deviation for the difference. Ti—total duration of the inspiratory cycle, Te—total duration of the expiratory cycle, Ttot—total duration of the respiratory cycle, Ti/Ttot—ratio of mean inspiratory time to the total time of the respiratory cycle, $PetCO_2$—end-tidal partial pressure of carbon dioxide.

In turn, between-group comparisons showed pre-intervention differences for the Te variable at 100 W workload ($\Delta = 0.41$; $p = 0.03$; $\eta_p^2 = 0.21$) and 150 W workload ($\Delta = 0.34$; $p = 0.02$; $\eta_p^2 = 0.23$) and for the Ti/Ttot variable at 150 W workload ($\Delta = -2.0$; $p = 0.03$; $\eta_p^2 = 0.22$) and 200 W workload ($\Delta = -3.0$; $p = 0.01$; $\eta_p^2 = 0.31$).

4. Discussion

The main finding of the study is that a six-week ARDS intervention of moderate intensity (HR: 125–140 beats min^{-1}) did not significantly change respiratory muscle strength (PImax, PEmax) or spirometric parameters (FVC, FEV_1, PEF, PIF), which did not confirm the assumed hypothesis. Interestingly, only in group E, maximal tidal volume increased by 5.5%.

Research on the use of ARDS to improve cardiopulmonary capacity in different exercise regimes and intensities is common [19–23,33]. However, to the best of our knowledge, this is the first study to analyse the effects of ARDS application during moderate-intensity swimming in recreational swimmers on changes in lung functional parameters and respiratory muscle strength. Studies suggest that swimming is an activity extremely demanding for inspiratory muscles since immersion in water forces swimmers to expand the chest wall under higher pressure and to increase both VT and the speed of muscle contraction, which can lead to premature appearance of fatigue symptoms [9]. We assumed that the use of ARDS during swimming would be a stronger stimulus for the development of respiratory muscle strength and lung function measured by spirometry.

In earlier research, the use of ARDS led to CO_2 accumulation above the physiological norm, triggering changes in the respiratory system, increasing VE by raising Rf and VT, and causing faster respiratory muscle fatigue [17,34]. This means that breathing with additional difficulty due to the increased respiratory resistance requires the involvement of greater respiratory muscle strength, which reduces lung susceptibility and, consequently, increases respiratory muscle endurance [35,36]. RMT and its variations employing high ventilation rates and generating high respiratory pressure improved PImax and VO_2max [37]. Resistance RMT (RRMT), involving application of efforts at increased respiratory resistance, led to improvements in PImax, PEmax, and VT [11]. Apnoea training, raising tolerance to hypoxaemia regardless of the genetic factor or muscle buffer capacity, shortened the time of 400-m front crawl [38]. In addition, Karaula et al. [39] revealed that the application of the hypercapnic-hypoxic respiratory pattern significantly improved the strength of inspiratory and expiratory muscles, by 14.9% and 1.9%, respectively, compared with the control group swimmers. Similarly, McEntire et al. [40] pointed out that the use of a device raising respiratory resistance and regular breathing exercises increased respiratory muscle strength. The results of our research are contrary to many experiments in which different RMT stimuli were used. Among the factors that may explain the lack of changes in spirometric parameters (FVC, FEV_1, PEF, PIF) and respiratory muscle strength parameters (PImax, PEmax) observed in our study, there is the application of too low a swimming intensity with 2.5-cm diameter ARDS, which did not generate sufficiently high inspiratory pressure. Enright et al. [41] suggest that most gains in inspiratory muscle strength occur at an intensity of PImax. We are unable to determine what inspiratory pressure was generated by the participants during the swimming sessions in the presented experiment. Therefore, further studies could be undertaken to clarify this issue.

High $PaCO_2$ (provoked by ARDS) irritates cardiovascular chemoreceptors and increases VE, mainly by raising VT [42]. Regular hypercapnia can also modify the reactivity of chemoreceptive areas and thus change the respiratory pattern [20]. McParland et al. [43] report that the application of ARDS (970 mL) increased VT, as opposed to Rf. Our results do not confirm these observations, indicating lack of differences in maximal and submaximal VE. However, during work with 100 W intensity, the progressive test in group E showed a decrease in VT without Rf changes. This may indicate an improvement in work economy as a result of applying similar intensity in training. This is in line with the findings provided by Michalik et al. [44], who implied an improvement in exercise economy in a progressive test with the intensity that had been used in the training process. After a six-week swimming training with ARDS, group E presented a decrease in VT accompanied by lower Ttot, Ti, and Ti/Ttot values. No such changes occurred in the control group. According to Buchler et al. [45], lowering Ti/Ttot increases blood flow in the diaphragm to provide more oxygen to the inspiratory muscles, which may also explain the increase in the maximum VT value as a result of a lower physiological cost of respiratory muscle work. The raised oxygen supply to the diaphragm can delay the occurrence of fatigue and thus improve exercise tolerance [3]. Unfortunately, we did not test blood $PaCO_2$ or the respiratory pattern during swimming sessions, and this knowledge could help interpret the results. It seems that even if hypercapnia was induced, the ventilation response was too weak a stimulus to induce long-term adaptation.

In group E, the value of $PetCO_2$ at an intensity of 100 and 150 W decreased. Similar results were observed in group C but at an intensity of 100 W. Changes in $PetCO_2$ during the progressive test may indicate a change in muscle metabolism and in chemoreceptor sensitivity to CO_2 and H^+ modifications [8]. In the previous study [24], we showed that CO_2 excretion did not change as a result of ARDS training. Thus, the lower $PetCO_2$ in the present study is associated with a more efficient CO_2 elimination by the lungs, as evidenced by the synergistic effect of the VE components mentioned above (VT, Rf). However, this conclusion requires further research and detailed verification in subsequent studies including measurements during training sessions.

Nevertheless, the presented results should be interpreted with caution. The study limitations include the small size of both groups. In addition, the progressive test was carried out in laboratory conditions on a cycle ergometer and therefore did not take into account the horizontal position of the body in water. Field tests similar to the training sessions will be a more accurate way to determine the aerobic capacity of swimmers. This approach can provide more sensitive data to enable a better direction of training, consequently facilitating improved performance. We applied the ARDS volume of 1000 mL and the tube diameter of 2.5 cm, as tested in previous studies, but these parameters were not adjusted to the individual vital capacity of the participants. The absence of significant changes in most of the measured characteristics may suggest that either the exercise stimulus was too small (low intensity) or the application time was too short. It is advisable to consider a higher intensity of training, e.g., second ventilatory (anaerobic) threshold, which would increase VE and respiratory muscle involvement. Dunham and Harms [28] proved that the stimulus to induce respiratory muscle adaptation required high-intensity work, as in the case of high-intensity interval training that they applied. Further changes to the ARDS training protocol, regarding frequency (number of training units per week) and volume (number of intervention weeks), may also cause other body reactions. In addition, the design of the device to increase the dead space can be altered, e.g., by reducing the tube diameter, in order to induce higher respiratory resistance and monitor the respiratory gas parameters in real time to determine changes in, among others, $PetCO_2$. Future studies should take these limitations into account.

5. Conclusions

Summing up, this study has shown for the first time that a six-week moderate-intensity training with the application of 1000-mL ARDS among recreational swimmers does not cause changes in respiratory muscle strength variables and pulmonary variables.

Author Contributions: Conceptualization, S.S. and K.Z.; Methodology, S.S.; Software, S.S. and Z.W.; Validation, S.S., and K.M.; Formal Analysis, S.S. and Z.W.; Investigation, S.S.; Resources, S.S.; Data Curation, S.S., K.M. and Z.W.; Writing—Original Draft Preparation, S.S., K.Z., K.M., N.D. and Z.W.; Writing—Review and Editing, S.S. and K.M; Visualization, S.S., K.M; Supervision, S.S.; Project Administration, S.S.; Funding Acquisition, S.S. and K.Z. All authors have read and agreed to the published version of the manuscript.

Funding: The research was funded by the Department of Swimming and the Department of Physiology and Biochemistry of the University School of Physical Education in Wroclaw, Poland, and by the "Young Scientists Research" grant (#65/20/M/2017) from the University School of Physical Education in Wroclaw, Poland.

Acknowledgments: The authors express their huge and sincere gratitude to Marek Zatoń for his support in aspects of applied exercise physiology during the implementation of this investigation. We also appreciate our volunteers for their enthusiastic participation.

Conflicts of Interest: The authors declare no conflict of interest. The study did not involve any commercial interest in any of the concepts discussed in the article. The experiment complies with the current laws of the country in which it was performed and the Declaration of Helsinki.

References

1. HajGhanbari, B.; Yamabayashi, C.; Buna, T.R.; Coelho, J.D.; Freedman, K.D.; Morton, T.A.; Palmer, S.A.; Toy, M.A.; Walsh, C.; Sheel, A.W.; et al. Effects of respiratory muscle training on performance in athletes: A systematic review with meta-analyses. *J. Strength Cond. Res.* **2013**, *27*, 1643–1663. [CrossRef] [PubMed]
2. ATS/ERS. Statement on respiratory muscle testing. *Am. J. Respir. Crit. Care Med.* **2002**, *166*, 518–624. [CrossRef] [PubMed]
3. Dempsey, J.A.; Romer, L.; Rodman, J.; Miller, J.; Smith, C. Consequences of exercise-induced respiratory muscle work. *Respir. Physiol. Neurobiol.* **2006**, *151*, 242–250. [CrossRef] [PubMed]
4. Dominelli, P.B.; Archiza, B.; Ramsook, A.H.; Mitchell, R.A.; Peters, C.M.; Molgat-Seon, Y.; Henderson, W.R.; Koehle, M.S.; Boushel, R.; Sheel, A.W. Effects of respiratory muscle work on respiratory and locomotor blood flow during exercise. *Exp. Physiol.* **2017**, *102*, 1535–1547. [CrossRef]
5. Vogiatzis, I.; Athanasopoulos, D.; Habazettl, H.; Kuebler, W.M.; Wagner, H.; Roussos, C.; Wagner, P.D.; Zakynthinos, S. Intercostal muscle blood flow limitation in athletes during maximal exercise. *J. Physiol.* **2009**, *587*, 3665–3677. [CrossRef]
6. Brown, S.J. Cardio-respiratory system efficiency in trained endurance cyclists. *Med. Sport.* **2010**, *14*, 176–181. [CrossRef]
7. Jones, N.L. An obsession with CO_2. *Appl. Physiol. Nutr. Metab.* **2008**, *33*, 641–650. [CrossRef]
8. Bussotti, M.; Magrì, D.; Previtali, E.; Farina, S.; Torri, A.; Matturri, M.; Agostoni, P. End-tidal pressure of CO_2 and exercise performance in healthy subjects. *Eur. J. Appl. Physiol.* **2008**, *103*, 727–732. [CrossRef]
9. Kilding, A.E.; Brown, S.; McConnell, A.K. Inspiratory muscle training improves 100 and 200 m swimming performance. *Eur. J. Appl. Physiol.* **2010**, *108*, 505–511. [CrossRef]
10. Illi, S.K.; Held, U.; Frank, I.; Spengler, C.M. Effect of respiratory muscle training on exercise performance in healthy individuals: A systematic review and meta-analysis. *Sports Med.* **2012**, *42*, 707–724. [CrossRef]
11. Held, H.E.; Pendergast, D.R. The effects of respiratory muscle training on respiratory mechanics and energy cost. *Respir. Physiol. Neurobiol.* **2014**, *200*, 7–17. [CrossRef] [PubMed]
12. Shei, R.J. Respiratory muscle training and aquatic sports performance. *J. Sports Sci. Med.* **2018**, *17*, 161–162.
13. Wylegala, J.A.; Pendergast, D.R.; Gosselin, L.E.; Warkander, D.E.; Lundgren, C.E.G. Respiratory muscle training improves swimming endurance in divers. *Eur. J. Appl. Physiol.* **2007**, *99*, 393–404. [CrossRef] [PubMed]
14. Cunha, M.; Mendes, F.; Paciência, I.; Rodolfo, A.; Carneiro-Leão, L.; Rama, T.; Rufo, J.; Delgado, L.; Moreira, A. The effect of inspiratory muscle training on swimming performance, inspiratory muscle strength, lung function, and perceived breathlessness in elite swimmers: A randomized controlled trial. *Porto Biomed. J.* **2019**, *4*, e49. [CrossRef]
15. Lemaitre, F.; Coquart, J.B.; Chavallard, F.; Castres, I.; Mucci, P.; Costalat, G.; Chollet, D. Effect of additional respiratory muscle endurance training in young well-trained swimmers. *J. Sports Sci. Med.* **2013**, *12*, 630–638. [PubMed]
16. Kido, S.; Nakajima, Y.; Miyasaka, T.; Maeda, Y.; Tanaka, T.; Yu, W.; Maruoka, H.; Takayanagi, K. Effects of combined training with breathing resistance and sustained physical exertion to improve endurance capacity and respiratory muscle function in healthy young adults. *J. Phys. Ther. Sci.* **2013**, *25*, 605–610. [CrossRef] [PubMed]
17. Koppers, R.J.; Vos, P.J.; Folgering, H.T. Tube breathing as a new potential method to perform respiratory muscle training: Safety in healthy volunteers. *Respir. Med.* **2006**, *100*, 714–720. [CrossRef]
18. Zatoń, M.; Smołka, Ł. Circulatory and respiratory response to exercise with added respiratory dead space. *Hum. Mov.* **2011**, *12*, 88–94. [CrossRef]
19. Hebisz, P.; Hebisz, R.; Zatoń, M. Changes in breathing pattern and cycling efficiency as a result of training with added respiratory dead space volume. *Hum. Mov.* **2013**, *14*, 247–253. [CrossRef]
20. Hebisz, R.; Hebisz, P.; Zatoń, M. Impact of training with additional respiratory dead space on spirometry and exercise respiratory pattern in cyclists. *Cent. Eur. J. Sport Sci. Med.* **2015**, *9*, 75–83.
21. Zatoń, M.; Hebisz, R.; Hebisz, P. The effect of training with additional respiratory dead space on haematological elements of blood. *Isokinet. Exerc. Sci.* **2010**, *18*, 137–143. [CrossRef]
22. Adam, J.; Zatoń, M.; Wierzbicka-Damska, I. Physiological adaptation to high intensity interval training with added volume of respiratory dead space in club swimmers. *Pol. J. Sports Med.* **2015**, *314*, 223–237. [CrossRef]
23. Michalik, K.; Zalewski, I.; Zatoń, M.; Danek, N.; Bugajski, A. High intensity interval training with added dead space and physical performance of amateur triathletes. *Pol. J. Sports Med.* **2018**, *34*, 247–255. [CrossRef]

24. Szczepan, S.; Michalik, K.; Borkowski, J.; Zatoń, K. Effects of swimming with added respiratory dead space on cardiorespiratory fitness and lipid metabolism. *J. Sports Sci. Med.* **2020**, *19*, 95–101. [PubMed]
25. Goodarzi-Ardakani, V.; Taeibi-Rahni, M.; Salimi, M.R.; Ahmadi, G. Computational simulation of temperature and velocity distribution in human upper respiratory airway during inhalation of hot air. *Respir. Physiol. Neurobiol.* **2016**, *223*, 49–58. [CrossRef] [PubMed]
26. Poon, C.S. Potentiation of exercise ventilatory response by airway CO_2 and dead space loading. *J. Appl. Physiol.* **1992**, *73*, 591–595. [CrossRef] [PubMed]
27. Michalik, K.; Danek, N.; Zatoń, M. Assessment of the physical fitness of road cyclists in the step and ramp protocols of the incremental test. *J. Sports Med. Phys. Fit.* **2019**, *59*, 1285–1291. [CrossRef]
28. Dunham, C.; Harms, C.A. Effects of high-intensity interval training on pulmonary function. *Eur. J. Appl. Physiol.* **2012**, *112*, 3061–3068. [CrossRef]
29. Thoma, J.R.; Nelson, J.K.; Silverman, S.J. *Research Methods in Physical Activity*, 7th ed.; Human Kinetics: Champaign, IL, USA, 2015; pp. 166–167.
30. Levine, T.R.; Hullett, C.R. Eta squared, partial eta squared, and misreporting of effect size in communication research. *Hum. Commun. Res.* **2002**, *28*, 612–625. [CrossRef]
31. Sullivan, G.M.; Feinn, R. Using effect size—Or why the p value is not enough. *J. Grad. Med Educ.* **2012**, *4*, 279–282. [CrossRef]
32. Faul, F.; Erdfelder, E.; Lang, A.G.; Buchner, A. G*Power 3: A flexible statistical power analysis program for the social, behavioral, and biomedical sciences. *Behav. Res. Methods.* **2007**, *39*, 175–191. [CrossRef] [PubMed]
33. Smołka, L.; Borkowski, J.; Zatoń, M. The effect of additional dead space on respiratory exchange ratio and carbon dioxide production due to training. *J. Sports Sci. Med.* **2014**, *13*, 36–43. [PubMed]
34. Jonville, S.; Delpech, N.; Denjean, A. Contribution of respiratory acidosis to diaphragmatic fatigue at exercise. *Eur. Respir. J.* **2002**, *19*, 1079–1086. [CrossRef] [PubMed]
35. Dicker, S.G.; Lofthus, G.K.; Thornton, N.W.; Brooks, G.A. Respiratory and heart rate responses to tethered controlled frequency breathing swimming. *Med. Sci. Sports Exerc.* **1980**, *12*, 20–23. [CrossRef]
36. Tzelepis, G.; McCool, F.D.; Leith, D.E.; Hoppin, F.G., Jr. Increased lung volume limits endurance of inspiratory muscles. *J. Appl. Physiol.* **1988**, *64*, 1796–1802. [CrossRef]
37. Turner, L.A.; Tecklenburg-Lund, S.L.; Chapman, R.F.; Stager, J.M.; Wilhite, D.P.; Mickleborough, T.D. Inspiratory muscle training lowers the oxygen cost of voluntary hyperpnea. *J. Appl. Physiol.* **2012**, *112*, 127–134. [CrossRef]
38. Robertson, C.; Lodin-Sundström, A.; O'Hara, J.; King, R.; Wainwright, B.; Barlow, M. Effects of pre-race apneas on 400-m freestyle swimming performance. *J. Strength Cond. Res.* **2020**, *34*, 828–837. [CrossRef]
39. Karaula, D.; Homolak, J.; Goran, L.E.K.O. Effects of hypercapnic-hypoxic training on respiratory muscle strength and front crawl stroke performance among elite swimmers. *Turk. J. Sport Exerc.* **2016**, *18*, 17–24. [CrossRef]
40. McEntire, S.J.; Smith, J.R.; Ferguson, C.S.; Brown, K.R.; Kurti, S.P.; Harms, C.A. The effect of exercise training with an additional inspiratory load on inspiratory muscle fatigue and time-trial performance. *Respir. Physiol. Neurobiol.* **2016**, *230*, 54–59. [CrossRef]
41. Enright, S.J.; Unnithan, V.B.; Heward, C.; Withnall, L.; Davies, D.H. Effect of high-intensity inspiratory muscle training on lung volumes, diaphragm thickness, and exercise capacity in subjects who are healthy. *Phys. Ther.* **2006**, *86*, 345–354. [CrossRef]
42. Toklu, A.S.; Kayserilioğlu, A.; Ünal, M.; Özer, Ş.; Aktaş, Ş. Ventilatory and metabolic response to rebreathing the expired air in the snorkel. *Int. J. Sports Med.* **2003**, *24*, 162–165. [CrossRef] [PubMed]
43. McParland, C.; Mink, J.; Gallagher, C.G. Respiratory adaptations to dead space loading during maximal incremental exercise. *J. Appl. Physiol.* **1991**, *70*, 55–62. [CrossRef] [PubMed]
44. Michalik, K.; Glinka, S.; Danek, N.; Zatoń, M. Interval training with active recovery and the physical capacity of recreational male runners. *Pol. J. Sport Tour.* **2018**, *25*, 15–20. [CrossRef]
45. Buchler, B.; Magder, S.; Roussos, C. Effects of contraction frequency and duty cycle on diaphragmatic blood flow. *J. Appl. Physiol.* **1985**, *58*, 265–273. [CrossRef] [PubMed]

International Journal of *Environmental Research and Public Health*

MDPI

Article

Effects of Six Weeks of High-Intensity Functional Training on Physical Performance in Participants with Different Training Volumes and Frequencies

Rômulo Vasconcelos Teixeira [1,2,*], Gilmário Ricarte Batista [3], Arnaldo Luis Mortatti [1,2], Paulo Moreira Silva Dantas [1,2] and Breno Guilherme de Araújo Tinôco Cabral [1,2]

1 Graduate Program on Physical Education, Federal University of Rio Grande do Norte, Natal, Rio Grande do Norte 59072970, Brazil; amortatti@gmail.com (A.L.M.); pgdantas@icloud.com (P.M.S.D.); brenotcabral@gmail.com (B.G.d.A.T.C.)

2 Department of Physical Education, Federal University of Rio Grande do Norte, Natal, Rio Grande do Norte 59072970, Brazil

3 Department of Physical Education, Federal University of Paraíba, João Pessoa, Paraíba 58051900, Brazil; cajagr@gmail.com

* Correspondence: romulovasconcelos11@hotmail.com; Tel./Fax: +55-85-987139879

Received: 6 July 2020; Accepted: 20 July 2020; Published: 20 August 2020

Abstract: High-intensity functional training (HIFT) is characterized by presenting high volumes and training intensities with constantly varied exercises. The aim of this study was to analyze the internal training load and the effects of high-intensity functional training on physical performance in subjects with different training volumes and frequencies. A total of 31 volunteers involved in high-intensity functional training (14 men and 17 women) were divided according to their training volumes and frequencies (high training-volume and frequency—HTVF; (n = 17) (nine women and eight men; age: 31.0 ± 6.3 years; height: 168.8 ± 8.1 cm, body weight: 73.6 ± 11.9 kg; BMI: 25.96 kg/m^2) and moderate training volume and frequency—MTVF; (n = 14) (eight women and six men; age: 26.6 ± 4.7 years; height: 167.2 ± 8.6 cm, body weight: 75.8 ± 18.0 kg; BMI: 27.33 kg/m^2)). The internal training load was determined using the session-rating of perceived exertion method. The monotony index (MI) and training strain (TS) were used to determine training variability during the training weeks. Countermovement vertical jump height, 20-m sprinting and handgrip strength were assessed at baseline and after six weeks of training. There was a time effect for MI (($F_{(5,\,145)} = 5.942$; $p = 0.0001$)), TS (($F_{(5,\,145)} = 5.734$; $p = 0.0001$)), weekly internal training load (($F_{(4.006,\,116.87)} = 4.188$; $p = 0.003$)) and mean weekly internal training load (($F_{(4.006,\,116.87)} = 4.188$; $p = 0.003$)). There was no increase in performance in either group for countermovement vertical jump height (($F_{(1,29)} = 6.081$; $p = 0.050$)), sprinting (($F_{(1,29)} = 1.014$; $p = 0.322$)), right handgrip strength (($F_{(1,29)} = 2.522$; $p = 0.123$)) or left handgrip strength (($F_{(1,29)} = 2.550$; $p = 0.121$)). The current findings suggest that six weeks of high-intensity functional training was not able to increase performance in either group. Therefore, different volumes and frequencies do not seem to influence the increase in physical performance of HIFT practitioners.

Keywords: perceived exertion; injury; physical training; workload; exercise

1. Introduction

High-intensity functional training (HIFT) is a modality characterized by presenting high volumes and training intensities [1] with constantly varied exercises [2] with or without any recovery interval between the series [3]. HIFT training sessions consist of Olympic weightlifting exercises (OWE) (e.g., clean and jerk, snatch), gymnastics (e.g., lunges and pull-ups) and metabolic conditioning (e.g., running and rowing) [2]. In addition to the diversity of functional movements performed in high intensity, HIFT aims to improve physical conditioning variables (i.e., strength, body composition, among others) and performance (i.e., speed, power, among others) [4]. Thus, HIFT has gained status in sports in recent years and investigations have consequently emerged around physical capabilities for success in the HIFT [5,6].

There are several determinants for success in sports such as vertical jumping [7], sprinting [8] and handgrip strength (HS) [9]. For example, the presence of short-haul running races (i.e., up to 800 m) which are constantly held in HIFT competitions are associated with success in HIFT [5]. In addition, the scientific literature has suggested that the training volume appears to be a determining factor in the magnitude of strength gains [10,11]. For example, it was observed that training protocols with equalized volume and different training frequencies (i.e., six times vs. three times) do not differ for gains in maximum strength in the bench press after six weeks of training [12]. Additionally, Saric et al. [13] did not observe differences between groups for strength gains in the upper and lower limbs in using a similar methodology and training time. Finally, Gomes et al. [14] analyzed the influence of an equalized and progressive training volume in highly trained men (i.e., ~7 years of experience). It was observed that there were no differences between groups for strength gains in the bench press and squat exercises after eight weeks of training. Although HIFT incorporates these capacities (i.e., vertical jumping, sprinting and handgrip strength) and high volumes and intensities of training, no studies to date have examined the impact of different volumes and training frequencies of HIFT on physical performance. This issue can be of great relevance for coaches and can give light to the science of HIFT.

Thus, understanding the influence of HIFT volume and training frequency can provide an efficient prescription with overload which enables adequate adaptation with less interference in the health status of practitioners, as it has been demonstrated that two consecutive days of HIFT may promote possible immunosuppression [15] and that training protocols with high volumes and absence of recovery intervals promote increased damage markers (i.e., creatinokinase and interleukin-6) [16]. In addition, training load management is of fundamental importance for performance enhancement [17], since long-term accumulated training loads, intensification periods and acute changes in the training load have been identified as potential causes for loss in performance [18], diseases and injuries [19]. On the other hand, it was observed that six months of HIFT is able to promote positive chronic responses in the immune and hormonal system [20]. Therefore, monitoring the internal training load (ITL) becomes necessary to better adapt to training along with minimizing the risk of injury [17].

The internal training load (ITL) reports the effects of loads on the body experienced by an athlete after training [21]. Due to the diversity of exercises applied in HIFT (i.e., gymnastics, strength and metabolic conditioning), the management of training loads is a challenge for coaches [17] who need efficient tools and with practical applicability. There are countless tools for controlling stress/recovery from training, such as creatine kinase, testosterone/cortisol ratio and immunological markers [22]. However, these tools are expensive, invasive and are not commonly used in daily training practice [17]. Thus, coaches need tools that reproduce the "real world" [17] and are effective and sensitive to variations in workloads, such as the session rating of perceived exertion (session-RPE) [23].

The session-RPE is one of the most used tools in sports for monitoring ITL [24,25] because it provides information about the physiological stress imposed by the training process [18]. The ITL control method based on session-RPE generates other important variables such as monotony index (MI) and training strain (TS) which can indicate training overload [26]. These indices were recently validated for HIFT [27,28], showing to be efficient with regard to ITL differentiation in different training phases [29]. Therefore, it is of fundamental importance to use efficient and validated tools in order to individualize the training and take into account the level of each subject.

Despite the exponential growth of both the modality and number of practitioners, there is a limited number of studies related to safety in HIFT practitioners. Studies have not performed ITL quantification or monitoring in order to analyze the stress/recovery ratio and the performance determinants for the sport [3] as measured through the session-RPE, MI and TS, nor a verification of physical performance between subjects with different training volumes and frequencies through performance tests after a 6-week training period. Hence, to our knowledge, this is the first study to examine the impact of different HIFT volumes and training frequencies on physical performance.

Thus, the aim of this study was to analyze the ITL during six weeks of HIFT and to verify the effects of HIFT on physical performance in subjects with different training volumes and frequencies. The hypothesis of the study is that the six weeks of HIFT may generate different ITL with increased physical performance, regardless of the training volumes and frequencies presented.

2. Materials and Methods

Participants

The study design is characterized as observational. An a priori power analysis was computed using G*Power 3.1.9.4. Thus, a significant variable from a previous study (i.e., back squatting) was used for presenting improvement after performing HIFT [30]. The lowest significant effect size of back squatting ($\eta^2p = 0.55$) was used for the power analysis. Thus, a sample size of 10 subjects in each group was calculated by inputting 0.55 as the effect size and setting the alpha significance level at 0.05 and power to 0.80. A total of 31 subjects (14 men and 17 women) of different training volumes and frequencies (high training-volume and frequency—HTVF (27.9 ± 9.2 months of training background), $n = 17$ (9 women and 8 men; age: 31.0 ± 6.3 years; height: 168.8 ± 8.1 cm, body weight: 73.6 ± 11.9 kg; BMI: 25.96 kg/m^2) and moderate training volume and frequency—MTVF (8.3 ± 3.7 months of training background), $n = 14$ (8 women and 6 men; age: 26.6 ± 4.7 years; height: 167.2 ± 8.6 cm, body weight: 75.8 ± 18.0 kg; BMI: 27.33 kg/m^2)) were followed for 6 weeks. The subjects were grouped by their training volumes and frequencies into HTVF and MTVF groups. The weekly frequency and training session time was configured into the following groups: HTVF (5 to 6 days; ~2 h) and MTVF (3 to 4 days; ~1 h). It is worth noting that all subjects participated in all the procedures inherent to the study, and therefore there was no sample loss. The project was explained to all subjects of the training center and those who volunteered to participate signed the free and informed consent form. The researchers spent a week at the training center's facilities explaining the study and aiming to recruit as many subjects as possible. The following inclusion criteria were adopted: (i) presenting a weekly minimum training frequency of 3 times; and (ii) over 18 years of age. All those with osteomioarticular injuries and who did not meet at least 75% of the training sessions were excluded from the sample. The adherence rate during the 6 weeks was 82.4% for the HTVF group and 84.3% for the MTVF group.

The study was approved by the local ethics research committee (No. 3,082,357) and followed all of the ethical standards set forth in the Helsinki Declaration 2013 (and the World Medical Association).

3. Procedures

Training Sessions

The subjects were familiar with all the adopted procedures and tests which were usually used during their training program. The schedule and training organization during the collection period were structured and programmed by the coaches responsible for the training center in order to provide a control between stress and recovery, thereby enabling subjects to handle the physical and physiological demands well throughout the collection period. All experimental procedures of the performance tests were performed at the beginning of each week (i.e., baseline and post 6 weeks). The subjects were instructed to maintain their usual diet and refrain from alcohol, caffeine and high-intensity exercise in the 72h preceding the test performance. In addition, all tests (i.e., countermovement vertical jump height (CVJH), sprints and handgrip strength (HS)) were performed indoors and at the same time of day to mitigate the climatic effects. The subjects were also submitted to a warm-up protocol proposed by the training center coaches for approximately 10 min prior to the tests consisting of different running speeds, jumps and specific HIFT activity. The subjects initially performed the CVJH, followed by sprints and HS.

The training sessions usually began with a general warm-up (i.e., squats, multi-joint exercises, among others) (~20 min for HTVF and ~10 min for MTVF). After the warm-up, the training session consisted of movement technique exercises and strength training (i.e., Olympic weightlifting, squats, bench-press, deadlift and their variations) (~40 min for HTVF and ~20 min for MTVF), and finally gymnastic exercises (hand stands, bar exercises, ring, among others) and metabolic conditioning (rowing, races, among others) (~60 min for HTVF and ~30 min for MTVF). The objective of the conditioning sessions was to conclude them in the shortest time possible, while the other conditioning sessions on later days (depending on the planning/organization of the weekly training) were intended to perform the highest number of repetitions within the subject's limit in a fixed time period. All subjects performed the same training program, however, the HTVF group performed higher training volumes and frequencies (i.e., higher weekly frequency and training session time), as mentioned above. In addition, as the individual capacity (for example, relative strength or ability to perform specific exercises) among subjects were distinct, all the loads and exercises were individualized (i.e., the load and exercises were modified by the coach when necessary so that each subject, regardless of the training volumes and frequencies, could complete all the proposed tasks). It is worth mentioning that the determination of the external training load was not carried out due to the modality characteristic which presents a wide variety of exercises in the same training session (i.e., strength, gymnastics and endurance), therefore constituting a challenge for coaches and future research [17]. However, monitoring was performed minimally through the session time.

The monitoring lasted 6 weeks with performance tests (i.e., CVJH, sprints and HS) before and after the training period. In addition, the session-RPE was calculated (i.e., RPE x session time) after each training session over the 6 weeks [26].

4. Instruments

Quantifying Training Load

The ITL was recorded using the session-RPE rating of perceived exertion scale [26]. The intensities of the training sessions were similar between the groups and proposed by the coach of the training center. However, according to the principle of individuality, each subject could respond differently to the intensity proposed by the coach. The subjects were asked how intense their training session was at around ~30 min after the end of each training session and responded based on a category ratio scale (CR-10) [26]. The subjects were already previously familiar with the CR-10 scale. The reported value was multiplied by the total duration of each training session in minutes, resulting in an arbitrary unit value (AU) (perceived internal training load) [26]. The training load was expressed in weekly internal training load (WITL) (the sum of 7 days). The mean weekly ITL (WMITL) was additionally performed by the sum of the weekly AU divided by 7 (number of days of the week). Finally, the session-RPE values (daily and weekly) were used for the analyses. The MI was calculated by the division of the WMITL by its respective standard deviation [26]. The TS was calculated by multiplying the sum of the weekly ITL (WITL) by MI of the same time interval [26].

5. Physical Performance

5.1. Countermovement Vertical Jump Height (CVJH)

The vertical jump height was verified from the use of CVJH. The subjects were familiar with performing the jump test and able to exert a downward movement followed by a complete extension of the legs and were free to establish the amplitude of the countermovement to avoid modifications in the jumps [31]. All attempts were performed with their hands fixed on their hips and subjects were encouraged to jump as high and as fast as possible [31]. A contact platform connected to the

Jump Test Pro 2.10 software program (Cefise®, São Paulo, Brazil) was used to measure CVJH, and five attempts with intervals of 15 s between them were granted [32]. Finally, the jump was considered valid for analysis if the takeoff and landing positions remained visually analogous. The best result of five attempts was subsequently used for data analysis. The intraclass correlation coefficient (ICCs) of the baseline and post CVJH were 0.99 in both.

5.2. Speed Test (20-m Sprint)

Prior to the speed tests and after the warm-up period proposed by the coach responsible for the training center, 1 photocell (Cefise®, São Paulo, Brazil) was allocated at 20 m from the starting point. A 20-m test was repeated (i.e., two times) from the standing position. All speed tests were performed at an indoor training center in order to mitigate weather effects. Recovery time between trials was 5 min and the best time was used for data analysis [32]. The ICCs of the baseline and post times of 0–20 m were 0.96 and 0.95, respectively.

5.3. Handgrip Strength (HS)

The subject was comfortably seated, positioned with their shoulder slightly adducted, elbow flexed at 90°, forearm in neutral position and the wrist positioning could oscillate from 0° to 30° long. These procedures are in accordance with the specifications of the American Society of Hand Therapists [33]. The dynamometer measurement (Jamar®, São Paulo, Brazil) was regulated according to the characteristics of each subject and the best results of three attempts in each hand were used for data analysis. ICCs were 0.99 for right HS (baseline and post) and 0.98 for left HS (baseline and post).

5.4. Statistical Analyses

Normality was tested using the Shapiro–Wilk test and Z-score analysis of asymmetry and kurtosis (−1.96 to 1.96). Continuous data are reported in mean and standard deviation. A mixed ANOVA of repeated measures (2 conditions and 6 times) was used to verify the MI, TS and magnitude of WITL and WMITL behavior within and between the different training volumes and frequencies (HTVF and MTVF) over 6 weeks of HIFT. A mixed ANOVA of repeated measures (2 conditions and 2 times) was adopted to verify differences in performance within and between training volumes and frequencies (HTVF and MTVF). Mauchly's sphericity test was adopted to verify the data measurement. The partial eta squared (η^2p) effect size (ES) was used for mixed ANOVA of repeated measures, being classified as: no effect (ES: < 0.04), minimum effect (ES: 0.04–0.25), moderate effect (ES: 0.25–0.64) and strong effect (ES: > 0.64) [34]. Bonferroni's post hoc was used to identify specific differences. A significance level of $p < 0.05$ was adopted for all analyses.

6. Results

An interaction effect was verified for MI (($F_{(5, 145)} = 2.912$; $p = 0.016$; $\eta^2p = 0.091$; power = 0.839, minimum effect)) and TS (($F_{(5, 145)} = 2.810$; $p = 0.019$; $\eta^2p = 0.088$; power = 0.824, minimum effect)). However, no interaction effect was verified for WITL (($F_{(4.006, 116.187)} = 1.855$; $p = 0.123$; $\eta^2p = 0.060$; power = 0.549, minimum effect)) or WMITL (($F_{(4.006, 116.187)} = 1.855$; $p = 0.123$; $\eta^2p = 0.060$; power = 0.549, minimum effect)). There was a time effect for MI (($F_{(5, 145)} = 5.942$; $p = 0.0001$; $\eta^2p = 0.170$; power = 0.994, minimum effect)), TS (($F_{(5, 145)} = 5.734$; $p = 0.0001$; $\eta^2p = 0.165$; power = 0.992, minimum effect)), WITL (($F_{(4.006, 116.87)} = 4.188$; $p = 0.003$; $\eta^2p = 0.126$; power = 0.914, minimum effect)) and WMITL (($F_{(4.006, 116.87)} = 4.188$; $p = 0.003$; $\eta^2p = 0.126$; power = 0.914, minimum effect)). There was only a difference in the MTVF group for MI from week 1 to week 4 (Δ% = 0.416; CI 95% = 0.097 to 0.735; $p = 0.004$), from week 1 to week 5 (Δ% = 0.551; CI 95% = 0.158 to 0.944; $p = 0.002$), from week 3 to week 4 (Δ% = 0.232; CI 95% = 0.020 to 0.444; $p = 0.022$) and between weeks 3 and 5 (Δ% = 0.367; CI 95% = 0.054 to 0.680; $p = 0.012$). There was only a difference in the MTVF group for TS from week 1 to week 4 (Δ% = 1476.3; CI 95% = 316.6 to 2635.9; $p = 0.005$), from week 1 to week 5 (Δ% = 1788.9; CI 95% = 477.8 to 3099.9; $p = 0.002$), from week 3 to week 4 (Δ% = 1023.1; CI 95% = 170.2 to 1875.9; $p = 0.009$) and between weeks 3 and 5 ($\Delta\%$ = 1335.7; CI 95% = 225.0 to 2446.3; p = 0.009). There was only a difference in the MTVF group for WITL from week 3 to week 4 ($\Delta\%$ = 558.9; CI 95% = 198.4 to 919.3; p = 0.0001) and between weeks 3 and 5 ($\Delta\%$ = 630.7; CI 95% = 6.1 to 1255.2; p = 0.046). There was only a difference in the MTVF group for WMITL from week 3 to week 4 ($\Delta\%$ = 79.8; CI 95% = 28.3 to 131.3; p = 0.0001) and between weeks 3 and 5 ($\Delta\%$ = 90.0; CI 95% = 0.8 to 179.3; p = 0.046). No group effect was verified for MI (($F_{(1,29)} = 0.095$; $p = 0.760$; $\eta^2p = 0.003$; power = 0.060, no effect)), TS (($F_{(1,29)} = 0.029$; $p = 0.865$; $\eta^2p = 0.001$; power = 0.053, no effect)), WITL (($F_{(1,29)} = 0.094$; $p = 0.761$; $\eta^2p = 0.003$; power = 0.060, no effect)) and WMITL (($F_{(1,29)} = 0.094$; $p = 0.761$; $\eta^2p = 0.003$; power = 0.060, no effect)) (see Table 1).

Table 1. Monotony index, training strain, weekly internal training load (ITL) and mean weekly ITL.

Variables	Groups	Week 1	Week 2	Week 3	Week 4	Week 5	Week 6
MI	HTVF	1.12 ± 0.25	0.99 ± 0.46	1.03 ± 0.38	1.08 ± 0.30	0.94 ± 0.27	1.16 ± 0.46
	MTVF	1.33 ± 0.42 †,∞	1.02 ± 0.30	1.15 ± 0.31 *,$	0.91 ± 0.22	0.78 ± 0.23	0.98 ± 0.18
TS	HTVF	2477.2 ± 1186.6	2072.3 ± 1653.1	2085.3 ± 1404.1	2310.5 ± 1310.3	1737.1 ± 911.3	2602.8 ± 1848.3
	MTVF	3143.4 ± 1422.2 †,∞	2123.5 ± 1366.9	2690.2 ± 1175.9 *,$	1667.1 ± 887.4	1354.5 ± 797.2	1966.9 ± 622.7
WITL	HTVF	2118.2 ± 775.6	1764.7 ± 992.6	1830.2 ± 741.3	1980.4 ± 778.1	1729.1 ± 642.5	1994.4 ± 802.9
	MTVF	2283.9 ± 558.2	1889.2 ± 750.8	2281.4 ± 789.4 *,$	1722.5 ± 675.0	1650.7 ± 620.6	1973.9 ± 442.7
WMITL	HTVF	302.5 ± 110.8	252.1 ± 141.8	261.4 ± 105.9	282.9 ± 111.1	247.0 ± 91.7	284.9 ± 114.7
	MTVF	326.2 ± 79.7	269.8 ± 107.2	325.9 ± 112.7 *,$	246.0 ± 96.4	235.8 ± 88.6	281.9 ± 63.2

MI—monotony index; TS—training strain; WITL—weekly internal training load; WMITL—mean weekly internal training load; HTVF—high training-volume and frequency; MTVF—moderate training volume and frequency; †—different from week 4 ($p < 0.05$); ∞—different from week 5 ($p < 0.05$); *—different from week 4 ($p < 0.05$); $—different from week 5 ($p < 0.05$); ITL—internal training load.

No interaction effect was verified for CVJH (($F_{(1,29)} = 0.232$; $p = 0.634$; $\eta^2p = 0.008$; power = 0.075, no effect)), sprinting (($F_{(1,29)} = 0.679$; $p = 0.417$; $\eta^2p = 0.023$; power = 0.125, no effect)), right HS (($F_{(1,29)} = 0.013$; $p = 0.909$; $\eta^2p = 0.0001$; power = 0.051, no effect)) or left HS (($F_{(1,29)} = 0.126$; $p = 0.725$; $\eta^2p = 0.004$; power = 0.064, no effect)). No time effect was verified for CVJH (($F_{(1,29)} = 6.081$; $p = 0.050$; $\eta^2p = 0.173$; power = 0.664, minimum effect)), sprinting (($F_{(1,29)} = 1.014$; $p = 0.322$; $\eta^2p = 0.034$; power = 0.164, no effect)), right HS (($F_{(1,29)} = 2.522$; $p = 0.123$; $\eta^2p = 0.080$; power = 0.336, minimum effect)) or left HS (($F_{(1,29)} = 2.550$; $p = 0.121$; $\eta^2p = 0.081$; power = 0.339, minimum effect)). No group effect was verified for CVJH (($F_{(1,29)} = 1.865$; $p = 0.183$; $\eta^2p = 0.060$; power = 0.262, minimum effect)), sprinting (($F_{(1,29)} = 0.085$; $p = 0.773$; $\eta^2p = 0.003$; power = 0.059, no effect)), right HS (($F_{(1,29)} = 0.771$; $p = 0.387$; $\eta^2p = 0.026$; power = 0.136, no effect)) or left HS (($F_{(1,29)} = 0.301$; $p = 0.587$; $\eta^2p = 0.010$; power = 0.083, no effect)) (see Figure 1).

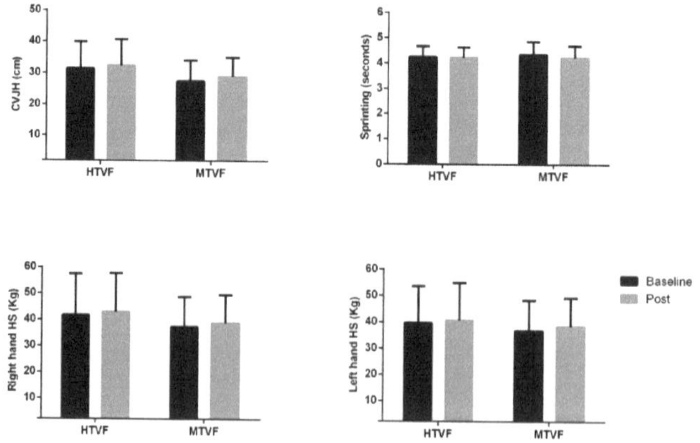

Figure 1. Countermovement vertical jump height (CVJH), sprinting, right and left handgrip strength between groups in HIFT. HTVF—high training-volume and frequency; MTVF—moderate training volume and frequency.

Figure 2 reports the individual values for the performance tests after 6 weeks of HIFT between groups. It was observed that 70.58% (i.e., 12 subjects) and 64.28% (i.e., 9 subjects) increased performance for the CVJH, 52.94% (i.e., 9 subjects) and 71.42% (i.e., 10 subjects) for sprinting, 41.17% (i.e., 7 subjects) and 71.42% (i.e., 10 subjects) for right HS and 52.94% (i.e., 9 subjects) and 71.42% (i.e., 10 subjects) for left HS of the HTVF group and of the MTVF group, respectively, after 6 weeks, although not significant.

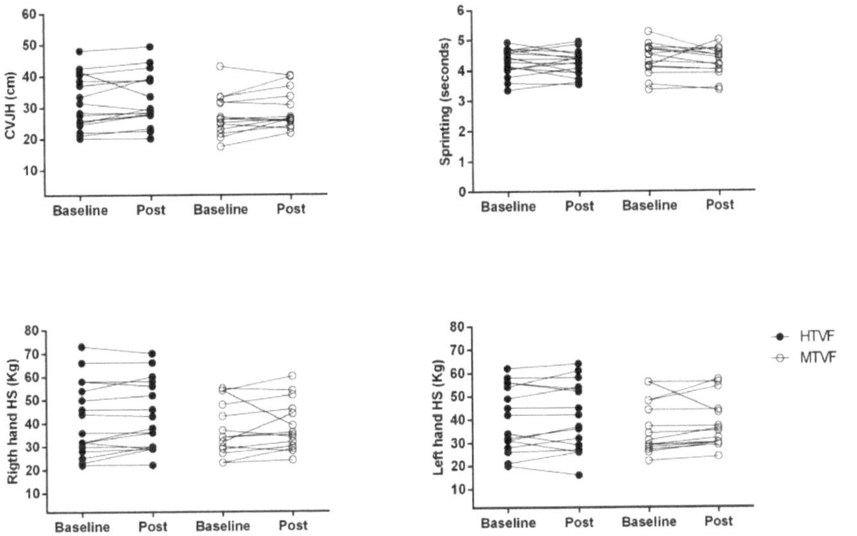

Figure 2. Individual values for countermovement vertical jump height (CVJH), sprinting, right and left handgrip strength between groups in HIFT. HTVF—high training-volume and frequency; MTVF—moderate training volume and frequency.

7. Discussion

The aim of this study was to analyze the ITL during six weeks of HIFT and to verify the effects of HIFT on physical performance in subjects with different training volumes and frequencies. No differences in MI, TS, WITL and WMITL in the HTVF group were observed over the six weeks. On the other hand, a variation of greater magnitude in MI, TS, WITL and WMITL in the MTVF group was observed over the six weeks (see Table 1). Regarding physical performance, six weeks of high-intensity functional training was not able to generally increase performance in either group (see Figure 1).

The arrangement of WITL and WMITL only differed during the six weeks of training in the MTVF group. The American College of Sports Medicine recently published a consensus on HIFT and suggested monitoring the training load to mitigate negative adaptations [35], since high training loads associated with low recovery is one of the main causes of overtraining [36]. These studies showed the relevance of applying a floating approach and periodic control of workloads for positive development of performance [37]. Thus, the willingness and adjustments of workloads in accordance with the state of readiness of subjects is shown to be a valuable strategy for efficient and safe prescription [38,39] in order to prevent detraining and promote increased performance [40].

Our data show a WMITL of 1903 AU for the HTVF group and 1967 AU for the MTVF group. The ITL values are in line with the values found by Tibana et al. [17] (2092 AU) and slightly below the values presented by Williams et al. [29] (2591 AU) who used session-RPE to quantify training loads in HIFT athletes. It is noteworthy that periods of load intensification, long-term accumulated loads, as well as strenuous competitions are possible predictors of injuries [19]. For example, weekly workloads between 3000 and 5000 AU revealed 50% to 80% more chances of injuries [41], as well as two subsequent weeks with weekly workloads greater than 2000 AU [42]. On the other hand, weekly workloads below 1250 AU also revealed potentiation in the risk of injury and did not promote increased fitness [42]. Therefore, session-RPE can assist coaches in performing "adjustments" of training loads when necessary, respecting the individuality of subjects, and in order to avoid high MI and TS [26] which constitute factors associated with larger chances of injury.

It is worth mentioning that no injuries were observed during the monitoring period in our study. This condition was consistent with the MI and TS values which were below the values that indicate a higher risk of injury or illness in both groups (see Table 1). Abrupt growth stemming from MI (i.e., above 2.0 AU) as well as high TS (i.e., above 8000 AU) were correlated with 77% and 89% in the occurrence of diseases, respectively [26]. In addition, high volumes and training intensities may have repercussions on the decline of the immune system and consequently increases in signs and symptoms of upper respiratory tract infection [43]. For example, Ferrari et al. [44] observed significant associations between upper respiratory tract infection and TS in the preparatory ($r = 0.72$; $p = 0.03$) and competitive phases ($r = 0.73$; $p = 0.03$) in trained cyclists. On the other hand, it was observed that six months of HIFT is able to promote positive chronic responses in the immune and hormonal systems [20]. In addition, performance tests are necessary for correct management of training loads and should be used in order to avoid non-functional overreaching and consequently overtraining [36].

Considering variations in training loads, it was observed that six weeks of high-intensity functional training was not able to generally increase performance in either group in our study. The literature suggests a dose–response relationship for training volume and increased performance [10,11]. For example, Brigatto et al. [45] compared different training volumes (i.e., number of sets) in strength gains in trained subjects (i.e., ~4 years of experience). The results suggest greater strength gains for the group which performed the highest training volumes. On the other hand, Jeffreys et al. [46] evaluated the effects on the performance of high volume protocols (i.e., 1920 ground contacts) vs. low volume (i.e., 480 ground contacts) of plyometric training in rugby players. It was observed that both groups increased performance in a similar way. However, the group with low training volume performed 75% less training volume. In addition, previous experience and the previously used training volume seem to be determining factors in decision making during the prescription of the training volume [47]. For example, Scarpelli et al. [47] compared standardized volumes (i.e., based on literature studies) vs. individualized volumes (i.e., based on previous experience). It was observed that muscle hypertrophy showed higher magnitudes for the group with individualized training volume (~10% vs. ~6%). Therefore, it is of fundamental importance that the principle of individuality be taken into account for assertive decision making in the training prescription.

CVJH has been widely adopted in order to verify adaptations and neuromuscular fatigue in relation to training [48]. Thus, training loads can be defined according to the vertical jump height oscillations and can be applied in training sessions (i.e., daily) with the objective of evaluating and effectively controlling neuromuscular responses and the readiness state of the subjects [31]. Studies have recently indicated associations between olympic weightlifting movements which are commonly used in HIFT [2] and increases in vertical jump height [49] and muscle power [50]. Increased muscle power provides valuable evolution in performance in sports [32]. Previous studies have shown that performing HIFT presents potential for maximizing performance [51,52], possibly due to the use of complex training (i.e., strength training paired with power exercises) [53], which in turn provides increases in vertical jump and sprint responses; however, the training program duration and subjects' profile should be considered [54].

The results regarding the sprinting test showed that there is no change in performance across the training period or among groups in general. Sprinting speed is of great importance for achieving success in sports [55]. For example, the presence of short-haul running races (i.e., up to 800 m) which are constantly held in HIFT competitions are associated with success in the sport [5]. Strong correlations were additionally observed between the best classifications of female athletes and the performance of sprints of 50 and 400 m (r = 0.77 and 0.69, respectively) presented in an official HIFT competition [8]. Therefore, sprinting should not be overlooked in the subject's training program in conjunction with maximum strength, especially when the modality requires these skills in training sessions and competitions [49]. Sprinting measured in the present study was short-distance (i.e., 20 m), which is considered the initial phase of acceleration [56]. Thus, it is possible that distinct results could have been found at greater distances.

There were no general differences verified in relation to handgrip strength (HS) after the 6-weeks of HIFT between groups. HS is of great importance in sports which require higher levels of HS to maximize performance and injury prevention [57]. Olympic weightlifting and gymnastics modalities [57] stand out among different sports which are often employed in HIFT [2]. For example, a varied relationship (r = 0.81; $p < 0.05$) between HS and endurance HS was observed in ring athletes [58]. Thus, high levels of HS are valuable for successful achievement in modalities which present exercises in rings and bars [57]. In addition, coaches need assessment tools that are sensitive, easy to handle and which replicate the sports movements, such as HS [57]. Therefore, HS can provide relevant information in order to identify possible changes in performance or during different periods of the rehabilitation process [9].

Although the results of this study are of great importance for coaches and sports scientists, some limitations need to be highlighted: (i) The external training load was not determined due to the modality characteristic which presents a wide variety of exercises in the same training session (i.e., strength, gymnastics and endurance), therefore constituting a challenge for coaches and future research [17]. However, monitoring was performed minimally through the session time; (ii) The absence of tapering (i.e., volume reduction with maintenance or increased training intensity); however, it is worth mentioning that the training was proposed by the training center coach, making it impossible to intervene in the prescription and training organization. On the other hand, all subjects were instructed to refrain from high-intensity exercise in the 72 h preceding the test performance. Nevertheless, this is the first study to examine the impact of different training volumes and frequencies of HIFT on physical performance. Therefore, further studies should be conducted to examine the impact of different training volumes and frequencies of HIFT with the inclusion of tapering and monitoring the external training load.

From a practical point of view, the present results indicate that coaches, sports scientists and other professionals in the field should manage workloads during the season with the aim to adjust and opt for consistent workloads respecting the individuality of subjects. Thus, tools which are accessible, efficient and non-invasive such as session-RPE provide simple and objective results on workloads and additionally on the readiness state of subjects. Therefore, daily and weekly controls can collaborate with the training planning and organization in order for athletes/subjects to reach the apex of physical form with lower risks of injury. Regarding performance tests, coaches can monitor adaptations in relation to the proposed training period and consequently opt for better training strategies in order to achieve superior results in training and subsequent competitions, since in our study it was observed that six weeks of high-intensity functional training was not able to increase performance, regardless of the training volume or frequency.

8. Conclusions

It was observed that the internal training load presented different magnitudes during the six weeks in both groups with differences only for the moderate training volume and frequency group. In addition, the current findings suggest that six weeks of high-intensity functional training were not able to increase performance in subjects with high training-volume and frequency or a moderate training volume and frequency. Therefore, coaches must opt for better training strategies in order to achieve superior results in training and subsequent competitions.

Author Contributions: Conceptualization, R.V.T., G.R.B., A.L.M., P.M.S.D. and B.G.d.A.T.C.; methodology, R.V.T. and B.G.d.A.T.C.; software, R.V.T.; validation, R.V.T., G.R.B., A.L.M., P.M.S.D. and B.G.d.A.T.C.; formal analysis, R.V.T.; investigation, R.V.T. and B.G.d.A.T.C.; resources, R.V.T.; data curation, R.V.T.; writing—original draft preparation, R.V.T. and B.G.d.A.T.C.; writing—review and editing, R.V.T., G.R.B., A.L.M., P.M.S.D. and B.G.d.A.T.C.; visualization, R.V.T., G.R.B., A.L.M., P.M.S.D. and B.G.d.A.T.C.; supervision, R.V.T., G.R.B., A.L.M., P.M.S.D. and B.G.d.A.T.C.; project administration, R.V.T. and B.G.d.A.T.C.; funding acquisition, R.V.T. All authors have read and agreed to the published version of the manuscript.

Funding: This research received external funding from *Coordenação de Aperfeiçoamento de Pessoal de Nível Superior* (*Capes*).

Acknowledgments: We acknowledge the *Coordenação de Aperfeiçoamento de Pessoal de Nível Superior* (*Capes*) for granting a postgraduate scholarship to Rômulo Vasconcelos Teixeira.

Conflicts of Interest: The authors declare no conflict of interest.

References

1. Fisker, F.Y.; Kildegaard, S.; Thygesen, M.; Grosen, K.; Pfeiffer-Jensen, M. Acute tendon changes in intense crossfit workout: An observational cohort study. *Scand. J. Med. Sci. Sports* **2017**, *27*, 1258–1262. [CrossRef]
2. Weisenthal, B.M.; Beck, C.A.; Maloney, M.D.; DeHaven, K.E.; Giordano, B.D. Injury rate and patterns among crossfit athletes. *Orthop. J. Sports Med.* **2014**, *2*. [CrossRef]
3. Claudino, J.G.; Gabbett, T.J.; Bourgeois, F.; Souza, H.S.; Miranda, R.C.; Mezêncio, B.; Soncin, R.; Cardoso Filho, C.A.; Bottaro, M.; Hernandez, A.J.; et al. CrossFit overview: Systematic review and meta-analysis. *Sports Med. Open* **2018**, *4*, 11. [CrossRef]
4. Feito, Y.; Heinrich, K.M.; Butcher, S.J.; Poston, W.S.C. High intensity functional training (HIFT): Definition and research implications for improved fitness. *Sports* **2018**, *6*, 76. [CrossRef]
5. Bellar, D.; Hatchett, A.; Judge, L.W.; Breaux, M.E.; Marcus, L. The relationship of aerobic capacity, anaerobic peak power and experience to performance in crossfit exercise. *Biol. Sport* **2015**, *32*, 315–320. [CrossRef]
6. Dexheimer, J.D.; Schroeder, E.T.; Sawyer, B.J.; Pettitt, R.W.; Aguinaldo, A.L.; Torrence, W.A. Physiological performance measures as indicators of crossfit®performance. *Sports* **2019**, *7*, 93. [CrossRef]
7. Rodríguez-Rosell, D.; Mora-Custodio, R.; Franco-Márquez, F.; Yáñez-García, J.M.; González-Badillo, J.J. Traditional vs. sport-specific vertical jump tests: Reliability, validity and relationship with the legs strength and sprint performance in adult and teen soccer and basketball players. *J. Strength Cond. Res.* **2017**, *31*, 196–206. [CrossRef]
8. Barbieri, J.F.; Correia, R.F.; Castaño, L.A.A.; Brasil, D.V.C.; Ribeiro, A.N. Comparative and correlational analysis of the performance from 2016 crossfit games high-level athletes. *Man. Ther. Posturology Rehabil. J.* **2017**, *15*, 1–4. [CrossRef]
9. Franchini, E.; Schwartz, J.; Takito, M.Y. Maximal isometric handgrip strength: Comparison between weight categories and classificatory table for adult judo athletes. *J. Exerc. Rehabil.* **2018**, *14*, 968–973. [CrossRef]
10. Figueiredo, V.C.; De Salles, B.F.; Trajano, G.S. Volume for muscle hypertrophy and health outcomes: The most effective variable in resistance training. *Sports Med.* **2018**, *48*, 499–505. [CrossRef]
11. Schoenfeld, B.J.; Contreras, B.; Krieger, J.; Grgic, J.; Delcastillo, K.; Belliard, R.; Alto, A. Resistance training volume enhances muscle hypertrophy but not strength in trained men. *Med. Sci. Sports Exerc.* **2019**, *51*, 94–103. [CrossRef] [PubMed]
12. Colquhoun, R.J.; Gai, C.M.; Aguilar, D.; Bove, D.; Dolan, J.; Vargas, A.; Couvillion, K.; Jenkins, N.D.M.; Campbell, B.I. Training volume, not frequency, indicative of maximal strength adaptations to resistance training. *J. Strength Cond. Res.* **2018**, *32*, 1207–1213. [CrossRef] [PubMed]
13. Saric, J.; Lisica, D.; Orlic, I.; Grgic, J.; Krieger, J.W.; Vuk, S.; Schoenfeld, B.J. Resistance training frequencies of 3 and 6 times per week produce similar muscular adaptations in resistance-trained men. *J. Strength Cond. Res.* **2019**, *1*, 122–129. [CrossRef] [PubMed]
14. Gomes, G.K.; Franco, C.M.; Nunes, P.R.P.; Orsatti, F.L. High-frequency resistance training is not more effective than low-frequency resistance training in increasing muscle mass and strength in well-trained men. *J. Strength Cond. Res.* **2019**, *33*, 130–139. [CrossRef] [PubMed]

15. Tibana, R.A.; Almeida, L.M.; Sousa, N.M.F.; Nascimento, D.C.; Sousa-Neto, I.V.; Almeida, J.A.; Souza, V.C.; Lopes, M.F.T.P.L.; Nobrega, O.T.; Vieira, D.C.L.; et al. Two consecutive days of extreme conditioning program training affects pro and anti-inflammatory cytokines and osteoprotegerin without impairments in muscle power. *Front. Physiol.* **2016**, *7*, 260. [CrossRef] [PubMed]
16. Heavens, K.R.; Szivak, T.K.; Hooper, D.R.; Dunn-Lewis, C.; Comstock, B.A.; Flanagan, S.D.; Looney, D.P.; Kupchak, B.R.; Maresh, C.M.; Volek, J.S.; et al. The effects of high intensity short rest resistance exercise on muscle damage markers in men and women. *J. Strength Cond. Res.* **2014**, *28*, 1041–1049. [CrossRef]
17. Tibana, R.A.; Sousa, N.M.F.; Prestes, J.; Feito, Y.; Ferreira, C.E.; Voltarelli, F.A. Monitoring training load, well-being, heart rate variability, and competitive performance of a functional-fitness female athlete: A case study. *Sports* **2019**, *7*, 35. [CrossRef]
18. Halson, S.L. Monitoring training load to understand fatigue in athletes. *Sports Med.* **2014**, *44*, 139–147. [CrossRef]
19. Jones, C.M.; Griffiths, P.C.; Mellalieu, S.D. Training load and fatigue marker associations with injury and illness: A systematic review of longitudinal studies. *Sports Med.* **2017**, *47*, 943–974. [CrossRef]
20. Poderoso, R.; Cirilo-Sousa, M.; Júnior, A.; Novaes, J.; Vianna, J.; Dias, M.; Leitão, L.; Reis, V.; Neto, N.; Vilaça-Alves, J. Gender differences in chronic hormonal and immunological responses to CrossFit®. *Int. J. Environ. Res. Public Health* **2019**, *16*, 2577. [CrossRef]
21. Drew, M.K.; Finch, C.F. The relationship between training load and injury, illness and soreness: A systematic and literature review. *Sports Med.* **2016**, *46*, 861–883. [CrossRef] [PubMed]
22. Antualpa, K.; Aoki, M.S.; Moreira, A. Salivary steroids hormones, well-being, and physical performance during an intensification training period followed by a tapering period in youth rhythmic gymnasts. *Physiol. Behav.* **2017**, *179*, 1–8. [CrossRef] [PubMed]
23. Gabbett, T.J. Debunking the myths about training load, injury and performance: Empirical evidence, hot topics and recommendations for practitioners. *Br. J. Sports Med.* **2020**, *54*, 58–66. [CrossRef] [PubMed]
24. Nakamura, F.Y.; Pereira, L.A.; Abad, C.C.C.; Franchini, E.; Loturco, I. Cardiac autonomic and neuromuscular responses during a karate training camp before to the 2015 pan american games: A case study with the brazilian national team. *Int. J. Sports Physiol. Perform.* **2016**, *11*, 833–837. [CrossRef] [PubMed]
25. Nakamura, F.Y.; Pereira, L.A.; Rabelo, F.N.; Flatt, A.A.; Esco, M.R.; Bertollo, M.; Loturco, I. Monitoring weekly heart rate variability in futsal players during the preseason: The importance of maintaining high vagal activity. *J. Sports Sci.* **2016**, *34*, 2262–2268. [CrossRef]
26. Foster, C. Monitoring training in athletes with reference to overtraining syndrome. *Med. Sci. Sports Exerc.* **1998**, *30*, 1164–1168. [CrossRef]
27. Tibana, R.A.; Sousa, N.M.F.; Cunha, G.V.; Prestes, J.; Fett, C.; Gabbett, T.J.; Voltarelli, F.A. Validity of session rating perceived exertion method for quantifying internal training load during high-intensity functional training. *Sports* **2018**, *6*, 68. [CrossRef]
28. Crawford, D.A.; Drake, N.B.; Carper, M.J.; DeBlauw, J.; Heinrich, K.M. Validity, reliability, and application of the session-RPE method for quantifying training loads during high intensity functional training. *Sports* **2018**, *6*, 84. [CrossRef]
29. Williams, S.; Booton, T.; Watson, M.; Rowland, D.; Altini, M. Heart rate variability is a moderating factor in the workload-injury relationship of competitive crossfit™ athletes. *J. Sports Sci. Med* **2017**, *16*, 443–449.
30. Cosgrove, S.J.; Crawford, D.A.; Heinrich, K.M. Multiple fitness improvements found after 6-months of high intensity functional training. *Sports* **2019**, *7*, 203. [CrossRef]
31. Cruz, I.F.; Pereira, L.A.; Kobal, R.; Kitamura, K.; Cedra, C.; Loturco, I.; Abad, C.C.C. Perceived training load and jumping responses following nine weeks of a competitive period in young female basketball players. *PeerJ* **2018**, *6*, e5225. [CrossRef] [PubMed]
32. Loturco, I.; Nakamura, F.Y.; Kobal, R.; Gil, S.; Pivetti, B.; Pereira, L.A.; Roschel, H. Traditional periodization versus otimum training load applied to soccer players: Effects on neuromuscular abilities. *Int. J. Sports Med.* **2016**, *37*, 1051–1059.
33. Marin, R.V.; Pedrosa, M.A.C.; Moreira-Pfrimer, L.D.F.; Matsudo, S.M.M.; Lazaretti-Castro, M. Association between lean mass and handgrip strength with bone mineral density in physically active postmenopausal women. *J. Clin. Densitom.* **2010**, *13*, 96–101. [CrossRef] [PubMed]
34. Ferguson, C. An effect size primer: A guide for clinicians and researchers. *Prof. Psy. Res. Prac.* **2009**, *40*, 532–538. [CrossRef]

35. Bergeron, M.F.; Nindl, B.C.; Deuster, P.A.; Baumgartner, N.; Kane, S.F.; Kraemer, W.J.; Sexauer, L.R.; Thompson, W.R.; O'Connor, F.G. Consortium for health and military performance and american college of sports medicine consensus paper on extreme conditioning programs in military personnel. *Curr. Sports Med. Rep.* **2011**, *10*, 383–389. [CrossRef]
36. Meeusen, R.; Duclos, M.; Foster, C.; Fry, A.; Gleeson, M.; Nieman, D.; Raglin, J.; Rietjens, G.; Steinacker, J.; Urhausen, A. Prevention, diagnosis, and treatment of the overtraining syndrome: Joint consensus statement of the european college of sport science and the american college of sports medicine. *Med. Sci. Sports Exerc.* **2013**, *45*, 186–205. [CrossRef]
37. Debien, P.B.; Mancini, M.; Coimbra, D.R.; Freitas, D.G.S.; Miranda, R.; Bara Filho, M.G. Monitoring training load, recovery, and performance of brazilian professional volleyball players during a season. *Int. J. Sports Physiol. Perform.* **2018**, *13*, 1182–1189. [CrossRef]
38. Aoki, M.S.; Ronda, L.T.; Marcelino, P.R.; Drago, G.; Carling, C.; Bradley, P.S.; Moreira, A. Monitoring training loads in professional basketball players engaged in a periodized training program. *J. Strength Cond. Res.* **2017**, *31*, 348–358. [CrossRef] [PubMed]
39. Gabbett, T.J.; Nassis, G.P.; Oetter, E.; Pretorius, J.; Johnston, N.; Medina, D.; Rodas, G.; Myslinski, T.; Howells, D.; Beard, A.; et al. The athlete monitoring cycle: A practical guide to interpreting and applying training monitoring data. *Br. J. Sports Med.* **2017**, *51*, 1451–1452. [CrossRef]
40. Bourdon, P.C.; Cardinale, M.; Murray, A.; Gastin, P.; Kellmann, M.; Varley, M.C.; Gabbett, T.J.; Coutts, A.J.; Burgess, D.J.; Gregson, W.; et al. Monitoring athlete training loads: Consensus statement. *Int. J. Sports Physiol. Perform.* **2017**, *12*, 161–170. [CrossRef]
41. Gabbett, T.J. The development and application of an injury prediction model for noncontact, soft-tissue injuries in elite collision sport athletes. *J. Strength Cond. Res.* **2010**, *24*, 2593–2603. [CrossRef] [PubMed]
42. Harrison, P.W.; Johnston, R.D. Relationship between training load, fitness, and injury over an australian rules football preseason. *J. Strength Cond. Res.* **2017**, *31*, 2686–2693. [CrossRef] [PubMed]
43. Nakamura, D.; Akimoto, T.; Suzuki, S.; Kono, I. Daily changes of salivary secretory immunoglobulin A and appearance of upper respiratory symptoms during physical training. *J. Sports Med. Phys. Fit.* **2006**, *46*, 152–157.
44. Ferrari, H.G.; Gobatto, C.A.; Manchado-Gobatto, F.B. Training load, immune system, upper respiratory symptoms and performance in well-trained cyclists throughout a competitive season. *Biol. Sport* **2013**, *30*, 289–294. [CrossRef] [PubMed]
45. Brigatto, F.A.; Lima, L.E.M.; Germano, M.D.; Aoki, M.S.; Braz, T.V.; Lopes, C.R. High resistance-training volume enhances muscle thickness in resistance-trained men. *J. Strength Cond. Res.* **2019**. Online ahead of print. [CrossRef]
46. Jeffreys, M.A.; De Ste Croix, M.B.A.; Lloyd, R.S.; Oliver, J.L.; Hughes, J.D. The effect of varying plyometric volume on stretch-shortening cycle capability in collegiate male rugby players. *J. Strength Cond. Res.* **2019**, *33*, 139–145. [CrossRef]
47. Scarpelli, M.C.; Nóbrega, S.R.; Santanielo, N.; Alvarez, I.F.; Otoboni, G.B.; Ugrinowitsch, C.; Libardi, C.A. Muscle hypertrophy response is affected by previous resistance training volume in trained individuals. *J. Strength Cond. Res.* **2020**. Online ahead of print. [CrossRef]
48. Loturco, I.; Pereira, L.A.; Kobal, R.; Kitamura, K.; Abad, C.C.C.; Marques, G.; Guerriero, A.; Moraes, J.E.; Nakamura, F.Y. Validity and usability of a new system for measuring and monitoring variations in vertical jump performance. *J. Strength Cond. Res.* **2017**, *31*, 2579–2585. [CrossRef]
49. Suchomel, T.J.; Nimphius, S.; Stone, M.H. The importance of muscular strength in athletic performance. *Sports Med.* **2016**, *46*, 1419–1449. [CrossRef]
50. Cormie, P.; McGuigan, M.R.; Newton, R.U. Developing maximal neuromuscular power: Part 2—Training considerations for improving maximal power production. *Sports Med.* **2011**, *41*, 125–146. [CrossRef]
51. Sousa, A.F.M.; Santos, G.B.; Reis, T.; Valerino, A.J.R.; Del Rosso, S.; Boullosa, D.A. Differences in physical fitness between recreational crossfit® and resistance trained individuals. *J. Exerc. Physiol. Online* **2016**, *19*, 112–122.
52. Hermassi, S.; Wollny, R.; Schwesig, R.; Shephard, R.J.; Chelly, M.S. Effects of in-season circuit training on physical abilities in male handball players. *J. Strength Cond. Res.* **2019**, *33*, 944–957. [CrossRef]
53. Neto, J.H.F.; Kennedy, M.D. The multimodal nature of high-intensity functional training: Potential applications to improve sport performance. *Sports* **2019**, *7*, 33. [CrossRef] [PubMed]

54. Freitas, T.T.; Martinez-Rodriguez, A.; Calleja-González, J.; Alcaraz, P.E. Short-term adaptations following complex training in team-sports: A meta-analysis. *PLoS ONE* **2017**, *12*, e0180223. [CrossRef] [PubMed]
55. Healy, R.; Smyth, C.; Kenny, I.C.; Harrison, A.J. Influence of reactive and maximum strength indicators on sprint performance. *J. Strength Cond. Res.* **2019**, *33*, 3039–3048. [CrossRef] [PubMed]
56. Contreras, B.; Vigotsky, A.D.; Schoenfeld, B.J.; Beardsley, C.; McMaster, D.T.; Reyneke, J.H.T.; Cronin, J.B. Effects of a six-week hip thrust vs. front squat resistance training program on performance in adolescent males: A randomized controlled trial. *J. Strength Cond. Res.* **2017**, *31*, 999–1008. [CrossRef]
57. Cronin, J.; Lawton, T.; Harris, N.; Kilding, A.; McMaster, D.T. A brief review of handgrip strength and sport performance. *J. Strength Cond. Res.* **2017**, *31*, 3187–3217. [CrossRef]
58. Ruprai, R.K.; Tajpuriya, S.V.; Mishra, N. Handgrip strength as determinant of upper body strength/physical fitness: A comparative study among individuals performing gymnastics (ring athletes) and gymnasium (powerlifters). *Int. J. Med. Sci. Public Health* **2016**, *5*, 1167–1172. [CrossRef]

International Journal of
Environmental Research and Public Health

MDPI

Article

Relationships between Linear Sprint, Lower-Body Power Output and Change of Direction Performance in Elite Soccer Players

Monika Papla, Michal Krzysztofik *, Grzegorz Wojdala, Robert Roczniok, Marcin Oslizlo and Artur Golas

Institute of Sport Sciences, The Jerzy Kukuczka Academy of Physical Education in Katowice, 40-065 Katowice, Mikolowska 72a, Poland; m.papla15@gmail.com (M.P.); wojdala.grzegorz@gmail.com (G.W.); r.roczniok@awf.katowice.pl (R.R.); m.oslizlo@awf.katowice.pl (M.O.); a.golas@awf.katowice.pl (A.G.)
* Correspondence: m.krzysztofik@awf.katowice.pl

Received: 17 July 2020; Accepted: 21 August 2020; Published: 22 August 2020

Abstract: The aim of this study was to investigate the relationship between linear sprint, power output obtained during a squat and change of direction (COD) performance. Fifteen elite soccer players participated in this study (age = 21.7 ± 0.72 years, body mass = 74.9 ± 9.11 kg, body height = 180.4 ± 7 cm, training experience = 9 ± 1.5 years). To examine these correlations a following battery of tests were carried out: 20-m linear sprint, one-repetition maximum (1RM) squat strength, peak power output obtained during a squat at 50% 1RM and time obtained in two 20-m COD tests with different angles of direction change (90° and 135°). In addition, COD deficits (90°-COD_{DEF} and 135°-COD_{DEF}) for both COD tests were calculated. The Spearman's rank order correlation showed a nearly perfect statistical relationship between the 90°-COD and the 90°-COD_{DEF} ($r = 0.9$; $p < 0.001$). In the case of 90°-COD_{DEF}, there was a large statistical relationship with 135°-COD_{DEF} ($r = 0.59$; $p = 0.021$). Moreover, there was a nearly perfect statistical relationship between 135°-COD and 135°-COD_{DEF} ($r = 0.91$; $p < 0.001$). The statistically insignificant ($p > 0.05$) relationship between 20-m linear sprint time, power output obtained during a squat at 50% 1RM, 1RM squat strength level and both COD test, as well as both COD deficits were found. Results of the present study showed that 20-m linear sprinting speed, 1RM squat strength, power output obtained during squat at 50% 1RM and COD ability at 90° and 135° angles, are separate physical qualities. Moreover, it seems that COD deficit provides a more isolated measure of COD ability than the COD tests alone and does not must be limited to a specific angle, but provides knowledge about the COD ability in a range of other angles, at least concerning 90° and 135° COD angles.

Keywords: agility; COD deficit; squat power; team sports; speed

---

1. Introduction

Most team sports require players to jump, sprint and change direction very frequently; such sports include American football, rugby and soccer [1,2]. During a soccer match, players make over 700 turns with different changes of direction (COD) [3], as well as numerous jumps and sprints [4]. During a COD, athletes' ability to accelerate, decelerate and reaccelerate in a new direction requires a rapid application of force. The acceleration phase in COD and linear sprint involves similar technical factors, so improving acceleration capability may be beneficial in terms of accelerating quickly after successive COD maneuvers and transition between them. Hence, it can be assumed that linear speed and lower-body power output may affect COD performance. Given that, many researchers examined the relationship between the performance of the above mentioned high-intensity actions and reached varying degrees of association, further studies seem justified [5–10]. Previous studies indicate a statistically significant large to very large relationships between linear sprints and different COD sprints (45°, 60°, 90° and 135° changes of direction) at various distances [7–9,11]. Additionally, Suarez-Arrones et al. [10] showed a statistically significant moderate and large relationship between 10-m linear sprint and equal distance different COD sprints (90° and 180°; respectively). At the same time, Loturco et al. [9] revealed no statistically significant relationship between 100° COD test and linear sprints at 5 m, as well as on 10 m.

Profiling of COD performance is difficult due to a variety of tests used in research. Certain COD tests differing in length, angle and a number of direction changes. Therefore, they may have different physical and mechanical requirements. In regards to the COD angles, as suggested by Falch et al. [12] and Bourgeuis et al. [13] angels below 90° are more velocity-oriented in contrast to the angles above 90°, which are more force-oriented. Consequently, it can be assumed that COD performance with the angles below 90° and that which exceeding 90° should be measured and trained separately. Regarding the number of direction change, a majority of COD tests consists of two or more turns [14], however in case of soccer players, it is rare to change direction more than three times during matches [15]. With respect to the fatigue caused by hundreds of COD during a soccer match, the use of COD tests with several or repeated COD tests seems warranted when the COD ability is assessed among soccer players.

The solution that can shed new light on the assessment of COD ability, is a measurement of COD deficit. However, to date little attention has been given to the relationship between COD deficit and the performance of the high-intensity actions and COD tests [2,10,15,16]. The COD deficit is an additional time that athletes need, to complete running with a COD in comparison to straight-line sprint at the same distance (e.g., athlete's 20-m sprint time is subtracted from the 20-m COD time). This difference in time allows to better isolate and identify an athlete's ability to change direction [2]. The lower the value, the greater the COD ability. A study by Nimphius et al. [2] showed a statistically significant positive relationship between COD deficit (measured as the difference between 10-m sprint time and 180° COD test) and COD test (505), but not with 10- and 30-m sprint time in male cricketers. In contrast, Loturco et al. [15] did not find a statistically significant relationship between COD deficit (measured as the difference between 20-m linear fly sprint and 100° COD test) and 100° COD test. However, the authors indicated a statistically significant positive moderate relationship between COD deficit and relative mean propulsive power obtained in the half-squat and sprint velocity at five meters. Furthermore, a large and nearly perfect relationship was found between 10- and 20-m linear flying sprint and COD deficit among elite soccer players. Moreover, Loturco and colleagues [15] found statistically significant positive large and nearly perfect relationship with 10-m and 20-m linear flying sprint, respectively. In reference to the Nimphius et al. [2], the COD deficit may be specific to the angle and, as shown by the results of previous studies, may also for the length of run, discipline and the type of start (standing vs. flying). Therefore, in order to increase the versatility of this measure, there is a need for research which compare the COD tests and COD deficits with different direction change and running length in the same group of athletes.

Therefore, the aims of this study were to examine the relationships between a 20-m linear sprint, 1RM squat strength, peak power output obtained during a squat at 50% 1RM, 90° and 135° COD tests. A second aim of this study was to analyze the possible relationships between the COD deficits (using 90° and 135° COD time and 20-m sprint time) with all considered tests. It was hypothesized that significant relationships between all measured variables will exist. The second hypothesis was that peak power output obtained in the squat and 20-m linear sprint would be positively correlated with the COD deficit and the magnitude of correlation will depend on the angle of change.

2. Materials and Methods

2.1. Experimental Design

To examine the relationship between linear sprint, lower-body maximum strength and power output as well as COD performance, the following tests were carried out: 20-m linear sprint, one-repetition maximum (1RM) squat strength, peak power output obtained during a squat at 50%1RM and two separate 20-m COD sprints, first with a 90° and the second with a 135° direction change angles. To assess a more isolated measure of the COD performance, the COD deficits for both conducted tests were calculated. Measurements were conducted on two different sessions, 72 h apart. Linear and COD sprints were performed during the first session, and 72 h later the lower-body power output was assessed.

2.2. Study Participants

Fifteen elite male soccer players from a professional team participated in the study (Second Polish League) (age = 21.7 ± 0.72 years, body mass = 74.9 ± 9.11 kg, body height = 180.4 ± 7 cm, training experience = 9 ± 1.5 years, 1RM squat = 200 ± 8.7 kg). The athletes were all full-time professionals who trained daily. All athletes had valid medical examinations and showed no contraindications to participate in physical fitness tests. The experimental sessions took place at the beginning of the pre-season. The athletes were instructed to maintain their normal dietary habits over the course of the study and not to use any supplements or stimulants for the duration of the experiment. Moreover, they were informed verbally and in writing about the experimental protocol, the possible risks and benefits of the study and the possibility to withdraw at any stage of the experiment. All players gave their written consent for participation. The study protocol was approved by the Bioethics Committee for Scientific Research (10/2018), at the Academy of Physical Education in Katowice, Poland and performed according to the ethical standards of the Declaration of Helsinki, 2013.

2.3. Testing Procedures

One week prior to starting the experimental sessions, all athletes were familiarized with the testing procedures and 1RM test for the Keiser Squat exercise. The experimental sessions were carried out at the same time of the day (between 9:00 and 11:00 a.m.) 72 h apart. Both sessions were preceded by the same warm-up protocol, which included 5 min of jogging, dynamic stretching, a single attempt of a 20-m linear sprint and two different COD sprints (90° and 135°) at submaximal intensity and 2 sets of body-weight squats. During the first experimental session, the athletes performed a 20-m linear sprint and 20-m COD sprints with two different turn angles (90° and 135°). All sprint tests were performed on an indoor court. The running times were recorded by two pairs of dual-beam Witty Gate photocells (Microgate, Bolzano, Italy) with the measuring precision of 0.01 s. The intraclass correlation coefficient for the test–retest reliability in times of linear sprinting and COD tests measured by used photocells ranged from 0.96 to 0.99. In the second experimental session peak power output obtained during a squat exercise at 50% 1RM was assessed using the Keiser Air 300 Squat pneumatic machine (Keiser Corporation, Fresno, CA, USA). This value of the external load was chosen because it is the lower value of the range that was indicated as optimal for obtaining the highest values of peak power outputs during a squat exercise [17]. The Keiser pneumatic resistance system utilizes air-pressurized resistance to maximize safety and allows for precision loading within one kilogram. The intraclass correlation coefficient for the test–retest reliability in the peak power output during a squat exercise measured by Keiser Air 300 Squat pneumatic machine was 0.97.

2.3.1. One-Repetition Maximum Test

One week before the first experimental session the 1RM squat exercise test was performed on the Keiser Squat air pneumatic machine. After a standardized warm-up, the athletes performed 10, 6, 4 and 3 repetitions, starting at a load of 20 kg and progressing to 60–80% of their estimated 1RM. The first testing load was set to an estimated 90% 1RM and was increased by 5–10 kg for each subsequent attempt until the athlete was unable to perform a proper lift with a correct technique. The 1RM test result was determined within 5 attempts, with 5 min of rest in between attempts. All testing was performed with a constant tempo of movement [18,19]. The strength coaches were present throughout the procedure of 1RM testing. The athletes started from an upright position, with the knees and hips fully extended, the stance approximately shoulder-width apart with both feet positioned flat on the floor in parallel or externally rotated to a maximum of 15° [20], hands were placed on the hand grips, and this setting was carefully replicated on every lift. From this position, they were required to descend until contact with the bench (without losing muscle tension) and then perform the concentric phase of the movement in an explosive manner. The height of the bench allowed each athlete to descend with the hips below the knee line to keep constant squat depth. No weight-lifting belts, shoes or other supportive garments were permitted.

2.3.2. Linear Sprint Test

Following the warm-up, all athletes performed 2 maximal 20-m linear sprints, interspersed with 5 min rest intervals. The athletes started with the front foot placed 0.5 m behind the first timing gate, to prevent any early triggering of the start gate. The athletes started when ready to eliminate the reaction time effect. The fastest time from both attempts was retained for further analysis.

2.3.3. Change of Direction Tests

Following the 20-m linear sprint test, the participants were provided with a 5 min rest interval before completing the COD tests. The two COD tests consisted of four 5-m sections marked with cones set at 90° (90°-COD) and 135° (135°-COD), requiring the athletes to decelerate and accelerate as fast as possible around each cone (Figures 1 and 2). The players executed two attempts of each COD test with 5 min rest intervals in between attempts and tests. The fastest time from each COD test was retained for further analysis.

2.3.4. Change of Direction Deficits

To provide a measure of each athletes' COD ability, an adapted COD deficit calculation was used. The COD deficit for both angles (90°-COD_{DEF} and 135°-COD_{DEF}) was calculated as follows: 20-m linear sprint time −90°-COD for 90°-COD_{DEF} and 20-m linear sprint time −135°-COD for 135°-COD_{DEF}.

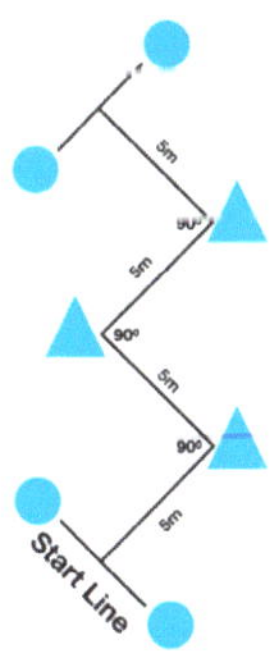

Figure 1. Schematic presentation of the 90° change of direction test. Circles represent the positions of the photocells.

2.3.5. Lower-Body Power Output

Following the warm-up, a lower-body power output test was assessed using the squat exercise performed on the Keiser Squat air pneumatic machine at 50% 1RM. The strength coaches were present throughout the test to ensure safety and to carefully replicate the setting on each lift. All athletes were instructed to perform the concentric phase of the movement as fast as possible. As during the 1RM test, no weight-lifting supportive garments were permitted. The players executed two attempts of lower-body power output with 5 min rest intervals in between. The best peak power output was considered for further analysis.

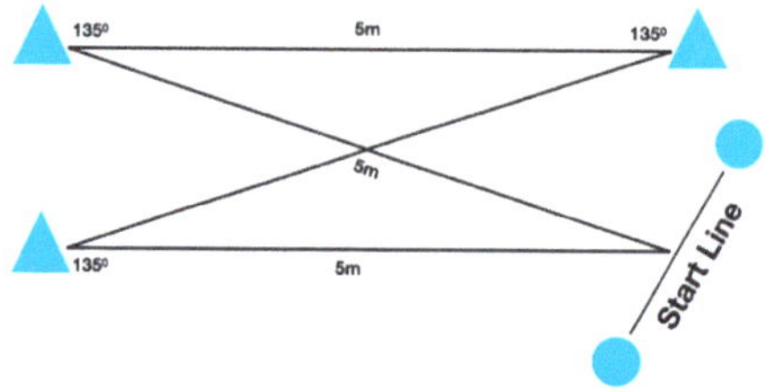

Figure 2. Schematic presentation of the 135° change of direction test. Circles represent the positions of the photocells.

2.4. Statistical Analysis

All statistical analyses were performed using Statistica 9.1 (Hillview, Palo Alto, CA, USA). The physical tests of this study were: 20-m linear sprint, 1RM squat strength, peak power output in squat, 90° and 135°-COD tests and 90° and 135°-COD_{DEF}. Data are presented as means and standard deviations (SD) with 95% confidence intervals. The normality of the data were examined by the Shapiro–Wilk test. Due to the lack of normal distribution of the studied variables (linear sprint and 135°-COD), the Spearman's rank order correlation was used to determine the relationship between all conducted tests. Correlations were evaluated as follows: trivial (0.0–0.09), small (0.10–0.29), moderate (0.30–0.49), large (0.50–0.69), very large (0.70–0.89), nearly perfect (0.90–0.99) and perfect (1.0) [21]. The significance level for the correlation analysis was set as $p < 0.05$.

3. Results

Descriptive data for all the tests is shown in Table 1, while the Spearman's rank order correlations between all measured variables are presented in Table 2. There were no statistically significant relationships between peak power output obtained during squat at 50% 1RM and all of the other measured variables. Further, there were no statistically significant relationships between squat 1RM and all of the other measured variables. Similarly, no statistically significant relationships between linear sprint and all of the other measured variables were found. In regards to the 90°-COD there was a nearly perfect statistically significant relationship with 90°-COD_{DEF} ($r = 0.9$; $p < 0.001$). In case of 90°-COD_{DEF}, there was a large statistically significant relationship with 135°-COD_{DEF} ($r = 0.59$; $p = 0.021$). Moreover, there was a nearly perfect statistically significant relationship between 135°-COD and 135°-COD_{DEF} ($r = 0.91$; $p < 0.001$).

Table 1. Descriptive data for all measured tests.

Test	Mean ± SD	95% CI
Squat 1RM (kg)	200 ± 8.7	192 to 208
Linear Sprint (s)	3.02 ± 0.1	2.97 to 3.08
90°-COD (s)	7.07 ± 0.25	6.93 to 7.2
135°-COD (s)	7.25 ± 0.28	7.09 to 7.4
90°-COD_{DEF} (s)	4.04 ± 0.21	3.93 to 4.16
135°-COD_{DEF} (s)	4.22 ± 0.24	4.09 to 4.35
Power Output Squat (W)	1408 ± 129	1337 to 1480

Mean ± standard deviation (SD); CI—confidence intervals; 1RM—one-repetition maximum; COD—change of direction; COD_{DEF}—change of direction deficit.

Table 2. Spearman's rank order correlations between all measured variables.

Test		Linear Sprint	Power Output Squat	90°-COD	90°-COD_{DEF}	135°-COD	135°-COD_{DEF}	Squat 1RM
Linear Sprint	r	/						
Power Output Squat	r	−0.30	/					
90°-COD	r	0.43	0.09	/				
90°-COD_{DEF}	r	0.15	0.07	0.90 **	/			
135°-COD	r	0.29	−0.30	0.33	0.38	/		
135°-COD_{DEF}	r	0.05	−0.27	0.42	0.59 *	0.91 **	/	
Squat 1RM	r	−0.16	−0.23	−0.17	−0.02	−0.05	−0.01	/

* statistically significant differences $p < 0.05$; ** statistically significant differences $p < 0.01$; r—Spearman's rank order correlation; COD—change of direction; COD_{DEF}—change of direction deficit.

4. Discussion

The main finding of this study was that 1RM squat strength, peak power output obtained during a squat at 50% 1RM and the 20-m linear sprint was not significantly correlated with each other and with any of the measured COD tests. However, there was a nearly perfect statistical relationship between the 90°-COD and 90°-COD_{DEF} as well as between 135°-COD and 135°-COD_{DEF}. Furthermore, there was a large statistical relationship between 90°-COD_{DEF} and 135°-COD_{DEF}. The results indicated that 20-m linear sprinting speed, 1RM squat strength and power output obtained during squat at 50% 1RM, as well as COD ability at 90° and 135° angles, are separate physical qualities. Moreover, it seems that the COD deficit does not must be limited to a specific angle but provides knowledge about the COD ability in a range of other angles, at least concerning 90° and 135° COD angles. Additionally, these data suggests that the COD deficit provides a more isolated measure of COD ability than the COD tests alone due to the reduced effect of linear sprinting speed within a COD test among elite soccer players.

A wide range of studies has been conducted to determine the applicability of a given exercise that leads to enhancement of specific athletic performance [22–25]. However, various resistance exercises are significantly related to performance of selected physical fitness tests. The lack of a statistically significant relationship between, 1RM squat strength and peak power output obtained in the squat exercise at 50% 1RM and 20-m linear sprint, as well as with COD performance may be explained by different mechanical demands of the hip and knee extensors executing these high-intensity actions. A study by Contreras et al. [24] found that 6-week hip thrust training could be more beneficial in improving 10- and 20-m linear sprint times compared with front squat training, which may be superior in vertical jump height enhancement. In addition, González-García et al. [25] revealed that strength improvement after 7-week hip thrust training showed greater improvements in 10- and 20-m sprint, as well as in COD test (90°) in comparison to back squat training [25]. It is possible that the hip thrust has a stronger transfer to sprint running, whereas the squat has more influence on vertical jump performance [24]. Furthermore, a lack of relationship between 20-m linear sprint time and peak power output obtained in the squat at 50% 1RM may be related to the used external load and measured variable. In the current study, the assessment of correlations is based only on a single value of external load (50% 1RM; 100 ± 4.35 kg) and on peak power output. In turn, a study by López-Segovia et al. [26] showed significant positive correlations with 10-, 20- and 30-m linear sprint time with mean power output obtained in a full squat, but not with peak power output among soccer players. That relationship was found only at 70 kg which was close to the body mass of participants (93%), but not at lower loads (from 20 to 60 kg with 10 kg increments). While in the present study, the external load used during the squat significantly exceeded the body mass of participants (~133%). These findings partially confirm the suggestion of López-Segovia et al. [26] that certain levels of neuromuscular activation, assessed by mean power output generated at loads to body may be related with linear sprint performance. Thus, future studies should examine the relationship between hip thrust and squat exercises at a wide range of external loads versus linear sprint, as well as COD performance.

To the best of the authors' knowledge, a limited number of studies have analyzed the relationship between linear sprint and the COD deficit among soccer players [15,27,28]. Findings of the current study revealed that 20-m linear sprint time was not statistically significant related to both COD deficits, what is contradict to findings of Loturco et al. [15]. The authors showed a statistically significant nearly perfect positive relationship between 100° COD deficit and 20-m flying start linear sprint in team-sport athletes. Moreover, Loturco et al. [15] found a statistically significant large positive relationship between 100° COD deficit and 10-m flying start linear sprint. Unfortunately, Loturco and colleagues [16] did not assess whether these results would be similar in the case of a linear sprint from the standing start. At the same time, Loturco et al. [28] revealed differences in the COD deficit between elite soccer players versus handball, rugby and futsal players. The COD deficit was significantly higher in soccer players in comparison with the remaining disciplines, which could be explained by the nature of these sports. It is important to note, that most COD-runs occur with angles between 0 and 90° (approximately 84%), with the next most common range of 90–180° (approximately 13%) in soccer players [3]. Therefore, the use of angles greater than 90° in COD tests should be considered with logical validity when the goal is to assess the relationships between high-intensity actions and COD performance among soccer players. However, angles greater than 90° occur much less frequently in a match, this should not be ignored, and players must also be prepared for such maneuvers. Therefore, the assessment of the relationship between COD tests and COD deficits with different angles, also exceeding 90°, seems justified from the training practice point of view. In the current investigation, there was a nearly perfect statistical relationship between performances in the COD tests and COD deficits for the same angles (90°-COD and 90°-COD_{DEF}; 135°-COD and 135°-COD_{DEF}). These results are in line with previous findings obtained by Nimphius et al. [2]. The authors revealed a large statistically significant relationship between the COD deficit and COD test time (505 test). Furthermore, there was a large statistically significant relationship between COD deficits between angles (90°-COD_{DEF} vs. 135°-COD_{DEF}), while it was not the case for COD test (90°-COD vs. 135°-COD). The rationale for that results may be similar mechanical requirement between COD angles suggested by the Falch et al. [12] and Bourgeuis et al. [13], that angles below 90° are more velocity-oriented, while angles above 90° are more force-oriented. These data provides further support for the use of a COD deficit to evaluate an athlete's COD ability, as it removes the influence of linear running speed on such tests. Therefore, it seems that the obtained relationship between the COD deficits indicates that this measure provides information about the athlete's COD ability regardless of the angle, at least for 90°- and 135°-COD. Thus, the COD deficits measure provides valuable information for the coaches, which allows the preparation of an individualized training program, e.g., whether the athletes require a complementary program aimed at improving the COD ability.

The present study has some limitations which must be addressed. The first limitation of the study is the assessment of relationships based only on a single value of external load during a squat exercise (50% 1RM). Hence, the results of the presented study do not translate to other loads. Moreover, only a single running length (20 m) for linear sprint and COD tests was examined, as well as the same number of direction changes (3 turns). In addition, these running tests were performed during one experimental session, so the impact of fatigue on the result cannot be ruled out. Taking into consideration the nature of soccer, relationships between high-intensity actions and angles below 90° during COD should be analyzed, however sharper angles should not be completely ignored. Thus, future studies should provide a detailed relationship between different exercises (e.g., hip thrust) at a wide range of external loads and COD performance with variety of angles and numbers of direction change, in a large number of soccer players.

5. Conclusions

The results of the present study showed that 20-m linear sprinting speed, 1RM squat strength, power output obtained during squat at 50% 1RM and COD ability at 90° and 135° angles, are separate physical qualities. Moreover, it seems that COD deficit provides a more isolated measure of COD ability than the COD tests alone and does not must be limited to a specific angle, but provides knowledge about the COD ability in a range of other angles, at least concerning 90° and 135° COD angles. Thus, the lower the deficit time in athletes, the more effective the COD or the higher the ability of an athlete to COD relative to their physical ability for linear speed. What indicates that COD deficits provides an isolated measure of athletes' COD ability and is not biased towards superior lower-body peak power output or 1RM squat strength level and 20-m linear sprint. Therefore, practitioners are recommended to evaluate COD performance based on COD deficits to detect the athlete's capacity to change direction.

6. Practical Applications

The findings from this study show that COD deficit is an easy way to evaluate the COD ability in athletes. Therefore, coaches should use the COD deficit to enable the prescription of more targeted and individualized training programs to enhance the athletes' capability to perform directional changes. Based on this, coaches can implement a more comprehensive training strategy depending on whether the athlete would benefit more from developing the ability to change direction or from improving linear sprint performance.

Author Contributions: Conceptualization, M.P. and A.G.; data curation, M.O. and G.W.; formal analysis, R.R.; investigation, M.P. and M.O.; methodology, M.P. and A.G.; supervision, M.K. and A.G.; writing—original draft, M.K. and M.P.; writing—review & editing, M.K. All authors have read and agree the published version of the manuscript.

Funding: The study was supported and funded by the statutory research of the Jerzy Kukuczka Academy of Physical Education in Katowice, Poland.

Conflicts of Interest: The authors declare that they have no conflicts of interest.

References

1. Lockie, R.G.; Murphy, A.J.; Spinks, C.D. Effects of resisted sled towing on sprint kinematics in field-sport athletes. *J. Strength Cond. Res.* **2003**, *17*, 760–767. [CrossRef]
2. Nimphius, S.; Callaghan, S.J.; Spiteri, T.; Lockie, R.G. Change of Direction Deficit: A More Isolated Measure of Change of Direction Performance Than Total 505 Time. *J. Strength Cond. Res.* **2016**, *30*, 3024–3032. [CrossRef]
3. Bloomfield, J.; Polman, R.; O'Donoghue, P. Physical Demands of Different Positions in FA Premier League Soccer. *J. Sports Sci. Med.* **2007**, *6*, 63–70.
4. Duthie, G.; Pyne, D.; Hooper, S. Time motion analysis of 2001 and 2002 super 12 rugby. *J. Sports Sci.* **2005**, *23*, 523–530. [CrossRef]
5. Vescovi, J.D.; Mcguigan, M.R. Relationships between sprinting, agility, and jump ability in female athletes. *J. Sports Sci.* **2008**, *26*, 97–107. [CrossRef]
6. Buchheit, M. Repeated-Sprint Performance in Team Sport Players: Associations with Measures of Aerobic Fitness, Metabolic Control and Locomotor Function. *Int. J. Sports Med.* **2012**, *33*, 230–239. [CrossRef]
7. Condello, G.; Minganti, C.; Lupo, C.; Benvenuti, C.; Pacini, D.; Tessitore, A. Evaluation of Change-of-Direction Movements in Young Rugby Players. *Int. J. Sports Physiol. Perform.* **2013**, *8*, 52–56. [CrossRef] [PubMed]
8. Sayers, M.G.L. Influence of Test Distance on Change of Direction Speed Test Results. *J. Strength Cond. Res.* **2015**, *29*, 2412–2416. [CrossRef] [PubMed]
9. Loturco, I.; Pereira, L.A.; Moraes, J.E.; Kitamura, K.; Cal Abad, C.C.; Kobal, R.; Nakamura, F.Y. Jump-Squat and Half-Squat Exercises: Selective Influences on Speed-Power Performance of Elite Rugby Sevens Players. *PLoS ONE* **2017**, *12*, e0170627. [CrossRef]
10. Suarez-Arrones, L.; Gonzalo-Skok, O.; Carrasquilla, I.; Asián-Clemente, J.; Santalla, A.; Lara-Lopez, P.; Núñez, F.J. Relationships between Change of Direction, Sprint, Jump, and Squat Power Performance. *Sports* **2020**, *8*, 38. [CrossRef] [PubMed]
11. Buchheit, M.; Haydar, B.; Ahmaidi, S. Repeated sprints with directional changes: Do angles matter? *J. Sports Sci.* **2012**, *30*, 555–562. [CrossRef] [PubMed]
12. Nygaard Falch, H.; Guldteig Rædergård, H.; van den Tillaar, R. Effect of Different Physical Training Forms on Change of Direction Ability: A Systematic Review and Meta-analysis. *Sports Med. Open* **2019**, *5*, 53. [CrossRef] [PubMed]
13. Bourgeuis, F.; McGuigan, M.R.; Gill, N.D.; Gamble, P. Physical characteristics and performance in change of direction tasks: A brief review and training considerations. *J. Aust. Strength Cond.* **2017**, *25*, 104–117.

14. Nimphius, S.; Callaghan, S.J.; Bezodis, N.E.; Lockie, R.G. Change of Direction and Agility Tests: Challenging Our Current Measures of Performance. *Strength Cond. J.* **2018**, *40*, 26–38. [CrossRef]
15. Loturco, I.; Nimphius, S.; Kobal, R.; Bottino, A.; Zanetti, V.; Pereira, L.A.; Jeffreys, I. Change-of direction deficit in elite young soccer players: The limited relationship between conventional speed and power measures and change-of-direction performance. *Ger. J. Exerc. Sport Res.* **2018**, *48*, 228–234. [CrossRef]
16. Cuthbert, M.; Thomas, C.; Dos'Santos, T.; Jones, P.A. Application of Change of Direction Deficit to Evaluate Cutting Ability. *J. Strength Cond. Res.* **2019**, *33*, 2138–2144. [CrossRef]
17. Siegel, J.A.; Gilders, R.M.; Staron, R.S.; Hagerman, F.C. Human muscle power output during upper- and lower-body exercises. *J. Strength Cond. Res.* **2002**, *16*, 173–178.
18. Wilk, M.; Golas, A.; Zmijewski, P.; Krzysztofik, M.; Filip, A.; Coso, J.D.; Tufano, J.J. The Effects of the Movement Tempo on the One-Repetition Maximum Bench Press Results. *J. Hum. Kinet.* **2020**, *72*, 151–159. [CrossRef]
19. Wilk, M.; Gepfert, M.; Krzysztofik, M.; Mostowik, A.; Filip, A.; Hajduk, G.; Zajac, A. Impact of Duration of Eccentric Movement in the One-Repetition Maximum Test Result in the Bench Press among Women. *J. Sports Sci. Med.* **2020**, *19*, 317–322.
20. Martínez-Cava, A.; Morán-Navarro, R.; Sánchez-Medina, L.; González-Badillo, J.J.; Pallarés, J.G. Velocity- and power-load relationships in the half, parallel and full back squat. *J. Sports Sci.* **2019**, *37*, 1088–1096. [CrossRef]
21. Hopkins, W.G. Measures of Reliability in Sports Medicine and Science. *Sports Med* **2000**, *30*, 1–15. [CrossRef] [PubMed]
22. Wisloff, U. Strong correlation of maximal squat strength with sprint performance and vertical jump height in elite soccer players. *Br. J. Sports Med.* **2004**, *38*, 285–288. [CrossRef] [PubMed]
23. Yetter, M.; Moir, G.L. The Acute Effects of Heavy Back and Front Squats on Speed during Forty-Meter Sprint Trials. *J. Strength Cond. Res.* **2008**, *22*, 159–165. [CrossRef] [PubMed]
24. Contreras, B.; Vigotsky, A.D.; Schoenfeld, B.J.; Beardsley, C.; McMaster, D.T.; Reyneke, J.H.T.; Cronin, J.B. Effects of a Six-Week Hip Thrust vs. Front Squat Resistance Training Program on Performance in Adolescent Males: A Randomized Controlled Trial. *J. Strength Cond. Res.* **2017**, *31*, 999–1008. [CrossRef]
25. González-García, J.; Morencos, E.; Balsalobre-Fernández, C.; Cuéllar-Rayo, Á.; Romero-Moraleda, B. Effects of 7-Week Hip Thrust Versus Back Squat Resistance Training on Performance in Adolescent Female Soccer Players. *Sports* **2019**, *7*, 80. [CrossRef] [PubMed]
26. López-Segovia, M.; Marques, M.; van den Tillaar, R.; González-Badillo, J. Relationships Between Vertical Jump and Full Squat Power Outputs With Sprint Times in U21 Soccer Players. *J. Hum. Kinet.* **2011**, *30*, 135–144. [CrossRef]
27. Rouissi, M.; Chtara, M.; Owen, A.; Chaalali, A.; Chaouachi, A.; Gabbett, T.; Chamari, K. Effect of leg dominance on change of direction ability amongst young elite soccer players. *J. Sports Sci.* **2016**, *34*, 542–548. [CrossRef]
28. Loturco, I.; Pereira, L.A.; Reis, V.P.; Abad, C.C.C.; Freitas, T.T.; Azevedo, P.H.S.M.; Nimphius, S. Change of Direction Performance in Elite Players From Different Team Sports. *J. Strength Cond. Res.* **2020**, 1. [CrossRef]

International Journal of
Environmental Research and Public Health

MDPI

Article

The Physical Characteristics of Elite Female Rugby Union Players

Logan Posthumus [1,2,3,*], Campbell Macgregor [1,4], Paul Winwood [1,5], Jamie Tout [3], Lillian Morton [3], Matthew Driller [6] and Nicholas Gill [2,3]

1 Faculty of Health, Education and Environment, Toi Ohomai Institute of Technology, Tauranga 3112, New Zealand; campbell.macgregor@toiohomai.ac.nz (C.M.); paul.winwood@toiohomai.ac.nz (P.W.)
2 Te Huataki Waiora School of Health, The University of Waikato, Hamilton 3216, New Zealand; nicholas.gill@nzrugby.co.nz
3 New Zealand Rugby, Wellington 6011, New Zealand; jt@xlr8.co.nz (J.T.); lillianmortonnutrition@gmail.com (L.M.)
4 School of Applied and Social Sciences, Central Queensland University, Rockhampton 4701, Australia
5 School of Sport and Recreation, Auckland University of Technology, Auckland 0627, New Zealand
6 School of Allied Health, Human Services and Sport, La Trobe University, Melbourne 3086, Australia; m.driller@latrobe.edu.au
* Correspondence: logan.posthumus@toiohomai.ac.nz

Received: 4 July 2020; Accepted: 31 August 2020; Published: 4 September 2020

Abstract: This study explored the anthropometric and body composition characteristics of elite female rugby union players, comparing between and within different playing positions. Thirty elite female rugby union players (25.6 ± 4.3 y, 171.3 ± 7.7 cm, 83.5 ± 13.9 kg) from New Zealand participated in this study. Physical characteristics were assessed using anthropometric (height, body mass, skinfolds) and body composition (dual-energy X-ray absorptiometry) measures. Forwards were significantly taller ($p < 0.01$; $d = 1.34$), heavier ($p < 0.01$; $d = 2.19$), and possessed greater skinfolds ($p < 0.01$; $d = 1.02$) than backs. Forwards also possessed significantly greater total ($p < 0.01$; $d = 1.83$–2.25) and regional ($p < 0.01$; $d = 1.50$–2.50) body composition measures compared to backs. Healthy bone mineral density values were observed in both forwards and backs, with significantly greater values observed at the arm ($p < 0.01$; $d = 0.92$) and femoral neck ($p = 0.04$; $d = 0.77$) sites for forwards. Tight-five players were significantly heavier ($p = 0.02$; $d = 1.41$) and possessed significantly greater skinfolds ($p < 0.01$; $d = 0.97$) than loose-forwards. Tight-five also possessed significantly greater total body composition measures ($p < 0.05$; $d = 0.97$–1.77) and significantly greater trunk lean mass ($p = 0.04$; $d = 1.14$), trunk fat mass ($p < 0.01$; $d = 1.84$), and arm fat mass ($p = 0.02$; $d = 1.35$) compared to loose-forwards. Specific programming and monitoring for forwards and backs, particularly within forward positional groups, appear important due to such physical characteristic differences.

Keywords: bone mineral density; lean mass; fat mass; fat percentage; skinfolds

1. Introduction

Rugby union (RU) is a high contact field-based team sport which is played all over the world at junior, senior, sub-elite, and elite levels by both males and females. In recent years, RU has become increasingly popular with more elite competitions and matches being contested by female RU players each year [1]. The same rules apply for both sexes, in which a game is contested over two 40 min halves by two teams consisting of 15 players aside comprised of eight forwards (numbers 1–8) and seven backs (numbers 9–15), with eight reserves on the bench (side-line). The game is intermittent in nature which is characterized by repeated bouts of high-intensity exercise (running, sprinting, tackling, scrummaging, rucking, and mauling) interspersed with periods of lower intensity exercise (standing, walking, and jogging). Both provincial [2] and elite [3] female RU players have been shown to cover approximately 5500 to 6400 m during a game, with elite female players demonstrating an average heart rate ~161 bpm and ~700 impacts during a game [3].

Specific anthropometric (height, body mass, skinfold) and body composition (lean mass, fat mass, bone mass) characteristics are required for specific positions in order to meet the physical demands of the sport [4]. Specifically, adequate amounts of body mass in the form of lean mass, fat mass, and bone mass appear to be crucial in order to withstand the frequency and intensity of collisions during offensive and defensive match-play [5]. Meanwhile, an optimal body composition that promotes lean mass and reduces fat mass are also desired to support the development of power, speed, and aerobic fitness, which are important factors to repeatedly perform and complete tasks at a high level [6].

Despite the known positional differences regarding anthropometrics and body composition within elite male RU players [5,7–12], body composition research within elite female RU players is limited. Elite female RU forwards have been shown to be significantly taller, heavier, and possess greater skinfolds and predicted fat percentage compared to backs [13–15]. However, a more recent study [16] demonstrated that forwards were larger and possessed more lean and fat mass than backs, but no significant differences were reported. Further research is required to understand the positional differences within these athletes, as it is well understood that specific roles between and within forwards and backs vary greatly due to the demands of the sport [4,17].

Body composition within elite female RU players has been predominantly determined using skinfolds and predictive equations to provide an estimated body fat percentage [13–15]. More advanced methods have also been implemented to assess body composition within these athletes, such as air displacement (BodPod) [16]. However, a method that has gained popularity for body composition analysis within elite male RU players is the use of dual-energy X-ray absorptiometry (DXA) [5,7–12,18]. Implementing DXA to assess body composition allows the measurement of lean, fat, and bone mass for both total and regional body compartments [19]. Moreover, DXA is the gold standard for measuring bone mineral content (BMC) and bone mineral density (BMD), which provide valuable information regarding the bone health of an athlete [20], which is particularly important among elite female athletes due to associations with female athlete triad [21].

Although a recent study has investigated the body composition of elite female rugby league (RL) players using DXA [22], no study has investigated the body composition and BMD of elite female RU players using DXA. Due to the differences in match-play demands observed between RU and RL [23,24], and between female and male RU [3,25], specific body composition information is required for elite female RU players. This information would be beneficial for talent identification purposes, and for practitioners developing female RU players by providing body composition benchmarks to inform training and nutrition programs. Therefore, the purpose of this study was to investigate the anthropometric and body composition characteristics of New Zealand (NZ) elite female RU players. Comparisons between forwards and backs, including differences within both forward and back positional groups, were explored. It was hypothesized that forwards would possess significantly greater anthropometric, total, and regional body composition measures compared to backs, and significant differences would be observed among forward and back positional groups.

2. Materials and Methods

2.1. Participants and Study Design

Thirty elite female RU players (25.6 ± 4.3 y, 171.3 ± 7.7 cm, 83.5 ± 13.9 kg) from NZ were recruited for this study. Players were first categorized into forwards (n = 15) and backs (n = 15) for analysis and comparison, followed by positional groups within forwards (tight-five (TF) and loose-forwards (LF)) and backs (inside-backs (IB) and outside-backs (OB)). The TF (n = 9) were comprised of hookers (n = 3), props (n = 4), and locks (n = 2), while LF (n = 6) were comprised of flankers and no. 8's. The IB (n = 8) were comprised of half-backs ($n = 2$), first-fives ($n = 3$), and second-fives ($n = 3$), while OB ($n = 7$) were comprised of centers ($n = 2$), wingers, and full backs ($n = 5$). All testing took place during the middle of the in-season period and all participants provided informed consent. The research was approved by the University of Waikato Human Research Ethics Committee (HREC 2019#02).

2.2. Anthropometrics

All anthropometric measures were collected using methods previously described [12]. Body mass was assessed using electronic scales (SECA, Birmingham, UK) to 0.1 kg accuracy upon waking with bladder voided. Height was then immediately assessed using a stadiometer (SECA, Birmingham, UK) to 0.5 cm accuracy. A Level 3 International Society for the Advancement of Kinanthropometry (ISAK) accredited anthropometrist with a technical error of measurement of 1.8% carried out sum of eight site skinfold measurements on all players. Skinfolds were taken using Harpenden callipers (British Indicators, Hertfordshire, UK) to 0.1 mm accuracy. Sum of eight site skinfold measurements from the following sites; biceps, triceps, subscapular, abdominal, supraspinale, iliac crest, mid-thigh and medial calf were made on the right side of the body using ISAK techniques previously described by Norton and Colleagues [26]. All anthropometric equipment was calibrated as recommended by the manufacturer's guidelines.

2.3. Body Composition

Using previously described methods [12], total and regional body composition (lean mass, fat mass, fat percentage, BMC, and BMD), were measured with a fan-beam DXA scanner (Hologic Discovery A, Hologic, Bedford, MA), with analyses performed using Apex 4.5.2 software (Hologic, Bedford, MA) using a whole-body scan protocol. The following clinical site measures for BMD; anterior-posterior lumbar spine (L2–L4) and left hip (femoral neck, trochanter, intertrochanter, and total hip) were included. All scanning procedures were standardized for all participants following the guidelines of the DXA manufacturer and the standards outlined by the International Society for Clinical Densitometry (ISCD). The scanner was tested for consistent calibration daily as per manufacturer guidelines for quality control purposes.

The quality control, acquisition, analysis, and interpretation of all scans were performed by the same experienced and Certified Clinical Densitometrist (CCD), therefore maintaining consistency and reliability of the scan results [27]. The head was included in the analysis for all total body measures and all scans were undertaken using the array mode. Scanned data was separated into axial, appendicular, and whole-body bone values. In the Bone Density Research Laboratory site, coefficients of variation (CV) for precision and accuracy for the spine phantom were 0.3% and 0.4%, respectively. The in vivo precision CV for the CCD technician are 0.9% for total body, 0.6% for lumbar spine (L2–L4), and 0.2% for left total hip BMD sites. The prevalence of osteoporosis and osteopenia were estimated based on the World Health Organization (WHO) classifications (t-score > -1.0 = normal; t-score -1.1 to -2.4 = osteopenia; t-score < -2.5 = osteoporosis) using the young adult reference database.

All participants were scanned on the same day within a five-hour window (1000–1500 h), with all participants consuming breakfast and fluids (~500 g) at the same time (0830 h). Participants were required to remove all metal items from their body and were scanned wearing tight-fitting sport shorts and top that were free from zips, studs, and/or metal objects. Participants were then instructed to lay supine on the scanning bed as still as possible for the duration of the scan. All protocols followed previously described techniques to maximize technical reliability and minimize error [19,28], however, players were unable to be scanned in a fasted state.

2.4. Statistical Methods

All data expressed as means and standard deviation (SD). A 95% confidence interval (95% CI) was presented alongside mean difference and standard error (SE) for all variables. Tests of normality (Shapiro–Wilk) were carried out, which revealed normally distributed data. Differences between forwards and backs and within positional groups (TF vs LF and IB vs OB) were compared using an independent *t*-test. Statistical significance was set as $p < 0.05$ for analyses. Henceforth, when the term 'significant' and 'significantly' is stated, it denotes a statistically significant difference. Effect sizes were calculated using the Cohen's *d* method with the following thresholds: d = *small* 0.20–0.49, *medium* 0.50–0.79, and *large* > 0.80 [29]. All statistical analyses were conducted using SPSS v24 for Windows (IBM, New York, NY, USA).

3. Results

3.1. Analysis between Forwards and Backs

The demographics, anthropometrics, and total body composition for all players and by position can be observed in Table 1. Forwards were significantly taller ($p < 0.01$; $d = 1.34$), heavier ($p < 0.01$; $d = 2.19$), and had significantly greater skinfold totals ($p < 0.01$; $d = 1.02$) than backs. Forwards possessed significantly greater total lean mass ($p < 0.01$; $d = 1.83$), fat mass ($p < 0.01$; $d = 2.25$), fat percentage ($p < 0.01$; $d = 1.87$), and BMC ($p < 0.01$; $d = 1.40$) than backs.

Regional body composition for all players and by position can be observed in Table 2. Forwards possessed significantly greater measures across the trunk, arms, and legs for lean mass ($p < 0.01$; d = 1.77, 1.53, 1.50, respectively), fat mass ($p < 0.01$; d = 1.75, 1.87, 2.50, respectively), and BMC ($p < 0.01$; d = 0.88, 1.51, 1.48, respectively) compared to backs. No clear differences were observed for age between forwards and backs.

Table 1. Demographics, anthropometrics and total body composition characteristics of elite female rugby union (RU) players.

	All Players	Position		Mean Diff	95% CI	% Diff; ES
		Forwards	Backs			
	(n = 30)	(n = 15)	(n = 15)	(± SE)		
Age (y)	25.6 ± 4.3	25.3 ± 3.6	25.8 ± 5.0	−0.5 ± 1.6	−3.7, 2.8	−1.8; −0.11
Height (cm)	171.3 ± 7.7	175.6 ± 6.3 *	167.0 ± 6.6	8.6 ± 2.4	3.8, 13.5	5.2; 1.34
Body Mass (kg)	83.5 ± 13.9	93.7 ± 10.9 *	73.3 ± 7.5	20.5 ± 3.4	13.5, 27.5	27.9; 2.19
Sum8SF (mm)	111.3 ± 36.7	128.2 ± 36.6 *	94.4 ± 29.0	33.8 ± 12.1	9.1, 58.5	35.8; 1.02
Lean Mass (kg)	60.9 ± 7.8	66.2 ± 6.3 *	55.6 ± 5.3	10.6 ± 2.1	6.3, 14.9	19.0; 1.83
Fat Mass (kg)	20.3 ± 6.6	25.3 ± 5.4 *	15.4 ± 3.1	9.9 ± 1.6	6.6, 13.2	64.5; 2.25
Fat % (%)	23.6 ± 4.2	26.5 ± 3.1 *	20.8 ± 3.0	5.8 ± 1.1	3.5, 8.1	27.7; 1.87
BMC (kg)	2.9 ± 0.3	3.1 ± 0.3 *	2.7 ± 0.2	0.4 ± 0.1	0.2, 0.5	13.1; 1.40
BMD (g/cm^2)	1.24 ± 0.08	1.26 ± 0.08	1.23 ± 0.07	0.03 ± 0.03	−0.03, 0.08	2.1; 0.33

Mean ± standard deviation (SD) reported for all players, forwards and backs. Mean Diff (±SE) = mean difference ± standard error of mean difference, 95% CI = 95% confidence interval (lower limit, upper limit), % Diff = percentage difference, ES = effect size, BMC = bone mineral content, BMD = bone mineral density, Sum8SF = sum of eight-site skinfolds. * Statistically significant difference ($p < 0.05$) compared to backs.

Table 2. Regional body composition characteristics of elite female RU players.

		All Players	Position		Mean Diff	95% CI	% Diff; ES
			Forwards	Backs			
		(n = 30)	(n = 15)	(n = 15)	(± SE)		
Trunk	Lean Mass (kg)	29.4 ± 4.2	32.2 ± 3.7 *	26.6 ± 2.5	5.6 ± 1.2	3.3, 7.9	21.0; 1.77
	Fat Mass (kg)	8.5 ± 3.5	10.8 ± 3.4 *	6.2 ± 1.6	4.6 ± 1.0	2.6, 6.6	75.3; 1.75
	BMC (kg)	0.90 ± 0.12	0.94 ± 0.12 *	0.85 ± 0.10	0.10 ± 0.04	0.01, 0.18	11.2; 0.88
Arms	Lean Mass (kg)	6.9 ± 0.9	7.5 ± 0.8 *	6.3 ± 0.7	1.1 ± 0.3	0.6, 1.7	17.9; 1.53
	Fat Mass (kg)	2.3 ± 0.9	2.9 ± 0.8 *	1.7 ± 0.4	1.2 ± 0.2	0.7, 1.7	71.7; 1.87
	BMC (kg)	0.40 ± 0.06	0.44 ± 0.05 *	0.37 ± 0.04	0.07 ± 0.02	0.04, 0.11	19.5; 1.51
Legs	Lean Mass (kg)	21.5 ± 3.0	23.3 ± 2.4 *	19.6 ± 2.5	3.7 ± 0.9	1.8, 5.5	18.6; 1.50
	Fat Mass (kg)	8.5 ± 2.6	10.5 ± 1.8 *	6.5 ± 1.4	4.0 ± 0.6	2.8, 5.2	62.2; 2.50
	BMC (kg)	1.08 ± 0.14	1.17 ± 0.13 *	1.00 ± 0.10	0.17 ± 0.04	0.08, 0.26	17.0; 1.48

Mean ± SD reported for all players, forwards and backs. Mean Diff (± SE) = mean difference ± standard error of mean difference, 95% CI = 95% confidence interval (lower limit, upper limit), % Diff = percentage difference, ES = effect size, BMC = bone mineral content. * Statistically significant difference ($p < 0.05$) compared to backs.

3.2. BMD between Forwards and Backs

The BMD for all players and by position can be observed in Table 3. No significant differences were observed between forwards and backs for total body ($p = 0.63$, $d = 0.33$) and total hip ($p = 0.73$, $d = 0.50$) BMD. However, forwards demonstrated significantly greater BMD in the arms ($p < 0.01$, $d = 0.92$) and femoral neck ($p = 0.04$; $d = 0.77$) compared to backs. There were no significant differences between forwards and backs for total body and clinical site BMD t-scores.

Table 3. Total and clinical site BMD (g/cm^2) of elite female RU players.

	All Players	Position		Mean Diff	95% CI	% Diff; ES
		Forwards	Backs			
	(n = 30)	(n = 15)	(n = 15)	(SE)		
Arms	0.84 ± 0.06	0.87 ± 0.07 *	0.82 ± 0.05	0.05 ± 0.02	0.01, 0.10	6.5; 0.92
Legs	1.29 ± 0.09	1.31 ± 0.10	1.27 ± 0.07	0.05 ± 0.03	−0.02, 0.11	3.7; 0.54
Ribs	0.77 ± 0.07	0.78 ± 0.07	0.76 ± 0.06	0.02 ± 0.02	−0.03, 0.07	3.1; 0.36
Spine	1.17 ± 0.13	1.19 ± 0.14	1.15 ± 0.12	0.04 ± 0.05	−0.05, 0.14	3.7; 0.34
Pelvis	1.55 ± 0.18	1.56 ± 0.17	1.55 ± 0.19	0.01 ± 0.07	−0.12, 0.15	0.7; 0.06
Head	2.19 ± 0.24	2.20 ± 0.27	2.18 ± 0.21	0.03 ± 0.09	−0.16, 0.21	1.2; 0.11
Total	1.24 ± 0.08	1.26 ± 0.08	1.23 ± 0.07	0.03 ± 0.03	−0.03, 0.08	2.1; 0.33
Total t-score	1.58 ± 0.97	1.80 ± 1.03	1.31 ± 0.86	0.49 ± 0.39	−0.32, 1.30	37.5; 0.51
Clinical Sites						
Lumbar (L2–L4)	1.31 ± 0.15	1.36 ± 0.14	1.25 ± 0.13	0.10 ± 0.05	0.00, 0.21	8.1; 0.73
Femoral Neck	1.12 ± 0.11	1.16 ± 0.10 *	1.07 ± 0.12	0.08 ± 0.04	0.00, 0.16	7.8; 0.77
Trochanter	0.94 ± 0.10	0.95 ± 0.10	0.94 ± 0.11	0.01 ± 0.04	−0.07, 0.09	0.8; 0.07
Intertrochanter	1.39 ± 0.14	1.42 ± 0.13	1.35 ± 0.14	0.07 ± 0.05	−0.03, 0.17	5.3; 0.53
Total hip	1.21 ± 0.11	1.24 ± 0.10	1.18 ± 0.12	0.06 ± 0.04	−0.03, 0.14	4.7; 0.50
Clinical site t-score	1.99 ± 1.46	2.46 ± 1.41	1.44 ± 1.37	1.03 ± 0.57	−0.16, 2.21	71.4; 0.74

Mean ± SD reported for all players, forwards and backs. Mean Diff (±SE) = mean difference ± standard error of mean difference, 95% CI = 95% confidence interval (lower limit, upper limit), % Diff = percentage difference, ES = effect size. * Statistically significant difference ($p < 0.05$) compared to backs.

3.3. Analysis within Forward and Back Positional Groups

Within position differences for forwards and backs can be observed in Table 4. The TF possessed significantly greater body mass ($p = 0.02$; $d = 1.41$) and skinfolds ($p < 0.01$; $d = 2.01$) compared to LF. The TF demonstrated significantly greater total lean mass ($p = 0.04$; $d = 0.97$), fat mass ($p < 0.01$; $d = 1.75$), and fat percentage ($p < 0.01$; $d = 1.77$) than LF. Regarding regional body composition, TF presented significantly greater trunk lean mass ($p = 0.04$; $d = 1.14$), trunk fat mass ($p < 0.01$; $d = 1.84$), and arm fat mass ($p = 0.02$; $d = 1.35$) compared to LF. No significant differences were observed between IB and OB for all measures.

Table 4. Demographics, anthropometrics, total and regional body composition within forward and back positional groups.

	Forward Positional Groups (n = 15)					Back Positional Groups (n = 15)				
	TF (n = 9)	LF (n = 6)	Mean Diff (± SE)	95% CI	% Diff; ES	IB (n = 8)	OB (n = 7)	Mean Diff (± SE)	95% CI	% Diff; ES
Age (y)	25.2 ± 3.0	25.5 ± 4.8	−0.3 ± 2.0	−4.6, 4.0	−1.1; −0.07	26.8 ± 4.9	24.7 ± 5.3	2.0 ± 2.6	−3.6, 7.7	8.2; 0.40
Anthropometrics										
Height (cm)	174.8 ± 7.6	176.8 ± 3.9	−2.1 ± 3.4	−9.4, 5.3	−1.2; −0.32	168.8 ± 8.0	164.9 ± 4.3	3.8 ± 3.4	−3.5, 11.2	2.3; 0.58
Weight (kg)	98.8 ± 10.9 *	86.0 ± 4.9	12.8 ± 4.8	2.5, 23.1	14.9; 1.41	73.6 ± 5.8	72.9 ± 9.6	0.7 ± 4.0	−8.0, 9.4	0.9; 0.09
Sum8SF (mm)	149.2 ± 28.8 *	96.8 ± 20.9	52.4 ± 13.7	22.8, 82.1	54.2; 2.01	95.5 ± 31.2	93.2 ± 28.9	2.3 ± 15.6	−31.4, 36.0	2.5; 0.08
Body Composition										
Total Lean Mass (kg)	68.5 ± 7.1 *	62.9 ± 2.3	5.6 ± 3.1	−1.0, 12.2	8.9; 0.97	55.5 ± 4.9	55.8 ± 6.0	−0.3 ± 2.8	−6.4, 5.8	−0.5; −0.05
Total Fat Mass (kg)	28.2 ± 4.7 *	21.0 ± 3.2	7.3 ± 2.2	2.5, 12.0	34.6; 1.75	15.8 ± 2.1	14.9 ± 4.0	0.9 ± 1.6	−2.5, 4.5	6.6; 0.31
Total Fat % (%)	28.2 ± 2.4 *	24.0 ± 2.3	4.2 ± 1.3	1.5, 6.9	17.5; 1.77	21.4 ± 2.4	20.1 ± 3.7	1.3 ± 1.6	−2.1, 4.8	6.6; 0.43
Trunk Lean Mass (kg)	33.7 ± 3.7 *	29.9 ± 2.6	3.8 ± 1.8	0.2, 7.6	12.7; 1.14	27.2 ± 2.2	25.9 ± 2.7	1.3 ± 1.3	−1.4, 4.1	5.1; 0.54
Trunk Fat Mass (kg)	12.7 ± 2.9 *	8.0 ± 1.9	4.7 ± 1.3	1.8, 7.6	58.6; 1.84	6.2 ± 1.3	6.1 ± 2.0	0.1 ± 0.9	−1.8, 1.9	0.4; 0.02
Arm Lean Mass (kg)	7.7 ± 0.8	7.2 ± 0.6	0.5 ± 0.4	−0.4, 1.3	6.7; 0.65	6.2 ± 0.6	6.5 ± 0.9	−0.3 ± 0.4	−1.1, 0.6	−3.8; −0.33
Arm Fat Mass (kg)	3.2 ± 0.8 *	2.3 ± 0.6	0.9 ± 0.4	0.2, 1.8	41.5; 1.35	1.8 ± 0.2	1.5 ± 0.4	0.3 ± 0.2	−0.1, 0.7	19.0; 0.86
Leg Lean Mass (kg)	23.8 ± 2.8	22.6 ± 1.5	1.2 ± 1.3	−1.5, 3.9	5.2; 0.50	19.1 ± 2.3	20.3 ± 2.8	−1.2 ± 1.3	−4.0, 1.7	−5.7; −0.46
Leg Fat Mass (kg)	11.1 ± 1.5	9.5 ± 1.9	1.6 ± 0.9	−0.3, 3.5	16.6; 0.96	6.8 ± 1.0	6.1 ± 1.8	0.7 ± 0.7	−0.9, 2.3	11.6; 0.50

Mean ± SD reported for all positions. TF = tight-five, LF = loose-forwards, IB = inside-backs, OB = outside-backs, Mean Diff (± SE) = mean difference ± standard error of mean difference, 95% CI = 95% confidence interval (lower limit, upper limit), % Diff = percentage difference, ES = effect size, Sum8SF = sum of eight-site skinfolds. * Statistically significant difference ($p < 0.05$) compared to LF.

4. Discussion

The purpose of this study was to investigate the anthropometric and body composition characteristics of NZ elite female RU players. Comparisons were made between forward and back positions, including analysis of within position differences. As hypothesized, forwards demonstrated significantly greater values across all anthropometric, total, and regional body composition measures than backs. Additionally, forwards presented greater BMD across all sites with significant differences present at the arms and femoral-neck compared to backs. Interestingly, only forward positional groups demonstrated significant differences, in which TF possessed significantly greater anthropometric, total, and regional body composition measures compared to LF. This study is the first to assess the body composition characteristics of elite female RU players using DXA, and the first to explore differences between forward and back positional groups.

The anthropometric and body composition differences between forwards and backs are consistent with previous research within both elite female [13–16] and elite male RU players [5,7–12]. Irrespective of sex, forwards require these specific physical characteristics to meet match demands where being taller is desirable in order to gain and retain possession of the ball during line outs, while greater body mass may assist in gaining and retaining ball possession during scrums, rucks, and mauls [4]. Meanwhile, backs are generally shorter, lighter, and leaner in order to achieve higher speeds in more open spaces in an attempt to outmaneuver opponents to create scoring opportunities [4]. Studies within male RU players have also demonstrated that as playing level increases, players are generally heavier with greater lean mass, whilst possessing lower skinfold and body fat percentage [17]. Researchers have also suggested that being taller and heavier appear to be important key performance indicators for World Cup success in elite male RU players [30,31]. More research is required to determine whether such trends exist within elite female RU players.

Within the current study, both forwards and backs were taller and heavier than elite female RU players reported in previous studies [13–16]. Although forwards and backs within the current study were substantially heavier compared to other elite female RU players [13–16], the current players possessed noticeably lower skinfolds, even when comparing sum of eight-site skinfolds within this study, with sum of seven-site skinfolds within previous studies [14,15]. The measured fat percentage using DXA for forwards and backs within this study were considerably lower than the predicted fat percentage reported for elite South African players [14] but were similar to elite English players [13]. Additionally, forwards within the current study demonstrated greater total body lean and fat mass, but lower fat percentage compared to elite Scottish female forwards. Meanwhile, backs demonstrated greater total body lean mass and considerably less fat mass and fat percentage compared to elite Scottish female RU backs [16].

It is important to note that considerably less body mass was reported within the previous studies [14, 16], but particularly within English players [13] compared to the current study. These comparisons highlight the substantial increases in size and in particular body mass within elite female RU players as the sport has progressed throughout the years [13–16]. Moreover, differences in size and body mass may also be attributed to cultural and ethnicity differences between countries [5,7,8,18]. Increases in body mass, but particularly lean mass, are desired due to the contractile element of muscle mass aiding force production, thus positively influencing power to weight ratio and the expression of strength, power, speed and momentum [7]. These are all important factors for attacking and defending within RU and may be further enhanced by limiting/reducing the amount of non-functional fat mass [12]. Too much fat mass may also negatively influence energy expenditure, thermoregulation, and the ability to repeatedly perform tasks within RU match-play [6]. This information supports the need for more current studies reporting the physical and fitness profiles of elite female RU players.

Until now, no research has been available regarding the regional body composition of elite female RU players. The results of this study align with previous research within elite male RU players which demonstrated significantly greater amounts of regional lean mass, fat mass, and BMC in forwards compared to backs [5,7]. When compared to elite female RL players, elite female RU forwards possess greater lean mass at all regional sites, while possessing similar amounts of fat mass at the arms and legs, but less fat mass at the trunk compared to elite female RL forwards [22]. Meanwhile, elite female RU backs demonstrated greater lean mass while possessing lower amounts of fat mass at all regional sites compared to elite female RL backs [22].

When comparing the positional differences within forwards and backs, only forward positional groups demonstrated significant differences. These findings suggest that positional groups within backs are more homogeneous than within forward positional groups. Therefore, more individualized training and nutrition programs may be required for forwards compared to backs. Moreover, TF forwards could potentially aim to decrease fat mass, particularly in the trunk and arms to improve power to weight ratio and acceleration capability [7]. However, further research is required to understand whether or not this extra fat mass demonstrated by TF players is important for the demands of the position. A general consensus is that greater fat mass within collision-based athletes may be required to better deal with impacts due to the "cushioning" effect of fat tissue [22]. Therefore, determining how much fat mass is optimal within female RU players would be valuable.

Interestingly, when comparing the percentage difference for all measures between forwards and backs within the current study to NZ elite male RU players [12], similar differences can be observed. The percentage difference for anthropometric and total body composition measures between forwards and backs within elite females were very similar to elite males [12]. This information suggests that regardless of sex, RU may produce similar positional differences in relation to anthropometrics and body composition. However, it is important to note that females possess unique physiological differences compared to males such as, constant changes in the female sex hormone milieu throughout the menstrual cycle and therefore, across the training program [32]. Due to the effect's hormones have on the body, training, and adaptation, these areas within female athletes need to be carefully considered when developing training and nutrition plans [32].

Future research could assess the physical characteristics derived from DXA alongside fitness measures in order to examine the associations between body composition and physical performance within elite female RU players. Furthermore, exploring the body composition changes using DXA and changes in fitness measures during pre-season and in-season phases would provide valuable information regarding seasonal changes in physical and fitness characteristics. Carrying out DXA scans to track longitudinal changes in body composition to inform training and nutrition programs also allows for the analysis of BMD. Although low BMD does not appear to be a concern within this group of elite athletes, DXA is valuable to identify any athletes with low BMD. Greater insight into the movement demands, training load, and energy requirements of elite female RU players would also be valuable due to the associations between training and nutrition for optimizing body composition [33,34].

A limitation within the current study was the relatively small sample size of elite players, particularly when exploring the within position differences for forwards and backs. A larger sample size would have provided a greater representation of the within position differences and would have allowed further exploration into forward (front row, second row, back row) and back (inside-back, midfield, outside-back) positions. However, this sample size should be appropriate to provide valuable information for talent identification, coaching, and sport science staff. Another limitation within this study was the fact that participants could not be in a fasted state before DXA scans. Researchers should strive to carry out DXA protocols in a fasted state, however within elite sporting environments this can be a challenging task. Although not optimal, all participants consumed less than 500 g of food and fluids which has been shown to maintain low biological measurement error when using DXA [35].

5. Conclusions

In conclusion, forwards were significantly larger than backs, possessing greater stature, body mass, skinfolds, and total and regional body composition measures. Total and regional BMD values are within normal ranges, with forwards demonstrating significantly greater arm and femoral neck BMD.

This study presented novel findings regarding the significant differences between forward positional groups, in which TF were significantly larger than LF. However, no significant differences were observed between back positional groups. This information may be useful for coaches and sport science staff when developing training and nutrition programs for female RU players. It may also provide useful benchmarks that can assist talent identification staff and the development of future female RU players.

Author Contributions: Conceptualization, L.P., C.M., P.W., J.T., L.M., M.D., and N.G.; Methodology, L.P., C.M., P.W., J.T., L.M., M.D., and N.G.; Software, L.P., C.M., and P.W.; Validation, L.P., C.M., P.W., J.T., L.M., M.D., and N.G.; Formal analysis, L.P., C.M., P.W., M.D., and N.G.; Investigation, L.P., C.M., J.T., L.M., and N.G.; Resources, L.P., C.M., J.T., L.M., M.D., and N.G.; Data curation, L.P., C.M., P.W., J.T., L.M., M.D., and N.G.; Writing—original draft preparation, L.P.; Writing—review and editing, L.P., C.M., P.W., J.T., L.M., M.D., and N.G.; Visualization, L.P., C.M., P.W., J.T., L.M., M.D., and N.G.; Supervision, M.D. and N.G.; Project administration, L.P., C.M., P.W., J.T., L.M., M.D., and N.G. All authors have read and agreed to the published version of the manuscript.

Funding: This research received no external funding.

Acknowledgments: The authors wish to thank the players and coaches for their participation and cooperation during this study.

Conflicts of Interest: The authors declare no conflict of interest.

References

1. King, D.A.; Hume, P.; Cummins, C.; Pearce, A.; Clark, T.; Foskett, A.; Barnes, M. Match and training injuries in women's rugby union: A systematic review of published studies. *Sports Med.* **2019**, *49*, 1559–1574. [CrossRef] [PubMed]
2. Busbridge, A.R.; Hamlin, M.J.; Jowsey, J.A.; Vanner, M.H.; Olsen, P.D. Running demands of provincial women's rugby union matches in New Zealand. *J. Strength Cond. Res.* **2020**. [CrossRef]
3. Suarez-Arrones, L.; Portillo, J.; Pareja-Blanco, F.; de Villareal, E.S.; Sánchez-Medina, L.; Munguía-Izquierdo, D. Match-play activity profile in elite women's rugby union players. *J. Strength Cond. Res.* **2014**, *28*, 452–458. [CrossRef]
4. Duthie, G.; Pyne, D.B.; Hooper, S. Applied physiology and game analysis of rugby union. *Sports Med.* **2003**, *33*, 973–991. [CrossRef]
5. Zemski, A.J.; Slater, G.J.; Broad, E.M. Body composition characteristics of elite Australian rugby union athletes according to playing position and ethnicity. *J. Sports Sci.* **2015**, *33*, 970–978. [CrossRef]
6. Smart, D.; Hopkins, W.G.; Quarrie, K.L.; Gill, N. The relationship between physical fitness and game behaviours in rugby union players. *Eur. J. Sport Sci.* **2011**, *14*, S8–S17. [CrossRef]
7. Zemski, A.J.; Keating, S.E.; Broad, E.M.; Marsh, D.J.; Hind, K.; Slater, G.J.; March, D.J. Preseason body composition adaptations in elite white and polynesian rugby union athletes. *Int. J. Sport Nutr. Exerc. Metab.* **2019**, *29*, 9–17. [CrossRef]
8. Zemski, A.J.; Keating, S.E.; Broad, E.M.; Slater, G.J. Longitudinal changes in body composition assessed using DXA and surface anthropometry show good agreement in elite rugby union athletes. *Int. J. Sport Nutr. Exerc. Metab.* **2019**, *29*, 24–31. [CrossRef]
9. Zemski, A.J.; Keating, S.E.; Broad, E.M.; Marsh, D.J.; Slater, G.J. Abdominal adiposity distribution in elite rugby union athletes using magnetic resonance imaging. *Sport Sci. Health* **2018**, *15*, 99–107. [CrossRef]
10. Higham, D.; Pyne, D.B.; Anson, J.; Dziedzic, C.; Slater, G.J. Distribution of fat, non-osseous lean and bone mineral mass in international rugby union and rugby sevens players. *Int. J. Sports Med.* **2014**, *35*, 575–582. [CrossRef]
11. Lees, M.; Oldroyd, B.; Jones, B.; Brightmore, A.; O'Hara, J.P.; Barlow, M.J.; Till, K.; Hind, K. Three-compartment body composition changes in professional rugby union players over one competitive season: A team and individualized approach. *J. Clin. Densitom.* **2017**, *20*, 50–57. [CrossRef] [PubMed]
12. Posthumus, L.; MacGregor, C.; Winwood, P.; Darry, K.; Driller, M.W.; Gill, N. Physical and fitness characteristics of elite professional rugby union players. *Sports* **2020**, *8*, 85. [CrossRef] [PubMed]
13. Kirby, W.; Reilly, T. Anthropometric and fitness profiles of elite female rugby union players. In *Science and Football II*; Reilly, T., Clarys, J., Stibbe, A., Eds.; E and FN Spon: London, UK, 1993; pp. 27–30.
14. Hene, N.; Bassett, S.; Andrews, B. Physical fitness profiles of elite women's rugby union players: Physical fitness and training programme. *Afr. J. Phys. Health Educ. Recreat. Danc.* **2011**, *17*, 1–8.

15. Hene, N.M.; Bassett, S. Changes in the physical fitness of elite women's rugby union players over a competition season. *S. Afr. J. Sports Med.* **2013**, *25*, 47–50. [CrossRef]
16. Nyberg, C.; Penpraze, V. Determination of anthropometric and physiological performance measures in elite scottish female rugby union players. *Int. J. Res. Exerc. Physiol.* **2016**, *12*, 10–16.
17. Smart, D.J.; Hopkins, W.G.; Gill, N.D. Differences and changes in the physical characteristics of professional and amateur rugby union players. *J. Strength Cond. Res.* **2013**, *27*, 3033–3044. [CrossRef]
18. Zemski, A.J.; Broad, E.M.; Slater, G.J. Skinfold prediction equations fail to provide an accurate estimate of body composition in elite rugby union athletes of caucasian and polynesian ethnicity. *Int. J. Sport Nutr. Exerc. Metab.* **2018**, *28*, 90–99. [CrossRef]
19. Nana, A.; Slater, G.J.; Stewart, A.D.; Burke, L.M. Methodology review: Using dual-energy X-Ray Absorptiometry (DXA) for the assessment of body composition in athletes and active people. *Int. J. Sport Nutr. Exerc. Metab.* **2015**, *25*, 198–215. [CrossRef]
20. Bilsborough, J.C.; Greenway, K.A.; Opar, D.; Livingstone, S.; Cordy, J.; Coutts, A.J. The accuracy and precision of DXA for assessing body composition in team sport athletes. *J. Sports Sci.* **2014**, *32*, 1821–1828. [CrossRef]
21. Bellver, M.; Del Rio, L.; Jovell, E.; Drobnic, F.; Trilla, A. Bone mineral density and bone mineral content among female elite athletes. *Bone* **2019**, *127*, 393–400. [CrossRef]
22. Jones, B.; Emmonds, S.; Hind, K.; Nicholson, G.; Rutherford, Z.; Till, K. Physical qualities of international female rugby league players by playing position. *J. Strength Cond. Res.* **2016**, *30*, 1333–1340. [CrossRef] [PubMed]
23. Austin, D.; Gabbett, T.J.; Jenkins, D.G. The physical demands of Super 14 rugby union. *J. Sci. Med. Sport* **2011**, *14*, 259–263. [CrossRef]
24. Austin, D.J.; Kelly, S.J. Positional differences in professional rugby league match play through the use of global positioning systems. *J. Strength Cond. Res.* **2013**, *27*, 14–19. [CrossRef] [PubMed]
25. Ziv, G.; Lidor, R. On-field performances of rugby union players—A review. *J. Strength Cond. Res.* **2016**, *30*, 881–892. [CrossRef] [PubMed]
26. Norton, K.; Whittingham, N.; Carter, L.; Kerr, D.; Gore, C.; Marfell-Jones, M. Measurement techniques in anthropometry. *Anthropometrica* **1996**, *1*, 25–75.
27. Lewiecki, E.M.; Binkley, N.; Morgan, S.L.; Shuhart, C.R.; Camargos, B.; Carey, J.J.; Gordon, C.M.; Jankowski, L.G.; Lee, J.-K.; Leslie, W.D. Best practices for dual-energy X-ray absorptiometry measurement and reporting: International society for clinical densitometry guidance. *J. Clin. Densitom.* **2016**, *19*, 127–140. [CrossRef]
28. Nana, A.; Slater, G.J.; Hopkins, W.G.; Halson, S.; Martin, D.T.; West, N.P.; Burke, L.M. Importance of standardized dxa protocol for assessing physique changes in athletes. *Int. J. Sport Nutr. Exerc. Metab.* **2016**, *26*, 259–267. [CrossRef]
29. Cohen, J. *Statistical Power Analysis for the Behavioral Sciences*, 2nd ed.; Lawrence Erlbaum Associates: Hillsdale, NJ, USA, 1988.
30. Barr, M.J.; Newton, R.U.; Sheppard, J.M. Were height and mass related to performance at the 2007 and 2011 Rugby World Cups? *Int. J. Sports Sci. Coach.* **2014**, *9*, 671–680. [CrossRef]
31. Sedeaud, A.; Marc, A.; Schipman, J.; Tafflet, M.; Hager, J.-P.; Toussaint, J.-F. How they won Rugby World Cup through height, mass and collective experience. *Br. J. Sports Med.* **2012**, *46*, 580–584. [CrossRef]
32. Sims, S.T.; Heather, A.K. Myths and Methodologies: Reducing scientific design ambiguity in studies comparing sexes and/or menstrual cycle phases. *Exp. Physiol.* **2018**, *103*, 1309–1317. [CrossRef]
33. Argus, C.K.; Gill, N.; Keogh, J.; Hopkins, W.G.; Beaven, C.M. Effects of a short-term pre-season training programme on the body composition and anaerobic performance of professional rugby union players. *J. Sports Sci.* **2010**, *28*, 679–686. [CrossRef] [PubMed]
34. Black, K.; Hindle, C.; McLay-Cooke, R.; Brown, R.C.; Gibson, C.; Baker, D.F.; Smith, B. Dietary intakes differ by body composition goals: An observational study of professional rugby union players in New Zealand. *Am. J. Mens Health* **2019**, *13*. [CrossRef] [PubMed]
35. Kerr, A.; Slater, G.J.; Byrne, N. Impact of food and fluid intake on technical and biological measurement error in body composition assessment methods in athletes. *Br. J. Nutr.* **2017**, *117*, 591–601. [CrossRef] [PubMed]

International Journal of
Environmental Research and Public Health

MDPI

Article

Grip Strength-Endurance in Ambitious and Recreational Climbers: Does the Strength Decrement Index Serve as a Feasible Measure?

Berit Kristin Labott [1], Steffen Held [2] and Lars Donath [2,*]

1 Institute of Sport Science, Otto-von-Guericke University, Zschokkestr. 32, D-39106 Magdeburg, Germany; berit.labott@ovgu.de

2 Department of Intervention Research in Exercise Training, Institute of Exercise Training and Sport Informatics, German Sport University Cologne, Am Sportpark Müngersdorf 6, D-50933 Cologne, Germany; s.held@dshs-koeln.de

* Correspondence: l.donath@dshs-koeln.de

Received: 13 November 2020; Accepted: 14 December 2020; Published: 19 December 2020

Abstract: The present study investigated the time course of repetitive maximal isometric grip strength, depending on the arm position, laterality (dominant vs. non-dominant side), and climbing level. The intervention aimed to provide a feasible indicator of maximal strength-endurance in climbing. Seventeen recreational (climbing level (CL): 6.8 (SD 0.5) on the Union Internationale des Associations d'Alpinisme (UIAA) metric scale) and eleven ambitious (CL: 8.7 (SD 0.6) UIAA metric scale) climbers (age: 27 (8) years; BMI: 21.6 (1.9) kg/m^2; ape index (arm span divided by body height): 1.05 (0.18); training volume: 2.2 (1.0) h/week). Participants completed maximal isometric handgrip strength (F_{max}) tests in four positions (left and right hand beside the trunk as well as left and right hand above the shoulder) plus twelve repetitive work-relief cycles, lasting 4 and 1 s where isometric strength, heart rate, and perceived exertion were recorded. F_{max} differed between groups in nearly all positions. A large side × position × time × group interaction was observed for repetitive isometric grip strength ($p = 0.009$, $\eta_p^2 = 0.71$). However, subsequent post-hoc tests did not reveal a significant difference between groups during each testing position. Additional correlation analysis between asymmetry and CL showed an inverse relationship for ambitious climbers ($r = -0.71$). In conclusion, the degree of grip strength decline did not relevantly differentiate between ambitious and recreational climbers. Thus, the time course of handgrip strength seems to mainly rely on maximal grip strength during the first contraction.

Keywords: hand; force decline; asymmetry; rock; boulder; power

1. Introduction

Recreational, ambitious, and elite sport climbing has gained notable popularity within the last two decades. A strong Olympic movement with its first recognition by the International Olympic Committee (IOC) in 2007 and the ongoing professionalization of sport climbing call for specific and valid measures to objectify individual performance levels in climbing. Such performance-determining parameters may then serve as relevant outcome measures following a progressively conducted climbing training, e.g., for performance monitoring during the training periods of climbers on various level.

Numerous studies in the past intended to derive and assess the performance parameters of climbing to contribute to a comprehensive sport climbing performance structure. A majority of these predominantly cross-sectional studies investigated, for example, aerobic energy costs [1,2], anthropometric determinants [3], anaerobic capacities of the forearm muscles [4], active and passive recovery [5], fingertip force [6], or work–relief ratio of load application [7].

Handgrip measures were also frequently considered in climbing-specific performance structure models. Although handgrip strength has been frequently regarded as a more general measure of local climbing strength mirroring less climbing-specific demands [8], finger and hand muscle strength testing was repeatedly reported to be the performance-limiting factor during climbing [6]. A review by Saul et al. in this regard underlined that the important elements in climbing are hand and forearm strength and endurance, also finding that handgrip strength is favorable for success in sport elite climbers [9]. Well-trained forearm flexors with high-aerobic capacities are thereby essential for an efficient climbing style [9].

Despite the available body of evidence on sex, age, laterality, and climbing level, climbing-specific relevance of different handgrip measures remain elusive. This is of greater importance because handgrip dynamometry does not reflect the heterogeneity of different hold positions [10] and is not specific enough to reflect performance of elite climbers [11].

Therefore, many efforts have been made to modify handgrip measures while considering climbing-specific hold position [6]. However, none of these studies investigated the left- and right-sided time course of handgrip strength in different positions depending on climbing level during a typical work–relief ratio of climbing as a grip strength-endurance surrogate [7,12].

Therefore, the present study investigated differences in maximal handgrip strength and handgrip strength-endurance in two groups of the dominant and non-dominant side during various arm–hand positions. The hypothesis is that the handgrip strength decline differs between ambitious and recreational climbers. The hypothesis was that the force decline is steeper and the maximal grip strength is lower in recreational compared to ambitious climbers. Thus, the intention of this study was to provide data on the time course of grip strength values depending on climbing level and arm position.

2. Materials and Methods

2.1. Participants

Twenty-eight right-handed young adult sport climbers were included in this study (Table 1). None of the participants reported any acute or chronic cardio-circulatory or metabolic diseases, health complaints, or previous injury. After a comprehensive study instruction, all subjects signed an informed consent to the study. The experimental setting of the study complied with the Declaration of Helsinki 2013. As the data were collected within standard handgrip screening, an ethical approval was obtained from the ethical committee of the German Sports university (127/2020). All included subjects practiced indoor sports climbing for at least one year. As a climbing-specific anthropometric measure, the ape index was calculated as arm span divided by body height [13]. Thereby, the largest tip-to-tip distance between the extended fingers was measured as arm span. Data were collected during upright stance. Climbing level was reported as the best redpoint ascent (complete ascent without falling with previously available information/inspections of the route) within the current year. A climbing level of 8.0 of the Union Internationale des Associations d'Alpinisme (UIAA) metric scale [14] was required to be allocated to the ambitious group.

Table 1. Anthropometric data of the included subjects.

Variable	Recreational (n = 17)	Ambitious (n = 11)	Total (n = 28)
Sex (f/m)	3/14	0/11	3/25
Age (years)	25.1 ± 7.4	30.6 ± 8.2	27.2 ± 8.0
Body mass (kg)	70.2 ± 9.2	72.2 ± 8.2	71.4 ± 8.8
Height (m)	1.78 ± 0.05	1.81 ± 0.09	1.79 ± 0.07
BMI (kg/m^2)	21.5 ± 2.0	21.8 ± 1.9	21.6 ± 1.9
Ape index	1.06 ± 0.23	1.01 ± 0.03	1.05 ± 0.18
Climbing level (UIAA metric)	6.8 ± 0.5 ***	8.7 ± 0.6	7.6 ± 1.0
Training frequency (times/week)	2.0 ± 0.9	2.5 ± 1.1	2.2 ± 1.0

BMI, body mass index; data are indicated as mean ± standard deviation (SD). Statistical significance level was, as intended, only present for the climbing level ($p < 0.001$ ***).

2.2. Testing

Before conducting the handgrip measures, the use of the 6–20-point rating of perceived exertion (RPE) Borg scale was introduced [15], and a heart rate monitor (Accurex Plus®, Polar Electro Oy, Kempele, Finland) was attached via a dampened chest strap. By performing some practice trials and hand mobilisations, all participants were able to familiarize themselves with the hydraulic handgrip dynamometer (Saehan®, Masan, Korea). The handgrip position had to be comfortable and the fingers needed to fully surround the device so that all the tips of the fingers were on one side [16]. The order of the four arm positions for handgrip testing was inter-individually randomly assigned.

Testing Positions

In total, four testing positions were applied, two testing positions with the left and two testing positions with the right hand from a seated position: upper arm straight beside the trunk, without abduction or rotation and with an elbow angle of 90°; and, lifted arm position, 90° abducted and 90° external rotation (Figure 1). As mentioned in the testing paragraph, the order of the arm positions was random.

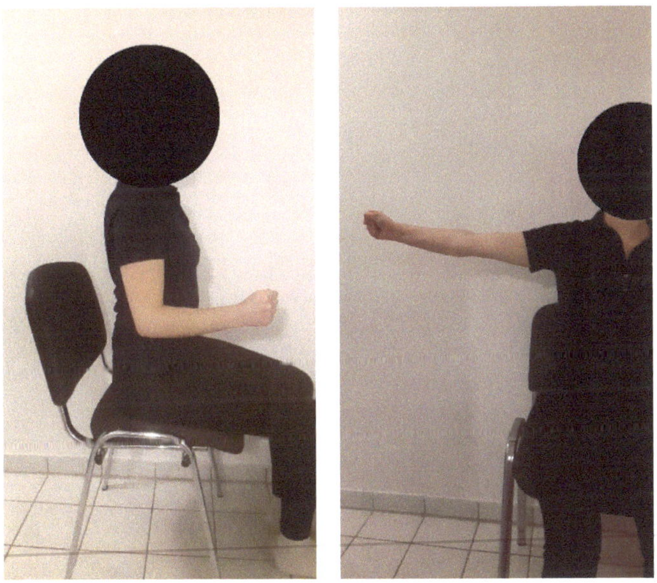

(a) (b)

Figure 1. Visualization of testing positions (here demonstrated for the right hand): (**a**) upper arm straight beside the trunk, without abduction or rotation and with an elbow angle of 90°; (**b**) lifted arm position, 90° abducted and 90° external rotation.

Two sets of the four positions were allowed. The four positions were tested one after the other. A 5 min break between each testing position was guaranteed. Then, all testing positions were measured a second time. Between the first and second rounds of testing, a complete break of 10 min was provided. The best trial of each position was included in further analysis. Before the repetitive strength endurance testing started, maximal isometric handgrip strength was assessed in each of the respective four arm positions. Then, each strength-endurance attempt consisted of 12 consecutive work–relief cycles with maximal effort. In accordance with a climbing-specific strain character, the work period lasted four seconds and the relief phase lasted one second [7]. An acoustic signal indicated the work and relief pattern. Verbal encouragement during the work period was also given by shouting out "go, go, go, go". Relief was initiated by commanding "relax". Work and relief periods alternated. The analogue gauge needle amplitude of the handgrip device was recorded by a 100 Hz sampling digital video camera (HandyCam DCR-DVD 201E PAL, Sony, Tokyo, Japan).

2.3. Statistical Analysis

The highest peak value within the four second work period was analysed. Force values of the handgrip device are provided in kilograms. The relative force values were adjusted to the individual's bodyweight in kilograms. Before and after the twelve repetitions, heartrate increases were recorded during each of the four positions. RPE levels were requested after the final repetition. As a measure of handgrip strength-endurance, the strength decrement index (SDI) was assessed according to Jones et al. [17]. Therefore, the first three ($mean_{first}$) and last three ($mean_{last}$) work phases were separately averaged. Then, the percentage decline of handgrip strength was calculated using the following formula: SDI [%] = $((mean_{first} - mean_{last})/ mean_{first})\cdot 100$.

Statistical analyses were conducted using SPSS 20 (IBM SPSS, Chicago, IL, USA). Data were tested for normal distribution (Kolmogorov–Smirnov test) and homogeneity of variances (Levene test). Demographic baseline data were analysed via multivariate analyses of variances (MANOVA) and follow-up univariate analyses for each parameter.

Differences between the left and right side of the upper and lower hold positions were calculated for maximal grip strength, SDI, and RPE. Therefore, separately 2 (group: recreational vs. ambitious) × 2 (side: left vs. right) repeated measures analyses of variances (rANOVA) were conducted for the upper and lower hold positions.

Concerning the consecutive time course of maximal grip strength, a complex rANOVA was performed. Thereby, a 2 (side: left vs. right) × 2 (position: upper hold vs. lower hold) × 12 (time: 12 grip strength cycles) was calculated. Tukey's honestly significant difference (HSD) post-hoc tests were applied in case of significant main and interaction effects. This procedure was analogously conducted for heartrate analysis.

Spearman correlation coefficients were calculated between the difference in the right and left side (degree of asymmetry level) during the upper and lower position for recreational and ambitious climbers separately.

To estimate the corresponding main or interaction effect sizes, partial eta squares (η_p^2) were additionally calculated. Thereby, $\eta_p^2 \geq 0.01$ indicates a small effect, $\eta_p^2 \geq 0.059$ a medium effect, and $\eta_p^2 \geq 0.138$ a large effect [18]. Cohen's d effect sizes were provided for pairwise comparison (trivial: $d < 0.2$, small: $0.2 \leq d < 0.5$, moderate: $0.5 \leq d < 0.8$, large $d \geq 0.8$) [19].

3. Results

3.1. Relative Force

A significant main effect of the factor side was found for both grip positions (lower grip positions: $F_{1,26} = 22.7$, $p < 0.001$, $\eta_p^2 = 0.47$, upper grip positions: $F_{1,26} = 11.4$, $p = 0.002$, $\eta_p^2 = 0.30$) with higher consecutive strength values on the dominant (right) side. Irrespective of the time course, a side × group interaction effect with a large effect size was found only for lower grip positions ($F_{1,26} = 4.6$, $p < 0.04$, $\eta_p^2 = 0.15$). Post-hoc testing for the interaction effect revealed significant differences between the left and right side for both the ambitious (left: 0.76 kg (SD 0.09) vs. right: 0.86 (0.08), $p = 0.01$) and recreation groups (left: 0.69 kg/kg bodyweight (SD 0.12) vs. right: 0.74 (0.09), $p = 0.04$). The upper grip position did not significantly differ for the ambitious (left: 0.74 (SD 0.10) vs. right: 0.84 (0.08), $p = 0.11$) and the recreation groups (left: 0.71 (SD 0.09) vs. right: 0.75 (0.11), $p = 0.34$). (Figure 2).

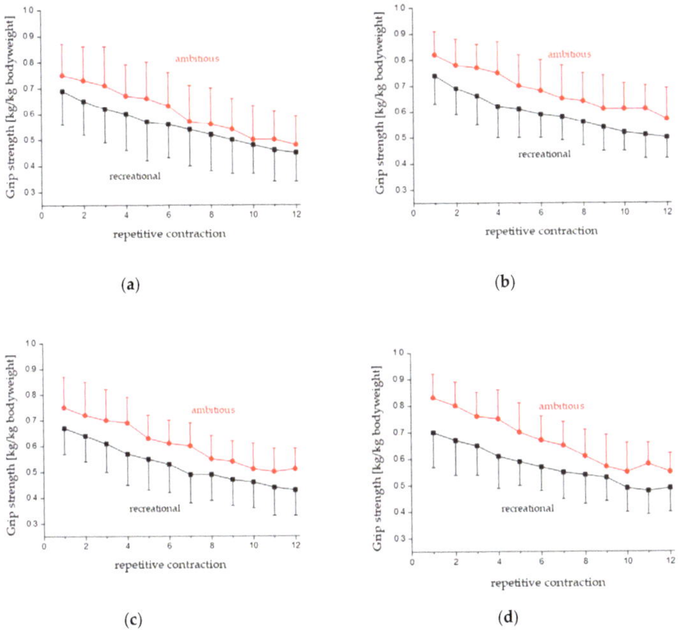

Figure 2. Relative force decline (kg/kg bodyweight) within the 12 repetitive contractions for ambitious (circles) and recreational (squares) climbers during the upper grip positions on the left (**a**) and right (**b**) side as well as the lower positions left (**c**) and right (**d**).

With notably high effect sizes, significant side effects with higher values on the dominant (right) side ($F_{1,26} = 41.5$, $p < 0.001$, $\eta_p{}^2 = 0.62$) and time effects ($F_{1,26} = 44.6$, $p < 0.001$, $\eta_p{}^2 = 0.97$) were found for the relative force decline (Figure 2). However, interaction effects were not observed ($p > 0.45$).

3.2. Strength Decrement Index (SDI)

Concerning percentage SDI, a side effect with a lower strength decline was only observed for the upper grip positions ($F_{1,\,26} = 7.4$, $p = 0.01$, $\eta_p{}^2 = 0.22$). The lower grip position did not reveal a side effect ($F_{1,\,26} = 0.28$, $p = 0.60$, $\eta_p{}^2 = 0.01$) (Figure 3c,d). Group x side interactions were not observed ($p > 0.32$). Pairwise Cohen's d effect sizes indicated merely a small effect ($0.15 < d < 0.47$).

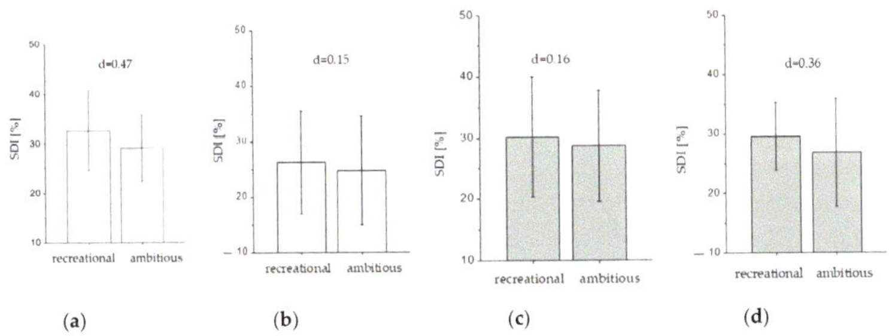

Figure 3. Strength decrement index (SDI) in percent for recreational and ambitious climbers during the upper grip positions on the left (**a**) and right (**b**) side as well as the lower position left (**c**) and right (**d**). Cohen's d was provided as a measure of effect size estimation between groups for each position (trivial: $d < 0.2$, small: $0.2 \leq d < 0.5$, moderate: $0.5 \leq d < 0.8$, large $d \geq 0.8$).

3.3. Asymmetry Levels

When comparing asymmetry levels between the left and right side for the upper and lower handgrip position, weak and non-significant inverse correlations were found for recreational climbers (low position, r = −0.05; $p = 0.67$, upper position, r = −0.31; $p = 0.13$). In contrast, a moderate and significant correlation was found between lower position asymmetry levels in ambitious climbers (r = −0.70; $p = 0.03$). For the upper position, a weak and non-significant correlation, similar to the recreational climbers, was found (r = −0.30; $p = 0.21$).

3.4. Heartrate

With a significant time × group interaction effect ($F1,26 = 6.51$, $p = 0.017$, $\eta_p{}^2 = 0.20$), heartrates only increased differently between groups from the 1st to the 12th consecutive handgrip trial during the left-sided position bottom beside the body (ambitious, pre: 91 min−1 (SD 19) to post: 106 (24); recreational, pre: 91 (21) to post: 124 (32)). All other positions showed solely a time effect ($p < 0.001$) but no group × time interactions ($0.23 < p < 0.76$).

3.5. Perceived Exertion

No significant side × position × group interaction was found for subjective perceived exertion levels after the 12 consecutive trials ($F4,23 = 0.40$, $p = 0.53$, $\eta_p{}^2 = 0.015$). Post exercise, RPE values increased to: left-sided, bottom recreational: 13.8 (SD 1.5); ambitious: 14.6 (2.1), $p > 0.05$; left-sided, top recreational: 14.5 (SD 1.6); ambitious: 15.5 (1.4), $p = 0.43$; right-sided, bottom recreational: 14.9 (SD 2.5); ambitious: 14.7 (1.9), $p = 0.73$; and right-sided, top recreational: 14.2 (SD 2.1); ambitious: 14.8 (1.9), $p = 0.56$.

4. Discussion

The hypothesis that handgrip decline varies with climbing level can be refuted. To the best of our knowledge, for the first time the present study investigated time-series data of maximal isometric handgrip strength within a climbing-specific work–relief cycle in recreational and ambitious climbers. Thereby, different arm–hand positions for the left and right side were compared in both groups. Mainly maximal isometric handgrip strength differed between the dominant (right) and non-dominant hand as well as between ambitious and recreational climbers in nearly all testing positions. Percentage decrease in grip strength following repetitive maximal grip contractions did not differentiate between groups, though it did between the left and right side for the upper position. Perceived exertion levels and heartrate response did not relevantly differ between groups, sides, or positions.

Compared to age-related norm values of grip strength in younger [20] and middle-aged adults [21], climbers of both levels in the present study showed notably higher absolute maximal grip strength values (at least >15%). With higher force values on the dominant side, the occurring side difference of maximal handgrip is fairly in line with previous findings [22]. However, it has been previously observed that the amount of difference between the left and right side tend to decrease from recreational to elite climbers [23]. Disappearance of asymmetry level has been attributed to a more symmetric load application induced by the training of elite climbers. A more symmetric load application in better climbers during an axial-symmetric climbing tour was corroborative found previously [7]. Interestingly, the present study also revealed that the better climbers showed less pronounced grip strength asymmetry between the left and right side.

Although ambitious climbers showed consistently higher grip strength values compared to the recreational climbers at each contraction cycle, grip strength-endurance capacity did not reveal notable group differences. It seemed more likely that climbing level is mainly determined by maximal isometric strength capacity. Since a comparatively higher maximal strength led to enhanced neuromuscular function, type 2a fiber recruitment and movement economy, it seems also plausible to assume that higher local maximal strength capacities also trigger higher local endurance performance [24] throughout the training process. This is of more importance, since climbing can be regarded as a clear maximal-strength-endurance sport discipline [1,23,25]. Concerning the relationship between maximal grip strength and grip strength-endurance, concordant observations have been made over the last years in healthy young subjects [13,26,27]. These findings might, thus, be transferable to climbers. From a training-related point of view, it appears to be required to first develop a high amount of local maximal strength in climbing-specific muscles (for grip strength, the brachioradialis muscles and the musculus flexor digitorum superficialis) with a subsequent endurance-specific emphasis. As boulder athletes showed higher maximal voluntary contraction (MVC) forces and rate of force development (RFD) compared to climbers [28], high intensity boulder exercises may serve as an appropriate training routine to enhance maximal strength. Endurance capacity can then be trained by extending the required time frames of climbing.

Regarding heartrate and perceived exertion levels, no relevant differences between groups have been observed. Interestingly, the non-dominant (left) lower position led to a steeper increase in heartrate in recreational climbers than in ambitious climbers from the beginning to the end of the twelve repetitive contractions. This specific finding might be attributed to a less pronounced intermittent recovery of the left-hand side of the recreational group. However, this assumption cannot be addressed with certainty within the present approach. Due to the high relative strength demands of both groups, the perceived exertion level did not differ. It seems of interest whether a certain sub-maximal climbing tour (e.g., two degrees below the maximal climbing level) would lead to differences in perceived exertion level between recreational and ambitious climbers.

Limitations

Some limitations need to be addressed. The threshold between ambitious and recreational climbers can be regarded as arbitrary. The assignment to the groups was conducted according to previous investigations [7]. Additionally, the sample size of groups differed and was lower for the more trained climbers. No statistical differences of training frequencies were found. Thus, the total training volume did not differ adequately between recreational and ambitious climbers. The applied handgrip dynamometer was not able to record the force–time kinetics for each contraction. A comparison of the force–time integral between both groups was not feasible. It could have been likely that the repetitive peak values occurred at the beginning, the middle, or the end of the 4 s contraction. To better distinguish between different force kinetics, future research should focus on the force–time relationship.

5. Conclusions

Maximal grip strength clearly distinguished between recreational and ambitious climbers independent of arm position during repetitive maximal grip strength cycles. The percentage decrease in maximal grip strength is not an adequate measure of climbing specific strength-endurance capacity. Since side differences occurred in all outcome measures, maximal grip strength and grip strength-endurance sufficiently address asymmetry level in climbing. Despite asymmetry level being difficult to measure in climbing, it is unclear whether grip strength asymmetry persists in climbing-related testing tasks. The exercise position of handgrip did not relevantly differentiate between groups. Future research should focus on increasing maximal grip strength as a basic performance requirement after climbing versus boulder exercises. Strength-endurance should be better tested employing climbing specific tests. Grip strength tests should also focus on a comprehensive strength testing approach, considering different hold shapes.

Practical Applications

Maximal grip strength is feasibly applicable to differentiate between ambitious and recreational climbers. Compared to recreational climbers, disappearing handgrip asymmetry might indicate better climbers. The strength decrement index (SDI) does not appropriately reflect grip strength-endurance in climbers, and repetitive strength decline mainly depends on maximal strength. However, the SDI and repetitive strength testing should be mandatorily employed in a therapeutic and diagnostic setting after hand injuries.

Author Contributions: Conceptualization, L.D.; study conduction, L.D.; manuscript drafting and revising, S.H. and B.K.L. All authors have read and agreed to the published version of the manuscript.

Funding: This research received no external funding.

Acknowledgments: We appreciatively acknowledge all participants who enthusiastically took part in the present study.

Conflicts of Interest: The authors declare no conflict of interest.

References

1. Billat, V.L.; Palleja, P.; Charlaix, T.; Rizzardo, P.; Janel, N. Energy specificity of rock climbing and aerobic capacity in competitive sport rock climbers. *J. Sports Med. Phys. Fit.* **1995**, *35*, 20–24.
2. Booth, J.; Marino, F.; Hill, C.; Gwinn, T. Energy cost of sport rock climbing in elite performers. *Br. J. Sports Med.* **1999**, *33*, 14–18. [CrossRef] [PubMed]
3. Mermier, C.M.; Janot, J.M.; Parker, D.L.; Swan, J.G. Physiological and anthropometric determinants of sport climbing performance. *Br. J. Sports Med.* **2000**, *34*, 359–365. [CrossRef]
4. Schoffl, V.R.; Mockel, F.; Kostermeyer, G.; Roloff, I.; Küpper, T. Development of a performance diagnosis of the anaerobic strength endurance of the forearm flexor muscles in sport climbing. *Int. J. Sports Med.* **2006**, *27*, 205–211. [CrossRef]
5. Watts, P.B.; Daggett, M.; Gallagher, P.; Wilkins, B. Metabolic response during sport rock climbing and the effects of active versus passive recovery. *Int. J. Sports Med.* **2000**, *21*, 185–190. [CrossRef] [PubMed]
6. Quaine, F.; Vigouroux, L. Maximal resultant four fingertip force and fatigue of the extrinsic muscles of the hand in different sport climbing finger grips. *Int. J. Sports Med.* **2004**, *25*, 634–637. [CrossRef] [PubMed]
7. Donath, L.; Rösner, K.; Schöffl, V.; Gabriel, H.H.W. Work-relief ratios and imbalances of load application in sport climbing: Another link to overuse-induced injuries? *Scand. J. Med. Sci. Sports* **2011**, *23*, 406–414. [CrossRef]
8. Cutis, A.; Bollen, S.R. Grip strength and endurance in rock climbers. *Proc. Inst. Mech. Eng. H* **1993**, *207*, 87–92.
9. Saul, D.; Steinmetz, G.; Lehmann, W.; Schilling, A.F. Determinants for success in climbing: A systematic review. *J. Exerc. Sci. Fit.* **2019**, *17*, 91–100. [CrossRef]
10. Draper, N.; Dickson, T.; Blackwell, G.; Priestley, S.; Fryer, S.; Marshall, H.; Shearman, J.; Hamlin, M.; Winter, D.; Ellis, G. Sport-specific power assessment for rock climbing. *J. Sports Med. Phys. Fit.* **2011**, *51*, 417–425.
11. Ozimek, M.; Staszkiewicz, R.; Rokowski, R.; Stanula, A. Analysis of tests evaluating sport climbers' strength and isometric endurance. *J. Hum. Kinet.* **2020**, *53*, 249–260. [CrossRef] [PubMed]
12. White, D.J.; Olsen, P.D. A time motion analysis of bouldering style competitive rock climbing. *J. Strength Cond. Res.* **2010**, *24*, 1356–1360. [CrossRef] [PubMed]
13. Watts, P.B.; Martin, D.T.; Durtschi, S. Anthropometric profiles of elite male and female competitive sport rock climbers. *J. Sports Sci.* **1993**, *11*, 113–117. [CrossRef] [PubMed]
14. Schoffl, V.; Morrison, A.; Hefti, U.; Ullrich, S.; Küpper, T. The UIAA Medical Commission injury classification for mountaineering and climbing sports. *Wilderness Environ. Med.* **2011**, *22*, 46–51. [CrossRef]
15. Borg, G. *Perceived Exertion and Pain Scales*; Human Kinetics: Champaign, IL, USA, 1998.
16. Trampisch, U.S.; Franke, J.; Jedamzik, N.; Hinrichs, T.; Platen, P. Optimal Jamar dynamometer handle position to assess maximal isometric hand grip strength in epidemiological studies. *J. Hand Surg.* **2012**, *37*, 2368–2373. [CrossRef]
17. Jones, D.W.; Robertson, L.D.; Figoni, S.F. A strength-endurance index for power grip. *J. Occup. Rehabil.* **2009**, *19*, 56–63. [CrossRef]
18. Cohen, J. *Statistical Power Analysis for the Behavior Sciences*; Lawrence Erlbaum Associates: Hillsdale, NJ, USA, 1988.
19. Cohen, J. A power primer. *Psychol. Bull.* **1992**, *112*, 155–159. [CrossRef]
20. Montalcini, T.; Migliaccio, V.; Yvelise, F.; Rotundo, S.; Mazza, E.; Liberato, A.; Pujia, A. Reference values for handgrip strength in young people of both sexes. *Endocrine* **2012**, *43*, 342–345. [CrossRef]
21. Budziareck, M.B.; Duarte, R.R.P.; Barbosa-Silva, M.C. Reference values and determinants for handgrip strength in healthy subjects. *Clin. Nutr.* **2008**, *27*, 357–362.

22. Giles, L.V.; Rhodes, E.C.; Taunton, J.E. The physiology of rock climbing. *Sports Med.* **2006**, *36*, 529–545. [CrossRef]
23. Grant, S.; Hynes, V.; Whittaker, A.; Aitchison, T. Anthropometric, strength, endurance and flexibility characteristics of elite and recreational climbers. *J. Sports Sci.* **1996**, *14*, 301–309. [CrossRef] [PubMed]
24. Aagaard, P.; Andersen, J.L. Effects of strength training on endurance capacity in top-level endurance athletes. *Scand. J. Med. Sci. Sports* **2010**, *20*, 39–47. [CrossRef] [PubMed]
25. Sheel, A.W. Physiology of sport rock climbing. *Br. J. Sports Med.* **2004**, *38*, 355–359. [CrossRef] [PubMed]
26. Burke, W.E.; Tuttle, W.W.; Thompson, C.W.; Janney, C.D.; Weber, R.J. The relation of grip strength and grip-strength endurance to age. *J. Appl. Physiol.* **1953**, *5*, 628–630.
27. Tuttle, W.W.; Janney, C.D.; Thompson, C.W. Relation of maximum grip strength to grip strength endurance. *J. Appl. Physiol.* **1950**, *2*, 663–670. [CrossRef]
28. Fanchini, M.; Violette, F.; Impellizzeri, F.M.; Maffiuletti, N.A. Differences in Climbing-Specific Strength between Boulder and Lead Rock Climbers. *J. Strength Cond. Res.* **2012**, *27*, 310–314. [CrossRef]

International Journal of
Environmental Research and Public Health

MDPI

Article

Muscle Tone and Body Weight Predict Uphill Race Time in Amateur Trail Runners

César Berzosa, Héctor Gutierrez *, Pablo Jesús Bascuas, Irela Arbones and Ana Vanessa Bataller-Cervero

Facultad de Ciencias de la Salud, Universidad San Jorge, Autov. A-23 Zaragoza-Huesca, km 299, 50830 Villanueva de Gállego, Zaragoza, Spain; cberzosa@usj.es (C.B.); pbascuas@usj.es (P.J.B.); iarbones@usj.es (I.A.); avbataller@usj.es (A.V.B.-C.)
* Correspondence: hgutierrez@usj.es

Abstract: Background: Vertical kilometer is an emerging sport where athletes continuously run uphill. The aims of this study were to assess changes in vertical impacts caused by uphill running (UR) and the relation between the anthropometric and lower limb muscular characteristics with speed. Methods: Ten male experienced runners (35 ± 7 years old) participated in this study. In the racetrack (4.2 km long, 565 m high), seven sections were stablished. Mean speed and impact value of sections with similar slope (≈21%) were calculated. The gastrocnemius stiffness (GS) and tone (GT); and the vastus lateralis stiffness (VS) and tone (VT) were assessed before the race. Results: Pearson's correlation showed a linear relationship between vs. and VT (r = 0.829; p = 0.000), GT and GS (r = 0.792; p = 0.001). Mean speed is correlated with weight (r = −0.619; p = 0.024) and GT (r = 0.739; p = 0.004). Multiple linear regressions showed a model with weight and GT as dependent variables of mean speed. Mean impacts decreased significantly between sections along the race. Conclusions: The vertical impacts during UR were attenuated during the race. Moreover, body weight and GT were associated with the time-to-finish, which supports that low weight alone could not be enough to be faster, and strength training of plantar flexors may be a determinant in UR.

Keywords: fatigue; vertical impacts; stiffness; GPS

Citation: Berzosa, C.; Gutierrez, H.; Bascuas, P.J.; Arbones, I.; Bataller-Cervero, A.V. Muscle Tone and Body Weight Predict Uphill Race Time in Amateur Trail Runners. *Int. J. Environ. Res. Public Health* **2021**, *18*, 2040. https://doi.org/10.3390/ijerph18042040

Academic Editor: Shaher A.I. Shalfawi

Received: 14 January 2021
Accepted: 16 February 2021
Published: 19 February 2021

1. Introduction

Trail running or mountain running is a sport that has become very popular in the last years, and the research associated with this long run discipline has also increased [1–4]. One of the modalities of trail running is the vertical kilometer, where the whole track is uphill. In this type of event, athletes must complete an uphill route of 1 km vertical elevation increase. In addition, a minimum average of 20% positive slope must exist and one or more sections of 5% positive slope of the total distance race must be included. Regarding the length and type of terrain, the maximum length must be 5 km and the terrain can vary between different races [5].

Uphill running is a very demanding activity. The athlete must perform positive mechanical power in order to displace their body upward against gravity. This generated mechanical power increases with increasing slope.

Compared to level running, in uphill running, due to the lower limb position, hip joint muscles increase their work, whereas the work of knee and ankle remains similar than in level running [6]. The use of elastic energy also changes during uphill running. While most of the energy stored in tendons is recovered in level running [7], running uphill with steeper slopes entails the necessity of raising the center of mass, causing an increase in the positive network generated by the body, considering that the elastic energy stored cannot be used due to the increase in ground contact time. Analyzing the mechanical efficiency, previous studies have proven than uphill runners show around 25% of efficiency, this value corresponds only to muscle contraction [8,9]. Uphill running cost could explain running performance because this parameter differs from level running. Balducci et al.

(2016) [10] studied the influence of stride length, stride frequency, and body mass index, and no correlation was found between these parameters with the cost of uphill running compared to level running. Nevertheless, influence of these anthropometric measures was not studied directly in uphill runners. For example, body weight has been shown to be a predictor in the performance of marathon runners [11] and it seems plausible that this factor also influences the performance of a modality in which it is necessary to raise your body on every step.

During running, the foot strikes the ground decelerating the body to zero and generating large ground reaction forces (GRF) [12]. Step by step, impacts are transmitted through the musculoskeletal system. Both passive and active mechanisms act in order to attenuate the shock, minimizing the damage. Although running impacts do not reach extreme values, the quantity of running impacts can be significant. Impact peak is very sensitive to leg stiffness and the damping effect of foot (pads) and leg [13].On one hand, the impacts received by the body in each step are attenuated by the bone bending, heel pads, and intervertebral discs as passive dampers; on the other hand, lower limb muscles work actively in order to absorb the impacts.

In order to assess running impact acceleration magnitude, several methods could be used, one of them is the tibial acceleration peak, assessed through the placement of an accelerometer in the shank [14], whose value is approximately 8 g [15]. Another method could be accelerometry measurement in the sacrum, presenting smaller values [16]. Through these measurements, the role of active and passive mechanisms to reduce the impact received during running from the shank to the head could be determined [17].

Several studies have analyzed the effect of fatigue on impacts, but their results have not offered a clear conclusion [18]. The possible cause of these discrepancies may be the existence of differences in the way of assessing running impacts between studies. Research articles that have analyzed the ground reaction forces disagree on the effect that fatigue has on running impacts [19], finding both increases [20] and decreases [21], and offering different explanations for it. The rise could be explained by an increased lower limb stiffness [22]. In addition, another study found a correlation between the pre-activation of gastrocnemius and GRF [23]. The regulation of the lower limb stiffness and the reduced storage of elastic energy could be a possible explanation for the decrease in GRF due to fatigue [24].

Researchers that measured the impacts with accelerometers found an increase in peak impact due to fatigue [25]. The different strategies used to face the fatigue could influence the responses. In long-distance runners, the global fatigue increases the impacts as well as the local fatigue due to the muscle activity imbalance [26]. Changes in lower limb stiffness can also have an influence in peak accelerations [14] as well as running technique. Crowell and Davis (2011) [27] found a relationship between running technique and the impacts.

The objective of this study was to assess the relationship between anthropometric and the lower limb muscular characteristics with speed, and to analyze the changes in vertical impacts caused by uphill running.

2. Materials and Methods

2.1. Participants

Ten male recreationally trained runners participated in the study (age 35 $\pm$ 7 years old, mass 68.2 $\pm$ 5.3 kg, height 1.77 $\pm$ 0.03 m, BMI 21.6 $\pm$ 1.4 kg/m^2). The inclusion criterion were, at least, one year of experience in trail running races and not suffered from lower limb injuries in the last three months. All the subjects were participants in the uphill race "TurrónSkyrace Pico Las Calmas", celebrated in Arguis, Huesca (Spain). The participants signed a written consent previous tothe data collection and this study was approved by the Ethics Committee of the University. All procedures followed the Declaration of Helsinki on the use of human subjects.

2.2. Procedure

The uphill race was 4.2 km long and had a 565 m positive slope. In this time-trial race, the runners started to run every 30 s and attempted to complete the racetrack as quickly as possible. In the racetrack, seven sections were distinguished, defined by six control points (Figure 1). For each section, the mean speed of the runners was calculated from the time in each control point and the official distance track. The GPS device was synchronized to the official race start time by means of the detection of the first change in velocity after a long period of standing.

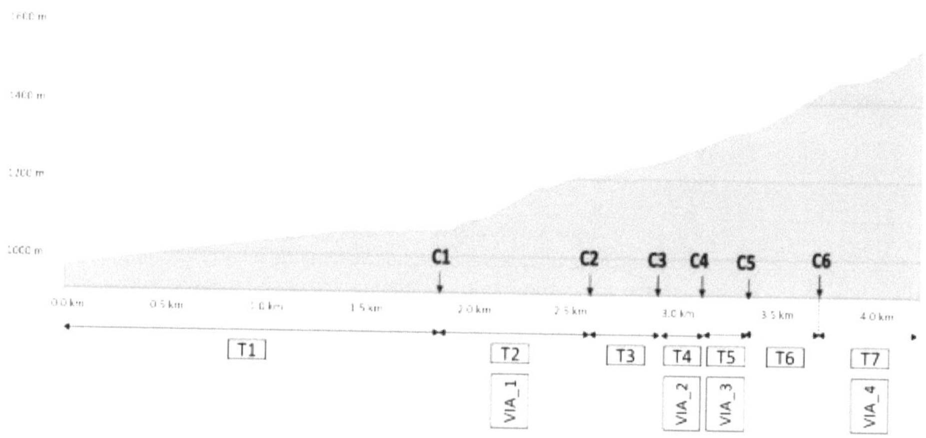

Figure 1. Track of the race with control points (C1–C6), sections (T1–T7), and vertical impact acceleration (VIA_1-VIA_4).

The measurements of the skeletal muscle tone and stiffness were taken in a tent provided by the organizer, near the race start zone.

2.3. Measurements

Muscle stiffness and tone were collected in lying position (both prone and supine position depending on the muscle evaluated) by a hand-held myometer (Myoton-Pro, Myoton AS, Tallinn, Estonia). Surface Electromyography for the Non-Invasive Assessment Muscle (SENIAM) guidelines [28] were followed to draw on the skin at the testing locations. Medial head of gastrocnemius (MG), lateral head of gastrocnemius (LG), vastus lateralis (VL) tone and stiffness were analyzed in the relaxed position. The probe of the Myoton-Pro was placed perpendicular to the skeletal muscle surface in each measurement. Five consecutive measurements were taken at each site, giving the mean stiffness in N/m and the mean tone measured in Hz [29].To ensure validity of the data, a measurement with a coefficient of variation fewer than 3% was accepted, and any measurement above this value was rejected and measured again. The Myoton-Pro offers good to excellent test-retest reliability for lower body tone and stiffness assessment [30].

Muscle tone is calculated using the following formula:

$$F = fmax \tag{1}$$

Muscle stiffness is calculated using the following formula:

$$S = \frac{amax \times mprobe}{\Delta l} \tag{2}$$

Raw data were grouped together in order to mitigate the effect of the asymmetries between both limbs (left and right) and to consider possible synergies between muscles (the medial and lateral gastrocnemius, the vastus medialis, and lateralis). Four parameters of the participants' muscle mechanical properties emerged out of this procedure: the gastrocnemius muscle stiffness (GS), the gastrocnemius muscle tone (GT), the vastus lateralis stiffness (VS), and the vastus lateralis tone (VT). Body weight was assessed using a Tanita BC-1000 scale.

The runners wore a vest during the race with a pocket located in the back (at the height of vertebrae C7) where an Apex GPS device (STATSport Group, Newry, Ireland, UK) was placed. This device includes a 18 Hz GPS and 100 Hz accelerometer in three axes, 100 Hz gyroscope, and 10 Hz magnetometer.

The accelerometer signal of the first 30 s of every race section was evaluated in a custom MAATLAB routine (The Mathworks Inc, Natick, MA, USA) in order to analyze the vertical impact acceleration (VIA) in each slope section. The magnitude of the accelerometer signal was low-pass filtered with a fourth order Butterworth filter with a cut-off frequency of 10 [16]. The mean value of the 15 first peaks, corresponding to the first 15 steps was calculated [31]. The mean impacts of sections with similar slope were compared in order to check the fatigue effect changes on the impact magnitude as a marker of fatigue. In this way, Sections 2, 4, 5, and 7 (Table 1) were analyzed (VIA_1, VIA_2, VIA_3, VIA_4, respectively).

Table 1. Slope and horizontal distance of every section of the race besides the type of surface.

	T1	T2	T3	T4	T5	T6	T7
Distance (m)	1800	800	250	200	220	390	380
Slope (%)	11	22	11	20	21	34	23
Terrain	Track	Canyon	Path	Path	Path	Path	Track/path

Aside from the impacts, the mean speed (MS) of each section was obtained from the GPS devices' software (Apex Software, STATSport Group, Newry, Ireland, UK).

2.4. Statistical Analysis

Statistical analyses were performed using SPSS version 21.0 for Windows (SPSS Inc., Chicago, IL, USA). Descriptive statistics mean, standard deviation (SD), lower 95% confidence limit (LCIL95%) and upper 95% confidence limit (UCIL95%) were calculated for weight, mean speed, VIA, GS, VS, GT, and VT. Normality of datasets was checked with the Shapiro–Wilk test. Pearson's correlation was calculated and used to determine lineal relationships between all measures.

A repeated measures one-way ANOVA were performed to compare VIA along the race (VIA_1, VIA_2, VIA_3, VIA_4) for all participants. The W de Mauchly test was used as sphericity criteria. Regression model (lineal, quadratic or cubic) with the highest order among all those that presented statistical significance was considered as the ideal model [32]. Eta square value (η^2) was used for effect size calculation. Bonferroni's post-hoc procedure was applied to locate pair-wise differences [33].

Multiple linear regressions were calculated using a "stepwise" method. Mean speed was considered the dependent variable and weight, VIA, GS, VS, GT, and VT as possible independent variables. Entry and exit criteria were an F probability greater than 0.05 and 0.10, respectively. Residual linearity and independence assumptions were checked with the Durbin–Watson test; values between 1 and 3 in the Durbin–Watson test were considered an acceptable criterion. Homoscedasticity was studied in a standardized residual-standardized prediction plot. Normality of residuals was checked with the Shapiro–Wilk test. Multicollinearity was estimated by a variance inflation factor (VIF), values greater than 10 were considered as excessive multicollinearity. Cases with Cook's distance greater than 1 were indicated as influential cases and removed fromthe data analysis [34].

All tests were performed with a level of significance of $p < 0.05$.

3. Results

A summary of the descriptive statistics of the sample can be studied in Table 2.

Table 2. Descriptive statistics of the participants. Standard deviation (SD), lower 95% confidence limit (LCIL95%); upper 95% confidence limit (UCIL95%), vertical impact acceleration (VIA),mean speed (MS), finishing time (min), gastrocnemius stiffness (GS), gastrocnemius tone (GT), vastus lateralis stiffness (VS), vastus lateralis tone (VT).

N = 13	Mean	SD	LCIL 95%	UCIL 95%	*p*
MS (m/s)	1.81	0.30	1.63	1.98	0.168
Weight (kg)	68.85	4.79	65.95	71.74	0.140
Finishing Time(min)	37.2	6.20	33.45	40.95	0.168
VIA_1 (9.8 m/s^2)	2.77	0.34	2.57	2.97	0.570
VIA_2 (9.8 m/s^2)	2.34	0.34	2.14	2.54	0.299
VIA_3 (9.8 m/s^2)	2.08	0.41	1.83	2.33	0.099
VIA_4 (9.8 m/s^2)	1.88	0.32	1.69	2.07	0.099
VT (Hz)	14.80	1.71	13.77	15.84	0.787
GT (Hz)	15.65	1.01	15.04	16.26	0.945
VS (N/m^2)	284.87	28.42	267.69	302.04	0.267
GS (N/m^2)	280.38	15.09	271.26	289.50	0.211

Pearson's correlation (Table 3) showed a linear relationship between VT and vs. (r = 0.829; p = 0.000), and GT and GS (r = 0.792; p = 0.001). Furthermore, mean speed was correlated with weight (r = −0.619; p =0.024) and GT (r = 0.739; p = 0.004).

Table 3. Pearson's correlation calculated to determine lineal relationships between all measures. Vertical impact acceleration (VIA), mean speed (MS) (m/s), gastrocnemius stiffness (GS) (N/m^2), gastrocnemius tone (GT) (Hz), vastus lateralis stiffness (VS) (N/m^2), vastus lateralis tone (VT) (Hz)* $p < 0.05$; ** $p < 0.01$.

	Weight	VIA_1	VIA_2	VIA_3	VIA_4	GT	VT	GS	VS
MS	−0.619 *	0.169	0.198	0.200	0.041	0.739 **	0.006	0.483	0.231
Weight		−0.288	−0.485	−0.370	−0.484	−0.279	0.063	−0.030	−0.095
VIA_1			0.423	−0.114	0.256	0.031	0.035	−0.201	0.162
VIA_2				0.113	0.113	0.106	0.460	−0.354	0.365
VIA_3					0.544	0.233	0.082	0.248	−0.010
VIA_4						−0.117	−0.432	0.021	−0.450
GT							0.265	0.792 **	0.356
VT								−0.008	0.829 **
GS									0.104

Variables included in the repeated measures one-way ANOVA showed an adequate sphericity (W de Mauchly = 0.546; p = 0.263). Only a linear model presented statistical significance (p = 0.000). Quadratic (p = 0.193) and cubic (p = 0.758) could not be considered. The effect size of the time factor over vertical impact acceleration was η^2 = 0.621. Bonferroni's post-hoc procedure revealed mean differences (MD) statistically significant between VIA_1 toVIA_2 (MD = 0.429; p = 0.006), VIA_1 to VIA_3 (MD = 0.688; p = 0.005), VIA_1 to VIA_4 (MD = 0.891; p = 0.000), andVIA_2 toVIA_4 (MD = 0.462; p = 0.015). These differences can be observed in Figure 2.

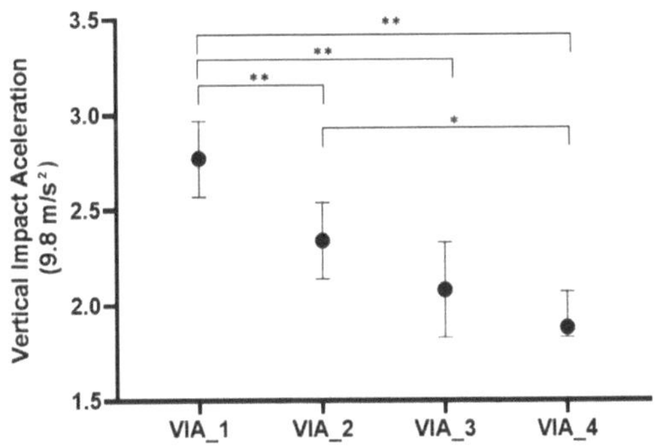

Figure 2. Vertical impact acceleration in four consecutive sectors with a similar slope of a vertical race. VIA: Vertical impact acceleration. * $p < 0.05$; ** $p < 0.01$ in Bonferroni's post-hoc test.

Multiple linear regressions showed a model with weight and GT as dependent variables of mean speed (Equation (3)). This model presented a R^2 = 0.732 and an adjusted R^2 = 0.678 (p = 0.025). Model predictive capacity was statistically significant (p =0.001). The model's coefficients were statistically significant (A = 0.179, p = 0.05; B = −0.028, p = 0.025); however, the model's constant was not (C = 0.907, p = 0.468).Standardized coefficients were A_{beta} = 0.615 and B_{beta} = -0.448,respectively.

$$MS = 0.179 \times GT - 0.028 \times weight + 0.907 \quad (3)$$

A Durbin–Watson test value of 2496 confirmed residual linearity and independence assumption. The standardized residual–standardized prediction plot did not show any relationship confirming homoscedasticity. The Shapiro–Wilk test confirmed normality of the residuals (p = 0.221). Multicollinearity between the dependent variables was not observed (VIF = 1.084). Excessive influential cases were not observed (max Cook's distance = 0.819; min Cook's distance = 0.004).

4. Discussion

The main objective of this study was to analyze the relationship between anthropometric and muscular characteristics of the lower limb with the speed in an uphill running race, while the second aim was to assess changes in the vertical impacts caused by uphill running. The main findings of this study were as follows: (1) There was a positive correlation in mean speed and gastrocnemius muscle tone and between tone and stiffness of leg and thigh muscles, and (2) a progressive decrease in vertical impacts along the race was observed.

In addition, an inverse correlation between race speed and weight was found. It has been observed that faster athletes weighed less. According to that, a study with marathon runners showed that race speed was correlated with body fat, but not with the total weight [11]. Contrary to what happens in level races, uphill runners have to raise their own weight step by step, which could explain these controversial results.

According to the multivariate model including weight and gastrocnemius tone, 68% of the variance in race speed could be explained. This finding suggests the importance of these variables in uphill running performance, although other parameters as metabolic values (e.g., oxygen uptake) [35] or tone of different muscles (e.g., gluteus maximus) [36] could be very important and explain part of the other 27% of the variance in race times. The predicted race speeds were explained by only two variables (weight and GT), showing a strong predictive capacity ($p = 0.001$) and $R^2 = 0.73$ with the real registered race times. This equation should be validated in a different group of participants and could be applied only to runners with the same characteristics (age, gender, years of experience, and training status).

Weight is the first of the parameters to consider in these types of races. It could seem obvious that, if you must lift your body to the top of a mountain, the smaller your weight, the faster you are. Saunders et al. (2004) [37] found an inverse correlation between running economy and body weight, with the lightest runners also being the most economical. Pate et al. (1992) [38] studied several variables (physiological, anthropometric, and training load) and their relationship to running economy, showing that the lightest runners were the fastest. Running economy is a key factor in running performance, obtaining better race times, as has been reported in this study. However, another study observed that there was no relationship between these aspects [11,39,40]. Perhaps this disagreement could be due to the differences in the level of body fat of runners. Lower levels of body fat are a variable predictive of running performance in terms of running speed [11] or performance in treadmill tests [41].

The gastrocnemius muscle tone is the second of the variables included in the predictive model. It is the only parameter of the muscle properties that fit in the multivariate regression analysis, although other parameters are clearly related to it. In this way, the GT and GS are significantly correlated as well as the VT and VS. All these facts could be explained, at least partially, because there is a higher ankle joint moment and a decrease in the knee moment associated with increasing slope [6]. The higher moment in ankle joint is mainly produced by gastrocnemius muscle action, and it is in accordance with the correlation found between gastrocnemius muscle tone and mean velocity during the running race segments analyzed. In another study, it was also described that stiffness is important in activities like jumping or sprinting [29], and according to the results found, it could also be important during uphill running. As previously mentioned, there is a positive correlation between muscle tone and stiffness, both in gastrocnemius and vastus medialis. Maybe training muscle tone and stiffness through strength training could be beneficial in order to improve uphill running performance.

Related to strength training, it could also be important in order to increase the attenuation of VIA along the race when comparing sectors with similar slopes. These results are quite interesting and suggest that during uphill running, the neuromuscular behavior is similar to previous studies [18]. Other studies have shown increases or similar vertical impacts and Zadpoor and A Nikooyan (2012) [19] concluded in their review that no significant changes could be found in ground reaction forces due to fatigue during running, although they reported studies that showed increases and decreases in GRF. It is also interesting that while level running increases vertical impacts possibly because of the change to rearfoot running strike pattern [25], in our study, VIA is attenuated while the running race is going on. These results are similar in both fast and slow athletes, so VIA attenuation is not related to race speed as could be thought, and the reduction in vertical impacts is common, so more studies should be performed to clarify this aspect. In our study, a slower speed in T2 (related to VIA1) was also observed than in T4 and T5 (related to VIA2 and 3). This could be explained due to the characteristics of the terrain as T2 is a canyon, while T3 and T4 are paths and are easier terrain to run.

5. Conclusions

In conclusion, the vertical impacts generated during uphill running are attenuated during the race, maybe because of the fatigue accumulated and the running technique changes linked to it. Even more, body weight and gastrocnemius tone were associated with the time-to-finish during an uphill running race in amateur athletes. It supports the idea that a greater muscle tone in ankle plantar flexors and a low body weight are determinant to achieve performance in these kinds of trail running races. Low body weight alone could not be enough to reach a faster race time, maybe accompanying body weight control with a strength training program focused on plantar flexors, emphasizing the eccentric and plyometric work to increase muscle stiffness may be determinant in uphill running.

Author Contributions: Conceptualization, A.V.B.-C. and C.B.; Methodology, A.V.B.-C. and C.B.; Performed experiments, P.J.B., A.V.B.-C., I.A., and C.B.; Formal analysis, H.G., A.V.B.-C., and C.B.; Investigation, P.J.B., H.G., and C.B.; Resources, P.J.B., H.G., and C.B.; Data curation, P.J.B., H.G., and C.B.; Writing—original draft preparation, H.G. and C.B.; Writing—review and editing, P.J.B., A.V.B.-C., I.A., and C.B. All authors have read and agreed to the published version of the manuscript.

Funding: This research received no external funding.

Institutional Review Board Statement: The study was conducted according to the guidelines of the Declaration of Helsinki, and approved by the Ethics Committee of the University.

Informed Consent Statement: Informed consent was obtained from all subjects involved in the study. Written informed consent was obtained from the patients to publish this paper.

Data Availability Statement: The data presented in this study are available on request from the corresponding author. The data are not publicly available due to legal and privacy issues.

Acknowledgments: This work was supported by the Operative Program ERDF Aragon 2014-2020, "Building Europe from Aragon", Research Group ValorA, under grant no. S08_20R, and by Fondo Social Europeo "Construyendo Europa desde Aragón.

Conflicts of Interest: The authors declare that the research was conducted in the absence of any commercial or financial relationships that could be construed as potential conflicts of interest.

References

1. Balducci, P.; Clémençon, M.; Trama, R.; Blache, Y.; Hautier, C. Performance Factors in a Mountain Ultramarathon. *Int. J. Sports Med.* **2017**, *38*, 819–826. [CrossRef] [PubMed]
2. Vernillo, G.; Savoldelli, A.; Skafidas, S.; Zignoli, A.; La Torre, A.; Pellegrini, B.; Giardini, G.; Trabucchi, P.; Millet, G.P.; Schena, F. An Extreme Mountain Ultra-Marathon Decreases the Cost of Uphill Walking and Running. *Front. Physiol.* **2016**, *7*. [CrossRef]
3. Vernillo, G.; Savoldelli, A.; Zignoli, A.; Skafidas, S.; Fornasiero, A.; La Torre, A.; Bortolan, L.; Pellegrini, B.; Schena, F. Energy cost and kinematics of level, uphill and downhill running: Fatigue-induced changes after a mountain ultramarathon. *J. Sports Sci.* **2015**, *33*, 1998–2005. [CrossRef]
4. Millet, G.Y.; Tomazin, K.; Verges, S.; Vincent, C.; Bonnefoy, R.; Boisson, R.-C.; Gergelé, L.; Féasson, L.; Martin, V. Neuromuscular Consequences of an Extreme Mountain Ultra-Marathon. Tarnopolsky M, editor. *PLoS ONE* **2011**, *6*, e17059. [CrossRef]
5. International Skyrunning Federation Rules. Available online: http://www.skyrunning.com (accessed on 6 February 2021).
6. Roberts, T.J.; Belliveau, R.A. Sources of mechanical power for uphill running in humans. *J Exp. Biol.* **2005**, *208*, 1963–1970. [CrossRef]
7. Snyder, K.L.; Kram, R.; Gottschall, J.S. The role of elastic energy storage and recovery in downhill and uphill running. *J. Exp. Biol.* **2012**, *215*, 2283–2287. [CrossRef] [PubMed]
8. Margaria, R.; Cerretelli, P.; Aghemo, P.; Sassi, G. Energy cost of running. *J Appl. Physiol.* **1963**, *18*, 367–370. [CrossRef]
9. Minetti, A.E.; Ardigò, L.P.; Saibene, F. Mechanical determinants of the minimum energy cost of gradient running in humans. *J. Exp. Biol.* **1994**, *195*, 211–225.
10. Balducci, P.; Clémençon, M.; Morel, B.; Quiniou, G.; Saboul, D.; Hautier, C.A. Comparison of level and graded treadmill tests to evaluate endurance mountain runners. *J. Sports Sci. Med.* **2016**, *15*, 239–246.
11. Barandun, U.; Knechtle, B.; Knechtle, P.; Klipstein, A.; Rüst, C.A.; Rosemann, T.; Lepers, R.; Knechtle, P. Running speed during training and percent body fat predict race time in recreational male marathoners. *J. Sports Med.* **2012**, *3*, 51–58.
12. Whittle, M.W. Generation and attenuation of transient impulsive forces beneath the foot: A review. *Gait Posture.* **1999**, *10*, 264–275. [CrossRef]
13. Heise, G.D.; Martin, P.E. "Leg spring" characteristics and the aerobic demand of running. *Med. Sci. Sports Exerc.* **1998**, *30*, 750–754. [CrossRef]

14. Sheerin, K.R.; Reid, D.; Besier, T.F. The measurement of tibial acceleration in runners: A review of the factors that can affect tibial acceleration during running and evidence-based guidelines for its use. *Gait Posture* **2019**, *67*, 12–24. [CrossRef] [PubMed]
15. Valiant, G.A. Transmission and attenuation of heel-strike accelerations. In *Biomech. Distance Run*; Human Kinetics Books: Champaign, IL, USA, 1990; pp. 225–248.
16. Wundersitz, D.W.T.; Gastin, P.B.; Richter, C.; Robertson, S.J.; Netto, K.J. Validity of a trunk-mounted accelerometer to assess peak accelerations during walking, jogging and running. *Eur. J. Sport Sci.* **2015**, *15*, 382–390. [CrossRef] [PubMed]
17. Shorten, M.R.; Winslow, D.S. Spectral analysis of impact shock during running. *J. Appl. Biomech.* **1992**, *8*, 288–304. [CrossRef]
18. Dickinson, J.A.; Cook, S.D.; Leinhardt, T.M. The measurement of shock waves following heel strike while running. *J. Biomech.* **1985**, *18*, 415–422. [CrossRef]
19. Zadpoor, A.; ANikooyan, A. The effects of lower-extremity muscle fatigue on the vertical ground reaction force: A meta-analysis. *P I MECH ENG H.* **2012**, *226*, 579–588. [CrossRef]
20. Christina, K.; White, S.; McCrory, J. The effects of dorsiflexor fatigue on kinetic measures during running. In Proceedings of the NACOB'98: The Third North American Congress on Biomechanics, Canadian Society for Biomechanics, Waterloo, ON, Canada, 14–18 August 1998; pp. 311–312.
21. Brüggemann, G.-P.; Arndt, A.; Kersting, U.; Knicker, A. Influence of fatigue on impact forces and rear foot motion during running. In Proceedings of the XVth congress of the International Society of Biomechanics, Jyväskylä, Finland, 2–6 July 1995; pp. 132–133.
22. Nicol, C.; Komi, P.; Marconnet, P. Fatigue effects of marathon running on neuromuscular performance. *Scand J. Med. Sci. Sports* **2007**, *1*, 10–17. [CrossRef]
23. Komi, P.V.; Gollhofer, A.; Schmidtbleicher, D.; Frick, U. Interaction between man and shoe in running: Considerations for a more comprehensive measurement approach. *Int. J. Sports Med.* **1987**, *8*, 196–202. [CrossRef]
24. James, C.R.; Scheuermann, B.W.; Smith, M.P. Effects of two neuromuscular fatigue protocols on landing performance. *J. Electromyogr. Kinesiol.* **2010**, *20*, 667–675. [CrossRef]
25. Verbitsky, O.; Mizrahi, J.; Voloshin, A.; Treiger, J.; Isakov, E. Shock transmission and fatigue in human running. *J. Appl. Biomech.* **1998**, *14*, 300–311. [CrossRef] [PubMed]
26. Mizrahi, J.; Voloshin, A.; Russek, D.; Verbitsky, O.; Isakov, E. The influence of fatigue on EMG and impact acceleration in running. *BAM* **1997**, *7*, 111–118.
27. Crowell, H.P.; Davis, I.S. Gait retraining to reduce lower extremity loading in runners. *Clin. Biomech.* **2011**, *26*, 78–83. [CrossRef] [PubMed]
28. Hermens, H.J.; Freriks, B.; Disselhorst-Klug, C.; Rau, G. Development of recommendations for SEMG sensors and sensor placement procedures. *J. ElectromyogrKinesiol.* **2000**, *10*, 361–374. [CrossRef]
29. Pruyn, E.C.; Watsford, M.; Murphy, A. The relationship between lower-body stiffness and dynamic performance. *Appl. Physiol. Nutr. Metab.* **2014**, *39*, 1144–1150. [CrossRef]
30. Bizzini, M.; Mannion, A.F. Reliability of a new, hand-held device for assessing skeletal muscle stiffness. *Clin. Biomech.* **2003**, *18*, 459–461. [CrossRef]
31. Boey, H.; Aeles, J.; Schütte, K.; Vanwanseele, B. The effect of three surface conditions, speed and running experience on vertical acceleration of the tibia during running. *Sports Biomech.* **2017**, *16*, 166–176. [CrossRef] [PubMed]
32. Park, E.; Cho, M.; Ki, C.-S. Correct use of repeated measures analysis of variance. *Korean J. Lab. Med.* **2009**, *29*, 1–9. [CrossRef]
33. Zghal, F.; Colson, S.S.; Blain, G.; Behm, D.G.; Granacher, U.; Chaouachi, A. Combined resistance and plyometric training is more effective than plyometric training alone for improving physical fitness of pubertal soccer players. *Front Physiol.* **2019**, *10*, 1026. [CrossRef]
34. Hammami, M.; Hermassi, S.; Gaamouri, N.; Aloui, G.; Comfort, P.; Shephard, R.J.; Chelly, M.S. Field tests of performance and their relationship to age and anthropometric parameters in adolescent handball players. *Front Physiol.* **2019**, *10*, 1124. [CrossRef]
35. Rüst, C.A.; Knechtle, B.; Knechtle, P.; Barandun, U.; Lepers, R.; Rosemann, T. Predictor variables for a half marathon race time in recreational male runners. *J. Sports Med.* **2011**, *2*, 113–119.
36. Lieberman, D.E.; Raichlen, D.A.; Pontzer, H.; Bramble, D.M.; Cutright-Smith, E. The human gluteus maximus and its role in running. *J. Exp. Biol.* **2006**, *209*, 2143–2155. [CrossRef] [PubMed]
37. Saunders, P.U.; Pyne, D.B.; Telford, R.D.; Hawley, J.A. Factors affecting running economy in trained distance runners. *Sports Med.* **2004**, *34*, 465–485. [CrossRef]
38. Pate, R.R.; Macera, C.A.; Bailey, S.P.; Bartoli, W.P.; Powell, K.E. Physiological, anthropometric, and training correlates of running economy. *Med. Sci. Sports Exerc.* **1992**, *24*, 1128–1133. [CrossRef]
39. Knechtle, B.; Knechtle, P.; Rosemann, T. Race Performance in Male Mountain Ultra-Marathoners: Anthropometry or Training? *Percept Mot. Skills* **2010**, *110*, 721–735. [CrossRef]
40. Tanda, G.; Knechtle, B. Marathon performance in relation to body fat percentage and training indices in recreational male runners. *J. Sports Med.* **2013**, *4*, 141–149.
41. Hetland, M.L.; Haarbo, J.; Christiansen, C. Regional body composition determined by dual-energy x-ray absorptiometry. Relation to Training, Sex Hormones, and serum lipids in male long-distance runners. *Scand. J. Med Sci. Spor.* **1998**, *8*, 102–108. [CrossRef] [PubMed]

International Journal of
Environmental Research and Public Health

MDPI

Article

Factors Related to the Performance of Elite Young Sailors in a Regatta: Spatial Orientation, Age and Experience

Israel Caraballo [1,2], Alejandro Lara-Bocanegra [3,*] and M. Rocío Bohórquez [4]

1 GALENO Research Group, Department of Physical Education, Faculty of Education Sciences, University of Cádiz, Cádiz, 11519 Puerto Real, Spain; israel.caraballo@uca.es
2 Research Unit, Biomedical Research and Innovation Institute of Cádiz (INiBICA), 11519 Puerto Real, Spain
3 Department of Physical Activity and Sport, Faculty of Education, University of Seville, 41013 Seville, Spain
4 Department of Social Psychology, Faculty of Psychology, University of Seville, 41013 Seville, Spain; rociobohorquez@us.es
* Correspondence: alejandrolarboc@us.es

Abstract: The objective of this study was to examine the role of spatial orientation in the performance of sport sailors. Participants were 30 elite male sailors from classes 420, Laser, Windsurfing RS:X and Windsurfing Techno, grouped into two categories: Monohull (18 sailors) and Windsurfing (12 sailors). Ages ranged between 13 and 18 years old (M = 15.7, SD = 1.05). To assess spatial orientation, the Perspective Taking/Spatial Orientation Test was used, and performance was inferred from the final classification at the regatta. In addition, the influence of experience and age on the performance was analyzed. The results show that in the Monohull group, the performance is determined by the spatial orientation (18% of the explained variance), while in the Windsurfing group, the variables that are related to performance are sailing experience and age (60% of the explained variance). Spatial orientation seems to be the more important variable for performance in the Monohull group, while in classes belonging to the Windsurfing group, this variable does not seem to be decisive for obtaining good results in the regatta.

Keywords: spatial orientation; performance; sport sailing; special ability

Citation: Caraballo, I.; Lara-Bocanegra, A.; Bohórquez, M.R. Factors Related to the Performance of Elite Young Sailors in a Regatta: Spatial Orientation, Age and Experience. *Int. J. Environ. Res. Public Health* **2021**, *18*, 2913. https://doi.org/10.3390/ijerph18062913

Academic Editor: Shaher A. I. Shalfawi

Received: 3 March 2021
Accepted: 9 March 2021
Published: 12 March 2021

1. Introduction

Research in sports science has been extensively concerned with the study of the factors that influence performance in the different sports modalities. At present, the most developed lines of research in sailing are the influence of physiological, anthropometric, biomechanical, and training factors [1].

Sports performance is also determined by psychological training, so that, through the evaluation of psychological skills in the athlete, it is possible to predict their potential for success [2,3]. According to Olmedilla, Ortega, González and Serpa [4], sailing is a complex sport and psychological skills are key in learning this sport discipline. Authors such as Araújo, Davids and Serpa [5] or Brandt, Da Silva, Segato and Andrade [6] state that the most important psychological skills in this sport are attention span and decision making, and both skills are directly related to navigation tactics. Studies such as those carried out by Araújo and Serpa [7], Manzanares [8], and Manzanares, Menayo and Segado [9] show that elite sailors have a better visualization capacity and a greater number of fixations in relevant stimuli compared to amateur sailors. These two characteristics allow them to reduce the time taken to obtain relevant information, so they increase their chances to place themselves in optimal places, both at the exits and during the journey made [7–9]. In sport sailing, including all types of boats, perceptual skills are highly required, and this is mainly due to its high complexity. The sailor must anticipate his rivals and capture as much information as possible from them to carry out the most appropriate actions according to each circumstance [10]. The ability of anticipation seems to be a fundamental element within sports sailing because the environment in which it develops is characterized by being highly unstable. This instability is produced both by the weather conditions and by the different actions carried out by opponents. It must be taken into account that the sailor obtains the information to orient himself in a dynamic way; in addition, competitors become a dynamic reference because they are also at continuous movement, and buoys are the only static referents, making the action of orientation even more complex [11]. The sources of information that will determine the sailor's orientation are the virtual representation of their position in space (rival sailors and buoys) and the cognitive map [12]. Through the cognitive map, the sailor is able to internally construct the context that surrounds him, thus being able to anticipate everything that is outside his visual field; this allows a more correct programming of the route to be followed [13]. Authors like Gómez, Rousset and Baciu [14] and Montello [15] affirm that a continuous updating of the spatial information received from the environment is necessary, because it allows the subject to be aware of their current position at all times. While the subject performs the task, the orientation process is automatic, but when the information is updated, the effort made by the athlete increases [16].

For Maier [17] the main components of spatial ability are spatial rotations, spatial perception, spatial visualization, mental rotation and spatial orientation. In spatial rotation, the reference frame used can be intrinsic or relative to an object; this frame of reference is defined by the upper/lower, anterior/posterior and right/left intrinsic axes [18].

Spatial perception, the information processing approach, has mainly been used to analyze spatial skills on a small scale; these skills use the speed of encoding and transformation of spatial information, memory capacity and spatial work strategies as differentiation elements [19,20]. Spatial visualization is more complex than relationship or orientation tasks; this circumstance occurs because the tasks that comprise it have a spatial figurative component in which movement or displacement of the figure's elements occurs [21]. Mental rotation is defined as the ability to rotate figures quickly and accurately in the mind [22]. Spatial orientation refers to the subject's ability to have a different perspective on an object when the observer is redirected [23]. Different systems for evaluating spatial ability have been used, although the most widespread are those that differentiate between large-scale and small-scale spatial abilities proposed by Ittelson [24], and endorsed and specified by Voyer, Voyer and Bryden [25]. Despite this differentiated classification, research demonstrates that small-scale spatial abilities predict performance on large-scale tasks, because spatial abilities at different scales are partially but not totally dissociated [26–28].

Spatial orientation—a large-scale ability—is the most commonly used component for the evaluation of spatial ability and is considered the most important component [29,30]. The literature on spatial orientation often differentiates between egocentric and allocentric representations, also called exocentric or geocentric [31]: egocentric representations are self-to-object-centered, while the allocentric anchor on environmental information uses object-to-object references. Recent studies have shown that both are related, since egocentric sensory information can be transformed into allocentric representations [32]; specifically, some studies affirm that the performance of the subjects in orientation capacity, in relation to the different elements that surround them, are related to the score they obtain in perspective-taking tasks [33,34]. For various tasks, navigators profit from both kinds of representation [35].

Regarding to experience, small differences in time of practice can make a huge difference, as is well known in the expertise literature [36,37]. The influence on performance of a multitude of personal (time of practice, physiognomy), social (influence of third parties) and contextual (culture, access to practice) factors has been postulated. Specifically, athletic preparation is capable of developing spatial ability [38], so athletes with more experience are able to extract critical information from a greater number of spatial references than novices [39]. Specifically, sailing experience has proven to be decisive for the development of strength, resistance and speed-oriented motor coordination and, therefore, for better sports performance [1,40,41]. In this sense, but in relation to psychological variables, experienced sailor decision-making is characterized by the cumulative non-linear effects of exploring and using information constraints in a regatta, making their performance better than the less experienced sailors [5]. Regarding the indicators of attention management, the time of recurrence of the fixation of the gaze is less in the less experienced sailors, whether they are relevant or irrelevant stimuli for the regatta [42]. Related to spatial ability, experience was shown to significantly influence performance in specific tests [43].

Age has not always been shown to generate differences in the spatial skills of the general population: sometimes, it has been postulated as a consequence of experience in different tasks or contexts [44], while, other times, it has been pointed out that the maturation of evolutionary development generates differences in spatial ability [45]. Those authors who propose that age influences the development of spatial orientation skills only because of its relationship with experience demonstrated that experts, unlike novices, showed a progression towards the extraction of more information early as a function of age [38,39], although it was only at the adult level that the anticipatory performance of the expert players significantly outperformed that of their novice counterparts (Abernethy). On the other hand, other authors have postulated a direct effect of age on the development of spatial orientation: the literature suggests that 3- to 10-year-old children develop their ability to combine egocentric and allocentric forms of spatial coding, and show adult-level performance on cognitive mapping tasks at around 10 or 12 years of age [45,46]. Regarding the decline in spatial orientation skills, some studies found that adults between 46 and 67 years of age performed worse than younger participants (18–30 or 31–45 years) in all the orientation skills evaluated [47], while other investigations pointed out that the egocentric spatial orientation progressively improves from 8 to 60 years old [48]. To our knowledge, the relationship between age and performance in spatial orientation tasks hasn't been studied with sport sailors.

Following what has been developed in the literature, the main objective of this study is to verify whether spatial orientation, experience and age are related to the performance of the sailors in a regatta. The following hypotheses emerge from this objective:

Hypothesis 1 (H1). *The better the spatial orientation of the sailors, the better performance they will obtain in competition.*

Hypothesis 2 (H2). *The more years of sailing experience, the better performance sailors will obtain in competition.*

Hypothesis 3 (H3). *The age of the sailors will not allow predicting their performance in competition.*

2. Materials and Methods

2.1. Participants

The investigation involved 30 elite sailors belonging to classes 420, Laser, Windsurfing RS:X and Windsurfing Techno which took part of the competition circuit of the Andalusian Sailing Federation (Spain) and participated regularly in national and international competitions. All sailors were male and their ages ranged from 13 to 18 years (M = 15.70, SD = 1.06). Regarding their sportive experience, they have been sailing between 2 and 11 years (M = 6.50, SD = 2.78).

2.2. Instruments

A sociodemographic questionnaire was designed including questions related to age, sex, class to which they belonged and years of experience in sailing.

The test designed by Kozhevinikov and Hegarty [21] was used to evaluate spatial orientation, as a modified version of Hegarty and Waller [23]. It includes 12 items in paper and pencil format (Figure 1). Each reactive is composed of a matrix with seven objects and a circle in which one direction is marked; participants should imagine their position in the circle and mark the direction towards one of the seven objects determined in the question.

The result of each question is calculated by the absolute deviation in degrees between the response of the participant and the correct address of the assigned object. Each reactive may be scored between 0 and 180°. To obtain the final score, the average deviation of the 12 items must be calculated. The items that were not answered were assigned a value of 90°. To finish the test, there is a maximum time of five minutes. The established reliability for this test was 0.83 in its original formulation [49].

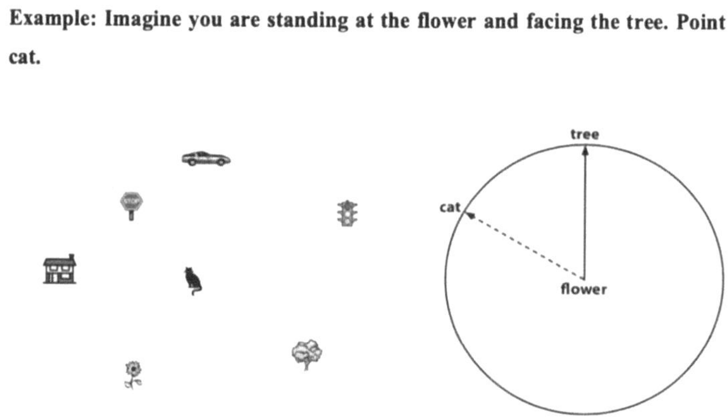

Figure 1. Spatial orientation test.

2.3. Procedure

Two weeks before the competition, the Andalusian Sailing Federation and the coaches of the different sailing clubs that participated in the regatta were contacted and informed about the objectives of the study, and invited to participate voluntarily. The day before the competition, a room was set up at the headquarters of the Andalusian Sailing Federation in which the tests were realized.

All sailors who participated voluntarily in this study had to sign an authorization form. Participants under 18 also required authorization from their parents and/or guardians by signing informed consent.

2.4. Regatta

To assess the performance, results from the final ranking at the XV New Year´s Race "X Memorial Kim Lythgoe" were used [50]. The ranking was determined with the sum of the positions obtained in each of the tests, in which a better classification meant a lower result in the final ranking. The race was held at the headquarters of the Specialized Center for Sailing Sports Technification "Bahía de Cádiz" from 27–30 December 2018. This regatta is of an international category. In the evaluated classes, a total of 83 sailors competed, so the study represents 31% of the total participants in the competition in classes 420 (14 sailors), Laser (38 sailors) and windsurfing (38 sailors). During the competition days, the 420 class made a total of four races and the Laser and Windsurfing classes performed six. In each length of the race, sailors complete a tour that was previously established by the organizing committee.

2.5. Data Analysis

The data obtained were reviewed for outliers and other anomalies; no adjustment or modification of the database was necessary. After that, two groups of sailors were created: classes 420 and Laser were united in a group called Monohull, and classes RS:X and Techno joined the group called Windsurfing. The justification for dividing these boats into two groups is because the boats that belong to each group share a series of similar characteristics in their structure as in their handling; however, these characteristics are totally different from the other group. In addition, the Windsurfing class, due to their characteristics, can develop faster than the monohull group boats; therefore, the way the racecourse is organized is very different between the classes that belong to each group.

Linear regression analyses were performed for Monohull and Windsurfing classes to examine the association between spatial orientation, experience, age and performance. The method used to perform the linear regression analysis was Stepwise in order to find the strongest predictor for ranking. To check the prediction value of the performance of the equations obtained, the Student's *t*-test was performed between the variables' real ranking and predicted ranking with this equation.

3. Results

Descriptive analysis and the results obtained in the spatial orientation test by the sailors of the Monohull and Windsurfing classes are shown in Table 1.

Table 1. Participants' age, experience and score obtained in the Spatial Orientation Test by groups and classes.

	Monohull			Windsurfing		
	All (n = 18)	420 (n = 6)	Laser (n = 12)	All (n = 12)	RS:X (n = 5)	Techno (n = 7)
Sailing experience (years)	7.33 ± 2.35	6.83 ± 1.94	7.58 ± 2.57	5.25 ± 2.99	6.20 ± 3.35	4.57 ± 2.76
Age (years)	15.78 ± 1.22	15.17 ± 0.75	16.08 ± 1.31	15.58 ± 0.79	16.40 ± 0.55	15.00 ± 0.00
Spatial Orientation Test	35.12 ± 22.98	50.03 ± 31.75	27.66 ± 13.25	60.04 ± 50.08	62.86 ± 60.89	58.03 ± 45.98

Note: Data presented in Mean ± SD.

Table 2 shows the linear regression analysis. We obtain a model in one step to find the optimal model, which has a linear relationship of 47% and a goodness of the fit = 0.18. This model includes the constant and the score variable in the spatial orientation test, excluding the navigation experience and age variables. The value of Durbin–Watson (1.51) indicates that our error variance is independent; therefore, it would be appropriate to use a linear model. The multicollinearity analysis shows high tolerance values in the variable spatial orientation test (0.88), the years of navigation experience (0.90) and the age (0.83). These results indicate that these variables do not show collinearity. The equation obtained with this model for the prediction of performance is the following: performance = 20.48 + (−0.20 * orientation test). When checking the value of the prediction of the performance obtained with this equation, using the Student's *t*-test to compare the relationship between the ranking variable and the ranking variable estimated, we observe that the error was −0.01.

Table 2. Coefficients of the linear regression models in Monohull and Windsurfing groups.

Model		Non-Standardized Coefficients	Typified Coefficients		t	Sig.	Confidence Interval 95% for B	
		B	Std. Error	Beta			Lower Bound	Upper Bound
Monohull	Constant	20.48	3.94		5.19	0.00 **	12.12	28.84
	S. O. T.	−0.20	0.09	−0.47	−2.16	0.04 *	−0.40	−0.00
Windsurfing	Constant	−88.19	33.96		−2.59	0.02 *	−163.87	−12.51
	Age	6.25	2.17	0.67	2.87	0.01 *	1.40	11.10
	Constant	−104.68	28.21		−3.71	0.00 **	−168.51	−40.85
	S. E.	−1.23	0.49	−0.50	−2.51	0.03 *	−2.35	−0.12
	Age	7.72	1.85	0.83	4.16	0.00 **	3.53	11.92

Note: S. O. T. = Spatial orientation Test; S. E. = sailing experience. Method used: "Stepwise". ** $p < 0.01$; * $p < 0.5$.

In the linear regression analysis for the Windsurfing group, we obtain two models in two steps and choose Model 2, which has a linear relationship of 82% and a goodness of 0.6 fit (Figure 2). This model excludes the spatial orientation test variable but includes the constant and the navigation experience and age variables of the sailor (Table 2). It would be appropriate to use this model since the value of Durbin–Watson (2.29) indicates that the residuals are independent. The most important variable in this model would be the age, since it contributes 83%, while the navigation experience would contribute 50%. The high tolerance values in the multicollinearity analysis of the variable spatial orientation test (0.95), the years of navigation experience (0.88) and the age (0.861) indicate that there is no collinearity for these variables.

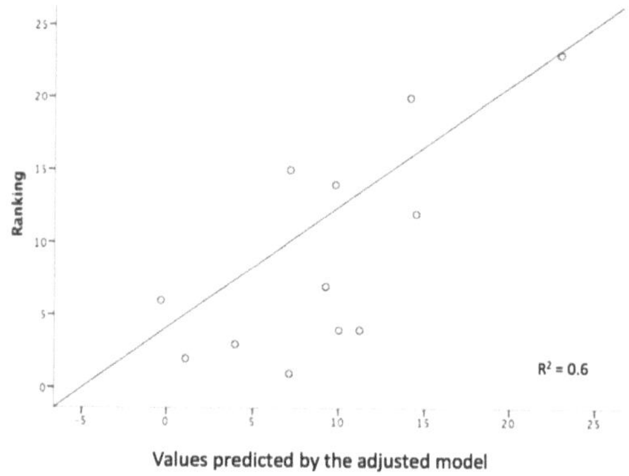

Figure 2. Fitted linear regression graph of model 2 for the Windsurfing group. Method of successive steps. Variables: age and sailing experience.

The equation obtained to predict the performance in the Windsurfing group would be determined as follows: performance = −104.68 + (7.72 * Age) + (−1.23 * Sailing experience). Checking the prediction value of this equation indicates that the error made is very low, its value being 0.00.

4. Discussion

The main objective of this study was to verify whether the spatial orientation, experience and age are related to the performance of the sailor in a regatta. First, it was hypothesized that the better the spatial orientation of the sailors, the better their performance in competition. The results only allow us to partially accept this hypothesis, since the spatial orientation predicted the performance of the sailors of the Monohull group, but not of the Windsurfing group. The correlation between spatial orientation and performance found in Monohull was also described with sailors of the Optimist class by Manzanares [8]. The spatial ability–performance relationship is based on the need of sailors to anticipate the behavior of their rivals [10], as well as the influence of environmental factors at each moment of the regatta [11], aspects directly related to performance in sailing, allowing a competitive advantage to be exploited [7–9]. It is possible to infer that both large- and small-scale spatial skills are involved in the sports behavior of sailors, and that they are closely related to each other [26–28] and to performance in real outdoor tasks [35]. We must also consider that, during the competition, sailors must pay attention to a visual field in motion and this may interfere with the cognitive tasks he is performing. Therefore, if the subject has a good spatial orientation, their attention resources will not be diverted by the movement that occurs in the objects of their visual field, thus they will not lose cognitive resources that attend to postural control and could affect the execution of sports technical gestures [51].

A priori, spatial orientation should be important for both Monohull and Windsurf groups, but our results only confirm its influence on the Monohull group. It is possible that the characteristics of each of these groups, and the navigation peculiarities that characterize them, may explain the differences found between both groups [52]. The sailors of the Windsurfing class, due to the difference between the large size of the sail surface and the reduced length/beam of the boat, perform a specific action after each turn to recover the speed, which is very efficient when the wind speed is less than fifteen knots, and is called rowing with the sail (sail-pumping) [53]. Monohull-type vessels, such as 420 and Laser, do this at very specific times, but, in the windsurfing class, it is done both when it goes against the wind and when it goes upwind, although when it is against the wind the physical demands on the Sailor are higher [54]. Therefore, it is logical to think that the lower the number of maneuvers performed during the tour, the lower the number cognitive demands required. However, we do not have information to ensure those aspects, so future research should address them and other possible hypotheses.

The second hypothesis predicted that the more years of sailing experience, the better sailors' performance in competition. The results prevent us from fully accepting this hypothesis, since experience allowed us to predict the performance of athletes in the windsurfing group, but not in the monohull group. The influence of experience on performance has been demonstrated both in the general literature [36,37] and the literature specific to navigation [5,42,43]. It is likely that the most expert sailors have a greater orientation, which is demonstrated in a better analysis of the positions of the buoys in the racecourse and the route chosen to approach them [55], as well as their ability to obtain the most relevant information on the racecourse and thus be able to execute efficient motor actions according to the characteristics of the situation [56–58]. The most experienced sailors were placed in a better position with respect to their rivals to obtain a more favorable wind and reduce the number of maneuvers they had to perform when exceeding the buoy. This tangent point seems to be critical when it comes to rounding on the windward buoy, and a bad choice would make the maneuvers come forward or backward with respect to the maneuvers performed by their opponents, with expert sailors reacting differently compared to inexperienced sailors [55]. Another aspect related to the spatial orientation is the perception of the wind direction and the orientation that the boat has with respect to this, which is key when differentiating between expert sailors and beginners [59]. That differentiation in the orientation with respect to the wind is more prominent in situations in which the wind speed is weak, highlighting even more the sailors with great experience [60]. Moreover, indirect effects of experience on performance are possible: having more experience could benefit the orientation skills, making the sailors more comfortable in general in those situations in which this skill is required, and therefore obtaining better sport performance [43].

Despite that general agreement, our results only confirm the hypothesis for the Winsurf group. We do not have information that allows us to create hypotheses about the origin of this contradictory result, so future studies should address this problem by accessing both personal, social and contextual variables.

Finally, it was hypothesized that the age of the sailors would not allow for prediction of their performance in competition. This hypothesis is accepted only for the Monohull group; for the Windsurf group, age—alone or in combination with experience—makes it possible to predict performance in the regatta. From the theoretical perspective, which defends that age influences spatial ability, this result is consistent with that provided by Ruggiero et al. [48], who found that the egocentric spatial orientation progressively improves from 8 to 60 years old as a consequence of maturation [35]. For our Windsurf sailors, older age probably implies better ability to visualize, allowing for the most relevant information of the competition environment and, therefore, better performance [61].

We do not have a hypothesis that allows us to explain or suppose why age influences the performance of Windsurfers, but not that of Monohulls. The sailors in both groups are homogeneous in terms of age and experience, so these variables could act in the same way in both groups. Some personal, social or contextual variables of these groups must mediate the relationship between age and performance. Future research should delve into these possible modulating variables.

In our study, we can consider some limitations. Only one test was used in this study to assess spatial orientation; it would have been very interesting to obtain data from a Mental Rotation test or Spatial Anxiety Scale to compare and corroborate our results. In the same way, performance was measured by a single event, so it is necessary to assume that it may not reflect the average performance of the sailors, but only that of this test. Moreover, due to the small number of the sample, it is not possible to extrapolate these results to the sailor population. However, to our knowledge, this is the first study analyzing the influence of spatial orientation ability, age and experience on sailors´ performance when belonging to different classes.

5. Conclusions

The results of this study demonstrate that, for sailors in the Monohull group (classes 420 and Laser), spatial orientation predicts competitive performance in a given regatta. In addition, for the athletes of the Windsurf group (classes RS:X and Techno), both the sailing experience and the age, and the combination of both, allow for prediction of the performance in a certain competition. Thus, it seems that, between both groups of navigators, there are personal, social or, more likely, contextual differences that explain dissimilar results.

Author Contributions: Conceptualization, I.C. and M.R.B.; methodology, I.C. and M.R.B.; software, I.C., A.L.-B. and M.R.B.; validation, I.C. and M.R.B.; formal analysis, I.C., A.L.-B. and M.R.B.; investigation, I.C. and A.L.-B.; resources, I.C.; data curation, I.C. and M.R.B.; writing—original draft preparation, I.C. and M.R.B.; writing—review and editing, I.C., A.L.-B. and M.R.B.; visualization, I.C. and M.R.B.; supervision, I.C. and M.R.B.; project administration, I.C.; funding acquisition, I.C. All authors have read and agreed to the published version of the manuscript.

Funding: This research received no external funding.

Institutional Review Board Statement: The study was conducted according to the guidelines of the Declaration of Helsinki.

Informed Consent Statement: Informed consent was obtained from all subjects involved in the study.

Data Availability Statement: No new data were created or analyzed in this study. Data sharing is not applicable to this article.

Conflicts of Interest: The authors declare no conflict of interest.

References

1. Callewaert, M.; Boone, J.; Celie, B.; De Clerq, D.; Bourgois, J.G. Indicators of sailing performance in youth dinghy sailing. *Eur. J. Sport Sci.* **2015**, *15*, 213–219. [CrossRef] [PubMed]
2. Gould, D.; Maynard, I. Psychological preparation for the Olympic games. *J. Sports Sci.* **2009**, *27*, 1393–1408. [CrossRef]
3. Serpa, S.; Castro, T. Psychology of the Olympic Games: The perception of coaches. *J. Sport Psychol.* **2006**, *15*, 183–199.
4. Olmedilla, A.; Ortega, E.; González, J.; Serpa, S. Psychological training in sailing: Performance improvement for the Olympic classification phase. *Univ. J. Psychol.* **2015**, *3*, 122–131. [CrossRef]
5. Araújo, D.; Davids, K.; Serpa, S. An ecological approach to expertise effects in decision-making in a simulated sailing regatta. *Psychol. Sport Exerc.* **2005**, *6*, 671–692. [CrossRef]
6. Brandt, R.; Da Silva, M.; Segato, L.; Andrade, A. Atençâo em velejadores conceitos e aplicaçâo. *Rev. Bras. Ciências Esporte* **2012**, *1*, 69–80. [CrossRef]
7. Araújo, D.; Serpa, S. Dynamic decision making at different levels of experience in sailing sport. *J. Sport Psychol.* **1999**, *8*, 103–115.
8. Manzanares, A. Analysis of Visual Behavior and Performance Achieved at the Star of Simulated Races: Differences Base on Experience. Ph.D. Thesis, San Antonio Catholic University, Murcia, Spain, 2013.
9. Manzanares, A.; Menayo, R.; Segado, F. Visual search strategy during regatta starts in a sailing simulation. *Motor Control* **2017**, *21*, 413–424. [CrossRef]
10. Ward, P.; Williams, A.M.; Bennett, S. Visual search and biological perception in tennis. *Res. Quart. Sport Exerc.* **2002**, *73*, 107–112. [CrossRef] [PubMed]
11. Anne, L. Spatial orientation skills and mathematical problem solving. *J. Res. Math. Educ.* **1990**, *21*, 216–229.

12. Wolbers, T.; Wiener, J.M. Challenges for identifying the neural mechanisms that support spatial navigation: The impact of spatial scale. *Front. Hum. Neurosci.* **2014**, *8*, 571. [CrossRef]
13. Boccia, M.; Piccardi, L.; D´Alessandro, A.; Nori, R.; Guariglia, C. Restructuring the navigational field: Individual predisposition towards field independence predicts preferred navigational strategy. *Exp. Brain Res.* **2017**, *235*, 1741–1748. [CrossRef]
14. Gómez, A.; Rousset, S.; Baciu, M. Egocentric-updating during navigation facilities episodic memory retrieval. *Acta Psychol.* **2009**, *132*, 221–227. [CrossRef] [PubMed]
15. Montello, D.R. Navigation. In *The Cambridge Handbook of Visuospatial Thinking*; Shan, P., Miyake, A., Eds.; Cambridge University Press: Cambridge, UK, 2005; pp. 257–294.
16. Wang, R.; Brockmole, J. Simultaneous spatial updating in nested environments. *Psychon. Bull. Rev.* **2003**, *10*, 981–986. [CrossRef] [PubMed]
17. Maier, P. Spatial Geometry and Spatial Ability: How to Make Solid Geometry Solid. In *Selected Papers from the Annual Conference of Didactics of Mathematics*; Osnabrück, E., Cohors-Fresenborg, K., Reiss, G., Toener, G., Weigand, H., Verlag-Franzbecker, K.G., Eds.; Franzbecker: Hildesheim, Germany, 1998; pp. 63–75.
18. Wraga, M.; Creem, S.; Proffitt, D. The influence of spatial reference frames on imagined object and viewer rotations. *Acta Psychol.* **1999**, *102*, 247–264. [CrossRef]
19. Hegarty, M.; Waller, D. Individual differences in spatial abilities. In *The Cambridge Handbook of Visuospatial Thinking*; Shah, P., Miyake, A., Eds.; Cambridge University Press: Cambridge, UK, 2005; pp. 121–169.
20. Just, M.A.; Carpenter, P.A. Cognitive coordinate systems: Accounts of mental rotation and individual differences in spatial ability. *Psychol. Rev.* **1985**, *92*, 137–172. [CrossRef]
21. Kozhevnikov, M.; Hegarty, M. A dissociation between object manipulation spatial ability and spatial orientation ability. *Mem. Cogn.* **2001**, *29*, 745–756. [CrossRef] [PubMed]
22. Hines, M.; Fane, B.A.; Pasterski, V.L.; Mathews, G.A.; Conway, G.S.; Brook, C. Spatial abilities following prenatal androgen abnormality: Targeting and mental rotations performance in individuals with congenital adrenal hyperplasia. *Psychoneuroendocrinology* **2003**, *28*, 1010–1026. [CrossRef]
23. Hegarty, M.; Waller, D. A dissociation between mental rotation and perspective-taking spatial abilities. *Intelligence* **2004**, *32*, 175–191. [CrossRef]
24. Ittelson, W.H. *Environment and Cognition*; Seminar: New York, NY, USA, 1973; pp. 1–19.
25. Voyer, D.; Voyer, S.; Bryden, M.P. Magnitude of Sex Differences in Spatial Abilities: A Meta-Analysis and Consideration of Critical Variables. *Psychol. Bull.* **1995**, *117*, 250–270. [CrossRef]
26. Hegarty, M.; Burte, H.; Boone, A.P. Individual differences in large-scale spatial abilities and strategies. In *Handbook of Behavioral and Cognitive Geography*; Montello, D.R., Ed.; Elgaronline: Northampton, MA, USA, 2008.
27. Hegarty, M.; Montello, D.R.; Richardson, A.E.; Ishikawa, T.; Lovelace, K. Spatial abilities at different scales: Individual differences in aptitude-test performance and spatial-layout learning. *Intelligence* **2006**, *34*, 151–176. [CrossRef]
28. Wang, L.; Carr, M. Working Memory and Strategy Use Contribute to Gender Differences in Spatial Ability. *Educ. Psychol.* **2004**, *49*, 261–282. [CrossRef]
29. Linn, M.; Petersen, A. Emergence and Characterization of Sex differences in Spatial Ability: A Meta-Analysis. *Child Dev.* **1985**, *56*, 1479–1498. [CrossRef] [PubMed]
30. Mafalda, R. Efeitos do uso de Diferentes Métodos de Representacao Gráfica no Desenvolmimento da Habilidade de Visualizacao Espacial. Ph.D. Thesis, Universidade de Sao Paulo, San Paolo, Portugal, 2000.
31. Klatzky, R.L. Allocentric and Egocentric Spatial Representations: Definitions, Distinctions, and Interconnections. In *Spatial Cognition. Lecture Notes in Computer Science*; Freksa, C., Habel, C., Wender, K.F., Eds.; Springer: Berlin/Heidelberg, Germany, 1998.
32. Wang, C.; Chen, X.; Knierim, J.J. Egocentric and allocentric representations of space in the rodent brain. *Curr. Opin. Neurobiol.* **2020**, *60*, 12–20. [CrossRef] [PubMed]
33. Fields, A.; Shelton, A. Individual skill differences and large-scale environmental learning. *J. Exp. Psychol.* **2006**, *32*, 506–515. [CrossRef]
34. Kozhevnikov, M.; Motes, M.A.; Rasch, B.; Blajenkova, O. Perspective-taking vs. mental rotation transformations and how the predict spatial navigation performance. *Appl. Cogn. Psychol.* **2006**, *20*, 397–417. [CrossRef]
35. Meilinger, T.; Vosgerau, G. Putting Egocentric and Allocentric into Perspective. In *Lecture Notes in Computer Science*; Hölscher, C., Shipley, T.F., Olivetti Belardinelli, M., Bateman, J.A., Newcombe, N.S., Eds.; Spatial Cognition VII; Springer: Berlin/Heidelberg, Germany, 2010; p. 6222.
36. Baker, J.; Farrow, M. *Routledge Handbook of Sport Expertise*; Routledge: Oxfordshire, UK, 2017.
37. Williams, A.M.; Ericsson, K.A. Perceptual-cognitive expertise in sport: Some considerations when applying the expert performance approach. *Hum. Mov. Sci.* **2005**, *24*, 283–307. [CrossRef]
38. Abernethy, B. The Effects of Age and Expertise upon Perceptual Skill Development in a Racquet Sport. *Res. Q. Exerc. Sport* **1988**, *59*, 210–221. [CrossRef]
39. Notarnicola, A.; Maccagnano, G.; Pesce, V.; Tafuri, S.; Novielli, G.; Moretti, B. Visual- spatial capacity: Gender and sport differences in young volleyball and tennis athletes and non-athletes. *BMC Res. Notes* **2014**, *7*, 57. [CrossRef] [PubMed]
40. Castagna, O.; Brisswalter, J. Assessment of energy demand in Laser sailing: Influences of exercise duration and performance level. *Eur. J. Appl. Physiol.* **2007**, *99*, 95–101. [CrossRef] [PubMed]

41. Vangelakoudi, A.; Vogiatzis, I.; Geladas, N. Anaerobic capacity, isometric endurance, and Laser sailing performance. *J. Sports Sci.* **2007**, *25*, 1095–1100. [CrossRef]
42. Sjøgaard, G.; Inglés, E.; Narici, M. Science in sailing: Interdisciplinary perspectives in optimizing sailing performance. *Eur. J. Sport Sci.* **2015**, *15*, 191–194. [CrossRef] [PubMed]
43. Devlin, A.S. Sailing Experience and Sex as Correlates of Spatial Ability. *Percept. Motor Ski.* **2004**, *98*, 1409–1421. [CrossRef]
44. Schoenfeld, R.; Lehmann, W.; Leplow, B. Effects of Age and Sex in Mental Rotation and Spatial Learning from Virtual Environments. *J. Individ. Differ.* **2010**, *31*, 78–82. [CrossRef]
45. Lehnung, M.; Leplow, B.; Friege, L.; Herzog, A.; Ferstl, R.; Mehdorn, M. Development of spatial memory and spatial orientation in preschoolers and primary school children. *Br. J. Psychol.* **1998**, *89*, 463–480. [CrossRef] [PubMed]
46. Newcombe, N.S. Navigation and the developing brain. *J. Exp. Biol.* **2019**, *222*, jeb186460. [CrossRef] [PubMed]
47. Liu, I.; Levy, R.M.; Barton, J.J.S.; Iaria, G. Age and gender differences in various topographical orientation strategies. *Brain Res.* **2011**, *1410*, 112–119. [CrossRef] [PubMed]
48. Ruggiero, G.; D´Errico, O.; Iachini, T. Development of egocentric and allocentric spatial representations from childhood to elderly age. *Psychol. Res.* **2016**, *80*, 259–272. [CrossRef] [PubMed]
49. Lin, C.H.; Chen, C.M.; Lou, Y.C. Developing Spatial Orientation and Spatial Memory with a Treasure Hunting Game. *Educ. Technol. Soc.* **2014**, *17*, 79–92.
50. XV New Year's Race "X Memorial Kim Lythgoe". Available online: https://andaluza.fav.es/default/events/event/text/xv-new-year\T1\textquoterights-race-x-memorial-kim-lythgoe (accessed on 12 March 2021).
51. Ehrenfierd, T.; Guerraz, M.; Thilo, K.V.; Yardley, L.; Gresty, M.A. Posture and mental task performance when viewing a moving visual field. *Cogn. Brain Res.* **2003**, *17*, 140–153. [CrossRef]
52. Bojsen-Moller, J.; Larsson, B.; Magnusson, P.; Aagaard, P. Yacht type and crew-specific differences in anthropometric, aerobic capacity, and muscle strength parameters among international Olympic class sailors. *J. Sports Sci.* **2007**, *25*, 1117–1128. [CrossRef] [PubMed]
53. Vogiatzis, I.; De Vito, G. Physiological assessment of Olympic windsurfers. *Eur. J. Sport Sci.* **2015**, *15*, 228–234. [CrossRef] [PubMed]
54. Vogiatzis, I.; De Vito, G.; Radio, A.; Marchetti, M. Comparison of the physiological responses to upwind and downwind sail-pumping in windsurfers. *N. Zeal. J. Sport Med.* **2005**, *33*, 66–67.
55. Pluijms, J.; Cañal-Bruland, R.; Bergmann-Tiest, W.M.; Mulder, F.A.; Savelsbergh, G.J.P. Expertise effects in cutaneous wind perception. *Atten. Percept. Psychophys.* **2015**, *77*, 2121–2133. [CrossRef]
56. Tenebaum, G. Expert athletes: An integrated approach to decision making. In *Expert Performance in Sport, Advances in Research on Sport Expertise*; Starkes, J., Ericsson, K., Eds.; Human Kinetics: Champaing, IL, USA, 2003; pp. 201–218.
57. Vickers, J. *Perception, Cognition and Decision Training. The Quiet Eye in Action*; Human Kinectics: Champaing, IL, USA, 2007.
58. Manzanares, A.; Menayo, R.; Segado, F.; Salmerón, D.; Cano, J.A. A probabilistic model for analysing the effect of performance levels on visual behaviour patterns of young sailors in simulated navigation. *Eur. J. Sports Sci.* **2015**, *15*, 203–212. [CrossRef] [PubMed]
59. Prlenda, N.; Oreb, I.; Vujcic, D. Buoys as a tool in teaching basic elements of sailing. *Sportlogia* **2018**, *14*, 47–58. [CrossRef]
60. Pluijms, J.P.; Cañal-Bruland, R.; Hoozemans, M.J.; Savelsbergh, G.J. Visual search, movement behavior and boat control during the windward mark rounding in sailing. *J. Sports Sci.* **2015**, *33*, 398–410. [CrossRef] [PubMed]
61. Newcombe, N.; Bandura, M.M. Effect of age at puberty on spatial ability in girls: A question of mechanism. *Dev. Psychol.* **1983**, *19*, 215–224. [CrossRef]

International Journal of
Environmental Research and Public Health

MDPI

Article

Effect of a Shock Micro-Cycle on Biochemical Markers in University Soccer Players

Diana García-Cardona [1,*], Patricia Landázuri [2] and Oscar Sánchez-Muñoz [3]

1 Biomedical Sciences Program, Research Group on Cardiovascular and Metabolic Diseases (GECAVYME) and Research Group on Physical Activity and Health Physiology (GIFAS), University of Quindío, Armenia 63000, Colombia
2 Medicine Program, Research Group on Cardiovascular and Metabolic Diseases (GECAVYME), University of Quindío, Armenia 63000, Colombia; plandazu@uniquindio.edu.co
3 Sánchez-Muñoz OE, Physical Education and Sports Program, Research Group on Physical Activity and Health Physiology (GIFAS), University of Quindío, Armenia 63000, Colombia; oesanchez@uniquindio.edu.co
* Correspondence: dmgarcia@uniquindio.edu.co; Tel.: +57-735-9300 (ext. 1132)

Abstract: This study aimed to examine various biochemical biomarkers changes during a shock micro-cycle in soccer players from a university team. The study had 22 players (age: 22 ± 3 years; body mass: 68.6 ± 7.1 kg; height: 1.73 ± 0.07 m). The study measured total cholesterol (TC), triglycerides (TG), cholesterol linked to high-density lipoproteins (HDL), low-density lipoproteins (LDL), very low density lipoproteins (VLDL), arterial index (AI), creatine kinase (CK), glutamate-oxalacetate-transaminase (GOT), glutamate-pyruvate-transaminase (GPT), creatinine (Cr), catalase (CAT), superoxide dismutase (SOD), cytokines IL6 and TNFα, total antioxidant capacity (Cap antiox tot), hemolysis percentage and glomerular filtration rate (GFR); measurements were conducted during a shock micro-cycle. The lipid profile variables had no statistical significance when compared on day 1 with day 14. Except for TNFα, the other biomarkers compared with day one had progressive increments until day seven, with a subsequent reduction on day 14; however, none of the biomarkers returned to baseline values despite this decrease. The data shown herein suggest the need to research these biomarkers in distinct types of mesocycles, exercise, intensity, load, and duration to diminish fatigue and improve athlete performance.

Keywords: biomarkers; soccer; oxidative stress; lipids

Citation: García-Cardona, D.; Landázuri, P.; Sánchez-Muñoz, O. Effect of a Shock Micro-Cycle on Biochemical Markers in University Soccer Players. *Int. J. Environ. Res. Public Health* **2021**, *18*, 3581. https://doi.org/10.3390/ijerph18073581

Academic Editor: Shaher A. I. Shalfawi

Received: 8 February 2021
Accepted: 25 March 2021
Published: 30 March 2021

1. Introduction

Soccer players are subject to an organizational structure of their training called mesocycle, within which the shock micro-cycle can be found, which is characterized by a large overall volume of work and a high level of incitement; its purpose is to stimulate the processes adaptation of the organism [1]. The high load of physical exercise and psychological stress can trigger an imbalance between the production of reactive oxygen species and other free radicals and the antioxidant defense mechanisms of the organism. This can cause molecular damage that can be measured through: biological markers, such as proteins; the activity of enzymes or their metabolites; lipid peroxidation; and nucleic acids, among others [2,3]. Several of these biomarkers have been studied concerning exercise, for example, biomarkers of: cardiac hypoxia [4], the immune system such as immunoglobulins [5], tissue damage or muscle activity [6], and some enzymes of the Redox system (catalase, peroxidase) [7].

Therefore, several biochemical markers could be used as indicators of physical stress, systemic inflammation, muscle damage, and physiological adaptation to sports activity [8]. Among the biomarkers that can be found, creatinine is a final product of muscle metabolism [9] and its activity (CK) is related to the intensity of the load to which the muscle is subjected [10]. In addition, its serum concentration is higher in athletes than in the population of people who are not physically active. Glutamate-oxaloacetate transaminase (GOT) and glutamate-pyruvate transaminase (GPT) serve as markers of liver disease. However, they could also be valuable tools to assess people's metabolic responses to exercise [11].

Regarding inflammation, muscle damage initiates a local inflammatory response that involves the production of cytokines [12] such as IL6 and TNFα. In soccer studies such as that of Souglis et al. [13], increases were detected in IL-6 and TNF-α between two and four times higher than the values at rest, with the maximum values being those obtained immediately after the game. Regarding the lipid profile, specifically high-density lipoproteins (HDL), it is considered a protective factor [14] due to its role in the reverse transport of cholesterol. It is also described how exercise increases this lipoprotein.

In soccer during matches, players perform a large number of high intensity non-linear activities based on running [15]. In addition, acceleration and deceleration during direction changes produce high levels of mechanical and metabolic stress, which increases the demands of metabolic power and total energy expenditure during training and matches [16]. Specifically, they are necessary between 48–72 h to restore metabolic alterations after a match [17,18], although 3–4 days of recovery between successive matches may be insufficient to restore homeostasis [19].

Commonly, most of the studies investigating biochemical markers in soccer have been done through follow-up in one game, three games, or under the development of tests. In Colombian university soccer, specifically in the university zonal competitions, they play between three and five games with a short recovery time (about 24 h between matches). In this context, there is little information about it in the formal bibliography that studies and analyzes the behavior of said markers in Colombian college soccer. In this sense, the purpose of this study was to examine changes in various biochemical biomarkers during a shock micro-cycle in a university soccer team.

2. Materials and Methods

2.1. Subjects

A total of 22 (mean ± SD: age, 22 ± 3 years; body mass, 68.6 ± 7.1 kg; height, 1.73 ± 0.07 m) male students of the Universidad del Quindío soccer team took part voluntarily in this trial. These students train about 10 to 14 h per week for regional competitions. The study excluded athletes with diseases proven through their clinical history and excluded injured athletes and those with less than one year of training in the sports discipline.

2.2. Ethics

This research was carried out according to the Helsinki Declaration and Resolution 8430 by the Colombian Ministry of Health and Social Protection, and it was approved by the Bioethics Committee of the Physical Education Program at Universidad del Quindío.

2.3. Variables

The studied variables were divided into three groups: biochemical, anthropometric, and physical condition.

Biochemical: total cholesterol (TC), triglycerides (TG), cholesterol linked to high-density lipoproteins (HDL), low-density lipoproteins (LDL), very low density lipoproteins (VLDL), arterial index (AI), creatine kinase (CK), glutamate-oxalacetate-transaminase (GOT), glutamate-pyruvate-transaminase (GPT), creatinine (Cr), catalase (CAT), superoxide dismutase (SOD), cytokines IL6 and TNFα, total antioxidant capacity (Cap antiox tot), hemolysis percentage and glomerular filtration rate (GFR).

Anthropometric: age, mass, height, body mass index (BMI), adipose percentage, and muscle percentage.

Physical condition: maximal oxygen uptake (VO_{2max}).

2.4. Procedure

The subjects participated in a 7-day shock micro-cycle.

Blood sampling: a blood sample was collected by venipuncture in a dried tube. Samples on days 1 and 14 were collected in the laboratory. Samples on days 4 and 7 were collected on the soccer field. Then, they were held in a portable freezer and transported to the laboratory. The serum was obtained through a centrifuge at 1000 g for 15 min, at 4 °C, separated in 1.5 mL micro-tubes, and stored until use (within two days).

Four blood samples were taken in the following manner:

Day 1: The blood sample was collected after 48 h without exercise and 12 h of fasting.

Day 4: The blood sample was collected once the training ended. Test subjects were under no fast conditions.

Day 7: The blood sample was collected once the training ended. Test subjects were under no fast conditions.

Day 14: Seven days after finishing the micro-cycle. The blood sample was collected after 48 h without exercise and 12 h of fasting. The measures of the 14th day aimed to determine if one week after of microcycle, biomarkers get the first day's values.

2.4.1. Biochemical Measurements

The TC and TG were quantified via colorimetric enzymatic methods (Human®, Wiesbaden, Germany), HDL was assessed through initial selective separation with phosphotungstic acid/magnesium chloride (Human®), CK, GOT, GPT, and Cr were quantified via colorimetric enzymatic methods (Wiener Lab®, Rosario, Argentina), CAT and SOD were quantified via colorimetric enzymatic methods (Invitrogen®, Frederick, USA), cytokines IL6 and TNFα were determined through sandwich ELISA by reading the spectrophotometer results (Genesis 5) at 450 nm for both proteins following manufacturer's instructions (BioLegend®, San Diego, USA), Cap antiox tot was quantified through the TBARS (Thiobarbituric Acid Reactive Substance) method, and hemolysis percentage was quantified via spectrophotometry.

The LDL, VLDL, and AI were calculated through formulas described for each.

The GFR was measured through the Cockcroft-Gault formula adjusted for body surface.

2.4.2. Anthropometric Evaluation

Body mass was determined with the least clothing possible using a calibrated electronic scale (Tanita Bc-585f), and height was measured with a stadiometer (Seca Ref 216). To obtain the fat percentage, subcutaneous body fat was evaluated by using a skinfold caliper (Harpende) in six sites [20] (triceps, pectoral, subscapular, abdominal, suprailiac, quadriceps).

2.4.3. Maximal Oxygen Uptake (VO_{2max})

The VO_{2max} was determined through the Course Navette (CN) test. The CN test was conducted based on the methodology described elsewhere [21]. Briefly, the participants were asked to run back and forth for 20 m, and in a straight line, and the running distance was defined by two cones at each end. The CN test ended when the participant stopped due to fatigue or when the participant did not reach the line defined before the beep signal. To determine VO_{2max}, the equation proposed by Paradisis et al., [22] was used (Equation (1)).

$$\mathrm{VO2}_{\max}(\mathrm{mL/kg/min}) = 0.2761x + 27.504 \quad (1)$$

2.4.4. Shock Micro-Cycle

The study subjects participated within their preparation period in a 7-day shock micro-cycle. Players did low-intensity training 72 h previous to this study. The micro-cycle was characterized by the increase in volume and intensity of the load. In such a way, micro-cycle development was carried out under the competition (regionals) simulation where the athletes had to perform for five games, the highest possible performance capacity. The characteristics of the micro-cycle are shown below.

Developer mesocycleShock Micro-cycle

Day 1: Smooth jog, joint movement, muscle activation, active stretching.
Day 2: Tactical training.
Day 3: Match 1.
Day 4: Match 2.
Day 5: Match 3.
Day 6: Match 4.
Day 7: Match 5.

For the soccer game, the coach formed two teams, which remains during microcycle with a 1-4-4-2 formation. A total of five games were played during the experimental period (one each day), all at the same time (08:30 h) on a natural grass surface. Each of the games lasted 90 min distributed in two halves of 45 min, and before each game they warmed up for 20 min.

The players were shown Borg's perceived exertion scale upon ending each training session. All the subjects were familiar with this scale, as part of the regular monitoring of the training.

2.5. Statistical Analyses

Initially, a descriptive analysis was conducted in the laboratory of the results obtained from the biomarkers during the four days evaluated. Likewise, normality assumptions were verified. Then, a paired means test on the lipidic profiles was conducted to determine any difference in the measured variables on days 1 and 14. Additionally, a repeated measures ANOVA was performed, followed by the post-hoc test by Bonferroni. The sphericity assumption was verified through the Mauchly test. A p-value < 0.05 was considered as a statistical significance.

Analysis of the data obtained was performed with the SPSS software 22.0 (IBM).

3. Results

Table 1 shows the anthropometric and physical condition variables of the study subjects. It displays, concerning adipose and muscle percentage, that the athletes were within the adequate standards for age and sport; besides, the BMI is normal. Finally, the VO_{2max} was at an excellent level (46.50–52.40 mL/kg/min).

Table 1. Physical characteristics of participants.

Variables	$n = 22$
BMI (kg/m^2)	23.66 ± 2.14
Body fat (%)	8.90 ± 0.93
Muscle percentage	46.84 ± 3.8
VO_{2max} (mL/kg/min)	51.66 ± 2.24

Mean ± SD. BMI: body mass index.

Table 2 shows the lipid profile results, and shows that the variables were within the values considered to be normal (TC < 200 mg/dL, TG < 150 mg/dL, HDLc > 40 mg/dL, LDL < 100 mg/dL, VLDL < 30 mg/dL, AI < 3.5 mg/dL) according to the ATPIII (Adult Treatment Panel III) [23]. Upon comparing these variables between days 1 and 14, no significant differences were evident despite their increase.

Table 2. Lipid profile.

VARIABLES	D1	D14	p-Value
TC (mg/dL)	153.80 ± 28.20	163.52 ± 32.3	0.495
HDL (mg/dL)	47.38 ± 7.10	48.55 ± 7.90	0.622
LDL (mg/dL)	88.58 ± 20.47	93.01 ± 21.56	0.666
VLDL (mg/dL)	16.66 ± 5.09	19.86 ± 4.67	0.101
TG (mg/dL)	78.62 ± 21.30	94.42 ± 21.49	0.051
AI	2.71 ± 0.84	2.90 ± 0.83	0.503

Mean ± SD. n = 22. D: day. TC: total cholesterol. HDL: high-density lipoprotein. LDL: low-density lipoprotein. VLDL: very low-density lipoprotein. TG: triglycerides. AI: arterial index. Note: No differences were observed among groups. Comparisons were tested via Student's t-test.

Table 3 presents the transaminase levels and hemolysis percentage. These variables had no statistically significant differences, although three variables (GPT, GOT, and hemolysis) increased progressively from days one to seven and decreased on day 14.

Table 3. Biomarkers without statistically significant changes.

VARIABLES	D1	D4	D7	D14	p-Value	
GPT (U/L)	16.26 ± 3.2	17.49 ±2.30	21.27 ± 3.60	17.74 ± 3.50	D1 vs. D4	0.563
					D4 vs. D7	0.076
					D7 vs. D14	0.400
					D1 vs. D14	0.435
GOT (U/L)	19.50 ± 2.78	21.06 ± 3.10	24.37 ± 4.26	22.55 ±3.15	D1 vs. D4	0.586
					D4 vs. D7	0.086
					D7 vs. D14	0.290
					D1 vs. D14	0.296
Hemolysis (%)	80.24 ± 3.90	81.74 ±3.60	81.95 ± 2.54	81.25 ± 3.10	D1 vs. D4	0.204
					D4 vs. D7	0.833
					D7 vs. D14	0.429
					D1 vs. D14	0.107
CAT (U/mL)	28.64 ± 3.50	29.39 ±0.30	29.31 ± 0.26	29.4 ± 0.15	D1 vs. D4	0.341
					D4 vs. D7	0.403
					D7 vs. D14	0.217
					D1 vs. D14	0.345

Mean ± SD. D: day. GPT: glutamate-pyruvate-transaminase. GOT: glutamate-oxalacetate-transaminase. CAT: catalase.

Figure 1 shows the levels of the oxidative stress biomarkers, showing that SOD and Cap antiox tot behaved similar to the prior variables, that is, with progressive increase from days one to seven. However, the SOD had significant differences from day one to day four (p-value = 0.001) (26.53% increase) and from day seven to day 14 (p-value = 0.001) (19.77% decrease), while in the Cap antiox tot, the decrease was only significant (23.36%) from days seven to 14 (p-value = 0.01).

Figure 2 displays the IL6 and TNFα, with respect to IL6, with statistically significant differences in all days evaluated, while the TNFα had no differences between decreased concentrations from days four to seven (p-value = 0.068).

For creatinine (Figure 3a), significant differences were evident, except for the increase from days four to seven (p-value = 0.801). Moreover, the GFR (Figure 3b) showed a decrease, from days one to seven, finding days four and seven with values (85.91 and 81.68 mL/min/1.73 m^2, respectively) below the value considered normal ($\geq$90 mL/min/1.73 m^2).

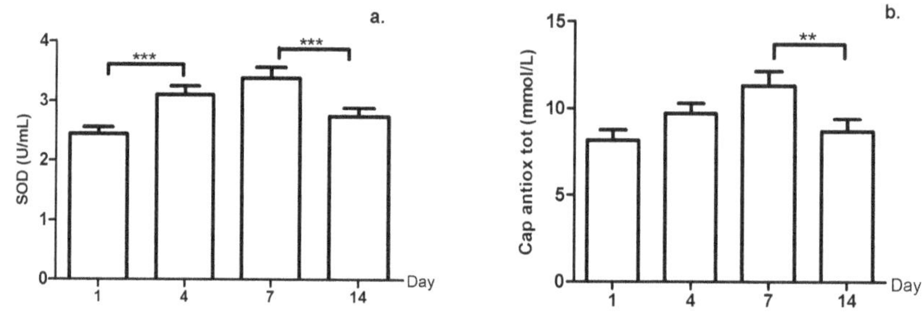

Figure 1. (**a**) Superoxide dismutase (SOD) levels. (**b**) Total antioxidant capacity (Cap antiox tot) during the micro-cycle, **: p-value < 0.01, ***: p-value < 0.001.

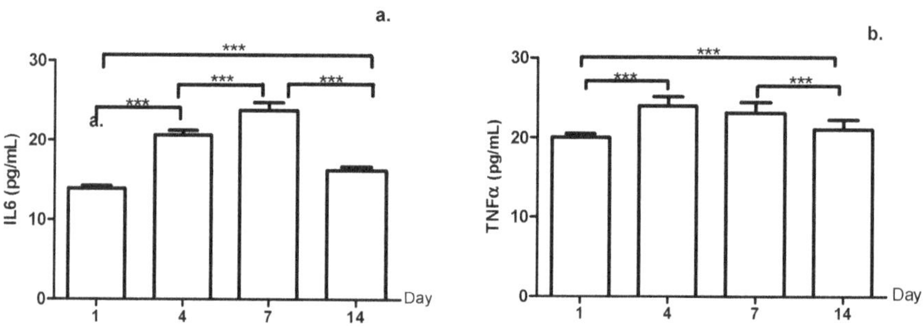

Figure 2. (**a**) Levels of Interleukin-6 (IL6); (**b**) levels of Tumor Necrosis Factor-alfa (TNFα) during the micro-cycle, ***: p-value < 0.001.

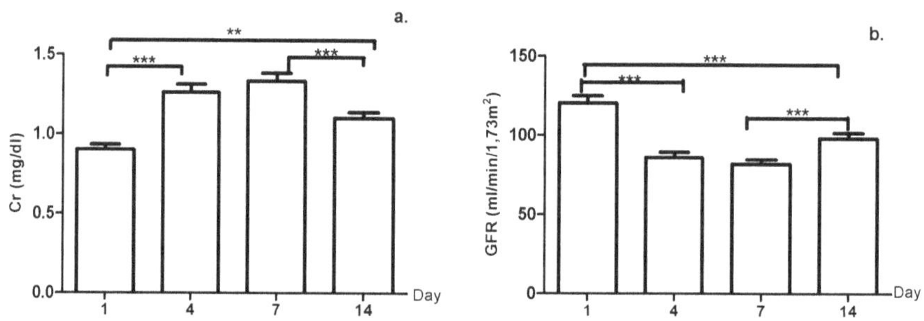

Figure 3. (**a**) Creatinine (Cr) levels; (**b**) Glomerular filtration rate (GFR) during the micro-cycle, **: p-value < 0.01, ***: p-value < 0.001.

The CK (Figure 4) showed increased concentration (105.9%) from day 1 to day 4 (p-value = 0.001); from day 4 to day 7 (p-value = 0.001) (51.3%); and from day 7 to day 14 (p-value = 0.0002), a 53.37% decrease, all with statistical significance.

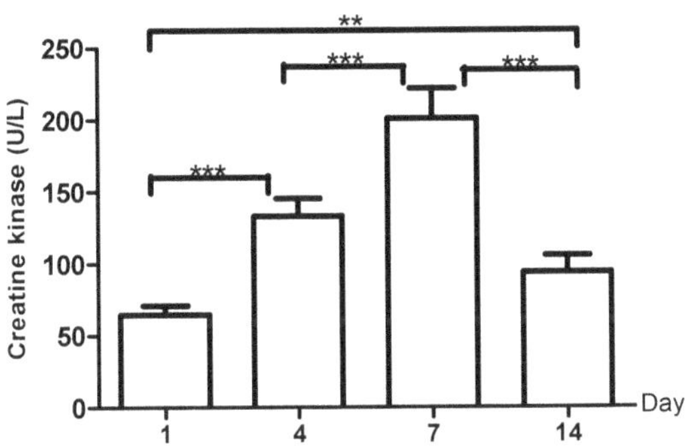

Figure 4. Creatine kinase levels during the micro-cycle, **: p-value < 0.01, ***: p-value < 0.001.

4. Discussion

This work studied some biochemical biomarkers during a shock micro-cycle of university soccer players.

Besides being subjected to academic stressors, the university soccer players were also subjected to other stressors due to their physical, technical, and tactical training to assume competition. High-level competitive sport requires the athletes to engage in high training loads, like a shock micro-cycle, which is characterized by a large overall volume of work and high level of incitement [1]. These high training loads and competitive stress produce changes in the body structure and metabolism to adapt to the physiological demands of training and competition [7].

The present study's main finding was that the biochemical markers were affected by the micro-cycle, which was developed by simulating a college zonal competition. The effect was reflected in the increase in the athletes oxidative stress evaluated through SOD and Cap antiox tot. Likewise, the variation in the cytokines concentration, where the rise in IL6 (anti-inflammatory) appeared to influence the decrease in TNFα (pro-inflammatory), showed the anti-inflammatory effect of training. High muscle damage was also observed, evidenced by the increase in CK and Cr levels. Although there were variations in the level of transaminases during the micro-cycle, they were not statistically significant.

From the point of view of their body composition, soccer players constitute a differentiated population group due to their lower level of fat and higher muscle development. In this regard, this work found the BMI within the normal range [24] and percentage of body fat at 8.9%, that is, a good percentage for high-performance athletes. These results are similar to the elite soccer players reported in the study by Slimani et al., [25] and lower concerning the Greek soccer players (age 18–37 years) evaluated by Leão et al., [26]. The variable percentage of muscle mass was higher than that reported by García-Cardona et al. [27], who evaluated this same team in 2016 and found, on average, a percentage of muscle mass of 43.07%; in this respect, this average is consistent with results shown at fat percentage level, which was higher in 2016. The present study found similar values to that reported (46.18%) by Gil and Vedoy [28] in Spanish university soccer players. Concerning the VO_{2max} found in our study (51.66 $\pm$ 2.24), the result places them at an excellent level, which means they have an excellent physical condition for their sports performance.

The present study also measured lipid profile as a measurement of the athletes' general health conditions; these variables were within the ranges considered normal for the lipid profile variables [23], as expected for individuals who practice a high-performance sport and take care of their health. These results are similar to those reported by Apostolidi et al. in Greek soccer players [29].

This work also assessed the hepatic function through transaminases; these enzymes indicate liver damage from disease or intake of medications or alcohol. The increase of these enzymes may be related to intense exercise [19]. Accelerated metabolic demands due to muscular exercise cannot be satisfied without a robust response by the liver [30].

In this work, transaminases increased on days four and seven of the shock micro-cycle; similar results were found by Nowakowska et al. [11]. Although these authors conducted an 11-month follow-up, and this work did so for only 14 days, the results show that on day 14 the transaminases had not returned to the baseline values of day one. In this regard, Pettersson et al. [31] state that intense muscular exercise can increase liver function at least seven days after exercise. In this same sense, Sjogren et al. [32] hold that individuals who engage in vigorous exercise (for example, weight lifters, marathon runners, and others] can have abnormal levels of transaminases due to a normal process of muscle tissue repair that causes inflammation and raises the levels of transaminases. The same authors indicate that transaminases can remain high for up to one week after stopping the exercise [32], as seen in the present research. Moreover, Chinedu et al., [33] also found increased GPT and other hepatic function markers, but not of GOT in soccer players subjected to training for 30 min, three times per week for three weeks. These findings suggest that vigorous exercise, like a shock microcycle affects transaminase levels.

It is known that exercise induces hemolysis [34] and although—at times—it is associated exclusively to impact sports, it is common in most sports modalities [35]. As potential sources of exercise-induced hemolysis, there are direct mechanical lesions caused by strong contact on the ground, repeated contractile muscle activity or vasoconstriction in internal organs, while pre-existing erythrocyte disorders or metabolic anomalies developed during exercise (for example, hyperthermia, dehydration, hypoxia, lactic acidosis, oxidative damage, increased catecholamine concentration) can contribute actively to triggering, accelerating, or amplifying this phenomenon [36]. It seems that the average life span of red blood cells in athletes is shorter, which is beneficial for performance [37]; different studies have identified significant hemolysis levels in long-distance runners and cyclists, among others. Our study also showed increased hemolysis on days four and seven of the micro-cycle without statistical significance; this non-significance likely is because, during the first phases of the exercise, hemolysis is stronger due to rapid destruction of the oldest population of erythrocytes, but these are renewed during the more advanced phases of training or competition, breaking down less, as shown by Yusof et al., in ultra-marathon runners [34].

Substantial evidence shows that exercise-induced hemolysis causes an increased inflammatory response and that it commonly occurs with increased IL6 [38], as with the results herein.

Although hemolysis could explain—in part—the increase of IL6, it is also known that exercise by itself can cause inflammatory states, such that IL6 and TNFα were also evaluated in this study. Cytokines are a diverse family of intercellular signaling molecules that regulate inflammation and immune response. According to Pussieldi et al. [39], intense acute exercise can induce muscle damage, producing cytokine release along with other local tissue factors related to the inflammatory phenomenon. In this study, IL6 levels increased continuously, while TNFα diminished as of day seven. In this respect, during exercise, muscle fibers release IL6 which also acts as a suppressor of TNFα production, like a pro-inflammatory cytokine [40]. The results agree with those reported by Stumpf et al., in elite soccer players [41], finding that after a stress test, pro-inflammatory cytokines IL-6, IL-8, TNF-a, and anti-inflammatory cytokine IL-10 were significantly high in all the soccer players.

Regarding the antioxidant capacity evaluated in this study during the shock microcycle, it was found that the CAT did not change significantly during the days considered. These results are similar to those reported by Jamurtas et al. [42] who assessed the effects of high-intensity interval training (HIIT) on the hematological profile and redox state in comparison with those following traditional continuous aerobic exercise. Although few indicators suggest that physical exercise provokes increased CAT activity in skeletal muscle, some studies describe a decrease or leveling of the catalase activity of the erythrocytes after exercising, [43].

Concerning the SOD enzyme, this is an important antioxidant defense that protects cells from ROS-induced oxidative stress [44]. The progressive increase of SOD found in this study was consistent with that reported by Silva et al. [45], who studied the biochemical impact of a sports season on professional soccer players and found that SOD increases, but then reaches its starting levels at the end of the season. Increased SOD can be explained by the increase in the superoxide radical during exercise. The superoxide radical is related to converting hemoglobin into meta-hemoglobin in erythrocytes during exercise and converted into H_2O_2 by the SOD enzyme [46]. Increased SOD in plasma could favor the accumulation of H_2O_2 and could indicate low efficiency of plasma elimination, which contributes to higher oxidative stress [47]. This is consistent with increased levels of lipid peroxidation (measured as TBARS) found until day seven in our study; during exercise, the process of supplying oxygen to active muscles can harm the polyunsaturated fatty acids in the membrane's structures. In other words, it causes lipid peroxidation [48], and increased TBARS suggests that ROS production exceeded antioxidant activity [49] despite the possible adaptation. In this sense, Zoppi et al. [50] demonstrated that supplementing with vitamins C and E reduces TBARS levels; this supplementation with antioxidants could be preventing the adverse effect on the oxide-reduction balance generated by training in professional soccer players.

As part of the biochemical markers of oxidative stress in athletes, creatinine and the creatine phosphate enzyme were also measured. Creatinine is a product of creatine metabolism. Prior studies have indicated that athletes and active individuals with higher muscle mass, also have more elevated serum creatinine levels. The Cr concentration in this study increased from days one to seven and diminished on day 14 with significant differences on all the days evaluated. These results agree with those reported by Nowakowska et al. [11] and Ekun et al. [51], which show variations in Cr level over time. Likewise, studies, such as that by Jacobs et al. [52], mention that after moderate- or high-intensity exercise, there is diminished urine volume and a marked reduction in renal plasma flow and filtering rate that lead to increased Cr. This study also noted a decrease in GFR time up to day seven, which would support this hypothesis.

Concomitant with plasma creatinine variations, the same changes were noted in creatine phosphate levels, which increased from days one to seven and diminished on day 14. Among the biochemical markers considered important as indicators of metabolic changes or adaptations made during physical training, CK and its serum activity has been widely studied and is considered a marker of muscle damage [53]. Increased CK from days one to seven may be attributed to mechanical damage of the muscle cell membranes as a result of a substantial force of muscle contraction and oxidative damage of the cell membranes [54]. However, our results showed that seven days after ending the shock micro-cycle, and although the sample from day 14 had been taken with 48 h without exercise, the CK did not return to baseline values. The difference was statistically significant with respect to studies, like that by Wilk et al. [55] in subjects with 6.1 years experience in strength training, which shows how after 24 h of recovery there is increased CK activity, indicating severe damage to the muscle cell membranes and a CK leak in the bloodstream during exercise and after ending it.

Finally, it was observed that seven days after finishing the micro-cycle, IL6, TNFα, Cr, GFR, and CK did not return to baseline values and this difference was statistically significant, which demonstrates that seven days of recovery after five successive matches like the ones developed during the micro-cycle can be insufficient to restore the homeostasis.

As a later work, it is proposed to use these results to determine the relationship between the evaluated markers and the performance according to the playing position.

5. Conclusions

In conclusion, this study demonstrates that the soccer team athletes face stressors during training that produce significant changes in biomarkers related to muscle damage, inflammation, and oxidative stress. Still, some values return to normality when training intensity is lowered, while others remain high. These last factors could be used as fatigue or extenuation markers that could indicate to the coach the need for a more prolonged rest or of complementary measures to avoid severe harm or lesions in athletes who do not recover quickly.

The data shown herein also suggest the need to research these biomarkers in different types of meso-cycles, exercise, intensity, load and duration to diminish fatigue and/or improve the performance of the athletes.

Author Contributions: Conceptualization, D.G.-C., and P.L.; data curation, D.G.-C. and O.S.-M.; formal analysis, D.G.-C.; methodology, D.G.-C., P.L., and O.S.-M.; writing—original draft, D.G.-C. and P.L.; writing—review and editing, D.G.-C., P.L., and O.S.-M. All authors have read and agreed to the published version of the manuscript.

Funding: This project was sponsored by the Department of Science, Technology and Innovation Colciencias, call for research proposals 727, 2015.

Institutional Review Board Statement: The study was conducted according to the Declaration of Helsinki. The protocol was approved by the Physical Education and Sports Program Council on Bioethics from Universidad del Quindio (Colombia) (No 01-2018 5 February 2018).

Informed Consent Statement: Informed consent was obtained from all subjects involved in the study.

Data Availability Statement: The data presented in this study are available on request from the corresponding author.

Acknowledgments: The authors thank the athletes and their coaches Elber Andrés Acosta, Jhon Iván Robledo and Jorge Iván Mejía for their cooperation during the study. In the same way, we thank the working group and the research groups GIFAS and GECAVYME. Thanks to Cristian Ramirez-Gutierrez from academic group of TICA-UPQ (México) for the manuscript reviewing support.

Conflicts of Interest: The authors declare no conflict of interest.

References

1. Padilla, J. *Planificación del Entrenamiento Deportivo: Un Enfoque Metodológico de la Estructura Clásica*, 1st ed.; Editorial Episteme: Barinas, Venezuela, 2017; 125p.
2. Pingitore, A.; Lima, G.P.P.; Mastorci, F.; Quinones, A.; Iervasi, G.; Vassalle, C. Exercise and oxidative stress: Potential effects of antioxidant dietary strategies in sports. *Nutrition* **2015**, *31*, 916–922. [CrossRef] [PubMed]
3. Fernández, J.; Da Silva-Grigoletto, M.; Túnez-Fiñana, I. Estrés oxidativo inducido por el ejercicio J.M. *Rev. Andal. Med. Del. Deport.* **2009**, *2*, 19–34.
4. Fernandez, E.; García, C.; de la Espriella, R.; Dueñas, C.; Manzur, F. Biomarcadores cardíacos: Presente y futuro. *Rev. Colomb. Cardiol.* **2012**, *19*, 300–311. [CrossRef]
5. Vendrell, E.; Lanau, P.; Salat, D.; Pérez, V.; Prat, M.S.; de Gracia Roldán, J.; Pujol, J.A. Influencia del medio y del ejercicio físico sobre las inmunoglobulinas séricas durante una carrera de trineos de nieve en montaña. *Arch. Med. Deport.* **2014**, *31*, 80–84.
6. Moreno-Perez, V.; Gallo-Salazar, C.; Del Coso, J.; Ruiz-Pérez, I.; Lopez-Valenciano, A.; Barbado, D.; Cabello-Manrique, D.; Fernandez-Fernandez, J. The influence of a badminton competition with two matches in a day on muscle damage and physical performance in elite junior badminton players. *Biol. Sport* **2020**, *37*, 195–201. [CrossRef] [PubMed]
7. Margaritelis, N.; Paschalis, V.; Theodorou, A.; Kyparos, A.; Nikolaidis, M. Redox basis of exercise physiology. *Redox Biol.* **2020**, *35*, 101499. [CrossRef]
8. Perroni, F.; Migliaccio, S.; Borrione, P.; Vetrano, M.; Amatori, S.; Sisti, D.; Rocchi, M.; Salerno, G.; Vescovo, R.; Cavarretta, E.; et al. Can Haematological and Hormonal Biomarkers Predict Fitness Parameters in Youth Soccer Players? A Pilot Study. *Int. J. Environ. Res. Public Health* **2020**, *17*, 6294. [CrossRef]
9. Bacallao, R.; Badell, A. La creatinina como indicador del tejido muscular esquelético y el estado nutricional. *Rev. Cuba. Aliment. Nutr.* **2015**, *25*, 4–23.
10. Mougios, V. Reference intervals for serum creatine kinase in athletes. *Br. J. Sports Med.* **2007**, *41*, 674–678. [CrossRef] [PubMed]
11. Nowakowska, A.; Kostrzewa-Nowak, D.; Buryta, R.; Nowak, R. Blood Biomarkers of Recovery Efficiency in Soccer Players. *Int. J. Environ. Res. Public Health* **2019**, *16*, 3279. [CrossRef] [PubMed]
12. Nédélec, M.; McCall, A.; Carling, C.; Legall, F.; Berthoin, S.; Dupont, G. Recovery in Soccer. *Sport Med.* **2012**, *42*, 997–1015.
13. Souglis, A.G.; Papapanagiotou, A.; Bogdanis, G.C.; Travlos, A.K.; Apostolidis, N.G.; Geladas, N.D. Comparison of Inflammatory Responses to a Soccer Match Between Elite Male and Female Players. *J. Strength Cond. Res.* **2015**, *29*, 1227–1233. [CrossRef]

14. Nieman, D.C.; Gillitt, N.D.; Knab, A.M.; Shanely, R.A.; Pappan, K.L.; Jin, F.; Lila, M.A. Influence of a Polyphenol-Enriched Protein Powder on Exercise-Induced Inflammation and Oxidative Stress in Athletes: A Randomized Trial Using a Metabolomics Approach. *PLoS ONE* **2013**, *8*, e72215. [CrossRef]
15. Bloomfield, J.; Polman, R.; O'Donoghue, P. Physical Demands of Different Positions in FA Premier League Soccer. *J. Sports Sci. Med.* **2007**, *6*, 63–70. [PubMed]
16. Osgnach, C.; Poser, S.; Bernardini, R.; Rinaldo, R.; Enrico, P.; Prampero, D.I. Energy cost and metabolic power in elite soccer: A new match analysis approach. *Med. Sci. Sport Exerc.* **2010**, *42*, 170–178. [CrossRef] [PubMed]
17. Nedelec, M.; McCall, A.; Carling, C.; Legall, F.; Berthoin, S.; Dupont, G. The Influence of Soccer Playing Actions on the Recovery Kinetics After a Soccer Match. *J. Strength Cond. Res.* **2014**, *28*, 1517–1523. [CrossRef] [PubMed]
18. Thorpe, R.; Sunderland, C. Muscle Damage, Endocrine, and Immune Marker Response to a Soccer Match. *J. Strength Cond. Res.* **2012**, *26*, 2783–2790. [CrossRef] [PubMed]
19. Fatouros, I.G.; Chatzinikolaou, A.; I Douroudos, I.; Nikolaidis, M.G.; Kyparos, A.; Margonis, K.; Michailidis, Y.; Vantarakis, A.; Taxildaris, K.; Katrabasas, I.; et al. Time-Course of Changes in Oxidative Stress and Antioxidant Status Responses Following a Soccer Game. *J. Strength Cond. Res.* **2010**, *24*, 3278–3286. [CrossRef] [PubMed]
20. Piñeda, A.; González, Y.; Álvarez, P.; Villareal, C. Selección y análisis de ecuaciones antropométricas para el cálculo de la composición corporal en adultos. *Rev. Ing. Matemáticas Cienc. Inf.* **2017**, *4*, 47–56. [CrossRef]
21. Mayorga-Vega, D.; Aguilar-Soto, P.; Viciana, J. Criterion-Related Validity of the 20-M Shuttle Run Test for Estimating Cardiorespiratory Fitness: A Meta-Analysis. *J. Sport Sci. Med.* **2015**, *14*, 536–547.
22. Paradisis, G.P.; Zacharogiannis, E.; Mandila, D.; Smirtiotou, A.; Argeitaki, P.; Cooke, C.B. Multi-Stage 20-m Shuttle Run Fitness Test, Maximal Oxygen Uptake and Velocity at Maximal Oxygen Uptake. *J. Hum. Kinet.* **2014**, *41*, 81–87. [CrossRef]
23. National Institutes of Health. *Adult Treatment Panel III. ATP III Guidelines At-A-Glance Quick Desk Reference*; NIH Publication: Bethesda, MD, USA, 2001.
24. Salas-Salvadó, J.; Rubio, M.; Moreno, B.; Grupo Colaborativo SEEDO. Consenso SEEDO 2007 para la evaluación del sobrepeso y la obesidad y el establecimiento de criterios de intervención terapéutica. *Med. Clin.* **2007**, *128*, 184–196. [CrossRef]
25. Slimani, M.; Znazen, H.; Hammami, A.; Bragazzi, N.L. Comparison of body fat percentage of male soccer players of different competitive levels, playing positions and age groups: A meta-analysis. *J. Sports Med. Phys. Fit.* **2017**, *58*, 857–866.
26. Leão, C.; Camões, M.; Clemente, F.M.; Nikolaidis, P.T.; Lima, R.; Bezerra, P.; Rosemann, T.; Knechtle, B. Anthropometric Profile of Soccer Players as a Determinant of Position Specificity and Methodological Issues of Body Composition Estimation. *Int. J. Environ. Res. Public Health* **2019**, *16*, 2386. [CrossRef]
27. Cardona, D.M.G.; Muñoz, O.E.S.; Arismendy, C.E.C.; Cortés, B.R. Perfil lipídico, antropométrico y condición física de estudiantes deportistas universitarios. *Univ. Salud* **2017**, *19*, 267. [CrossRef]
28. Gil, J.; Verdoy, P. Caracterización de deportistas universitarios de fútbol y baloncesto: Antropometría y composición corporal. e-balonmano.com. *Rev. Cienc. Deport.* **2011**, *7*, 39–51.
29. Apostolidis, N.; Bogdanis, G.C.; Kostopoulos, N.; Souglis, A.; Papadopoulos, C. Changes in the Lipid Profile of Elite Basketball and Soccer Players After a Match. *Res. Sports Med.* **2014**, *22*, 100–110. [CrossRef]
30. Trefts, E.; Williams, A.S.; Wasserman, D.H. Exercise and the Regulation of Hepatic Metabolism. *Prog. Mol. Biol. Transl. Sci.* **2015**, *135*, 203–225. [CrossRef]
31. Pettersson, J.; Hindorf, U.; Persson, P.; Bengtsson, T.; Malmqvist, U.; Werkström, V.; Ekelund, M. Muscular exercise can cause highly pathological liver function tests in healthy men. *Br. J. Clin. Pharmacol.* **2007**, *65*, 253–259. [CrossRef] [PubMed]
32. Sjogren, M. Transaminase Levels and Vigorous Ex. *Adv. Hepatol.* **2007**, *3*, 913–914.
33. Chinedu, I.A.; Chima, I.S.; Emmanuel, O.; Nwabunwanne, O.V.; Chinedu, M.S. Effects of regular exercise on the liver function tests of male subjects in college of health sciences, Nnamdi Azikiwe. *Int. J. Curr. Res. Med. Sci.* **2018**, *4*, 73–79.
34. Yusof, A.; Leithauser, R.M.; Roth, H.J.; Finkernagel, H.; Wilson, M.T.; Beneke, R. Exercise-induced hemolysis is caused by protein modification and most evident during the early phase of an ultraendurance race. *J. Appl. Physiol.* **2007**, *102*, 582–586. [CrossRef]
35. Domínguez, R.; Garnacho-Castaño, M.; Maté-Muñoz, J. Efecto de la hepcidina en el metabolismo del hierro en deportistas. *Nutr. Hosp.* **2014**, *30*, 1218–1231.
36. Lippi, G.; Sanchis-Gomar, F. Epidemiological, biological and clinical update on exercise-induced hemolysis. *Ann. Transl. Med.* **2019**, *7*, 270. [CrossRef]
37. Domínguez, R. Hemólisis en el deporte: Una revisión bibliográfica. *Rev. Entren. Deport.* **2013**, *27*, 1–8.
38. Sim, M.; Dawson, B.; Landers, G.; Trinder, D.; Peeling, P. Iron Regulation in Athletes: Exploring the Menstrual Cycle and Effects of Different Exercise Modalities on Hepcidin Production. *Int. J. Sport Nutr. Exerc. Metab.* **2014**, *24*, 177–187. [CrossRef]
39. Pussieldi, G.; Veneroso, C.; De Paz, J.; Teixeira, M. Respuesta inflamatoria y antiinflamatoria tras el esfuerzo agudo en natación. *Rev. Int. Med. Cienc. Act. Fís. Deporte.* **2018**, *18*, 413–421.
40. Ghafourian, M.; Ashtary-Larky, D.; Chinipardaz, R.; Eskandary, N.; Mehavaran, M. Inflammatory Biomarkers' Response to Two Different Intensities of a Single Bout Exercise Among Soccer Players. *Iran. Red Crescent Med J.* **2016**, *18*, e21498. [CrossRef] [PubMed]
41. Stumpf, C.; Simon, M.; Wilhelm, M.; Zimmermann, S.; Rost, C.; Achenbach, S.; Brem, M.H. Left atrial remodeling, early repolarization pattern, and inflammatory cytokines in professional soccer players. *J. Cardiol.* **2016**, *68*, 64–70. [CrossRef] [PubMed]

42. Jamurtas, A.Z.; Fatouros, I.G.; Deli, C.K.; Georgakouli, K.; Poulios, A.; Draganidis, D.; Papanikolaou, K.; Tsimeas, P.; Chatzinikolaou, A.; Avloniti, A.; et al. The Effects of Acute Low-Volume HIIT and Aerobic Exercise on Leukocyte Count and Redox Status. *J. Sports Sci. Med.* **2018**, *17*, 501–508. [PubMed]
43. Knez, W.; Jenkins, D.; Coombes, J. The Effect of an Increased Training Volume on Oxidative Stress. *Int. J. Sports Med.* **2013**, *35*, 8–13. [CrossRef]
44. Peternelj, T.; Coombes, J.S. Antioxidant Supplementation during Exercise Training: Beneficial or Detrimental? *Sport Med.* **2011**, *41*, 1043–1069. [CrossRef]
45. Silva, J.R.; Rebelo, A.; Marques, F.; Pereira, L.; Seabra, A.; Ascensão, A. Biochemical impact of socce: An analysis of hormonal, muscle damage, and redox markers during the season. *Appl. Physiol. Nutr. Metab.* **2014**, *39*, 432–438. [CrossRef]
46. Inal, M.; Akyüz, F.; Turgut, A.; Getsfrid, W.M. Effect of aerobic and anaerobic metabolism on free radical generation swimmers. *Med. Sci. Sports Exerc.* **2001**, *33*, 564–567. [CrossRef]
47. Gaeta, L.; Tozzi, G.; Pastore, A.; Federici, G.; Bertini, E.; Piemonte, F. Determination of superoxide dismutase and glutathione peroxidase activities in blood of healthy pediatric subjects. *Clin. Chim. Acta* **2002**, *322*, 117–120. [CrossRef]
48. Zivkovic, V.; Lazarevic, P.; Djuric, D.; Čubrilo, D.; Macura, M.; Vuletic, M.; Barudzic, N.; Nešić, M.; Jakovljevic, V. Alteration in basal redox state of young male soccer players after a six-month training programme. *Acta Physiol. Hung.* **2013**, *100*, 64–76. [CrossRef] [PubMed]
49. Viada Pupo, E.; Gómez Robles, L.; Campaña Marrero, I.R. Estrés oxidativo. *Correo Científico Médico* **2017**, *21*, 171–186.
50. Zoppi, C.C.; Hohl, R.; Silva, F.C.; Lazarim, F.L.; Neto, J.A.; Stancanneli, M.; Macedo, D.V. Vitamin C and E Supplementation Effects in Professional Soccer Players Under Regular Training. *J. Int. Soc. Sports Nutr.* **2006**, *3*, 37–44. [CrossRef]
51. Ekun, O.A.; Emiabata, A.F.; Abiodun, O.C.; Ogidi, N.O.; O Adefolaju, F.; Ekun, O.O. Effects of football sporting activity on renal and liver functions among young undergraduate students of a Nigerian tertiary institution. *BMJ Open Sport Exerc. Med.* **2017**, *3*, e000223. [CrossRef] [PubMed]
52. Jacobs, D.; Sluik, D.; Rokling-Andersen, M.; Anderssen, S.; Drevon, C. Association of 1-y changes in diet pattern with cardiovascular disease risk factors and adipokines: Results from the 1-y randomized Oslo Diet and Exercise Study. *Am. J. Clin. Nutr.* **2009**, *89*, 509–517. [CrossRef]
53. Baird, M.; Graham, S.; Baker, J.; Bickerstaff, G. Creatine-kinase- and exercise-related muscle damage implications for muscle performance and recovery. *J. Nutr. Metab.* **2012**, *2012*, 13. [CrossRef] [PubMed]
54. Fisher-Wellman, K.; Bell, H.K.; Bloomer, R.J. Oxidative Stress and Antioxidant Defense Mechanisms Linked to Exercise during Cardiopulmonary and Metabolic Disorders. *Oxidative Med. Cell. Longev.* **2009**, *2*, 43–51. [CrossRef] [PubMed]
55. Wilk, M.; Michalczyk, M.; Gołaś, A.; Krzysztofik, M.; Maszczyk, A.; Zając, A. Endocrine responses following exhaustive strength exercise with and without the use of protein and protein-carbohydrate supplements. *Biol. Sport* **2018**, *35*, 399–405. [CrossRef] [PubMed]

International Journal of
Environmental Research and Public Health

MDPI

Article

Upper Limb Strikes Reactive Forces in Mix Martial Art Athletes during Ground and Pound Tactics

Vaclav Beranek [1,2,*], Petr Stastny [2,*], Vit Novacek [3], Petr Votapek [4] and Josef Formanek [4]

1 Department of Rehabilitation Fields, Faculty of Health Care Studies, University of West Bohemia, 30100 Pilsen, Czech Republic
2 Department of Sport Games, Faculty of Physical Education and Sport, Charles University, 16252 Prague, Czech Republic
3 Biomechanical Human Body Models, New Technologies—Research Centre, University of West Bohemia, 30100 Pilsen, Czech Republic; vnovacek@ntc.zcu.cz
4 Department of Machine Design, Faculty of Mechanical Engineering, University of West Bohemia, 30100 Pilsen, Czech Republic; pvotapek@kks.zcu.cz (P.V.); formanek@kks.zcu.cz (J.F.)
* Correspondence: vberanek@kfe.zcu.cz (V.B.); stastny@ftvs.cuni.cz (P.S.); Tel.: +420-737480136

Received: 25 September 2020; Accepted: 20 October 2020; Published: 24 October 2020

Abstract: Athletes of mixed martial arts use a ground and pound strategy with the strikes in the dominant ground position. The aim of this study was to compare the average peak force (F_{peak}) among three punches and to estimate the probability of achieving a skull bone fracture force of 5.1 kN for each type of strike in male and female athletes. A total of 60 males and 31 females (26 ± 8 years, 75 ± 20 kg, 177 ± 11 cm) practicing professional self-defense at the advanced and professional levels performed 15 strikes on a force plate. The analyses of 1360 trials showed significant differences among the strikes F_{peak} in females ($p < 0.01$) and males ($p < 0.01$). Straight punches had lower F_{peak} than palm strikes and elbow strikes in both genders, and palm strikes had higher F_{peak} than elbow strikes in females. No difference was observed between palm strikes and elbow strikes in males ($p = 0.09$). The ground and pound strikes resulted in higher impacts than previously reported strikes in the standing position. Male athletes can deliver a F_{peak} above 5.1 kN with a probability of 36% with elbow and palm strikes. Such forces can cause head injury; therefore, the use of these strikes in competition should be carefully considered.

Keywords: mixed martial arts; system of self-defense; straight punch; palm strike; elbow strike; ground striking; head injuries

1. Introduction

Mixed martial arts (MMA) is surging in popularity worldwide [1] as a modern, full-contact sport discipline, where competitors utilize different styles of martial arts and combative sports. Because of this complexity, combat athletes use several kinds of tactics, where they fight out of standing on the ground or in the standing using various strikes and other movement actions. One of the combat strategies is called "ground and pound", where one athlete wants to obtain superior positioning over the opponent to execute strikes. Ground striking is a frequently used way of fighting when the dominant opponent sits on an athlete (mount) and uses upper limb strikes, such as a clenched fist, an open palm or an elbow [2]. Generally, the target is most often the opponent's head because hitting the head area is a determining factor for success in MMA [3]. MMA athletes can use almost any strike at its highest intensity [4], but there is currently a lack of evidence-based comparisons of different strikes that can be used in a position on the "mount".

Some types of strikes performed in standing stance have been compared in values of peak (F_{peak}) and mean forces (F_{mean}), where strikes with a clenched fist (straight punch) have been reported being higher in F_{mean} [5,6] and F_{peak} [6–11] than strikes with the open palm (palm strike) [6,12–14]. Conversely, the palm strikes have been reported for more effective force transferring to an object than straight punches [15]. Moreover, F_{peak} and F_{mean} may vary between genders [16,17] and level of experience [13,18,19]. In addition to a general comparison of strikes in reactive forces, it is also possible to estimate the strike potential and probability of causing bone fractures. Compilation of previous studies have reported that strikes exceeding 5.1 kN of F_{peak} would cause a skull bones fracture [6] and therefore, 5.1 kN has been defined as skull bone fracture force. This 5.1 kN threshold, represents the average load tolerance limit for bones of the skull, with the exception of the occipital region with higher load tolerance, where exact values are summarized in Table A1.

The usefulness of a strike might be represented by its velocity impact or other biomechanical advantage; the winners in elite boxing demonstrated higher strike impact represented by F_{peak} and F_{mean} than did their losing peers [8], and F_{mean} itself has been identified as one of the determinants of winning a boxing match [20]. Other studies have reported that F_{mean} is more important for success in combat sports than speed and accuracy of the strike [8,21,22]. This knowledge from boxing demonstrates that comparisons of F_{mean} and F_{peak} among different strikes is beneficial for individual combat tactics, e.g., in MMA combat where injury patterns are similar to those in professional boxing [23]. Moreover, the MMA rules allow the elbow strikes (elbow strike) for which force values reports lack in current literature.

Since ground and pound strikes have an important role in MMA tactics and might have high potential to cause injury, the aim of this study was to compare F_{peak} among kneeling straight punches with a clenched fist, palm strikes and elbow strikes in conditions close to the regular fight competition conditions in advanced male and female athletes. Furthermore, our aim also included a comparison between genders, comparison of our results with previously reported values of strikes performed in the standing stance position, calculation of the relation of F_{peak} with basic anthropometrics and calculation of the probability of achieving a skull bone fracture force of 5.1 kN for each type of strike. In the context of these aims, we hypothesized that straight punches with a clenched fist would reach higher F_{peak} values than palm strikes and elbow strikes. Another hypothesis was that the F_{peak} of ground strikes would be higher than those reported in the standing stance position, men would have higher F_{peak} than woman in each strike, and that the probability of skull bone fracture would be above 30% for all experimental strikes and in both genders.

2. Materials and Methods

2.1. Experimental Approach to the Problem

This cross-sectional study was performed during one familiarization session and one testing session separated by 48 h, where both sessions had the same schedule. The independent variables were the types of the strikes which were compared in dependent variable of F_{peak}. General warm-up consisted of 10 min of jogging and stretching with supervised bodyweight exercises followed by specific warm-up involving 15 strikes of variable intensity on the measuring device. Then, the athletes received a detailed explanation of how to strike during a measurement. The participants performed 5 straight punches with a clenched fist, 5 palm strikes (straight strikes with an open palm) and 5 elbow strikes (strikes using elbow olecranon) in a randomized order.

2.2. Participants

A total of 60 males and 31 females (n = 91, 26 ± 8 years of age, 75 ± 20 kg of body weight, 1.77 ± 11 m of body height) who were practicing professional self-defense at advanced or professional levels of experience participated in the study (Table 1). At the time of testing, all participants were older than 18 years, had no injuries or other medical restrictions and signed informed consent about the purpose and contend of the study. The study protocol was approved by the local ethical committee at the Faculty of Physical Education and Sport, Charles University, Prague, Czech Republic (No. 267/2019) and was in accordance with the Declaration of Helsinki (2013).

Table 1. Mean values with standard deviations of anthropometric characteristics of participants.

Sex	Experience	n	Age ± SD, y, [MIN, MAX]	Height ± SD, cm [MIN, MAX]	Weight ± SD, kg [MIN, MAX]
Female	Advanced	30	21 ± 1 [19, 23]	167 ± 6 [157, 179]	61 ± 7 [51, 77]
Male all		61	28 ± 9 [20, 48]	182 ± 9 [164, 205]	82 ± 20 [68, 186]
	Advanced	51	26 ± 8 [20, 45]	180 ± 7 [164, 198]	76 ± 11 [58, 105]
	Professional	10	37 ± 6 [29, 48]	195 ± 7 [175, 205]	113 ± 27 [75, 186]
All		91	26 ± 8 [19, 48]	177 ± 11 [157, 205]	75 ± 20 [51, 186]

2.3. Procedures of Striking Action

All data collection was carried out in a biomechanical laboratory by the same investigator and at the same hours in both sessions. Each athlete delivered 15 strikes to the force plate that was horizontally oriented with the longer side in front of the athlete. The strikes were performed from a kneeling position with a 15-s rest interval between strikes and a 5-min break between strike types.

The participants were tested with for their preferred dominant hand strikes. After adjustment the impact area of the force plate, they were asked to perform all strikes with the maximal energy that they felt comfortable with. The athletes executed an approximately perpendicular straight punch with the phalanges of the clenched fist and a palm strike in straight direction with the metacarpal area of an open palm. During the elbow strike, the athlete performed a perpendicular strike using the olecranon as the striking surface (Figure 1).

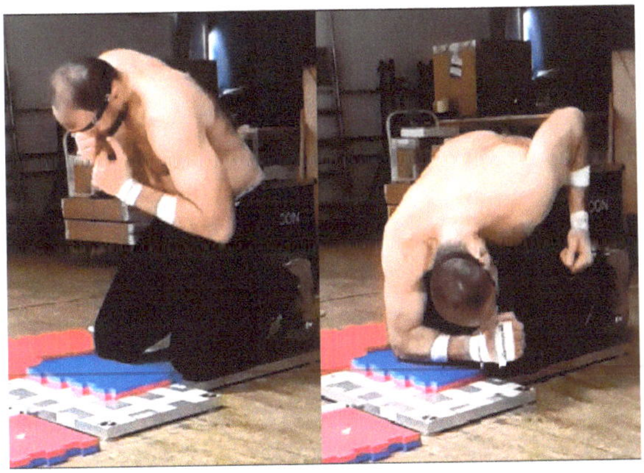

Figure 1. Start (left part) and finish (right part) positions for the elbow "ground" strike.

The athletes performed strikes using the specified starting position for each trial so that the results were directly comparable. The starting position of the striking hand was in contact with the lower jaw (standard defense cover). To avoid the nonstandard bending (above 40° hip flexion) of the athlete's body above the plate before the strike, the athlete had to maintain a vertical distance from the plate to the length of the stretched upper limb in each attempt. The athletes did not touch any part of the body of the measuring device during the experiment, and the distance between the athlete's knees from the edge of the plate was 10 cm. If the participants did not comply the specified measurement protocol, the trial was not recorded.

2.4. Instrumentation and Data Acquisition

All strikes were performed into a force plate (Kistler 9286B, Kistler Inc instrumente, GmbH, Winterthur, Switzerland) mounted to the floor with the participants kneeling on a raised surface next to the force plate. The apparatus consisted of a force plate with a built-in charge amplifier, Type 1758A connection cable, Type 5695B DAQ system and BioWare Type 2812A software. The sampling frequency was 10,000 Hz. The normalized weight was set to 80 kg. The measured force threshold was set to 10 N, and the default setting of the force plate for axis "z" (depth) was modified to account for the foam height from the default value of −22 mm to −40 mm. Each file contained the time, three force components Fx, Fy, Fz, and total force Ft. F_{peak} was defined as the maximum reached force during the recording interval for each trial.

The measurement plate was covered with densely dimensioned polyethylene 1.8 cm thick (Tatami Trocellen) covering because the athlete did not use any protective equipment during the measurement. Hardness was determined using a durometer (type A, DIN 53505; ASTM D 2240; ISO 7619) with different hardnesses for both sides: 20 and 35. Dynamic attenuation (accelerometer, amplifier, SW Spurt) was measured from its own frequency and relative attenuation measurements: 13.7%. The impact attenuation, which is dependent on the compressibility of the damping foam, was measured (load cell). The plate was deformed by a force of 500 N on an area of 20 cm2 from a width of 18 mm to a width of 1 mm, where further compression was no longer possible and the plate attenuation was negligible. The attenuation foam influences the measured force values with a dynamic attenuation of 20% and an impact attenuation of 500 N.

2.5. Statistical Analysis

The data were analyzed in MATLAB® R2019b (The Math Works, Inc., Natick, MA, USA), including Statistics and Machine Learning Toolbox™ used for statistical analysis, where the significance level for all statistical tests was set to 5%. Microsoft® Office Excel 2010 (Microsoft, Redmond, WA, USA) was used for the descriptive statistics and correlations between anthropometric and peak force values.

For comparisons among the strikes, the best and the worst F_{peak} performance was removed for each subject, and the mean from remaining trials were used for statistical analysis. Regarding comparisons with the literature and the probability assessment, all F_{peak} values were conserved for the statistical analysis.

The data normality for each analyzed subgroup was assessed using the Lilliefors test and one-sample Kolmogorov–Smirnov test. The F_{peak} values between the strikes for each gender were separately compared by Kruskal–Wallis test with Tukey's honestly significant difference post hoc test and were considered significant at $p < 0.01$. Additionally, a two-sample left-tailed Wilcoxon rank-sum test was used to compare female and male results for each of the three techniques. It tested the alternative hypothesis that the F_{peak} median of the strike technique in females was lower than the F_{peak} median of the strike technique in males.

A one-sided z-test was used to compare our values to those reported in strikes in the standing stance position from previous studies.

To be able to measure if a skull bone fracture force has been achieved, the probability P of achieving a threshold peak force $\overline{F}$ was calculated by the Rayleigh cumulative distribution function for each strike and gender as follows:

$$P = 1 - \int_{0}^{\overline{F}} \frac{x}{b^2} \exp\left(-\frac{x^2}{2b^2}\right) dx$$

where b is the corresponding Rayleigh scale parameter and x is the peak force data for a given data subset.

3. Results

The acquisition procedure resulted in 1360 successfully processed values of strikes, which were categorized for subsequent analyses (Table 2).

Table 2. Basic characteristics of strikes peak forces across the study subgroups (from all trials).

Gender	Technique	N	Mean [kN] (95% CI)	SD [kN]	CV [%] (95% CI)	*b* [kN] (95% CI)	Min [kN]	Max [kN]
Female	Straight Punch	149	1.66 (1.51; 1.82)	0.74	26.90 (22.68; 31.13)	1.29 (1.17; 1.43)	0.71	4.88
	Palm Strike	150	2.88 (2.70; 3.06)	0.87	17.55 (15.46; 19.63)	2.13 (1.93; 2.37)	1.12	5.55
	Elbow Strike	150	2.44 (2.24; 2.64)	0.96	23.24 (19.30; 27.18)	1.85 (1.68; 2.06)	0.82	5.84
Male	Straight Punch	301	3.55 (3.36; 3.74)	1.29	25.97 (22.34; 29.60)	2.67 (2.49; 2.88)	0.84	7.83
	Palm Strike	300	4.75 (4.51; 4.99)	1.61	18.85 (16.38; 21.32)	3.55 (3.30; 3.83)	2.01	8.83
	Elbow Strike	299	4.49 (4.19; 4.78)	2.02	28.15 (24.56; 31.73)	3.48 (3.24; 3.75)	0.90	10.80
Both Genders	Straight Punch	450	2.92 (2.75; 3.10)	1.45	26.28 (23.52; 29.04)	2.30 (2.17; 2.45)	0.71	7.83
	Palm Strike	450	4.12 (3.92; 4.32)	1.66	18.42 (16.65; 20.19)	3.14 (2.96; 3.34)	1.12	8.83
	Elbow Strike	449	3.80 (3.56; 4.04)	1.99	26.53 (23.80; 29.26)	3.03 (2.86; 3.23)	0.82	10.80

N = number of analyzed strikes; SD = standard deviation; CI = confidence interval; CV = mean individual co-efficient of variation; b = scale parameter of Rayleigh distribution; kN = kilonewtons; Min = minimum; Max = maximum.

Five strikes were removed due to improper execution, and eleven trials were discarded due to excessively high initial total force (>30 N) exceeding the established collection threshold. The anthropometric values of body height and weight did not correlate with F_{peak} values (Figure 2). The data normality was rejected for all subsets (all at $p < 0.01$); instead, the data met the characteristics of the Rayleigh distribution. These results and basic characteristics of strikes are summarized in Table 2.

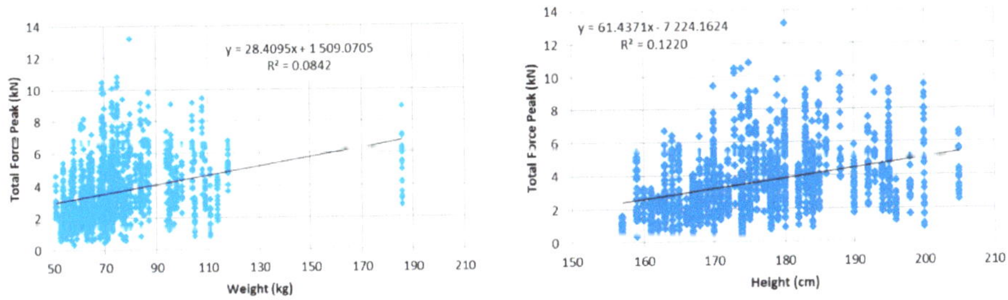

Figure 2. Correlation between peak force and participants weight and height.

The Kruskal–Wallis test indicated significant differences among the strikes for F_{peak} values in females (H = 92.85, $p < 0.01$) and males (H = 49.42, $p < 0.01$), where the post hoc tests showed that straight punches had lower F_{peak} values than palm strikes and elbow strikes in both genders (Figure 3), and palm strikes had higher F_{peak} values than elbow strikes in females. No difference was observed between palm strike and elbow strike in males ($p = 0.09$) (Figure 3).

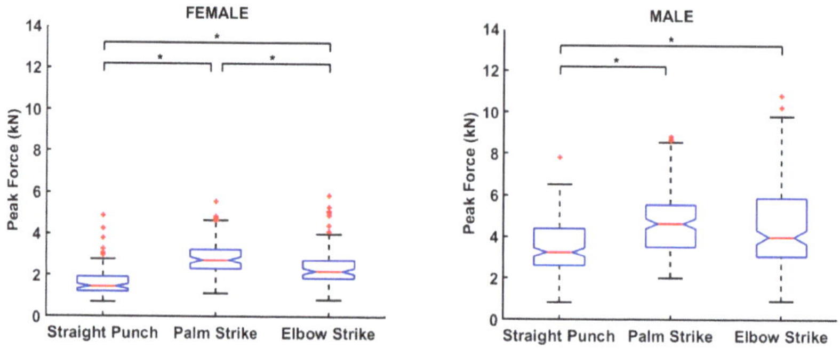

Figure 3. Peak force comparison of male and female strike techniques. * significantly different at $p < 0.01$.

The two-sample left-tailed Wilcoxon rank-sum test rejected the null hypothesis for all three techniques ($p < 0.01$) and confirmed that female F_{peak} median values were lower than male F_{peak} median values for all strikes.

The comparison of our strikes to the values reported for strikes in the standing stance position was possible only for straight punches and palm strikes. One-sided z-tests confirmed that our F_{peak} values did not differ from values (3.4 ± 0.8 kN) reported by Walilko et al. [5] and were greater than the F_{peak} values reported in other literature for both straight punches and palm strikes (Figure 4 and Table A1 and Table S1). Despite nonnormality of the collected data, the z-test was used for comparison because only means and standard deviations had been reported, thereby preventing the use of a nonparametric statistical test.

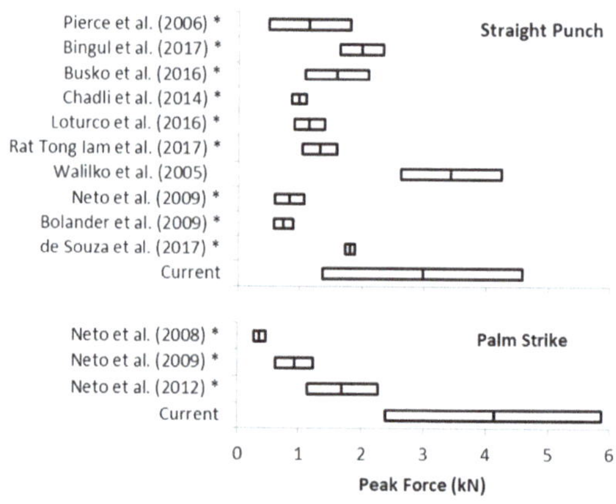

Figure 4. Comparison of straight punch and palm strike peak forces reported in previous studies. * significantly lower than current study. The bar present the means and standard deviations.

The threshold F_{peak} of 5.1 kN was selected with respect to the reported strength of various cranial bones (Appendix A). The comparison was performed for all techniques and for male, female, and all subjects. When considering all participants, there were 10.2%, 26.2%, and 27.4% probabilities of exceeding the selected force threshold with the straight punch, elbow strike and palm strikes, respectively. These are the probabilities that most of the cranial bones would suffer from serious injuries. When stratifying the data according to gender, these probabilities increased to 18.3%, 36.3%, and 36.1% with straight punches, elbow strikes and palm strikes, respectively, in the male group. In the female group, these percentages were much lower, with 0.1%, 2.5%, and 6.0% with straight punches, elbow strikes and palm strikes, respectively. These results are summarized in Figures 5 and 6.

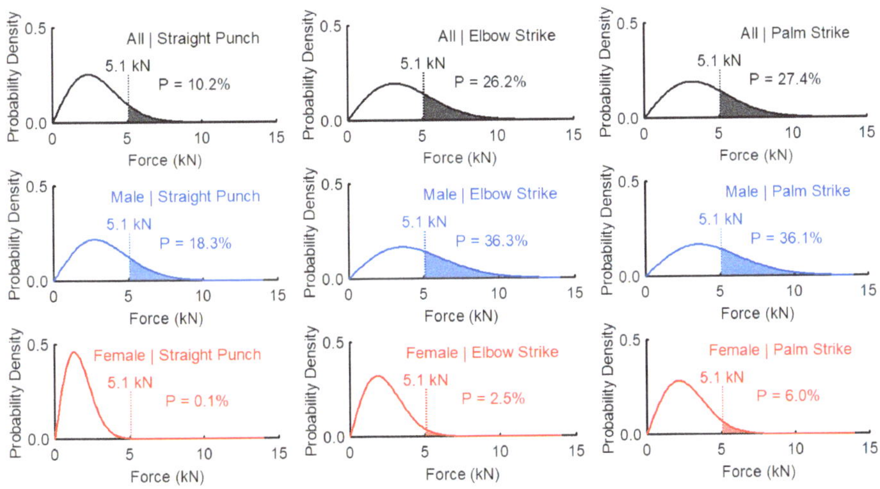

Figure 5. Probability of exceeding the 5.1 kN threshold force. The blue color–Male, the red color-Female.

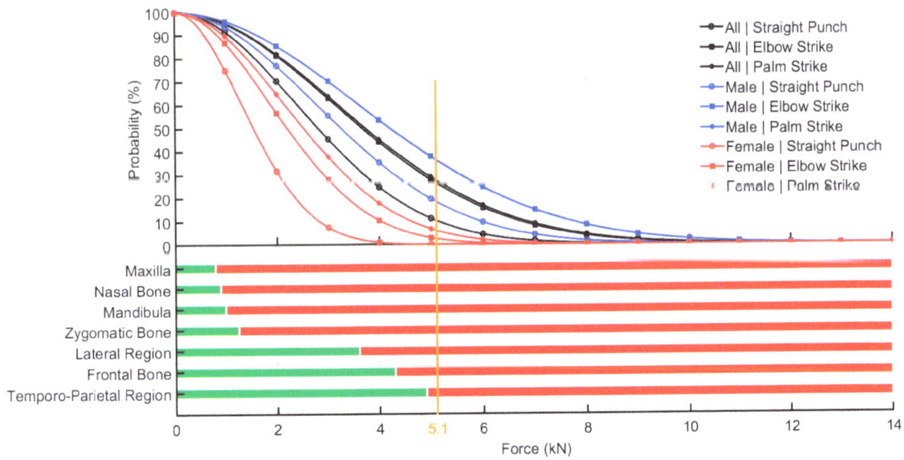

Figure 6. Probability of different strikes to exceed the 5.1 kN and bone tolerance. Green color–limits of allowed average load tolerance of bone fracture. Red color–over the limit of allowed average load tolerance of bone fracture.

4. Discussion

Our results did not confirm our hypotheses because palm strikes and elbow strikes have higher F_{peak} values than straight punches in men, and because palm strikes had higher F_{peak} values than straight punches and elbow strikes in women. On the other hand, our reported results are in accordance with the results of one previous study [15], where palm strikes in a standing stance proved to have the greatest average magnitude compared to a straight punch in a standing position. One explanation for this result is that the force and energy transfers through the forearm more efficiently than through the metacarpals, and palm strikes would be a better way to transfer force to the target. Regarding elbow strikes, it was assumed that athletes use a significantly greater weight of his or her body to deliver the elbow strike because the athlete does not reach the target area by simply extending the upper limb. The reason is that the olecranon impact area is farther from the target than the hand impact area; therefore, athletes must always deliver a strike along with movements of the whole trunk. A longer distance can increase the force of the strike [13,15,24]. In comparison to strikes in standing stance, the ground and pound strikes reach a significantly higher average F_{peak}. Therefore, we can conclude that different body positions during ground striking positively change how the attacker uses the substantial weight of his or her body to support the punch. The horizontal impact area on the ground provides biomechanical advantages, in that the upper limb is located under the mass of the upper torso and is moving the entire time while this movement is also enhanced by gravitational acceleration. Moreover, the ground and pound scenario decrease the submissive opponent head potential to move in free space to diminish strike impact. In worst case, the submissive opponent head might face the full impact absorption if in contact with the surface on strike impact.

The high reported kneeling strike forces, in particular, the greater than 36% probability for achieving a 5.1 kN F_{peak} value with palm strikes and elbow strikes in men, is alarming from a legal point of view. The value of 5.1 kN represents the average limit for skull bone load tolerance for the front and side regions (Appendix A). Upon reaching this value as a result of a strike, a high-risk fracture can be assumed for athletes during fight competitions, even in self-defense situations. Moreover, those results were not correlated with the participant's body weight and body height, and therefore, there are high risks of injury following kneeling palm and elbow strikes that might appear in any weight category. Although previous studies have agreed that there is lack of correlation of the impact or effective mass of a upper limb strike or kick with the height or weight category [8,13,25], this consequence in the kneeling position is surprising and may be related to the advanced combat skills of the selected participants. On the other hand, this is not consistent with the results of recent studies that confirmed a correlation between impact force and weight category in boxing competitions [5].

The results of our analysis confirmed the hypothesis that palm strikes and elbow strikes reach significantly higher F_{peak} values than straight punches with a clenched fist in women. The average F_{peak} values with palm strikes and elbow strikes were approximately 1000 N higher than those by straight punches. In the complete dataset that included extreme values, the highest strike force measured was for the elbow strike (13,188.2 N) and next for the palm strike (9804.2 N). However, the elbow strike showed a lower median than the palm strike. The reason may be that an elbow strike among the ground and pound tactics is not so familiar, unlike the hand strikes; this was similar to what was observed in a standing stance where the impact surface of the elbow may be subjectively more sensitive than the impact surface of the open palm, and thus, the athletes did not perform maximum strikes by elbow in all trials. Furthermore, in the case of an elbow strike, the athlete had to make a longer movement of the whole torso/upper part of the body, which makes it more difficult to perform, and the longer movement also means that it is more difficult to control the falling limb. As a result, the subjects could intentionally perform the movement with less force, and the strike area was also vertically lowered to the level of the measuring platform; however, the opponent's head was at a higher height during testing and training. The dominance of palm strikes and elbow strikes was also confirmed by the conclusions of our probability results, where a significantly higher probability of reaching a peak force of 5.1 kN occurred with elbow strikes and palm strikes than with straight punches. In the overall results across genders, only 10.2% of strikes reached the level of 5.1 kN for a straight punch with a clenched fist as opposed to elbow (26.2%) and palm (27.4%) strikes.

Significantly higher F_{peak} values for strikes in the combat style using "ground striking" compared to strikes in a standing stance confirmed the assumption that the position of body while ground striking positively affects the impact force of the strikes. Data from the literature allowed us to compare 7 sets of results with the straight punch and 4 sets of results with the palm strike (Table A2). In addition to the Walilko et al. [5] study of Olympic boxers, straight punches and palm strikes while ground striking achieved significantly higher average forces than straight punches and palm strikes in a standing. Only data from the literature that reported the F_{peak} with standard deviations could be included in the comparisons, while other studies were excluded. The included studies from the literature reported a lower number of subjects in total (up to 48 subjects) than the current study (91 subjects). Likewise, the literature studies reported data only from those with professional-level experience, while the current study reported data from 10 professionals and 81 advanced level athletes, which supports the evidence for the observed results regarding differences between ground and standing stance striking.

The results of the measurements also showed that the F_{peak} values for three types of punches significantly exceeded the load tolerance of bone tissue. Male athletes with an average weight of 75 kg and height 1.7 m can deliver sufficient F_{peak} values to break all bones of the front and side of the skull, with the exception of the occipital bone, with a probability of 36% for palm strikes and elbow strikes. Strikes on the spine and back of the head are not allowed in MMA competition; therefore, only the facial and lateral parietal parts of the head were rated. In MMA, all three punches are allowed during ground striking. Unlike fighting in a standing stance, a submissive opponent is at a disadvantage because this individual cannot mitigate the impact forces of the hit by changing distance. For this reason, it is possible to assume even greater likelihood of injuries for the combat athlete in a competition. On the other hand, our study provided the optimal time and distance conditions to produce the highest F_{peak} values, and these conditions do not necessarily happen during competition, especially due to the sudden timing of the strikes to hit opponents.

Generally, there has been significant scrutiny from medical associations regarding the high rates of trauma in MMA [26], where aggressive techniques present substantial injury risk [27]. MMA fighters were significantly more likely to experience injury (typically contusion/bruising) compared to boxers [27]. Because blows directly to the head are an effective way to achieve a win, MMA has reported even higher rates of traumatic brain injury than those assessed in American-style football, ice hockey or other contact sports [28,29], and the injury incidence in MMA appears to be greater than in most, if not all, other popular and commonly practiced combat sports [23]. In contrast to these findings, Curran-Sills and Abedin [30] reported that MMA does not confer the same exposure to concussion over a 10-year period as seen in other popular sports (e.g., ice hockey, American football, rugby union), but it is important to avoid this simplified derivation because of methodological differences across the studies [30]. A recent study found that head injuries dominate in MMA [23,30–33]. Professional mixed martial artists (MMA fighters) as such boxers are at risk of sustaining acute head and neck injury each time they engage in practice or competition [34]. These athletes are exposed to the cumulative long-term neurocognitive sequelae of repetitive insults [35]. Brain injury arising from head trauma is a major concern in MMA because knockout (KO) or technical knockout (TKO) are frequent fight outcomes, many movement combinations are targeted to hit the head area [36], and previous studies have shown a high incidence of matches ending due to strikes to the head. Strikes to the head are the major techniques used to end a match via KO/TKO, regardless of sex and weight class [28]. Based on an examination of 440 matches from 2002 to 2014, the main cause of injuries in doctor-stoppage situations was facial injuries (90%), with 87.1% occurring after striking actions. This report also showed higher values related to striking the head in stand-up actions as well as on-the-ground actions [4]. Rates of KOs and TKOs in MMA are higher than previously reported rates in other combative and contact sports. Competition data and video records for all KOs and TKOs from numbered Ultimate Fighting Championship MMA events (n = 844) between 2006 and 2012 identified that all KOs were the result of direct impact to the head, most frequently a strike to the mandibular region (53.9%) [29]. Similarly, head injuries were the most common injuries recorded in 285 championship fights between 2016 and 2018, where head injuries were significantly associated with KOs. Additional research should be extended to head-related injuries in MMA matches, especially those associated with KOs/TKOs [37], including an examination of injury prevention policies to limit injury risk in MMA [1].

A Limitation of the Study

A major limitation of the study is the use of only the dominant side, which we expected to be preferred by athletes and might be the main premise of future studies. The fact that participants did not wear competition hand protection was accounted for by the foam covering force plate. However, the inelastic approach to the measurement cause the impact hardness which may be a psychological barrier for the striker due to fear of injury. Therefore, it is necessary to use sufficient damping because the elasticity of the target has an influence on the measurement of the impact force [38]. Other option is the use of piezoelectric sensors as accelerometers [5,7,39], force sensors based on strain gauges [19], high-speed cameras [36,40,41], use of the dummy [42], or a combination of those techniques [14]. This article presents F_{peak} strikes comparison without the lower and upper extremes, which are typical for F_{peak} results and cause high individual co-efficient of variation (Table 2). However, the results are the same even for whole datasets including extremes. On the other hand, some results might slightly alternate if strikes comparison would be done only for highest F_{peak} values or other special selection, which is available in Supplementary material 2—raw data file.

5. Conclusions

Straight punches, palm strikes, and elbow strikes are effective solutions for victory in ground and pound tactics due to their high impact potential, but they should also be considered high injury-risk strikes. MMA athletes, trainers, self-defense or tactical coaches can expect a high F_{peak} (2900–4100 N) on average for both genders. No significant difference was found in the effectiveness of palm strikes and elbow strikes in men; therefore, both strikes should be preferred in men during ground and pound striking because they each have the advantage of high impact peak forces. In contrast, straight punches showed lower impact forces (to 3000 N) in both genders, and the impact force will probably be further attenuated during the match by gloves. Palm and elbow strikes also provided extreme reactive maximum peak forces (for men, 13 kN), which have a high probability of causing head injury. The elbow strike has the highest potential to reach extreme impact values and fracture skull bones.

Supplementary Materials: The following are available online at http://www.mdpi.com/1660-4601/17/21/7782/s1, Table S1: Results of one-sided z-test testing hypothesis that our Fpeak values come from normal distributions with means and standard deviations reported in literature for straight punch and palm strike against the alternative that the our Fpeak mean is greater. CI = confidence interval. Higher boundary of the confidence intervals is equal to infinity in one-sided test, Supplementary material 2: Raw data file.

Author Contributions: Conceptualization, V.B. and P.S.; methodology, V.B. and P.S.; software, P.S. and V.N.; validation, P.V. and J.F.; formal analysis, V.B. and P.S.; investigation, V.B. and P.S.; resources, V.B.; data curation, V.B.; writing—original draft preparation, V.B. and P.S.; writing—review and editing, V.B. and P.S.; visualization, V.N.; supervision, P.S.; project administration, V.B.; funding acquisition, P.S. All authors have read and agreed to the published version of the manuscript.

Funding: This research was funded by Charles University grant UNCE/HUM/032, European Regional Development Fund-Project "Application of Modern Technologies in Medicine and Industry" (No. CZ.02.1.01/0.0/0.0/17_048/0007280) and by SGS—2019—001 of the University of West Bohemia.

Acknowledgments: This study was supported by Charles University grant UNCE/HUM/032, European Regional Development Fund-Project "Application of Modern Technologies in Medicine and Industry" (No. CZ.02.1.01/0.0/0.0/17_048/0007280) and by SGS—2019—001 of the University of West Bohemia.

Conflicts of Interest: The authors declare no conflict of interest. The funders had no role in the design of the study; in the collection, analyses, or interpretation of data; in the writing of the manuscript, or in the decision to publish the results.

Appendix A

Table A1. Biomechanical tolerance of different regions/bones of the skull—contact force required for fracture.

Region Bone	Study	Force Tolerance (kN)	Force Tolerance (kg)	Impact Area (cm^2)	N mm^{-2}/MPa	Weight (kg)	Velocity ($m \cdot s^{-1}$)
Frontal (forehead)	Schneider and Nahum (1972)	4.0–6.2		6.5		1.1–3.8	3–6
	Advani et al. (1975)	4.0–6.2		6.45		9.1	5–10
	Nahum et al. (1968)	4.0–6.2					
	Voigt and Thomas (1974)	5.5					
	Allsop et al. (1988)	2.2–6.4	224–662				
	Gadd et al. (1968)		498		7.58		
	Tarriere et al. (1981)	7.7					
	Hodgson (1967)	4.6–8.7					2.5–3.3
	Cormier et al. (2011)	2.5–7.6		6.45		3.2	
Temporo-parietal	Nahum et al. (1968)	2.5–5.2		6.45			
	Allsop (1991)						
	Advani et al. (1975)	5.7				9.1	5–10
	Hodgson (1967)		159–454			0.9–7.2	4
	Gadd et al. (1968)		249				
	Raymond et al. (2009)	5.9		38.1 mm projectile		0.10	18–37
	Hodgson and Thomas (1971)	5.5					1.6–4.7
	Hodgson (1967)						
Lateral region	Schneider et al. (1972)	2.0–3.6		6.5		1.1–3.8	3–6
	Nahum et al. (1968)	2.0–3.6		6.45			
	Allsop et al. (1988)	5.2					
	Yoganandan et al. (2003)	5.5–9.9		5			4.8–7.7
Occipital region	Advani et al. (1982)	12.5					
	Allsop (1991)	12.5					
	Hodgson (1967)	15.9					3.7
	Stalnaker et al. (1977)	7.1		15.2 cm diameter		10	6.8–7.2
Os zygomaticum	Advani et al. (1982)	1.0		6.45			
	Nahum et al. (1968)	1.0			1.38–4.17		
	Nyquist et al. (1986)	0.4		2.54			2.7–7.2
	Hodgson (1967)		159–454	2.54–13.2 cm diameter		0.9–7.2	4
	Gadd et al. (1968)		225				
	Allsop et al. (1988)	0.8–2.4	90–244				
	Yoganandan et al. (1991)	1.1–1.3					4
	Gallup (1988)	3.2–3.8	335–394				
Mandibula	Nahum et al. (1968)	1.4		6.45			
	Hodgson (1967)		159–454	2.54–13.2 cm diameter		0.9–7.2	4
	Nyquist et al. (1986)	0.6		2.54			2.7–7.2
	Schneider and Nahum (1972)				2.76–6.20	1.1–3.8	3–6
Os nasale	Nyquist et al. (1986)	0.3	306	2.54			2.7–7.2
	Hodgson (1967)		159–454	2.54–13.2 cm diameter			2.5–3.7
	Gallup (1988) (nasal area)	1.9–2.9	200–299				
	Swearingen (1965)	0.3–4.5					
	Nahum et al. (1968)				0.13–0.34		
Maxilla	Nahum et al. (1968)	0.7–1.5		6.45			
	Advani et al. (1982)						
	Nyquist et al. (1986)	1.4		2.54			
	Hodgson (1967)	0.6–1.8	159–454	2.54–13.2 cm diameter			
	Allsop et al. (1988)	1.0–1.8	102–184				
	Nahum et al. (1968)				1.03–2.07	1.1–3.8	3–6
	Schneider and Nahum (1972)						

Table A2. Direct and palm strike peak force mean and standard deviation.

Name of Strike	Author	F MEAN (N)	SD	Number of Subjects	Experiences
Palm strike	Neto et al. (2012)	1706.14	557.03	7	EXPERT: 4 MALE, 3 FEMALE
	Neto et al. (2009)	930.00	301.00	13	MIX: 10 MALE, 3 FEMALE
	Neto et al. (2008)	355.00	96.50	13	EXPERT: 7 MALE; NOVICE: 6 MALE
	Bolander et al. (2009)	736	159	13	EXPERT: 10 MALE, 3 FEMALE
	This study (complete)	4131.20	1747.03	91	ADVANCED = 81
	This study (reduced)	4121.91	1658.01		PROFESSIONAL = 10
Straight punch	Walilko et al. (2005)	3427.00	811.00	7	EXPERT, MALE
	Rat Tong Iam et al. (2017)	1323.30	278.50	3	EXPERT, MALE
	Loturco et al. (2016)	1152.22	246.87	15	EXPERT: 9 MALE, 6 FEMALE
	Chadli et al. (2014)	989.00	116.70	11	EXPERT, MALE
	Busko et al. (2016)	1592.50	507.10	48	EXPERT: 21 MALE, 27 FEMALE
	Bingul et al. (2017)	1987.42	341.95	10	EXPERT, MALE
	Pierce et al. (2016)	1149.20	665.80	12	EXPERT, MALE
	This study (complete)	2971.85	1603.80	91	ADVANCED = 81
	This study (reduced)		1445.88		PROFESSIONAL = 10

References of Appendix

- Allsop, D.C.; Warner, M.W.; Schneider, D.; Nahum, A. Facial impact response—a comparison of the hybrid iii dummy and human cadaver. *J. Passeng. Cars* **1988**, *97*, 1224–1240.
- Allsop, D.; Perl, T.R.; Warner, C.Y. Force/deflection and fracture characteristics of the temporoparietal region of the human head. In Proceedings of the 35th Stapp Car Crash Conference, Detroit, MI, USA, 1991; pp. 269–278.
- Advani, S.; Powell, W.; Huston, J.; Ojala, S. Human head impact response-experimental data and analytical simulations. In Proceedings of the International Conference on the Biomechanics of Impact (IRCOBI), Berlin, Germany, 1975; pp. 153–162.
- Advani, S.H.; Ommaya, A.K.; Yang, W.J. *Human body dynamics*; Claredon: Oxford, UK, 1982.
- Adamec, J.; Mai, V.; Graw, M.; Schneider, K.; Hempel, J.-M.; Schöpfer, J. Biomechanics and injury risk of a headbutt. *Int. J. Legal Med.* **2013**, *127*, 103–110.
- Cormier, J.; Manoogian, S.; Bisplinghoff, J.; Rowson, S.; Santago, A.; McNally, C.; Duma, S.; Bolte, J. The Tolerance of the Frontal Bone to Blunt Impact. *J. Biomech. Eng.* **2011**, *133(2)*, 021004. doi: 10.1115/1.4003312, 2011.
- Schneider, D.C.; Nahum, A.M. Impact studies of facial bones and skull. In Proceedings of the 16th Stapp Car Crash Conference, Detroit, MI, USA, 1972; pp. 186–203.
- Swearingen, J.J. *Tolerances of the human face to crash impact*; Federal Aviation Agency, Civil Aeromedical Research Institute: Oklahoma City, OK, USA, 1965.
- Gallup, B.M.; Hallgrimson, B.H.; Cotton, C.E.; Smith, T.A.; Newman, J.A. *The development of an improved ATD bead form with a frangible facial insert*; LR.C.O.B.I.: Bergisch-Gladbach, Germany, 1988.
- Gadd, C.W.; Nahum, A.M.; Gatts, J.; Danford, J.P. A study of head and facial bone impact tolerances. In *Proc. G.M.*; Auto Safety Seminar: Detroit, USA, 1968.
- Nahum, A.M.; Gatts, J.D., Gadd, C.W.; Danforth, J.P. Impact tolerance of the face and skull. In Proceedings of the 12th Stapp Car Crash Conference, Detroit, MI, USA, 1968; pp. 302–317.
- Hampson, D. Facial injury: A review of biomechanical studies and test procedures for facial injury assessment. *J. Biomech.* **1995**, 28(1), 1–7. doi:10.1016/0021-9290(95)80001-8.
- Hodgson, V.R. Tolerance of facial bones to impact. *Am. J. Anat.* **1967**, *120*, 113–122.
- Hodgson, V.R.; Thomas, L.M. Comparison of head acceleration injury indices in cadaver skull fracture. *SAE Tech. Pap.* **1971**, *80*, 710619–710867. doi:10.4271/710854.

- Nyquist, G.W.; Cavanaugh, J.M.; Goldberg, S.J.; King, A.I. Facial impact tolerance and response. In Proceedings of the 30th Stapp Car Crash Conference, Detroit, MI, USA, 1986; pp. 379–400.
- Voigt, R.; Thomas, L.M. *Breaking strength of the human skull* vs. *impact surface curvature;* School of Medicine, Dept. of Neurosurgery, Wayne State University, Detroit, MI, USA, 1974.
- Tarriere, C.; Leung, Y.C.; Fayon, A.; Got, C.; Patel, A.; Banzet, P. Field facial injuries and study of their simulation with dummy. In Proc. 25th Stapp Car Crash Conf., San Francisco, USA, 1981.
- Raymond, D.; Van Ee, C.; Crawford, G.; Bir, C. Tolerance of the skull to blunt ballistic temporo-parietal impact. *J. Biomech.* **2009,** *42(15),* 2479–2485. doi:10.1016/j.jbiomech.2009.07.018.
- Stalnaker, R.L.; Melvin, J.W.; Nusholtz, G.S.; Alem, N.M.; Benson, J.N. Head Impact Response. *SAE Tech. Pap.* **1977**, 770921. doi.org/10.4271/770921.
- Svoboda, M.; Soukup, J.; Jelen, K.; Kubový, P. Measurement of force impact taekwondo athletes, assessing the possibility of injury of human head. *Procedia Engineering* **2016**, *136* 211–215. doi:10.1016/j.proeng.2016.01.199, 2016.
- Siswanto, W.A.; Hua, C.S. Strength analysis of human skull on high speed impact. *Int. Rev. Mech. Eng.* **2016**, *6(7)*, 1508–1514.
- Yoganandan, N.; Pintar, F.; Sances, A. Biodynamics of steering wheel induced facial trauma. *J. Safety Res.* 1991, *22*, 179–190.
- Yoganandan, N.; Zhang, J.; Pintar, F.A.; Gennarelli, T.A.; Kuppa, S.M.; Eppinger, R.H. Biomechanics of Lateral Skull Fracture, In Proceedings of the IRCOBI Conference, Lisbon, Portugal, 2003.
- Yoganandan, N.; Pintar, F.A. Biomechanics of temporo-parietal skull fracture. *Clin. Biomech.* **2004**, *19(3)*, 225-239. doi:10.1016/j.clinbiomech.2003.12.014.

References

1. Fares, M.Y.; Fares, J.; Fares, Y.; Abboud, J.A. Musculoskeletal and head injuries in the ultimate fighting championship (UFC). *Phys. Sportsmed.* **2019**, *47*, 205–211. [CrossRef]
2. Ruebusch, C. The Science of Ground and Pound: Introduction. 2014. Available online: https://www.bloodyelbow.com/2014/8/18/6030011/science-ground-and-pound-introduction-mma-technique-series-posture-guard-ko-gif (accessed on 1 February 2020).
3. Kirk, C. Does anthropometry influence technical factors in competitive mixed martial arts? *Hum. Mov.* **2018**, *19*, 46–59. [CrossRef]
4. Miarka, B.; Bello, F.D.; Brito, C.J.; Del Vecchio, F.B.; Amtmann, J.; Chamari, K.; Brito, J.C. A 12-year cohort study of DOC-stoppage in professional mixed martial arts. *Int. J. Sport Physiol.* **2019**, *14*, 606–611. [CrossRef] [PubMed]
5. Walilko, T.J.; Viano, D.C.; Bir, C.A. Biomechanics of the head for Olympic boxer punches to the face. *Brit. J. Sports Med.* **2005**, *39*, 710–719. [CrossRef] [PubMed]
6. Beranek, V.; Votapek, P.; Stastny, P. Force and velocity of impact during upper limb strikes in combat sports: A systematic review and meta-analysis. *Sports Biomech.* **2020**. [CrossRef]
7. Atha, J.; Yeadon, M.R.; Sandover, J.; Parsons, K.C. The damaging punch. *Brit. Med. J.* **1985**, *291*, 1756–1757. [CrossRef]
8. Pierce, J.D.; A Reinbold, K.; Lyngard, B.C.; Goldman, R.J.; Pastore, C.M. Direct Measurement of Punch Force During Six Professional Boxing Matches. *J. Quant. Anal. Sports* **2006**, *2*, 1–19. [CrossRef]
9. Halperin, I.; Chapman, D.W.; Martin, D.T.; Abbiss, C.R. The effects of attentional focus instructions on punching velocity and impact forces among trained combat athletes. *J. Sports Sci.* **2017**, *35*, 500–507. [CrossRef]
10. Dyson, R.; Smith, M.; Fenn, L.; Martin, C. Differences in lead and rear hand punching forces, delivered at maximal speed relative to maximal force, by amateur boxers. In Proceedings of the 23th International Symposium on Biomechanics in Sports Conference, Beijing, China, 22–27 August 2005.
11. Svoboda, M.; Soukup, J.; Jelen, K.; Kubový, P. Measurement of force impact taekwondo athletes, assessing the possibility of injury of human head. *Procedia Eng.* **2016**, *136*, 211–215. [CrossRef]

12. Neto, O.P.; Silva, J.H.; Marzullo, A.C.D.M.; Bolander, R.P.; Bir, C.A. The effect of hand dominance on martial arts strikes. *Hum. Mov. Sci.* **2012**, *31*, 824–833. [CrossRef]
13. Neto, O.P.; Magini, M.; Saba, M.M.F.; Pacheco, M.T.T. Comparison of force, power, and striking efficiency for a kungfu strike performed by novice and experienced practitioners: Preliminary analysis. *Percept. Mot. Ski.* **2008**, *106*, 188–196. [CrossRef] [PubMed]
14. Neto, O.P.; Pacheco, M.T.T.; Bolander, R.; Bir, C. Force, reaction time, and precision of kungfu strikes. *Percept. Mot. Ski.* **2009**, *109*, 295–303. [CrossRef]
15. Bolander, R.P.; Neto, O.P.; Bir, C.A. The effects of height and distance on the force production and acceleration in martial arts strikes. *J. Sports Sci. Med.* **2009**, *8*, 47–52.
16. Buśko, K.; Staniak, Z.; Szark-Eckardt, M.; Nikolaidis, P.T.; Mazur-Różycka, J.; Łach, P.; Michalski, R.; Gajewski, J.; Górski, M. Measuring the force of punches and kicks among combat sport athletes using a modified punching bag with an embedded accelerometer. *Acta Bioeng. Biomech.* **2016**, *18*, 47–54. [CrossRef]
17. LoTurco, I.; Nakamura, F.Y.; Artioli, G.G.; Kobal, R.; Kitamura, K.; Abad, C.C.C.; Cruz, I.F.; Romano, F.; Pereira, L.A.; Franchini, E. Strength and power qualities are highly associated with punching impact in elite amateur boxers. *J. Strength Cond. Res.* **2016**, *30*, 109–116. [CrossRef]
18. Daruis, D.D.I.; Ridzuan, M.M.; Ismail, S.J.; Deros, B.M.; Ramli, A.S. Female student-athletes' biomechanics and anthropometric profile of unarmed combat kicks. In Proceedings of the 2014 IEEE Conference on Biomedical Engineering and Sciences (IECBES), Kuala Lumpur, Malaysia, 8–10 December 2014; pp. 408–413. [CrossRef]
19. De Souza, V.A.; Marques, A.M. Relationship between age and expertise with the maximum impact force of a reverse punch by shotokan karate athletes. *Arch. Budo.* **2017**, *13*, 243–254.
20. Bingul, M.B.; Bulgan, C.T.; Aydin, M.; Bal, E. The effects of impact forces and kinematic of two different stance at straight punch techniques in boxing. *Arch. Budo.* **2017**, *13*, 35–39.
21. Lenetsky, S.; Harris, N.; Brughelli, M. Assessment and contributors of punching forces in combat sports athletes: Implications for strength and conditioning. *SCJ* **2013**, *35*, 1–7. [CrossRef]
22. Smith, M. Physiological profile of senior and junior England international amateur boxers. *J. Sport Sci. Med.* **2006**, *5*, 74–89.
23. Lystad, R.P.; Gregory, K.; Wilson, J. The epidemiology of injuries in mixed martial arts: A systematic review and meta-analysis. *Orthop. J. Sports Med.* **2014**, *2*. [CrossRef]
24. Gulledge, K.J.; Dapena, J.A. Comparison of the reverse and power punches in oriental martial arts. *J. Sports Sci.* **2007**, *26*, 189–196. [CrossRef]
25. Estevan, I.; Falco, C.; Álvarez, O.; Molina-García, J. Effect of olympic weight category on performance in the roundhouse kick to the head in taekwondo. *J. Hum. Kinet.* **2012**, *31*, 37–43. [CrossRef]
26. Thomas, R.E.; Thomas, B.C. Systematic review of injuries in mixed martial arts. *Phys. Sportsmed.* **2018**, *46*, 155–167. [CrossRef]
27. Karpman, S.; Reid, P.; Phillips, L.; Qin, Z.; Gross, D.P. Combative sports injuries: An edmonton retrospective. *Clin. J. Sport Med.* **2016**, *26*, 332–334. [CrossRef]
28. Follmer, B.; Dellagrana, R.A.; Zehr, E.P. Head trauma exposure in mixed martial arts varies according to sex and weight class. *Sports Health.* **2019**, *11*, 280–285. [CrossRef]
29. Hutchison, M.G.; Lawrence, D.W.; Cusimano, M.D.; Schweizer, T.A. Head trauma in mixed martial arts. *AMJ Sport Med.* **2014**, *42*, 1352–1358. [CrossRef]
30. Curran-Sills, G.; Abedin, T. Risk factors associated with injury and concussion in sanctioned amateur and professional mixed martial arts bouts in Calgary, Alberta. *BMJ Open Sport Exerc. Med.* **2018**, *4*. [CrossRef]
31. Demorest, R.A.; Koutures, C.; LaBella, C.R.; Council on Sports Medicine and Fitness. Youth participation and injury risk in martial arts. *Pediatrics* **2016**, *138*. [CrossRef]
32. Ji, M. Analysis of injury types for mixed martial arts athletes. *J. Phys. Ther. Sci.* **2016**, *28*, 1544–1546. [CrossRef]
33. Lockwood, J.; Frape, L.; Lin, S.; Ackery, A. Traumatic brain injuries in mixed martial arts: A systematic review. *Trauma* **2018**, *20*, 245–254. [CrossRef]
34. Bartsch, A.; Benzel, E.; Miele, V.; Morr, D.; Prakash, V. Impact fingerprints and preliminary implications for an intelligent mount guard head impact dosimeter. *Sports Eng.* **2012**, *15*. [CrossRef]
35. Miele, V.J.; Bailes, J.E. Objectifying when to halt a boxing match: A video analysis of fatalities. *Neurosurgery* **2007**, *60*, 307–315. [CrossRef]

36. Tong-Iam, R.; Rachanavy, P.; Lawsirirat, C. Kinematic and kinetic analysis of throwing a straight punch: The role of trunk rotation in delivering a powerful straight punch. *JPES* **2017**, *17*, 2538–2543. [CrossRef]
37. McClain, R.; Wassermen, J.; Mayfield, C.; Berry, A.C.; Grenier, G.; Suminski, R.R. Injury profile of mixed martial arts competitors. *Clin. J. Sport Med.* **2014**, *24*, 497–501. [CrossRef]
38. Falco, C.; Alvarez, O.; Castillo, I.; Estevan, I.; Martos, J.; Mugarra, F.; Iradi, A. Influence of the distance in a roundhouse kick's execution time and impact force in taekwondo. *J. Biomech.* **2009**, *42*, 242–248. [CrossRef]
39. Chiu, H.T.; Shiang, T.Y. A new approach to evaluate karate punch techniques. In Proceedings of the ISB Conference Proceedings Archive, Perth, Western Australia, 30 June–6 July 1999; pp. 61–64.
40. Gianino, C. Physics of Karate. Kinematics analysis of karate techniques by a digital movie camera. *J. Phys. Educ.* **2010**, *4*, 5.
41. Daniel, T.M.; Liviu-Razvan, P. Correlation between Plantar Pressure and Striking Speed in Karate-do. *Procedia Soc. Behav. Sci.* **2014**, *117*, 357–360. [CrossRef]
42. Clark, J.; Michio, T.; Blaine, H.; Gilchrist, M.D. Event-specific impact test protocol for ice hockey goaltender masks. *Sports Biomech.* **2018**. [CrossRef]

Publisher's Note: MDPI stays neutral with regard to jurisdictional claims in published maps and institutional affiliations.

International Journal of
Environmental Research and Public Health

MDPI

Article

Does Post-Activation Performance Enhancement Occur during the Bench Press Exercise under Blood Flow Restriction?

Michal Wilk [1,*], Michal Krzysztofik [1], Aleksandra Filip [1], Agnieszka Szkudlarek [2], Robert G. Lockie [3] and Adam Zajac [1]

1 Institute of Sport Sciences, The Jerzy Kukuczka Academy of Physical Education in Katowice, 40-065 Katowice, Poland; m.krzysztofik@awf.katowice.pl (M.K.); a.filip@awf.katowice.pl (A.F.); a.zajac@awf.katowice.pl (A.Z.)
2 Department of Physical Pharmacy, Faculty of Pharmaceutical Sciences in Sosnowiec, Medical University of Silesia in Katowice, 40-055 Katowice, Poland; aszkudlarek@sum.edu.pl
3 Center for Sports Performance, Department of Kinesiology, California State University, Fullerton, CA 92831, USA; rlockie@fullerton.edu
* Correspondence: m.wilk@awf.katowice.pl

Received: 23 April 2020; Accepted: 25 May 2020; Published: 26 May 2020

Abstract: *Background*: The aim of the present study was to evaluate the effects of post-activation performance enhancement (PAPE) during successive sets of the bench press (BP) exercise under blood flow restriction (BFR). *Methods*: The study included 10 strength-trained males (age = 29.8 ± 4.6 years; body mass = 94.3 ± 3.6 kg; BP 1-repetition maximum (1RM) = 168.5 ± 26.4 kg). The experiment was performed following a randomized crossover design, where each participant performed two different exercise protocols: under blood flow restriction (BFR) and control test protocol (CONT) without blood flow restriction. During the experimental sessions, the study participants performed 3 sets of 3 repetitions of the BP exercise at 70%1RM with a 5 min rest interval between sets. The differences in peak power output (PP), mean power output (MP), peak bar velocity (PV), and mean bar velocity (MV) between the CONT and BFR conditions were examined using 2-way (condition × set) repeated measures ANOVA. Furthermore, t-test comparisons between conditions were made for the set 2–set 1, set 3–set 1, and set 3–set 2 delta values for all variables. *Results*: The post hoc results for condition × set interaction in PP showed a significant increase in set 2 compared to set 1 for BFR ($p < 0.01$) and CONT ($p = 0.01$) conditions, a significant increase in set 3 compared to set 1 for the CONT ($p = 0.01$) condition, as well as a significant decrease in set 3 compared to set 1 for BFR condition occurred ($p < 0.01$). The post hoc results for condition × set interaction in PV showed a significant increase in set 2 compared to set 1 for BFR ($p < 0.01$) and CONT ($p = 0.01$) conditions, a significant increase in set 3 compared to set 1 for CONT ($p = 0.03$) condition, as well as a significant decrease in set 3 compared to set 1 for BFR condition ($p < 0.01$). The t-test comparisons showed significant differences in PP ($p < 0.01$) and PV ($p = 0.01$) for set 3–set 2 delta values between BFR and CONT conditions. *Conclusion*: The PAPE effect was analyzed through changes in power output and bar velocity that occurred under both the CONT and BFR conditions. However, the effects of PAPE have different kinetics in successive sets for BFR and for CONT conditions.

Keywords: upper limb resistance exercise; power output; bar velocity; occlusion; performance

1. Introduction

The ability to generate high power outputs is one of the most significant factors determining performance in numerous sport disciplines. The increase in power output observed during and directly after resistance exercises is termed post-activation performance enhancement (PAPE) [1]. Previous studies have shown a ergogenic effect of initial muscle activation on power output in consecutive sets of a single resistance exercise [2,3] in addition to a stimulating effect of initial muscle activation on effectiveness of throwing, jumping, and hitting movements as well on the time under tension during exercise performed to volitional failure [4–7]. The physiological rationale for PAPE is a greater contractibility and excitability of muscles due to several mechanisms [2,8]. The rationale for this phenomenon might be related to residual of post-activation potentiation (PAP) in its earliest stages after a conditioning activity (CA) and other mechanisms such as enhanced muscle activation, increased muscle temperature and muscle force, and/or increased shortening velocity triggered by fiber water content [8].

Most studies that have analyzed the acute effects of PAPE on power output have considered training components such as external load, number of sets and repetitions, as well as the duration of rest intervals between particular sets and between the conditioning and explosive exercise [5,9–11]. Regarding the intensity a wide range of loads have been found to potentiate subsequent performance (40–90% 1-repetition maximum (1RM)) [12–15]. In addition to the applied external load, the number of sets during the conditioning activity also have a significant impact on PAPE [3,16]. One of the newly introduced training means in resistance exercise includes occlusion, which is better known as blood flow restriction (BFR) [17]. The BFR technique involves the use of a tourniquet, inflatable cuff, or elastic wraps [18,19]. The compression is placed at the upper part of the limb to reduce arterial blood flow and to occlude venous blood flow during physical exercise [17]. The main mechanisms responsible for the adaptive responses related with exercise under BFR include increased mechanical tension and elevated metabolic stress [20]. Although the exact mechanisms remain unknown, most evidence seems to allude to a muscle cell swelling response and the indirect effect of metabolites, instigating an increased muscle activation through fatigue [21]. Further, the exercise under BFR resulted in greater muscle cross-sectional area, isometric strength, and 1RM performance [22]. Application of BFR acutely increases muscle swelling due to fluid shifts [18]. Given that myofibrillar fluid shifts can increase muscle fiber force and shortening velocity and, thus, power, this mechanism can increase effectiveness of PAPE [8]. Furthermore, Wilk et al. [23] suggest that not only the physiological responses but also mechanical work generated by the cuff can potentially cause acute positive changes during resistance exercise under BFR. Currently only few previous studies have compared the effects of high load resistance training under BFR conditions [23–26], and only one refers to acute changes in power output [23]. The study by Wilk et al. [23] showed that short-term BFR increases power output and bar velocity during the bench press (BP) exercise.

While PAPE alone offers an attractive and practical means for conditioning coaches to elicit an increase in performance, the additional use of BFR during resistance training can additionally enhance the PAPE effect. Considering this, numerous studies have attempted to determine optimal variables of resistance training that would maximize PAPE [3,27,28]. However, none of them relate to the acute changes in power output following successive sets of resistance exercise under BFR. Due to the fact that short-term BFR significantly increases the power output and bar velocity [23], the aim of the present study was to evaluate the effects of BFR on power output and bar velocity between successive sets of the BP exercise. We hypothesized that the PAPE effect occurs during successive sets of the BP exercise under BFR.

2. Methods

The experiment was performed following a randomized crossover design, where each participant performed two different exercise protocols: under BFR with a 10 cm cuff (BFR) and a control test protocol (CONT) without BFR. The entire research procedure lasted 4 weeks with a one-week interval between each trial. During the experimental sessions, the study participants performed 3 sets of the BP exercise of 3 repetitions at 70% of 1RM with a 5 min rest interval between sets at maximum speed. The following variables were registered: peak power output (PP), mean power output (MP), peak bar velocity (PV), and mean bar velocity (MV). All testing sessions were performed in the Strength and Power Laboratory at the Academy of Physical Education in Katowice.

2.1. Participants

Ten healthy males who were experienced in resistance training (12.7 ± 6.8 years) volunteered for the study (age = 29.8 ± 4.6 years; body mass = 94.3 ± 13.6 kg; BP 1RM = 168.5 ± 26.4 kg; mean ± SD). The inclusion criterion was a BP personal record with a load of at least 120% body mass. The participants were instructed to maintain their normal dietary habits over the course of the study and not to use any supplements or stimulants for the duration of the experiment. All participants were required to refrain from resistance training 72 h prior to each experimental session, and were informed about the benefits and potential risks of the study before providing their written informed consent for participation. The participants could withdraw from the experiment at any moment of the study. The study protocol was approved by the Bioethics Committee for Scientific Research at the Academy of Physical Education in Katowice, Poland (no. 02/2019), and performed according to the ethical standards of the latest version of the Declaration of Helsinki, 2013.

2.2. Familiarization Session and One Repetition Maximum Test

Two weeks before the main experiment, the participants took part in familiarization sessions consisting of 4 sets of 3 repetitions of the BP at 50%1RM with BFR with cuff pressure set to the value of ~60% full arterial occlusion pressure (AOP).

One week before the main experiment, all participants performed the 1RM BP test. The general warm-up before the 1RM test consisted of cycling on an ergometer for 5 min, followed by several push-ups, pull-ups, and dynamic stretching of the upper body. Next, the participants performed 15, 10, and 5 BP repetitions using 20%, 40%, and 60% of their estimated 1RM, respectively. For the evaluation of 1RM, the loading started at 80% estimated 1RM, and was increased by 2.5 to 10 kg for each subsequent attempt, and the process was repeated until failure. During the 1RM test, the participants executed single repetitions with a constant movement tempo (2 s duration of the eccentric phase, maximal speed in the concentric phase) [29,30] and a 5 min rest interval between successful attempts. Hand placement on the bar was set at 150% bi-acromial distance.

2.3. Experimental Sessions

In a randomized, crossover fashion, the participants performed the BP exercise at 70%1RM either with BFR (BFR) or without BFR (CONT). The general and specific warm-up for the experimental sessions was identical to the one used during the 1RM test. After the warm-up, the participants started the main protocol and performed 3 sets of 3 repetitions of concentric and eccentric contractions at maximal tempo of movement with a 5 min rest interval between sets. The repetitions were performed without intentionally pausing at the transition between the eccentric and concentric phases. A linear position transducer system (Tendo Sport Machines, Trencin, Slovakia) was used for the evaluation of bar velocity. The Tendo Power Analyzer is a reliable system for measuring movement velocity and power output (commercially calibrated) [31]. The measurement was made independently for each repetition and automatically converted into values of peak power output (PP), mean power output (MP), peak velocity (PV), and mean velocity (MV). The mean power output and bar velocity were obtained as the mean of the three repetitions. Peak power output and peak bar velocity were obtained from the best repetition.

2.4. Blood Flow Restriction

The participants wore occlusion cuffs at the most proximal region of both arms during experimental sessions. During the exercise protocol with BFR, Smart Cuffs (10 cm width) produced by Smart Tools Plus LLC, Strongsville, USA were applied to the upper limbs. In order to determine the individual occlusion pressure, the value of full AOP at rest was determined. The measurement was conducted twice on each limb, and the obtained differences were within 20 mmHg [32]. The average value was then used to set the cuff pressure for the exercise protocol. The pressure of the cuff for BFR condition was set to ~90% of full AOP (152 mmHg ± 11.4 for BFR) [23]. The level of vascular restriction was controlled by a handheld Edan SD3 Doppler (Edan Instruments, Shenzen, China). During the BFR condition, the restriction was set immediately before the onset of exercise and released following the completion of the third repetition [23].

2.5. Statistical Analysis

All statistical analyses were performed using Statistica 9.1 (Hillview, Palo Alto, CA, USA) and were presented as means with standard deviations. The Shapiro–Wilk and Mauchly's tests were used in order to verify the normality/homogeneity and sphericity of the sample data variances, respectively. Verification of differences between CONT and BFR conditions in PP, MP, PV, and MV was performed using a two-way 2 × 3 (condition × set) analysis of variance (ANOVA) with repeated measures. Statistical significance was set at $p < 0.05$. In the event of a significant main effect, post hoc comparisons were conducted using Tukey's test. Furthermore, t-test comparisons between conditions were made for the set 2–set 1, set 3–set 1, and set 3–set 2 delta values for all variables. Additionally, independent sample t-tests were used to verify the differences between successive sets independently for BFR and CONT conditions as well as differences in individual sets between BFR and CONT conditions. Percent changes and 95% confidence intervals were also calculated. Effect sizes (Cohen's d) were reported where appropriate. Parametric effect sizes (ES) were defined as large $d > 0.8$; moderate between 0.79 and 0.5; small between 0.49 and 0.20; and trivial as <0.2 [33].

3. Results

The two-way repeated measures ANOVA indicated significant condition × set interaction effect for PP ($p = 0.01$) and PV ($p = 0.03$). There was no significant condition × set interaction effect for MP ($p = 0.08$) and MV ($p = 0.11$). Furthermore, there was a significant main effect of condition in PP, MP, PV and MV.

The post hoc results for condition × set interaction in PP showed a significant increase in set 2 compared to set 1 for BFR ($p < 0.01$) and CONT ($p = 0.01$) conditions, a significant increase in set 3 compared to set 1 for the CONT ($p = 0.01$) condition, as well as a significant decrease in set 3 compared to set 1 for BFR condition ($p < 0.01$). The post hoc results for the condition × set interaction in PV showed a significant increase in set 2 compared to set 1 for BFR ($p < 0.01$) and CONT ($p = 0.01$) conditions, a significant increase in set 3 compared to set 1 for CONT ($p = 0.03$) condition, as well as a significant decrease in set 3 compared to set 1 for BFR condition ($p < 0.01$). Further, the post hoc results for the condition × set interaction in PP and PV showed a significant increase in set 1, set 2, and set 3 for BFR compared to CONT condition $p < 0.01$ for all; Table 1; Figures 1–4).

The post hoc results for the main effect of particular conditions showed a significant increase in PP (792 vs. 965 W), MP (559 vs. 667 W), PV (0.62 vs. 0.74 m/s), and MV (0.46 vs. 0.53 m/s) for BFR when compared to the CONT ($p < 0.01$ for all).

The t-test comparisons for delta values showed significant differences in PP ($p < 0.01$) and PV ($p = 0.01$) for set 3–set 2 between BFR and CONT conditions (Table 2).

The results of the t-test used to compare differences between sets and between conditions are presented in Tables 3 and 4.

Table 1. Power output and bar velocity in 3 successive sets of the bench press exercise under CONT and BFR conditions.

	Set 1	Set 2	Set 3
	Peak Power Output (W)		
CONT	753 ± 6	809 ± 100	813 ± 93
(95% CI)	(708 to 799)	(738 to 880)	(746 to 879)
BFR	938 ± 82	1011 ± 103	946 ± 105
(95% CI)	(879 to 996)	(938 to 1085)	(871 to 1021)
	Mean Power Output (W)		
CONT	546 ± 55(	570 ± 6	561 ± 79
(95% CI)	507 to 585)	(522 to 617)	(505 to 617)
BFR(95% CI)	657 ± 92	687 ± 105	658 ± 86
	(591 to 723)	(611 to 762)	(596 to 719)
	Peak Bar Velocity (m/s)		
CONT	0.58 ± 0.09	0.64 ± 0.10	0.63 ± 0.09
(95% CI)	(0.52 to 0.64)	(0.56 to 0.71)	(0.56 to 0.69)
BFR	0.73 ± 0.06	0.78 ± 0.08	0.73 ± 0.10
(95% CI)	(0.68 to 0.77)	(0.72 to 0.83)	(0.65 to 0.80)
	Mean Bar Velocity (m/s)		
CONT	0.42 ± 0.08	0.43 ± 0.07	0.43 ± 0.06
(95% CI)	(0.36 to 0.48)	(0.38 to 0.48)	(0.38 to 0.47)
BFR	0.52 ± 0.07	0.55 ± 0.08	0.51 ± 0.08
(95% CI)	(0.47 to 0.57)	(0.49 to 0.60)	(0.46 to 0.57)

CONT—control condition; BFR—blood flow restriction condition.

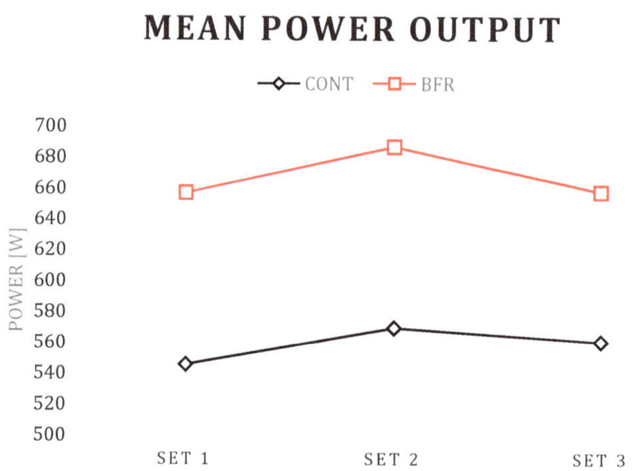

Figure 1. Mean power output for the BFR and CONT conditions during three successive sets of the bench press exercise.

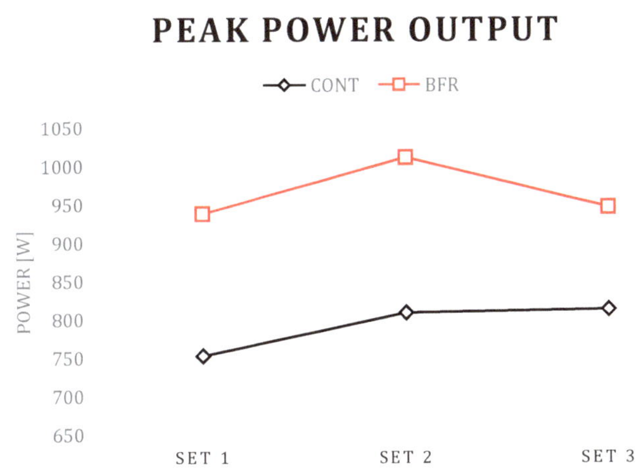

Figure 2. Peak power output for the BFR and CONT conditions during three successive sets of the bench press exercise.

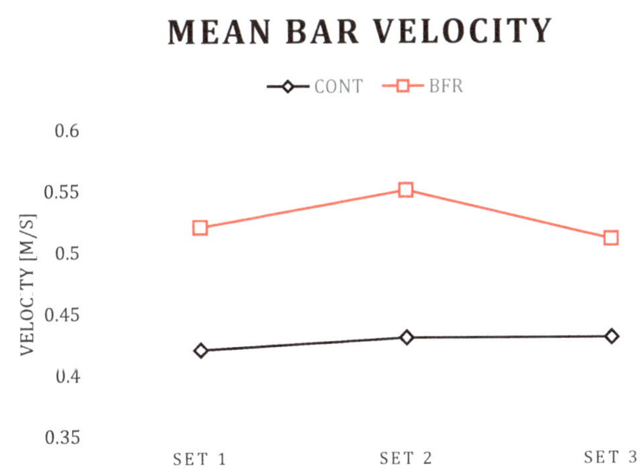

Figure 3. Mean bar velocity for BFR and CONT conditions during three successive sets of the bench press exercise.

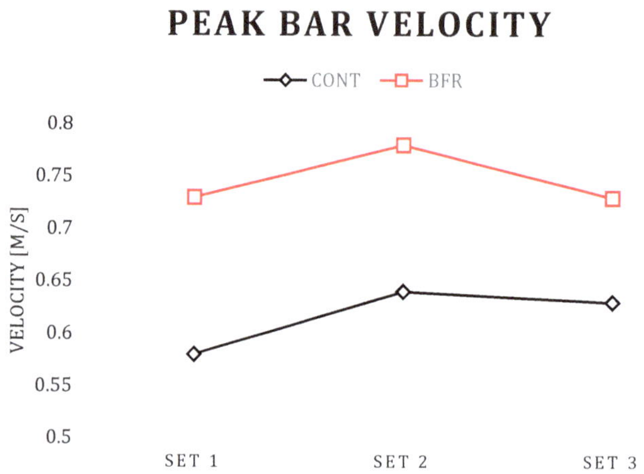

Figure 4. Mean bar velocity for BFR and CONT conditions during three successive sets of the bench press exercise.

Table 2. The comparison of differences in particular sets between BFR and CONT conditions.

Bench Press	**CONT**	**BFR**	**Mean Difference**	**95% CI for Difference**	***p***	**ES**
Differences between sets			Mean Power Output			
Set 2–set 1	23.7 ± 28.2	29.1 ± 16.5	5.4	−27.43 to 16.63	0.59	0.23
Set 3–set 1	15.1 ± 48.4	0.5 ± 27.3	14.6	−34.5 to 63.6	0.52	0.37
Set 3–set 2	−8.6 ± 24.8	−28.6 ± 34.8	20.0	−12.6 to 52.6	0.20	0.66
Differences between sets			Peak Power Output			
Set 2–set 1	55.7 ± 40.7	73.7 ± 56.8	18.0	−54.5 to 18.5	0.29	0.36
Set 3–set 1	59.2 ± 44.2	8.7 ± 71.1	50.5	−10.1 to 111.1	0.09	0.85
Set 3–set 2	3.5 ± 29.9	−65.0 ± 39.4	68.5	24.8 to 112.2	0.01*	1.96
Differences between sets			Mean Bar Velocity			
Set 2–set 1	0.015 ± 0.025	0.028 ± 0.019	0.013	−0.034 to 0.008	0.20	0.59
Set 3–set 1	0.007 ± 0.058	−0.007 ± 0.020	0.014	−0.039 to 0.067	0.57	0.32
Set 3–set 2	−0.008 ± 0.040	−0.035 ± 0.033	0.027	−0.014 to 0.068	0.17	1.15
Differences between sets			Peak Bar Velocity			
Set 2–set 1	0.054 ± 0.033	0.053 ± 0.029	0.001	−0.029 to 0.031	0.94	0.03
Set 3–set 1	0.042 ± 0.037	−0.001 ± 0.053	0.043	−0.004 to 0.089	0.07	0.94
Set 3–set 2	−0.012 ± 0.017	−0.054 ± 0.037	0.042	0.006 to 0.078	0.03 *	1.46

Mean ± standard deviation (SD); * statistically significant difference $p < 0.05$; CONT—control condition; BFR—blood flow restriction condition.

Table 3. A comparison between particular sets of the bench press exercise based on t-test results.

Bench Press	**Peak Power Output**			**Mean Power Output**			**Peak Velocity**			**Mean Velocity**		
	Mean Difference	***p***	**Effect Size**	**Mean Difference**	***p***	**Effect Size**	**Mean Difference**	***p***	**Effect Size**	**Mean Difference**	***p***	**Effect Size**
						CONT						
Set 2 vs. Set 1	74	0.01 *	0.67	24	0.03 *	0.40	0.06	0.01 *	0.63	0.01	0.09	0.13
Set 3 vs. Set 1	78	0.01 *	0.76	15	0.35	0.22	0.05	0.01 *	0.55	0.01	0.71	0.14
Set 3 vs. Set 2	4	0.72	0.04	9	0.30	0.12	0.01	0.06	0.10	0.00	0.54	0.00
						BFR						
Set 2 vs. Set 1	73	0.01 *	0.78	30	0.01 *	0.30	0.05	0.01 *	0.71	0.03	0.01 *	0.40
Set 3 vs. Set 1	8	0.71	0.08	1	0.95	0.01	0.00	0.95	0.00	0.01	0.30	0.13
Set 3 vs. Set 2	65	0.01 *	0.62	29	0.03 *	0.30	0.05	0.01 *	0.55	0.04	0.01 *	0.50

Mean ± standard deviation (SD); * statistically significant difference $p < 0.05$; CONT—control condition; BFR—blood flow restriction condition.

Table 4. A comparison in individual sets between conditions based on t-test results.

	Peak Power Output			Mean Power Output			Peak Velocity			Mean Velocity		
	Mean Difference	p	Effect Size	Mean Difference	p	Effect Size	Mean Difference	p	Effect Size	Mean Difference	p	Effect Size
	CONT vs. BFR											
Set 1	185	0.01 *	3.18	111	0.01 *	1.46	0.15	0.01 *	1.96	0.10	0.01 *	1.33
Set 2	202	0.01 *	1.99	117	0.01 *	1.57	0.14	0.01 *	1.55	0.12	0.01 *	1.60
Set 3	133	0.01 *	1.34	97	0.01 *	1.17	0.10	0.01 *	1.05	0.08	0.01 *	1.13

Mean ± standard deviation (SD); * statistically significant difference $p < 0.05$; CONT—control condition; BFR—blood flow restriction condition.

4. Discussion

The main finding of the study was that the PAPE effect can occur during the BP exercise under BFR. The results showed that the PAPE effect analyzed by changes in PP and PV occurred under both the CONT as well as BFR conditions. However, based on the direct analysis of changes between particular sets, significant differences were observed in result of set 3–set 2 between CONT and BFR conditions. Furthermore, the results of the present study show significant increases in power output and bar velocity during the BP exercise for the BFR condition compared to the CONT condition, which confirms previous results [23].

The main goal of this study was to evaluate the changes in power output and bar velocity between successive sets of the BP exercise, with and without BFR. This is the first study to address the effect of PAPE during high load resistance exercise under BFR which limits the possibility of comparing our results to other studies. Previous research has shown that resistance exercise under BFR increases metabolic stress compared to traditional resistance training [34]. However, most studies with BFR relate to chronic adaptive changes [34–36]. Only the study by Wilk et al. [23] analyzed acute changes in power output and bar velocity between exercises performed without and under BFR. The study of Wilk et al. [23] showed that short-term and high-pressure BFR increased power output and bar velocity during the BP compared to exercise without BFR. To date, two studies [37,38] examined the use of BFR on PAPE. In the study by Cleary and Cook [38], the use of BFR (60%AOP) led to diminished vertical jump performance after a CA at 30%1RM, while Miller et al. [37] showed increased vertical jump height after a 10 s maximal isometric deadlift combined with BFR. However, in both studies, BFR was used only during the CA and was removed for the post-activation exercise. Previous studies showed that the main adaptive changes during exercise with BFR are related to increased metabolic stress [35,36]. The increased metabolic stress following exercise with BFR results from the accumulation of metabolic products of physical activity in the part of the limb that is restricted from blood flow [24,39]. However, the increase in metabolic stress following exercise with BFR probably does not refer to short-term occlusion [23], as has been conducted in the present study. The occlusion applied in our experiment lasted only a few seconds (3 repetitions; maximal tempo of movement; ~5 s) during each set of the BP exercise. The short duration of the effort was dictated by the predominance of anaerobic metabolism; therefore, the metabolic stress associated with training under BFR conditions was probably not very intense.

Interestingly, a detailed analysis of the differences between particular sets indicated that the PAPE effect has different kinetics between particular sets for the BFR and CONT conditions. Significantly different kinetics for BFR and CONT conditions were observed in PP and PV values between set 3 and set 2. For the BFR condition, PP and PV were increased in set 2 compared to set 1, and decreased in set 3 compared to set 2. However, the decrease was not observed in the CONT condition. It is possible that benefits from a more pronounced PAPE in set 2 in the BFR condition could be counterbalanced by more pronounced muscle exhaustion in set 3. The short-term BFR increased the absolute value of power output and bar velocity during the BP exercise [23], however, such an increase of performance may promote greater fatigue which, as a consequence, may cause a decrease in power and related variables in subsequent sets of the exercise, as observed in the present study. However, despite the observed significant decrease in PP and PV in set 3–set 2 for the BFR condition, the absolute value of power output and bar velocity was still significantly higher when compared to the CONT condition, which suggests the BFR is an effective tool in acute enhancement of power output and bar velocity during several sets of the BP exercise.

These results indicated that short-term, high-pressure BFR has a significant impact on the level of acute changes during resistance exercise. The results of our study are partially consistent with findings presented by Morales-Artacho et al. [16] and Wilk et al. [3], who documented increases in power output during a resistance exercise in the second set compared to the first. However, contrary to Morales-Artacho et al. [16] and Wilk et al. [3], we also observed significant increases in power output and bar velocity in the third set compared to first and, thus, the BFR condition did not show such an significant advantage. The ratio of the duration of the effort during the rest interval is an important factor in PAPE exercise protocols [3,9,40]. An optimal rest interval should ensure the optimal balance between fatigue and potentiation [3,9]. Wilk et al. [3] showed that longer duration of repetitions limit PAPE effectiveness in successive sets due to insufficient rest and accumulated fatigue. Therefore, it can also be assumed that during the BFR condition, the lack of PAPE benefit in set 3–set 2 may be associated with an insufficient rest interval and fatigue. The higher absolute values of power output and bar velocity during the BFR condition as well as the fact that blood flow restriction may potentially promote greater fatigue may indicate the need for a longer rest interval between activation and potentiation [3,9]. Nevertheless, there are no data and guidelines for optimizing the rest interval for increased power performance during exercise under BFR, which requires further research.

To induce the PAPE effect, it is necessary to use high loads [9–12]. A combination of high loading (70%1RM) and BFR with high pressure (90%AOP) is not compatible with the recommendations of Patterson et al. [32]. Furthermore, Counts et al. [41] showed that higher relative pressures (90%AOP) may not be necessary when exercising under BFR. However, it should be noted that during the present study, we used intermittent and not continuous occlusion. Furthermore, the occlusion applied lasted only a few seconds during a set (~15 s for the whole training session), while the recommendations by Patterson et al. [32] for resistance exercise under BFR assume a restriction time of 5–10 min with reperfusion between exercises, not between sets. Currently, there are no guidelines for determining the optimal pressure as well as the time of restriction for exercise under BFR when the goal is acute increases of strength or power performance. Furthermore, a recent study by Wilk et al. [42] has shown the positive effect of extremely high pressure (150%AOP) on acute strength and strength endurance performance enhancement. This study suggested that not only BFR but also external muscle compression and mechanical energy generated by the cuff may be an important factor in the effectiveness of occlusion during the resistance exercise [23].

The type of exercise chosen for the study protocol may be a factor determining the level of acute changes during resistance exercise under BFR. In the present study, muscle occlusion was used at the upper limb (arms), while the main muscles involved in the BP are the pectoralis major and anterior deltoid [43]. The triceps brachii muscle shows high activity during BP [43], but BFR in this area does not affect the changes taking place in the pectoralis major and deltoid muscles, the two other primary muscles involved in the BP exercise. Despite the fact that Yasuda et al. [44] suggested that BP training under BFR also leads to an increase in muscle size in the area of the chest muscles, the presented results were related to acute and not chronic responses. Therefore, it can be assumed that the use of a long-term training program or another exercise, especially an exercise involving only those muscles that are occluded, could cause different, even conflicting results to those presented in this study.

The present study has some limitations which should be addressed. Although the results showed that the PAPE effect occurred during resistance exercise under BFR, the direct causes of these changes cannot be determined and explained. There was no analysis of direct physiological changes that would be the basis for explaining the obtained results. Furthermore, it is possible that the BFR increases local blood volume and therefore increases skin temperature [45], which may be related to performance enhancement [46,47]; however, skin temperature was not recorded in our study. Finally, the results of our study refer only to PAPE effects of the upper limbs during the BP exercise, and only to the cuff pressure used, and cannot be translated into other exercises, volumes, or intensities nor other occlusion pressures. Therefore, further research is required, especially in assessing the acute impact of continuous and intermittent BFR on the PAPE, during different training protocols as well as with different cuff pressures.

Practical Implications

The short-term BFR increases power output and bar velocity during the BP exercise compared to CONT conditions. Such an acute increase under BFR conditions compared to the CONT occurred in all three sets of the BP exercise. However, there are differences in the kinetics of power output and bar velocity changes between BFR and CONT conditions especially in the difference between set 3 and set 2. Under BFR, we observed an increase in the second set compared to the first, but in the third set, the power decreased compared to the second set. On the contrary, in the CONT condition, power output and bar velocity were maintained in the third set compared to the first. Therefore, given a real exercise program, the use of BFR and its effect on the increase in acute power performance should be controlled by measuring devices in order to individually adjust the optimal number of sets and time interval to the induced PAPE. Furthermore, even if an increase in power output and bar velocity occurs as a result of BFR, this effect may not necessarily translate into long-term effects or may even hinder performance. The frequent use of BFR can impair the muscle structure directly in the region under the cuff, which can decrease sport performance and increase the risk of injury [48,49]. Therefore, resistance exercise under BFR should be used occasionally and be well periodized.

5. Conclusions

This study demonstrated that the PAPE effect occurs during successive sets of the BP exercise under BFR at 70%1RM. However, compared to the CONT condition, we observed different kinetics of power output and bar velocity changes during successive sets of the BP exercise. Therefore, the application BFR during resistance training can introduce, a new, additional tool in the development of power output, which opens opportunities for modification of strength training programs, particularly in elite athletes.

Author Contributions: Conceptualization, M.W.; Data curation, M.K., A.F. and A.S.; Formal analysis, M.W.; Investigation, M.W., M.K., A.F. and A.S.; Methodology, M.W. and A.S.; Software, M.K. and A.F.; Supervision, M.W. and A.Z.; Writing—original draft, M.W., M.K. and A.F.; Writing—review & editing, M.W., R.G.L. and A.Z. All authors have read and agreed to the published version of the manuscript.

Funding: The study was supported and funded by the statutory research of the Jerzy Kukuczka Academy of Physical Education in Katowice, Poland.

Conflicts of Interest: The authors declare that they have no conflicts of interest.

References

1. Cuenca-Fernández, F.; Smith, I.C.; Jordan, M.J.; MacIntosh, B.R.; López-Contreras, G.; Arellano, R.; Herzog, W. Nonlocalized postactivation performance enhancement (PAPE) effects in trained athletes: A pilot study. *Appl. Physiol. Nutr. Metab.* **2017**, *42*, 1122–1125. [CrossRef] [PubMed]
2. Tillin, N.A.; Bishop, D. Factors Modulating Post-Activation Potentiation and its Effect on Performance of Subsequent Explosive Activities. *Sports Med.* **2009**, *39*, 147–166. [CrossRef] [PubMed]
3. Wilk, M.; Krzysztofik, M.; Drozd, M.; Zajac, A. Changes of Power Output and Velocity During Successive Sets of the Bench Press with Different Duration of Eccentric Movement. *Int. J. Sports Physiol. Perform.* **2020**, *15*, 162–167. [CrossRef] [PubMed]
4. Krzysztofik, M.; Wilk, M.; Filip, A.; Zmijewski, P.; Zajac, A.; Tufano, J.J. Can Post-Activation Performance Enhancement (PAPE) Improve Resistance Training Volume during the Bench Press Exercise? *Int. J. Environ. Res. Public Health* **2020**, *17*, 2554. [CrossRef] [PubMed]

5. Golas, A.; Wilk, M.; Stastny, P.; Maszczyk, A.; Pajerska, K.; Zając, A. Optimizing Half Squat Postactivation Potential Load in Squat Jump Training for Eliciting Relative Maximal Power in Ski Jumpers. *J. Strength Cond. Res.* **2017**, *31*, 3010–3017. [CrossRef] [PubMed]
6. Sale, D.G. Postactivation potentiation: Role in human performance. *Exerc. Sport Sci. Rev.* **2002**, *30*, 138–143. [CrossRef]
7. Marques, M.C.; van den Tillaar, R.; Vescovi, J.D.; González-Badillo, J.J. Relationship Between Throwing Velocity, Muscle Power, and Bar Velocity During Bench Press in Elite Handball Players. *Int. J. Sports Physiol. Perform.* **2007**, *2*, 414–422. [CrossRef]
8. Blazevich, A.J.; Babault, N. Post-activation Potentiation Versus Post-activation Performance Enhancement in Humans: Historical Perspective, Underlying Mechanisms, and Current Issues. *Front. Physiol.* **2019**, *10*, 1359. [CrossRef]
9. Gossen, E.R.; Sale, D.G. Effect of postactivation potentiation on dynamic knee extension performance. *Eur. J. Appl. Physiol.* **2000**, *83*, 524–530. [CrossRef]
10. Kilduff, L.P.; Owen, N.; Bevan, H.; Bennett, M.; Kingsley, M.I.C.; Cunningham, D. Influence of recovery time on post-activation potentiation in professional rugby players. *J. Sports Sci.* **2008**, *26*, 795–802. [CrossRef]
11. Chiu, L.Z.F.; Fry, A.C.; Weiss, L.W.; Schilling, B.K.; Brown, L.E.; Smith, S.L. Postactivation potentiation response in athletic and recreationally trained individuals. *J. Strength Cond. Res.* **2003**, *17*, 671–677. [CrossRef]
12. Farup, J.; Sørensen, H. Postactivation Potentiation: Upper Body Force Development Changes after Maximal Force Intervention. *J. Strength Cond. Res.* **2010**, *24*, 1874–1879. [CrossRef] [PubMed]
13. Hrysomallis, C.; Kidgell, D. Effect of heavy dynamic resistive exercise on acute upper-body power. *J. Strength Cond. Res.* **2001**, *15*, 426–430. [PubMed]
14. Tsoukos, A.; Brown, L.E.; Veligekas, P.; Terzis, G.; Bogdanis, G.C. Postactivation Potentiation of Bench Press Throw Performance Using Velocity-Based Conditioning Protocols with Low and Moderate Loads. *J. Hum. Kinet.* **2019**, *68*, 81–98. [CrossRef] [PubMed]
15. Liossis, L.D.; Forsyth, J.; Liossis, C.; Tsolakis, C. The Acute Effect of Upper-Body Complex Training on Power Output of Martial Art Athletes as Measured by the Bench Press Throw Exercise. *J. Hum. Kinet.* **2013**, *39*, 167–175. [CrossRef] [PubMed]
16. Morales-Artacho, A.J.; Padial, P.; García-Ramos, A.; Feriche, B. The Effect of the Number of Sets on Power Output for Different Loads. *J. Hum. Kinet.* **2015**, *46*, 149–156. [CrossRef] [PubMed]
17. Wilk, M.; Krzysztofik, M.; Gepfert, M.; Poprzecki, S.; Gołaś, A.; Maszczyk, A. Technical and Training Related Aspects of Resistance Training Using Blood Flow Restriction in Competitive Sport-A Review. *J. Hum. Kinet.* **2018**, *65*, 249–260. [CrossRef]
18. Loenneke, J.P.; Pujol, T.J. The Use of Occlusion Training to Produce Muscle Hypertrophy. *Strength Cond. J.* **2009**, *31*, 77–84. [CrossRef]
19. Scott, B.R.; Loenneke, J.P.; Slattery, K.M.; Dascombe, B.J. Exercise with Blood Flow Restriction: An Updated Evidence-Based Approach for Enhanced Muscular Development. *Sports Med.* **2015**, *45*, 313–325. [CrossRef]
20. Takarada, Y.; Takazawa, H.; Sato, Y.; Takebayashi, S.; Tanaka, Y.; Ishii, N. Effects of resistance exercise combined with moderate vascular occlusion on muscular function in humans. *J. Appl. Physiol.* **2000**, *88*, 2097–2106. [CrossRef]
21. Jessee, M.B.; Mattocks, K.T.; Buckner, S.L.; Dankel, S.J.; Mouser, J.G.; Abe, T.; Loenneke, J.P. Mechanisms of Blood Flow Restriction: The New Testament. *Tech. Ortho.* **2018**, *33*, 72–79. [CrossRef]
22. Allen, D.G.; Trajanovska, S. The multiple roles of phosphate in muscle fatigue. *Front. Physio.* **2012**, *3*. [CrossRef] [PubMed]
23. Wilk, M.; Krzysztofik, M.; Filip, A.; Zajac, A.; Bogdanis, G.C.; Lockie, R.G. Short-Term Blood Flow Restriction Increases Power Output and Bar Velocity During the Bench Press. *J. Strength Cond. Res.* **2020**, 5. [CrossRef] [PubMed]
24. Teixeira, E.L.; Barroso, R.; Silva-Batista, C.; Laurentino, G.C.; Loenneke, J.P.; Roschel, H.; Ugrinowitsch, C.; Tricoli, V. Blood flow restriction increases metabolic stress but decreases muscle activation during high-load resistance exercise. *Muscle Nerve.* **2018**, *57*, 107–111. [CrossRef]
25. Luebbers, P.E.; Fry, A.C.; Kriley, L.M.; Butler, M.S. The effects of a 7-week practical blood flow restriction program on well-trained collegiate athletes. *J. Strength Cond. Res.* **2014**, *28*, 2270–2280. [CrossRef]

26. Rawska, M.; Gepfert, M.; Mostowik, A.; Krzysztofik, M.; Wojdala, G.; Lulinska, A.; Wilk, M. Does blood flow restriction influence the maximal number of repetitions performed during the bench press? A pilot study. *Balt. J. Health Phys. Act.* **2019**, 9–17. [CrossRef]
27. Krzysztofik, M.; Wilk, M.; Golas, A.; Lockie, R.G.; Maszczyk, A.; Zajac, A. Does Eccentric-only and Concentric-only Activation Increase Power Output? *Med. Sci. Sports Exer.* **2020**, *52*, 484–489. [CrossRef]
28. Golas, A.; Maszczyk, A.; Zajac, A.; Mikolajec, K.; Stastny, P. Optimizing post activation potentiation for explosive activities in competitive sports. *J. Hum. Kinet.* **2016**, *52*, 95–106. [CrossRef]
29. Wilk, M.; Golas, A.; Zmijewski, P.; Krzysztofik, M.; Filip, A.; Coso, J.D.; Tufano, J.J. The Effects of the Movement Tempo on the One-Repetition Maximum Bench Press Results. *J. Hum. Kinet.* **2020**, *72*, 151–159. [CrossRef]
30. Wilk, M.; Gepfert, M.; Krzysztofik, M.; Mostowik, A.; Filip, A.; Hajduk, G.; Zajac, A. Impact of Duration of Eccentric Movement in the One-Repetition Maximum Test Result in the Bench Press among Women. *J. Sport Sci. Med.* **2020**, *19*, 317–322.
31. Goldsmith, J.A.; Trepeck, C.; Halle, J.L.; Mendez, K.M.; Klemp, A.; Cooke, D.M.; Haischer, M.H.; Byrnes, R.K.; Zoeller, R.F.; Whitehurst, M.; et al. Validity of the Open Barbell and Tendo Weightlifting Analyzer Systems Versus the Optotrak Certus 3D Motion-Capture System for Barbell Velocity. *Int. J. Sports Physiol. Perform.* **2019**, *14*, 540–543. [CrossRef] [PubMed]
32. Patterson, S.D.; Hughes, L.; Warmington, S.; Burr, J.; Scott, B.R.; Owens, J.; Abe, T.; Nielsen, J.L.; Libardi, C.A.; Laurentino, G.; et al. Blood Flow Restriction Exercise Position Stand: Considerations of Methodology, Application, and Safety. *Front. Physiol.* **2019**, *10*. [CrossRef]
33. Cohen, J. *Statistical Power Analysis for the Behavioral Sciences*, 2nd ed.; L. Erlbaum Associates: Hillsdale, NJ, USA, 1988.
34. Abe, T.; Kearns, C.F.; Sato, Y. Muscle size and strength are increased following walk training with restricted venous blood flow from the leg muscle, Kaatsu-walk training. *J. Appl. Physiol.* **2006**, *100*, 1460–1466. [CrossRef] [PubMed]
35. Lixandrão, M.E.; Ugrinowitsch, C.; Laurentino, G.; Libardi, C.A.; Aihara, A.Y.; Cardoso, F.N.; Tricoli, V.; Roschel, H. Effects of exercise intensity and occlusion pressure after 12 weeks of resistance training with blood-flow restriction. *Eur. J. Appl. Physiol.* **2015**, *115*, 2471–2480. [CrossRef]
36. Lowery, R.P.; Joy, J.M.; Loenneke, J.P.; de Souza, E.O.; Machado, M.; Dudeck, J.E.; Wilson, J.M. Practical blood flow restriction training increases muscle hypertrophy during a periodized resistance training programme. *Clin. Physiol. Funct. Imaging* **2014**, *34*, 317–321. [CrossRef]
37. Miller, R.M.; Keeter, V.M.; Freitas, E.D.S.; Heishman, A.D.; Knehans, A.W.; Bemben, D.A.; Bemben, M.G. Effects of Blood-Flow Restriction Combined with Postactivation Potentiation Stimuli on Jump Performance in Recreationally Active Men. *J. Strength Cond. Res.* **2018**, *32*, 1869–1874. [CrossRef] [PubMed]
38. Cleary, C.J.; Cook, S.B. Postactivation Potentiation in Blood Flow–Restricted Complex Training. *J. Strength Cond. Res.* **2020**, *34*, 905–910. [CrossRef]
39. Fujita, S.; Abe, T.; Drummond, M.J.; Cadenas, J.G.; Dreyer, H.C.; Sato, Y.; Volpi, E.; Rasmussen, B.B. Blood flow restriction during low-intensity resistance exercise increases S6K1 phosphorylation and muscle protein synthesis. *J. Appl. Physiol.* **2007**, *103*, 903–910. [CrossRef] [PubMed]
40. Chaouachi, A.; Poulos, N.; Abed, F.; Turki, O.; Brughelli, M.; Chamari, K.; Drinkwater, E.J.; Behm, D.G. Volume, intensity, and timing of muscle power potentiation are variable. *Appl. Physiol. Nutr. Metab.* **2011**, *36*, 736–747. [CrossRef] [PubMed]
41. Counts, B.R.; Dankel, S.J.; Barnett, B.E.; Kim, D.; Mouser, J.G.; Allen, K.M.; Thiebaud, R.S.; Abe, T.; Bemben, M.G.; Loenneke, J.P. Influence of relative blood flow restriction pressure on muscle activation and muscle adaptation: Relative BFR Pressure. *Muscle Nerve.* **2016**, *53*, 438–445. [CrossRef]
42. Wilk, M.; Krzysztofik, M.; Filip, A.; Lockie, R.G.; Zajac, A. The acute effects of external compression with blood flow restriction on maximal strength and strength-endurance performance of the upper limbs. *Front. Physiol.* **2020**, in press. [CrossRef]
43. Golas, A.; Maszczyk, A.; Stastny, P.; Wilk, M.; Ficek, K.; Lockie, R.; Zajac, A. A New Approach to EMG Analysis of Closed-Circuit Movements Such as the Flat Bench Press. *Sports* **2018**, *6*, 27. [CrossRef] [PubMed]
44. Yasuda, T.; Fujita, S.; Ogasawara, R.; Sato, Y.; Abe, T. Effects of low-intensity bench press training with restricted arm muscle blood flow on chest muscle hypertrophy: A pilot study: Bench press training with blood flow restriction. *Clin. Physiol. Funct. Imaging.* **2010**, *30*, 338–343. [CrossRef] [PubMed]

45. Chudecka, M. The use of thermal imaging in the evaluation of the body surface temperature in various physiological states and in patients with different body composition and varying levels of physical activity. *Cent. Eur. J. Sport Sci. Med.* **2013**, *2*, 15–20.
46. Abate, M.; Di Carlo, L.; Di Donato, L.; Romani, G.L.; Merla, A. Comparison of cutaneous termic response to a standardised warm up in trained and untrained individuals. *J. Sports Med. Phys. Fitness* **2013**, *53*, 209–215.
47. Formenti, D.; Ludwig, N.; Trecroci, A.; Gargano, M.; Michielon, G.; Caumo, A.; Alberti, G. Dynamics of thermographic skin temperature response during squat exercise at two different speeds. *J. Therm. Biol.* **2016**, *59*, 58–63. [CrossRef]
48. Ellefsen, S.; Hammarström, D.; Strand, T.A.; Zacharoff, E.; Whist, J.E.; Rauk, I.; Nygaard, H.; Vegge, G.; Hanestadhaugen, M.; Wernbom, M.; et al. Blood flow-restricted strength training displays high functional and biological efficacy in women: A within-subject comparison with high-load strength training. *Am. J. Physiol. Regul. Integr. Comp. Physiol.* **2015**, *309*, R767–R779. [CrossRef]
49. Kacin, A.; Strazar, K. Frequent low-load ischemic resistance exercise to failure enhances muscle oxygen delivery and endurance capacity: Ischemic training and muscle endurance. *Scand. J. Med. Sci. Sports* **2011**, *21*, e231–e241. [CrossRef]

International Journal of
Environmental Research and Public Health

MDPI

Article

The Factorial Validity of the Norwegian Version of the Multicomponent Training Distress Scale (MTDS-N)

Cathrine Nyhus Hagum * and Shaher A. I. Shalfawi

Department of Education and Sports Science, University of Stavanger, 4036 Stavanger, Norway; shaher.shalfawi@uis.no
* Correspondence: cathrine.n.hagum@uis.no; Tel.: +47-941-50-190

Received: 9 September 2020; Accepted: 12 October 2020; Published: 19 October 2020

Abstract: Background: Athlete self-report measures (ASRM) are methods of athlete monitoring, which have gained considerable popularity in recent years. The Multicomponent Training Distress Scale (MTDS), consisting of 22 items, is a promising self-report measure to assess training distress among athletes. The present study aimed to investigate the factorial validity of the Norwegian version of MTDS (MTDS-N) among student-athletes (n = 632) attending the optional program subject "Top-Level Sports" in upper secondary schools in Norway. Methods: A confirmatory factor analysis (CFA) was conducted to assess the six-factor model proposed by Main and Grove (2009). McDonald's omega (ω) along with confidence intervals (CIs) were used to estimate scale reliability. After examining the fit of the CFA model in the total sample, covariates were included to investigate group differences in latent variables of MTDS-N, resulting in the multiple indicators multiple causes (MIMIC) model. Further, direct paths between the covariates and the factor indicators were included in an extended MIMIC model to investigate whether responses to items differed between groups, resulting in differential item functioning (DIF). Results: When modification indices (MIs) were taken into consideration, the alternative CFA model revealed that MTDS-N is an acceptable psychometric tool with a good fit index. The factors in MTDS-N all constituted high scale reliability with McDonald's ω ranging from 0.725–0.862. The results indicated statistically significant group differences in factor scores for gender, type of sport, hours of training per week, school program, and school level. Further, results showed that DIF occurred in 13 of the MTDS-N items. However, after assessing the MIMIC model and the extended MIMIC model, the factor structure remained unchanged, and the model fit remained within acceptable values. The student-athletes' reports of training distress were moderate. Conclusion: The MTDS-N was found to be suitable for use in a Norwegian population to assess student-athletes' training distress in a reliable manner. The indications of group effects suggest that caution should be used if one is interested in making group comparisons when the MTDS-N is used among student-athletes in Norway until further research is conducted.

Keywords: confirmatory factor analysis; multiple indicators multiple causes; differential item functioning; athlete monitoring; student-athletes

1. Introduction

The combination of sport and education, also referred to as "dual-career" [1] can be challenging for young athletes between the ages of 10 and 18 years old [2] as it demands the development of their full potential in both areas [3]. In addition to training and school loads, athletes typically encounter additional stress from other external sources such as social, work-related, lifestyle, and the athlete–coach relationship [4]. Consequently, there is a unique interaction between physical and psychological stresses [5]. Increased stresses can potentially lead to fatigue and increase the risk of illness and injury [6,7]. Hence, the balance between stress and recovery is a key factor for continuous high-level of performance [8]. Therefore, without a sufficient balance between training load and recovery, non-functional overreaching (NFOR) can occur [9]. At this stage, the first signs and symptoms of extended training distress such as performance decrements, psychological disturbance, and hormonal disturbances could occur and require weeks or months for the athlete to recover [9].

Periods of accumulated training load and changes in acute training load have also been reported to increase the risk of injury and illness [6]. Research showed that training and competition load resulted in temporary decrements in physical performance and significant levels of post-competition fatigue [10]. These decrements have been explained by increased muscle damage [11], reduction in the effectiveness of the immune system [12], an imbalance in anabolic and catabolic processes in the body [13], athlete mood disturbance [14], and a reduction in the neuromuscular effectiveness [15]. Besides training load, non-sport events can impose further stress on athletes, which shifts their physical and psychological well-being along a continuum that starts with homeostasis and progress through the stages of acute fatigue, functional overreaching, NFOR, overtraining syndrome, subclinical tissue damage, clinical symptoms, and time-loss injury or illness [16]. In normal circumstances, it can take up to five days to return to a balanced physical state (homeostasis) [13], and with increased training load and non-training stressors, it might take up to several weeks to recover [9,17]. The additional stress is not only evident in athletes playing sport at a high-performance level but also in athletes at the lower representative standards, where external pressure from schoolwork, relationship tensions, and pressure from parents and coaches has been reported [18]. Hence, there can be a risk of NFOR and overtraining (OT) for all young athletes. Consequently, this is not only an important issue for those adults that are involved in sport but also for coaches and teachers [18].

One of the challenges for those involved with athletes is to carefully monitor and manage the stresses and recovery to be able to optimize their performance capacity and to avoid harmful outcomes [19–24]. Athlete self-report measures (ASRMs) are methods of athlete monitoring, which have gained considerable popularity in recent years [25] and will likely continue growing in popularity as a monitoring strategy [26]. The utility of ASRMs as a monitoring tool is well supported and has been reported to be useful [10,23,24,27]. Their popularity stems from their low cost, easy to use, and the growing body of literature which have emphasized ASRMs to be sensitive to the risk of illness and injury, compared to physiological biomarkers [28]. An ASRM that has been considered to be promising in monitoring athletes [28] is the Multicomponent Training Distress Scale (MTDS) [29]. The instrument has been used in different sports, including swimming [30], rowing [31], soccer [32,33], cycling [34], alpine skiing [35], and tennis [36]. The instrument combines measures of mood disturbances, perceived stress, and symptoms of acute overtraining over a small number of items (22 questions) [29], and provides an insight into the intensity and frequency of psycho-behavioral responses [37]. Thus, the purpose of the present study was to translate MTDS into Norwegian (MTDS-N) and investigate whether the Norwegian version of the questionnaire can be considered a valid measure in detecting training distress among young athletes attending the optional program subject "Top-Level Sports" in upper secondary schools in Norway. Further, the study aimed to investigate the effect of covariates on the factor structure and model fit.

2. Materials and Methods

2.1. Sample Size Estimation

For the validity of the MTDS-N, the sample size was estimated using the point of stability approach, which is described in Kretzschmar and Gignac [38], Schönbrodt and Perugini [39], and the study of Hirschfeld, et al. [40]. The latter gave a direction to estimate the sample size needed for the Big Five Inventory and the International Personality Item Pool Big Five measure. The point of stability ensures that the deviation between the estimated sample and the population parameter is stable (small) and is expected to remain small at a stable statistical power = 80% [38,39]. To ensure that the stability is small, Schönbrodt and Perugini [39] indicated that, according to Cohen [41], the corridor of stability should not exceed a small correlation of 0.10. The study of Schönbrodt and Perugini [39] suggested that 240–250 participants would be the minimum number needed to reach the point of stability. Kretzschmar and Gignac [38] continued the work of Schönbrodt and Perugini [39] and reported that with perfect reliability (omega, $\omega = 1.0$) of both latent factors and a population correlation of $p = 0.20$, the point-estimates of the correlation was stabilized at a sample size of 220 [38]. Since perfect reliability is almost never achieved, the authors suggested that the required sample at a population correlation of $p = 0.20$ and reliability of $\omega = 0.7$ would be ≥490 participants [38]. Similar results have been reported by Hirschfeld, Brachel and Thielsch [40], and the recommended sample size to reach a point of stability was > 500 participants [40]. Therefore, the total number of participants that was required in this study was to be more or equal to the recommendations from similar studies (i.e., $n \geq 500$).

2.2. Participants

The participants in the present study were 632 student-athletes attending the optional program subject Top-Level Sport from 23 different upper secondary schools in Norway. Seven covariates that characterize the profile of the respondents are presented in Table 1. The participants reported 35 different sports, which are shown in Table 2. This study was carried out according to the World Medical Association Declaration of Helsinki. Informed consent was obtained from all participants who agreed to take part in this study in accordance to the ethical approval from the Norwegian Social Science Data Services (NSD) (Project number 836079) and the Regional Committees for Medical and Health Research Ethics (REK) (Project number 54584).

Table 1. The profile of the 632 student-athletes in the present study.

Characteristics (Total) [1]	Modalities	Frequency or M ± SD	%
Gender (630)	Male	327	51.9
	Female	303	48.1
Type of sport (630)	Individual	207	32.9
	Team sport	423	67.1
Region (632)	West Norway	344	54.4
	East Norway	148	23.4
	Mid Norway	160	16.8
	Northern Norway	34	5.4
Age in years (631)	Male	17.37 ± 0.06	
	Female	17.23 ± 0.05	
Training hours (617)	Total	12.54 ± 4.99	
	Specialization in general studies	12.60 ± 4.95	
	Sports and physical education	12.45 ± 5.06	
School program [2] (632)	Specialization in general studies	369	58.4
	Sports and physical education	263	41.6
School level [3] (632)	First grade	232	36.7
	Second grade	239	37.8
	Third grade	161	25.5

Notes. M = mean; SD = standard deviation; % = percentage. [1] Values in brackets indicate total responses from the participants. There were 20 missing values, but the number of cases with missing values on the characteristics was 18. [2] In the education program specialization in general studies with Top-Level Sports, the student-athletes are attending regular specialization in general studies with Top-Level sports as an optional program subject. Thus, they have only theoretical subjects in addition to the physical Top-Level sports subject. In the education program sports and physical education, the student-athletes have many subjects that are related to sports, both theoretical and practical. The subjects are activity theory, theory of training, training management, sports and society, and the optional program subject Top-Level Sports. Hence, student-athletes connected to the program sports and physical education have more hours of training per week at school, compared to those connected to the program specialization in general studies. [3] In Norway, the ages of the students are 15–16 years in first grade, 16–17 years in second grade, and 17–18 years in third grade. These ages can be compared to sophomores, juniors, and seniors, respectively, in high schools in the United States.

Table 2. The different sports reported by the 630 participants (two missing).

Descriptive Statistics					
Type of Sport	Frequency	%	Type of Sport	Frequency	%
Soccer	306	48.6	Sailing	6	1.0
Handball	91	14.4	Martial art	9	1.4
Swimming	24	3.8	Badminton	5	0.8
Track field	21	3.3	Cheerleading	1	0.2
Gymnastics	11	1.7	Strength training	4	0.6
Ice hockey	19	3.0	Sky jumping	1	0.2
Cross-country skiing	34	5.4	Diving	1	0.2
Orienteering	8	1.3	Sports drill	4	0.6
Alpine skiing	15	2.4	Shooting	1	0.2
Cycling	12	1.9	Snowboard	1	0.2
Golf	5	0.8	Jet ski	1	0.2
Floorball	2	0.3	Dance	1	0.2
Volleyball	5	0.8	Motocross	2	0.3
Rowing	3	0.5	Triathlon	2	0.3
Biathlon	12	1.9	Freeski	1	0.2
Show jumping	12	1.9	Climbing	1	0.2
Ice skate	4	0.6	Figure skating	1	0.2
Tennis	4	0.6			

2.3. Instrument

The MTDS was developed by Main and Grove [29] using three different instruments; the 10-item version of the Perceived Stress Scale (PSS) [42], the 24-item Brunel Mood State Scale (BRUMS) [43], and a checklist of 19 symptoms of acute overtraining [44]. The initial validation conducted by Main and Grove [29] concluded 22 items, addressing six factors. Four factors (depression, vigor, stress, and fatigue) are measured in terms of their frequency and scored on a five-point Likert scale ranging from "never" (0)–"very often" (4). The factor vigor is reversed scored, indicating that higher scores reflect the greater frequency of experiencing higher levels of energy. Further, two factors (physical symptoms and sleep disturbances) are measured in terms of their intensity and scored on a five-point Likert scale ranging from "not at all" (0) –"an extreme amount" (4). From a psychometric standpoint, the questionnaire exhibited a theoretically relevant relationship with a similar distinct construct, namely; the risk of burnout using the Athlete Burnout Questionnaire (ABQ) [29,45]. The results indicated that low scores on the ABQ resulted in low scores on the five negative training distress factors (depression, perceived stress, fatigue, sleep disturbances, and physical symptoms) and a high score on the positive factor (vigor). Conversely, high scores on ABQ resulted in high scores on the five negative training distress factors and a low score on the positive factor [29].

2.4. Procedures

Translation of the MTDS from English to Norwegian

Figure 1 illustrates the process of translating MTDS to the Norwegian context. The translation of the original English version to Norwegian was accomplished with reference to Guillemin, Bombardier, and Beaton [46] four-step translation procedure. Further, the International Test Commission (ITC) Guidelines for Translating and Adapting Tests were taken into consideration during the translation process [47].

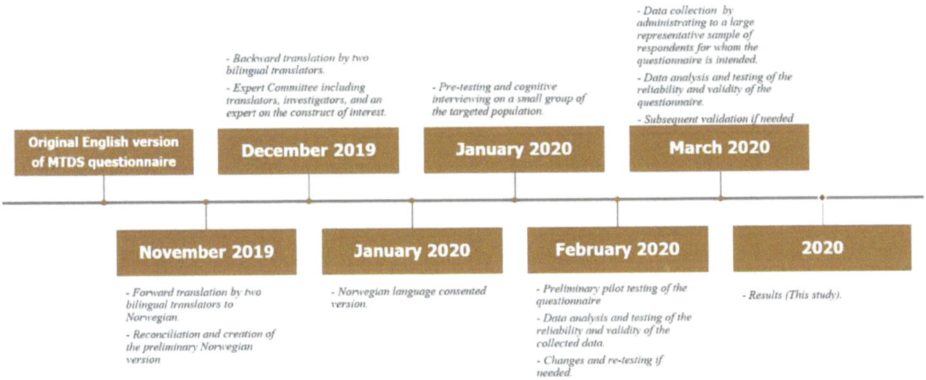

Figure 1. The process of translating Multicomponent Training Distress Scale (MTDS) to the Norwegian context.

In the first step, two independent bilingual, native Norwegian speakers forward translated the questionnaire from English to Norwegian. One of the translators was aware of the concepts the questionnaire intended to measure where the other was not aware of the objective of the questionnaire to offer more reliable restitution of the intended measurement [48]. A third translator compared the two versions and corrected differences to find the most appropriate words, expressions, and sentence structures to capture the meaning of the items.

In the second step, two different independent translators conducted the backward translation from Norwegian to English. To avoid bias, the translators were not familiar with the original version of the questionnaire. Both were bilingual and native English speakers. The original and backward translated versions of the questionnaire were then compared to ensure that the forward translation was precise and as complete as possible.

In the third step, an expert committee (consisting of one expert who was familiar with the construct of interest, a methodologist, one of the forward translators, and two which were not involved in the process of translations) were consulted to produce the final version of the Norwegian translation. All translated versions were reviewed with reference to achieve semantic, idiomatic, experiential, and conceptual equivalence, and any discrepancies were resolved [46].

In the fourth step, before conducting the pilot data collection of the final version of the MTDS-N, the items were tested on a small intended sample of respondents, following a probe technique [46]. Eight respondents completed the translated questionnaire and were asked verbally to elaborate on what they thought each item and their corresponding response meant. This was done in order to ensure that the final item was understood as having a meaning equivalent to that of the source item.

In the fifth step, a preliminary pilot testing of the questionnaire was carried out by distributing the questionnaire to a small group of the targeted population (n = 162) to measure its reliability and validity prior to the major data collection [47]. The results from the preliminary pilot testing demonstrated that the MTDS was successfully translated, culturally adapted, and reproduced the original reported psychometric properties (results of the preliminary pilot testing are attached in the Supplementary Materials). Therefore, a data collection to a larger group representing the targeted population was carried out (this study).

2.5. Data Collection

Invitations to participate were sent to all upper secondary schools that offer the optional program subject Top-Level Sports in Norway (n = 119). The final version of MTDS-N was then distributed electronically using SurveyXact version 8.0 [49] to all school management who agreed to participate in this study (n = 34, 28.6%). After that, the school management distributed the questionnaire electronically to the student-athletes at their respective schools (n = 23, 19.3%). In addition to completing the questionnaire, all participants completed questions regarding their age, gender, type of sport, hours of training per week, county, name of the school, study program, and grade level. The data collection started in March 2020 and ended in May 2020 (see Section 2.2).

2.6. Statistical Analysis

Prior to analyses, Microsoft Excel (version 2016) was used to prepare the data (source data are attached in the Supplementary Materials). Then, the factor vigor, with positive scores, was reversed. Demographic and descriptive data were analyzed using Statistical Package for the Social Sciences (SPSS) Version 25 (IBM Corporation, Armonk, NY, USA). Preliminary analyses investigating the normal distribution of the data were conducted using Mplus Version 8.4 (Muthén and Muthén, Los Angeles, CA, USA) [50]. The normality was examined using skewness and kurtosis (Table 3). Skewness and kurtosis values between ±1.0 were considered excellent, while values between ±1.0–2.0 were considered acceptable [51]. A non-normality test due to skewness and kurtosis was conducted to investigate if the data violated the multivariate normality assumption [52]. If the data were found not to violate the multivariate normality assumption, a Kolmogorov–Smirnov test (KS) and the Shapiro–Wilk test (SW) were further assessed to confirm that the data was normally distributed. A non-statistically significant ($p > 0.05$) Kolmogorov–Smirnov test (KS) and Shapiro–Wilk test (SW) would indicate normally distributed data [53].

Table 3. Descriptive statistics for 632 participants on the items of MTDS-N.

Items	Descriptive Statistics			
	M	SD	Skewness	Kurtosis
Depression (dep1–dep5)				
Miserable (dep1)	1.47	0.82	1.95	3.44
Unhappy (dep2)	1.75	0.94	1.27	1.09
Bitter (dep3)	1.64	0.86	1.49	2.16
Downhearted (dep4)	2.03	1.06	0.92	0.11
Depressed (dep5)	1.49	0.90	2.09	3.97
Vigor (vig1–vig4)				
Energetic (vig1)	2.70	0.99	0.38	−0.08
Lively (vig2)	2.61	0.95	0.54	0.03
Active (vig3)	2.52	0.90	0.32	−0.24
Alert (vig4)	2.87	0.94	0.30	−0.21
Physical symptoms (sym1–sym3)				
Muscle soreness (sym1)	2.52	1.03	0.18	−0.68
Heavy arms or legs (sym2)	2.43	0.98	0.38	−0.44
Stiff/sore joints (sym3)	2.11	1.03	0.73	−0.19
Sleep disturbances (sle1–sle3)				
Difficulties falling asleep (sle1)	2.15	1.18	0.84	−0.32
Restless sleep (sle2)	2.06	1.16	0.90	−0.21
Insomnia (sle3)	1.83	1.11	1.22	0.51
Stress (str1–str4)				
Stressed (str1)	3.06	1.11	−0.02	−0.65
Could not cope (str2)	2.76	1.02	0.10	−0.46
Difficulties piling up (str3)	2.12	0.96	0.68	0.08
Nervous (str4)	2.78	1.09	0.15	−0.56
Fatigue (fat1–fat3)				
Tired (fat1)	2.69	0.98	0.28	−0.42
Sleepy (fat2)	2.54	1.09	0.43	−0.55
Worn-out (fat3)	2.46	1.07	0.41	−0.59

Notes. M = mean; SD = standard deviation; Dep = depression; Vig = vigor; Sym = physical symptoms; Sle = sleep disturbances; Str = stress; Fat = fatigue.

All further analyses were carried out using Mplus [50]. To investigate the six-factor solution of the MTDS questionnaire proposed by Main and Grove [29], confirmatory factor analysis (CFA) was assessed. Considering a multivariate non-normality in the measures (Table 3), a maximum likelihood estimator (MLR) with robust standard errors using a numerical integration algorithm was used (Mplus codes used are attached in the Supplementary Materials).

The goodness of fit was assessed using χ^2, root mean square error of approximation (RMSEA), comparative fit index (CFI), Tucker-Lewis index (TLI), and the standardized root mean square residual (SRMR). A good fit was indicated if the corresponding *p*-value of $\chi^2 > 0.05$ [54], a RMSEA value close to 0.06 [55], or a stringent upper limit of 0.07 [56], CFI and TLI ≥ 0.90 [55,57], and SRMR of $\leq$0.07 to indicate a good model [58], and $\leq$0.08 to indicate an acceptable model [55]. The model fit was further examined based on factor loadings and the estimated squared standardized factor loading (R-squared, R^2). A factor loading of $\geq$0.30 was considered as the cut-off point [59,60]. To capture model misspecification, the model fit modification indices (MIs) were also taken into consideration, as CFA models with many indicators often do not fit the data [52]. High MI values would suggest freeing the corresponding parameter in the analysis if it were theoretically meaningful to do so. Together with MIs, also expected parameter change (EPC) provided information on model respecification [52]. Since the chi-square (χ^2) statistic of the MLR cannot be used for χ^2 difference tests, the Satorra–Bentler scaled χ^2 difference test was used for the comparison of nested models. Further details of this procedure are given in the Mplus Web site [61]. The interpretation of effect sizes was based on the guidelines proposed by Funder and Ozer [62], where an effect size *r* of 0.05 indicated a very small effect; an effect size *r* of 0.10 indicated a small effect; an effect size *r* of 0.20 indicated a medium effect; an effect size *r* of 0.30 indicated a large effect; an effect size *r* of $\geq$0.40 indicated a very large effect.

A popular measure that has been widely used in social sciences to investigate internal consistency is Cronbach's alpha (α). However, it does not provide a dependable estimate of scale reliability as it has been found to underestimate or overestimate the scale reliability depending on measurement parameters [63]. To overcome the disadvantage of Cronbach's α, the McDonald's omega (ω) with confidence intervals (CIs) has been recommended and applied in this study to estimate scale reliability based on the results of CFA [52,64–66]. The calculation of ω alongside a CI reflects the variability in the estimation process, which provides a more accurate degree of confidence in the consistency of the administration of a scale [67]. There are different reports about the acceptable values of reliability estimates, but a rule of thumb has been that it should reach 0.70 for an instrument to be acceptable [68,69]. However, very high values of α may suggest that some items are redundant as they are testing the same question but in a different way. Hence, a maximum value of reliability estimate <0.90 has been recommended [51,70] and was used as a guide in the interpretation of the ω in the preset study.

After establishing a well fitted CFA model for the total sample, covariates were included to investigate group differences in the factors from MTDS-N [71]. Such a model is referred to as multiple indicators and multiple causes (MIMIC) model [72]. The MIMIC model consists of two parts: (i) the measurement model, in which observed indicators (i.e., 22 items) measure six underlying latent factors (i.e., depression, vigor, physical symptoms, sleep disturbances, stress, and fatigue); (ii) structural equations, in which observed variables predict the six latent factors. Five covariates were included in the MIMIC model to estimate group differences on the factors, such as gender (1 = male; 2 = female), sport (1 = individual sport; 2 = team sport), hours of training per week (continuous), program (1 = specialization in general studies with Top-Level Sports; 2 = sports and physical education with Top-Level Sports), and school level (1 = first grade; 2 = second grade; 3 = third grade). Covariates labeled with the value one were considered as the reference group. Further, the MIMIC model was extended, which involved regressing the indicators and factors on the exogenous variables [73]. The purpose of the extended MIMIC model was to determine if there were any group differences in specific items, over and above differences in the latent variables [71]. Such a model is linked to differential item functioning (DIF). Differential item functioning occurs when an item has different measurement properties for one group versus another, irrespective of mean difference on the factor [74].

Detecting DIF is important since it can lead to an inaccurate conclusion about differences in groups and invalidate procedures for making decisions about individuals [75]. The factors (depression, vigor, physical symptoms, sleep disturbances, stress, and fatigue) and all endogenous indicators, except one of each latent variable, were regressed on the five covariates. This was done for the purpose of model identification [71,73]. If all direct effects between the covariates and indicators had been freely estimated at the same time, the model would be under-identified [60]. In the MIMIC models, the covariates served as grouping variables, and a significant direct effect of a covariate on a factor or item would indicate measurement non-invariance or measurement heterogeneity across the groups of the covariate (e.g., males and females).

3. Results

3.1. Item Analysis of MTDS-N

The statistical tests KS and SW yielded statistically significant ($p < 0.001$) results for all items, indicating not normally distributed data. However, in large samples, these tests can be statistically significant even when the scores are only slightly different from a normal distribution [53,76,77]. Hence, the KS and SW were interpreted in conjunction with the values of skewness (−0.02–2.09) and kurtosis (−0.08–3.97) which showed that the data were a little skewed and kurtotic. The items miserable, bitter, and depressed did not meet the criteria of ±2.0, showing kurtosis values of 3.44, 2.16, and 3.97, respectively. Furthermore, when testing for both multivariate skewness and kurtosis, the results indicate statistically significant ($p < 0.001$) results, indicating a violation of the multivariate normality assumption in the data under study.

3.2. Confirmatory Factor Analysis

In the first step, a CFA of the hypothesized six-factor model proposed by Main and Grove (2009) was run. The model did not fit the data well: $\chi^2 = 814.824$, p-value of $\chi^2 = <0.001$, RMSEA = 0.071 (90% CI: 0.066–.076), CFI = 0.873, TLI = 0.848, and SRMR = 0.057. As the hypothesized model yielded a poor fit, MIs was examined as a guide in search of model misspecification. A couple of high error covariances were specified in the model. Hence, a new alternative model was run where three error covariances (str4 with str1, MI = 147.57, EPC = 0.48; vig4 with vig3, MI = 84.13, EPC = 0.27; and fat2 with fat1, MI = 53.97, EPC = 0.33) were set as free parameters in model estimation. It appeared that the correlated items' measurement errors in the hypothesized model were due to somewhat similar wording in the corresponding questions of the MTDS-N. After the residual covariances were set as free parameters, factor loadings were basically unchanged. Still, all the fit indices were improved with higher CFI and TLI, as well as smaller RMSEA and SRMR. The fit indices from the two CFA models are presented in Table 4.

Table 4. The test of model fit from the six-factor solution proposed by Main and Grove (2009) and the alternative model taking three measurement errors into consideration.

Fit Indices	The Hypothesized Model	The Alternative Model
χ^2	814.824	523.017
df	194	191
p	<0.001	<0.001
RMSEA	0.071	0.052
CI	0.066–0.076	0.047–0.058
CFI	0.873	0.932
TLI	0.848	0.918
SRMR	0.057	0.050

Notes. χ^2 = chi-square value; Df = degree of freedom; p = probability value of χ^2; RMSEA = root mean square error of approximation; CI = confidence interval; CFI = comparative fit Index; TLI = Tucker–Lewis index; SRMR = standardized root mean square residual.

Using the robust estimator MLR for model estimation, a scaled difference in χ^2 was computed for nested model comparison (Table 5). The hypothesized CFA model was re-run with equality restrictions on the factor loadings to each factor, and a likelihood ratio (LR) test was conducted to test whether the indicators of each factor were equally loaded to the underlying factors. With these restrictions, the number of free parameters was reduced, the degrees of freedom of the model increased, as well as the MLR χ^2 statistics. To compare the restricted model with the alternative model, the following formula was used for calculating the scaled difference in χ^2 for model comparison [52]:

$$TRd = (T_0 \times c_0 - T_1 \times c_1)/c_d$$

where T_0 and T_1 are MLR χ^2 statistics, and c_0 and c_1 were the scaling correction factors for the restricted model and alternative model, respectively. For MLR, the products $T_0 * c_0$ and $T_1 * c_1$ were the same as the corresponding maximum likelihood (ML) χ^2 statistics. The denominator C_d in the equation was the difference test scaling correction, defined as:

$$C_d = [(d_0 \times c_0) - (d_1 \times c_1)]/(d_0 - d_1)$$

where d_0 and d_1 were the degrees of freedoms for the restricted model and the alternative model. Substituting the corresponding values, the following formula was:

$$\begin{aligned} TR_d &= (T_0 \times c_0 - T_1 \times c_1)(d_0 - d_1)/[(d_0 \times c_0) - (d_1 \times c_1)] \\ &= (1035.880 - 604.085)(204 - 191)/[204 \times 1.169) - (191 \times 1.155)] \\ &= 314.02 \end{aligned} \quad (1)$$

Table 5. Calculating the scaled difference in chi-square for nested model comparison using the robust estimator MLR.

MLR			ML	
Alternative model				
T_1	d_1	c_1	$T_1 \times c_1$	d_1
523.017	191	1.155	604.085	191
Restricted model				
T_0	d_0	c_0	$T_0 \times c_0$	d_0
886.125	204	1.169	1035.880	204

Note. MLR: robust maximum likelihood; ML: maximum likelihood; Alternative model: modified six-factor CFA of the MTDS-N; T_1: MLR chi-square statistic for the alternative model; d_1: the degree of freedom (df) for the alternative model; c_1: scaling correction factor for the alternative model. Restricted model: six-factor CFA with restricted factor loadings; T_0: MLR chi-square statistic for the restricted model; d_0: df for the restricted model; c_0: scaling correction factor for the restricted model.

Change in the model χ^2 statistics between the restricted model and the alternative model followed a χ^2 distribution: χ^2 = (886.125 − 523.017) = 363.108 with the degree of freedom (df) of (204 − 191) = 13. The χ^2 test was statistically significant ($p < 0.001$). The result indicated that restricting factor loadings equal made the model fit significantly worse than otherwise. Hence, the alternative model was preferred and retained. Standardized factor loadings and standardized R^2 values for the two models are presented in Table 6, while inter-factor correlations from the alternative model are shown in Table 7. All factors were highly correlated ($p < 0.001$), except for the correlation between vigor and physical symptoms ($r = 0.035$, $p = 0.535$).

Table 6. Standardized factor loadings and R^2 values for each item in the questionnaire for the hypothesized model and the alternative model.

Item	Hypothesized	R^2	Alternative	R^2
Miserable (dep1)	0.768	0.590	0.773	0.598
Unhappy (dep2)	0.782	0.611	0.777	0.604
Bitter (dep3)	0.632	0.400	0.631	0.399
Downhearted (dep4)	0.715	0.512	0.713	0.508
Depressed (dep5)	0.773	0.598	0.775	0.601
Energetic (vig1)	0.830	0.689	0.864	0.716
Lively (vig2)	0.798	0.637	0.805	0.648
Active (vig3)	0.498	0.248	0.451	0.204
Alert (vig4)	0.455	0.207	0.404	0.163
Muscle soreness (sym1)	0.614	0.377	0.613	0.376
Heavy arms or legs (sym2)	0.789	0.623	0.790	0.625
Stiff/sore joints (sym3)	0.650	0.423	0.650	0.422
Difficulty falling asleep (sle1)	0.803	0.645	0.805	0.649
Restless sleep (sle2)	0.855	0.732	0.856	0.732
Insomnia (sle3)	0.806	0.649	0.804	0.646
Stressed (str1)	0.627	0.393	0.534	0.285
Could not cope (str2)	0.699	0.489	0.726	0.527
Difficulties piling up (str3)	0.809	0.654	0.855	0.731
Nervous (str4)	0.601	0.361	0.507	0.257
Tired (fat1)	0.797	0.635	0.650	0.422
Sleepy (fat2)	0.809	0.655	0.664	0.440
Worn-out (fat3)	0.700	0.490	0.806	0.649

Note. R^2 = coefficient of determination.

Table 7. Standardized inter-factor correlations from the alternative model above the diagonal and inter-correlations from the initial study of MTDS are presented below the diagonal.

Factor	Depression	Vigor	Physical Symptoms	Sleep Disturbances	Stress	Fatigue
DEP	1	0.304 **	0.292 **	0.460 **	0.668 **	0.634 **
VIG	−0.194	1	0.035	0.207 **	0.269 **	0.207 **
SYM	−0.228	0.041	1	0.331 **	0.305 **	0.502 **
SLE	−0.394	0.110	0.247	1	0.441 **	0.541 **
STR	0.437	−0.259	−0.181	−0.273	1	0.667 **
FAT	−0.208	0.182	0.321	0.207	−0.311	1

Notes. ** = $p < 0.001$.

As presented in Figure 2 and Table 6, standardized factor loadings ranged from 0.404–0.864, and all factor loadings were statistically significant ($p < 0.001$) and in the expected direction. The high loadings in the measurement model indicate a strong association between each of the latent factors and their respective items. The estimated R^2 provides information about how much variance of each observed indicator variable is accounted for by its underlying factors. These values can be considered as a model estimated item reliability [52]. In the present study, sle2 has the highest R^2 (0.732), while vig4 has the lowest (0.163).

Scale Reliability

The McDonald's ω, along with CIs for the factors in MTDS-N, are presented in Table 8. The scale reliability estimate for depression and sleep disturbances was >0.80. The scale reliability for vigor, physical symptoms, stress, and fatigue ranged from 0.73–0.75. No estimations were above the maximum value of reliability estimate >0.90 [51,70].

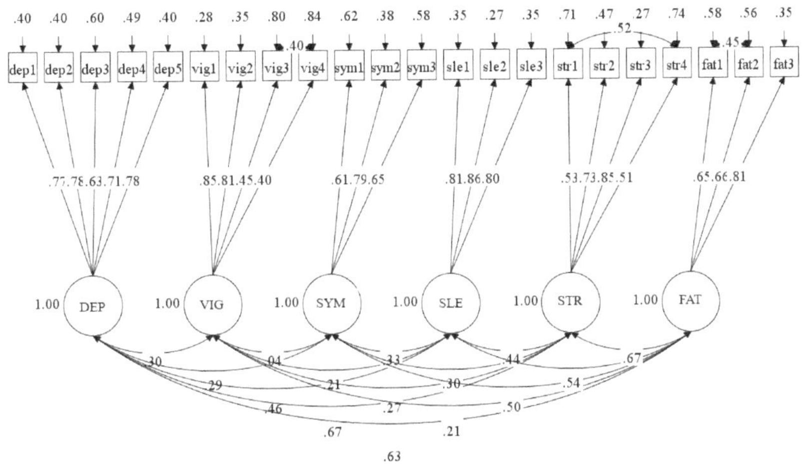

Figure 2. Standardized factor loadings, covariance estimates, and residual variances from the alternative model with three specified error covariances (vig3 with vig4; str1 with str4; fat1 with fat2).

Table 8. Calculated McDonald's ω along with confidence intervals (CIs) to estimate scale reliability.

Factor	Estimate	Lower 5% CI	Upper 5% CI
Depression	0.853	0.831	0.887
Vigor	0.747	0.714	0.799
Physical symptoms	0.725	0.690	0.779
Sleep disturbances	0.862	0.841	0.895
Stress	0.745	0.715	0.739
Fatigue	0.753	0.717	0.809

Note. CI = confidence interval.

To examine the extent to which athletes reported symptoms of psychophysiological stress related to training, scores from the MTDS-N were investigated. Taken collectively, as shown in Table 9, the student-athletes' reports of training distress were moderate. Most of the factors (i.e., vigor, physical symptoms, sleep disturbances, stress, and fatigue) mean scores were between the range of "moderate amount" and "quite a bit" from the Likert-scale. The only exception was depression (M = 1.67; SD = 0.92), scoring between "a little bit" and "moderate amount." The total score of the six factors was 13.96 (SD = 6.11).

Table 9. Mean scale scores for the six factors in MTDS-N.

Factor	Descriptive Statistics	
	M	SD
1. Depression (dep)	1.67	0.92
2. Vigor (vig)	2.67	0.94
3. Physical symptoms (sym)	2.35	1.01
4. Sleep disturbances (sle)	2.01	1.15
5. Stress (str)	2.68	1.05
6. Fatigue (fat)	2.56	1.05
Total score [a]	13.96	6.11

[a] Total score represents the sum of the six MTDS factors.

3.3. Estimating Group Differences in Latent Variables

In order to assess the effect of covariates on the factor structure, the MIMIC model was used. By conducting this model, the aim was to describe the relationship between the covariates and the training distress factors. Five covariates were included in the MIMIC model, such as gender (1 = male; 2 = female), type of sport (1 = individual sport; 2 = team sport), hours of training per week (continuous), school program (1 = specialization in general studies; 2 = sports and physical education), and school level (1 = first grade; 2 = second grade; 3 = third grade) were used to predict the latent variables. The same three error covariances specified in the alternative CFA model, were set as free parameters in model estimation (str4 with str1, MI = 133.12, EPC = 0.45; vig4 with vig3, MI = 94.10, EPC = 0.29; and fat2 with fat1, MI = 45.33, EPC = 0.30). Considering the multivariate non-normality in the measures, the MLR estimator was used for model estimation. Taken together, the covariates had 18 missing values (Table 1). Hence, the MIMIC model was based on a sample size of 614 participants. The model is specified in Figure 3.

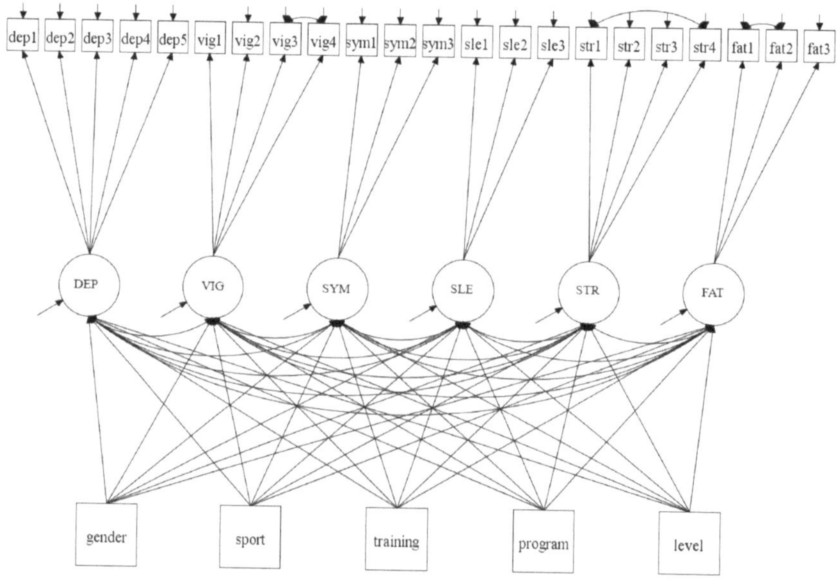

Figure 3. The multiple indicators multiple causes (MIMIC) model, where five covariates affect all the six factors. Gender (1 = male; 2 = female), sport (1 = individual sport; 2 = team sport), hours of training per week (continuous), program (1 = specialization in general studies; 2 = sports and physical education), and school level (1 = first grade; 2 = second grade; 3 = third grade).

After incorporating the five covariates, the factor structure remained unchanged and the model fit remained within acceptable values: $\chi^2 = 808.872$, p-value of $\chi^2 < 0.001$, RMSEA = 0.057 (90% CI: 0.052–0.061), CFI = 0.897, TLI = 0.871, and SRMR = 0.055. Further, the standardized (STD) results indicated that gender was a statistically significant positive predictor of the factor depression ($\beta = 0.269$, $p = 0.002$), physical symptoms ($\beta = 0.213$, $p = 0.022$), sleep disturbances ($\beta = 0.448$, $p < 0.001$), stress ($\beta = 0.502$, $p < 0.001$), and fatigue ($\beta = 0.235$, $p = 0.013$). The results suggest that male student-athletes tend to score lower on depression, physical symptoms, sleep disturbances, stress, and fatigue compared to female student-athletes. Participants in an individual sport tend to score lower on physical symptoms compared to team sports participants ($\beta = 0.231$, $p = 0.028$). Participants with fewer hours of training per week tend to score lower on physical symptoms compared to participants with more hours of training per week ($\beta = 0.024$, $p = 0.020$). Participants attending the school program specialization in general studies tend to score lower on depression ($\beta = 0.090$, $p = 0.020$), physical symptoms ($\beta = 0.110$,

$p = 0.007$), stress ($\beta = 0.105$, $p = 0.020$), and fatigue ($\beta = 0.094$, $p = 0.025$) compared to those attending the school program sport and physical education. Contrary, participants attending the school program specialization in general studies tend to score higher on vigor ($\beta = -0.237$, $p < 0.001$) compared to those attending the school program sport and physical education. Furthermore, student-athletes in first grade tend to score lower on depression ($\beta = 0.149$, $p = 0.008$) and vigor ($\beta = 0.141$, $p = 0.003$), compared to student-athletes in second- and third grade. The covariates that did not have a statistically significant effect on the six training distress factors indicate invariance in the means of the factors between the groups [52]. The explained variances in the six latent variables varied from 3.1–9.4%. In detail, the covariates accounted for 4.5%, 9.4%, 3.8%, 5.9%, 8.0%, and 3.1% of the variance in the factors of depression, vigor, physical symptoms, sleep disturbances, stress, and fatigue, respectively. Table 10 presents the standardized (STD) path coefficients for the effect of the covariates on the six factors in the MIMIC model. The score values of the covariances for the different groups can be found in Supplementary Materials Table S1.

Table 10. MIMIC model results of the covariates gender, age, type of sport, hours of training per week, county, school program, and school level on the factors depression, vigor, physical symptoms, sleep disturbances, stress, and fatigue.

Factor (Explained Variances)	Covariates	β	S.E.	p
Depression (0.045 = 4.5%)	Gender	0.269	0.086	0.002 *
	Sport	−0.172	0.103	0.096
	Training	−0.008	0.010	0.445
	Program	0.090	0.038	0.020 *
	Level	0.149	0.057	0.008 *
Vigor (0.094 = 9.4%)	Gender	0.135	0.079	0.089
	Sport	−0.062	0.092	0.501
	Training	−0.011	0.007	0.143
	Program	−0.237	0.038	0.000 **
	Level	0.141	0.048	0.003
Physical symptoms (0.038 = 3.8%)	Gender	0.213	0.093	0.022 *
	Sport	0.231	0.105	0.028 *
	Training	0.024	0.010	0.020 *
	Program	0.110	0.040	0.007 *
	Level	−0.008	0.061	0.895
Sleep disturbances (0.059 = 5.9%)	Gender	0.448	0.086	0.000 **
	Sport	−0.090	0.100	0.370
	Training	−0.012	0.008	0.163
	Program	0.044	0.034	0.193
	Level	0.073	0.055	0.186
Stress (0.080 = 8.0%)	Gender	0.502	0.089	0.000 **
	Sport	−0.042	0.105	0.686
	Training	−0.012	0.009	0.207
	Program	0.105	0.045	0.020 *
	Level	0.079	0.056	0.159
Fatigue (0.031 = 3.1%)	Gender	0.235	0.094	0.012 *
	Sport	0.048	0.106	0.650
	Training	−.016	0.009	0.090
	Program	0.094	0.042	0.025 *
	Level	0.066	0.064	0.306

Notes. S.E. = standard error; β = beta; * = $p < 0.05$; ** = $p < 0.001$.

3.4. Estimating Group Differences in Factor Indicators

The MIMIC model was extended by including direct paths between the covariates and the factor indicators (i.e., MTDS-N items). The purpose of the extended model was to investigate if differences in response to items between groups would have any effect on the factor structure and the model fit. In the extended MIMIC model testing for DIF, a dummy variable was created for the covariate load (1 = more than 10 h of training per week; 0 = less than 10 h of training per week). The factors (depression, vigor, physical symptoms, sleep disturbances, stress, and fatigue) and all endogenous indicators except one of each latent variable were regressed on the covariates gender (1 = male; 2 = female), type of sport (1 = individual sport; 2 = team sport), school program (1 = specialization in general studies; 2 = sports and physical education), school level (1 = first grade; 2 = second grade; 3 = third grade), and load. To be able to identify the model, the first indicators dep1 of depression, vig1 of vigor, sym1 of physical symptoms, sle1 of sleep disturbances, str1 of stress, and fat1 of fatigue were not regressed on the covariates [52,73]. Figure 4 illustrates the extended MIMIC model testing for DIF.

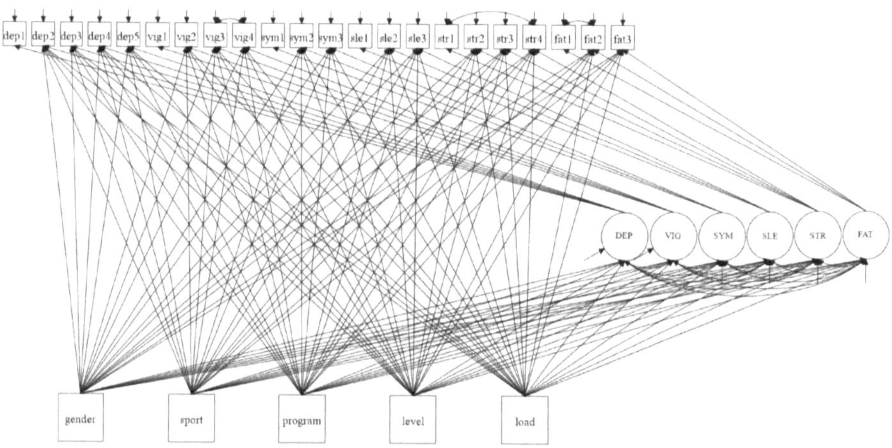

Figure 4. MIMIC model testing for differential item functioning (DIF). The five covariates affect all the six factors and all the items except one of each latent variable.

After incorporating the five covariates on the extended MIMIC model testing for DIF, the factor structure remained unchanged and the model fit remained within acceptable values: $\chi^2 = 414.661$, p-value of $\chi^2 < 0.001$, RMSEA = 0.043 (90% CI: 0.038–0.049), CFI = 0.958, TLI = 0.925, and SRMR = 0.036. The results indicated that there was DIF for 13 of the items in MTDS-N. The different items with DIF are presented in Table 11.

Results indicated that gender had a statistically significant positive effect on dep2 (unhappy), dep4 (downhearted), dep5 (depressed), and sle2 (restless sleep). This result suggests that male student-athletes tend to score lower on these items compared to female student-athletes, given the same level of depression and sleep disturbances. Contrary, gender had a statistically significant negative effect on str2 (cope), str3 (piling), and fat2 (sleepy), indicating that males tend to score higher on these items compared to females, given the same level of stress and fatigue. These results imply that there are statistically significant gender differences in response to seven items, controlling for the underlying factors. However, while DIF for these items is statistically significant, it appears variously in magnitude and does not accrue systematically across the seven items. The covariate type of sport had a statistically significant positive effect on dep3 (bitter), indicating that those in an individual sport tend to score lower on the item "bitter", compared to those in team sports, given the same level of depression. However, the magnitude of the effect was small. The covariate program had a statistically significant positive effect on vig2 (lively), vig3 (active), str2 (cope), str3 (piling), and str4 (nervous), indicating that those attending the school program specialization in general studies tend to score lower on these items compared to student-athletes attending the school program sports and physical education, controlling for the underlying factors vigor and stress. Further, the covariate program had a statistically significant negative effect on dep2 (unhappy), dep4 (downhearted), and fat3 (worn-out), indicating that those attending the school program specialization in general studies tend to score higher on these items compared to student-athletes participating the school program sports and physical education, considering the same level of depression and fatigue. The results appear variously in magnitude, from a small effect for vig3, fat3, dep2, and str4 to a very large effect for str2 and str3. Further, DIF does not accrue systematically across the eight items. The covariate level had a statistically significant negative effect on fat2 (sleepy) and fat3 (worn-out), indicating that those in first grade tend to score higher on these items compared to those in second- and third grade, controlling for the underlying factor fatigue. The effect was very small and small for the two items, respectively. Lastly, the covariate load had a statistically significant negative effect on vig3 (active) and vig4 (alert), indicating that student-athletes with less than 10 h of training per week tend to score higher on the item active and the item alert compared to student-athletes with more than 10 h of training per week, given the same level of vigor (effect was small to medium). The score values of the covariances for the different groups on the items can be found in Supplementary Materials Table S2.

Table 11. Standardized (STD) model results for the MIMIC model testing DIF with the interpretation of effect sizes.

Indicators	Covariates	β	S.E.	p	Effect Size
dep2 (unhappy)	Gender Program	0.255 −0.194	0.072 0.045	0.000 ** 0.000 **	M S
dep3 (bitter)	Sport	0.164	0.072	0.023 *	S
dep4 (downhearted)	Gender Program	0.287 −0.213	0.075 0.043	0.000 ** 0.000 **	M M
dep5 (depressed)	Gender	0.182	0.064	0.004 *	S
vig2 (lively)	Program	0.231	0.046	0.000 **	M
vig3 (active)	Program Load	0.143 −0.174	0.033 0.069	0.000 ** 0.012 *	S S
vig4 (alert)	Load	−0.200	0.072	0.006 *	M
sle2 (restless sleep)	Gender	0.181	0.075	0.016 *	S
str2 (cope)	Gender Program	−0.295 0.528	0.108 0.061	0.006 * 0.000 **	M VL
str3 (piling)	Gender Program	−0.369 0.559	0.111 0.062	0.001 * 0.000 **	L VL
str4 (nervous)	Program	0.151	0.044	0.001 *	S
fat2 (sleepy)	Gender Level	−0.212 −0.090	0.070 0.045	0.002 * 0.047 *	M VS
fat3 (worn-out)	Program Level	−0.107 −0.177	0.047 0.060	0.017 * 0.003 *	S S

Note. * = $p < 0.05$; ** = $p < 0.001$; VS = very small; S = small; M = medium; L = large; VL = very large; sym2, sym3 and sle3 were DIF-free and were not included in the table.

4. Discussion

The purpose of the present study was to translate MTDS to the Norwegian context and to test the measurement instruments factorial validity, which is a form of construct validity [78]. Construct validity is essential to be able to make assumptions from scale scores about the underlying construct of interest [79]. To our knowledge, this is the first study evaluating the factor structure of MTDS by CFA. The main finding from the present study indicated that the alternative model with three error covariances set as free, fitted the data very well showing a high representativeness of all the items concerning the underlying construct of training distress. Furthermore, the MTDS-N factors scale reliability were found to be acceptable with McDonald's ω ranging from 0.725–0.862. After incorporating the five covariates on the MIMIC model and the extended MIMIC model testing for DIF, the factor structure remained unchanged and the model fit remained within acceptable values. These results indicate that MTDS-N can be considered as an acceptable psychometric tool and appears to be a promising measure of training distress among Norwegian athletes.

4.1. Confirmatory Factor Analysis

Similar results can be observed when comparing the factor loadings from the present study with the results from Main and Grove [29]. For instance, the standardized factor loadings from the alternative model in Table 6 show a similarity in depression (0.631–0.777 vs. 0.636–0.747) and vigor (0.404–0.864 vs. 0.494–0.781). The factor alert had the lowest factor loading in both this study (0.404) and in the Main and Grove [29] study (0.494), which is in line with the low factor loading in studies where BRUMS were translated into Chinese (<0.19) [80], Malaysian (0.46) [81], and Spanish (0.16) [82]. Furthermore, factor loadings of physical symptoms (0.613–0.790 vs. −0.672–−0.790), sleep disturbances (804–0.856 vs. −0.636–−0.947), stress (0.507–0.855 vs. 0.411–0.776), and fatigue (0.650–0.806 vs. −0.502–−0.785), were also found to be quite similarly loaded. However, as shown in Table 7, the inter-factor correlations from this study were not consistent with the Main and Grove study [29]. In the Main and Grove study [29], the inter-factor correlations ranged from 0.041–0.437, with most correlations indicating medium effect sizes. In the present study, the correlations ranged from 0.035–0.668, with the most correlation indicating large to very large effect sizes. The correlations between depression and sleep disturbances (0.460), depression and stress (0.668), depression and fatigue (0.634), physical symptoms and fatigue (0.502), sleep disturbances and stress (0.441), sleep disturbances and fatigue (0.541), and stress and fatigue (0.667) were statistically significant ($p < 0.001$) and indicated very large effect sizes (Table 7). In the Main and Grove study [29], the only inter-factor correlation that yielded a very large effect size was between depression and stress (0.437). The fact that there were a few relatively high inter-factor correlations between some of the factors tells that the constructs measured can be interrelated. For example, the statistically significant ($p < 0.001$) correlation between depression and fatigue (0.634) indicates that when the value of depression increases, the value of fatigue also tends to increase. According to Puffer and McShane [83], depression and fatigue are symptoms that can be used interchangeably by athletes to describe their symptoms and feelings. Furthermore, fatigue and depression tend to be comorbid, and it has been reported that at least 30% of young people with chronic fatigue syndrome also have symptoms of depression [84]. A study by Boolani and Manierre [85] reported that depression is a predictor of long-standing feelings of fatigue in a non-athlete convenience sample [85]. Further, a statistically significant ($p < 0.001$) result was found between depression and stress (0.668). Previous studies have found statistically significant correlations between high levels of depressive symptoms and high levels of chronic stress in athletes [86,87] and women [88]. According to Brown [60], factor correlations that exceed 0.80 or 0.85 are often used as a criterion to define poor discriminant validity. In the present study, none of the correlations met this criterion; hence we can assume that the discriminant validity of the factors is good. The inter-factor correlations indicate that the domains of training distress should be regarded as factors measuring different but related aspects of training distress. This can be due to that MTDS is based on three different questionnaires, such as PSS [42], the 24-item Brunel Mood State Scale (BRUMS) [43], and a checklist of 19 symptoms of acute overtraining [44]. Nevertheless, the results from this study support the notion that the six factors can be regarded as substantially unique, as was described by Main and Grove [29], where they identified six conceptually distinct factors. In detail, the factors depression, vigor, and stress were representative of measures associated with psychological overload. The factors physical symptoms, sleep disturbances, and fatigue reflected physical and behavioral complaints associated with training distress. As such, the findings from Main and Grove [29] identified depressed mood, reduced vigor, and perceived stress as important psychological indicators of training distress. Further, their findings confirmed that physical symptoms, sleep disturbances, and general fatigue were behavioral correlates of training distress.

Scale Reliability

The scale reliability for the factors in MTDS-N was also acceptable with McDonald's ω ranging from 0.725–0.862. To our knowledge, no other studies have used McDonald's ω regarding scale reliabilities for the MTDS factors. However, other studies have reported Cronbach's α. The internal consistency presented by Main and Grove [29] showed values of α ranging from 0.72–0.86, and the six-factor solution accounted for 67.01% of the common item variance. The following Cronbach's α has been reported from a study on alpine skiers: depressed = 0.84, vigor = 0.76, physical symptoms = 0.50, sleep disturbances = 0.87, stress = 0.81, and fatigue = 0.80 [35]. Another study reported the overall internal consistency as $\alpha = 0.90$ [89]. Other studies that have used the MTDS have not reported values of α, or any other measure of scale reliability [31,33,34,36]. Collectively, the scale from the present study constitutes high scale reliability when compared with other studies that have used the same instrument. However, it is important to keep in mind the limitations that are associated with Cronbach's α as it has been found to underestimate or overestimate the scale reliability depending on measurement parameters [63]. Hence, it does not provide a dependable estimate of scale reliability, and for this reason, the McDonald's ω with CIs has been recommended and applied in this study to estimate scale reliability based on the results of CFA [52,64–66].

4.2. Estimating Group Differences in Latent Variables

The MIMIC model was conducted to investigate whether factor means were different between groups and to assess the effect of covariates on the factor structure and goodness of fit. The results from the present study indicated that the estimated factor structure remained unchanged and the model fit remained within acceptable values ($\chi^2 = 808.872$, p-value of $\chi^2 < 0.001$, RMSEA = 0.057 (90% CI: 0.052–0.061), CFI = 0.897, TLI = 0.871, and SRMR = 0.055) after incorporating the five covariates to the model. Further, the analysis indicated statistically significant differences in factor scores for *gender* on the factors of depression, physical symptoms, sleep disturbances, stress, and fatigue. The statistically significant effect of gender on the MTDS-N factors represent population heterogeneity; that is, the factor means are different at different levels of the covariate gender [60]. Population heterogeneity in MTDS has also been reported showing that females have overall higher scores than males, indicating differing mood disturbances between the genders [32,90]. The MTDS is a recently developed ASRM instrument and hence less investigated [28]; however, similar results regarding gender differences for PSS, which include some of the same symptoms as in the MTDS, have been reported. Those results indicate that women tend to score significantly higher on PSS scores compared to men [91]. Further, a prospective study on young elite athletes revealed that females reported more stress and more depressive symptoms, compared to males [92]. Interestingly, there were no statistically significant differences in vigor factor scores for gender, indicating invariance in the factor means. Hence, the probability of a student-athlete receiving an observed score is not dependent on the individuals' gender, but the individuals' true score [93]. Nevertheless, research shows that females most often score consistently higher than males on instruments measuring negative characteristics [94–96]. The finding from the present study corresponds with previous research [94–96], where population heterogeneity was found for the negative symptoms and not for the positive symptoms from the factor vigor. However, it is not clear whether this trend is a result of reasonable gender differences in terms of the latent constructs being measures or caused by other secondary factors [94]. According to Terry, et al. [97], there are a number of theories and empirical attempts to explain gender disparity, among others, these differences are artifacts of measurement bias and not true differences between males and females. An artifact explanation is based on the hypothesis that males may be less willing than females to admit negative symptoms [98]. Thus, rates of the negative symptoms may be equivalent in males and females; however, depressive symptoms are perceived as less masculine, which could result in males unwillingness to report such symptoms [99–101]. The indication of gender differences suggests that caution should be taken if group comparison is the intended purpose when using the MTDS-N among student-athletes.

The results of the present study showed a statistically significant difference in physical symptoms factor scores for the type of sport, suggesting that participants from individual sports tend to score lower on physical symptoms compared to participants from team sports. This finding is not in line with previous research where it has been reported that athletes from individual sports are more likely to report anxiety and depression compared to team sport athletes [102–104], which is explained by the fact that team sports athletes, throughout adolescence, tend to have a protective effect against depressive symptoms compared to individual sport athletes [105]. Conversely, no statistically significant differences were observed for depression, vigor, sleep disturbances, stress, and fatigue (Table 10), which are in line with findings from Birrer, et al. [106], indicating no statistically significant differences in the prevalence of training distress and overtraining syndrome between individual sport and team sports. A potential explanation for this finding can be linked to differences in the practice of sport in a given country. Differences between countries exist based on the nation's geographical, economic, social, historical, political, and cultural profile [107–109].

Regarding the covariate hours of training, results indicated statistically significant differences in factor scores of physical symptoms. There were no statistically significant differences in factor scores for the other factors in MTDS-N. Although the effect was small, this result suggests that participants with fewer hours of training per week tend to score lower on physical symptoms compared to participants with more hours of training per week. Previous research has indicated a clear effect of training load on soreness and neuromuscular fatigue in rugby athletes [110]. Another study revealed that muscle soreness is moderately related to the daily training load in professional soccer players [111]. Training and competition load results in temporary decrements in physical performance and significant levels of post-competition fatigue [10]. These decrements have been explained by increased muscle damage [11], reduction in the effectiveness of the immune system [12], an imbalance in anabolic and catabolic processes in the body [13], athlete mood disturbance [14], and a reduction in the neuromuscular effectiveness [15].

The covariate school program was a statistically significant positive predictor for the factors of depression, physical symptoms, stress, fatigue, and a statistically significant negative predictor of vigor. Hence, indicating that participants attending the school program specialization in general studies tend to score lower on depression, physical symptoms, stress, and fatigue compared to those attending the school program sport and physical education. Contrary, participants attending the school program specialization in general studies tend to score higher on vigor compared to those attending the school program sport and physical education. This could be explained by the fact that, in Norway, athletes attending the school program sport and physical education have more subjects involving physical training compared to students attending specialization in general studies. Further, the finding can be linked to the statistically significant result regarding the covariate hours of training, suggesting that participants with more hours of training per week tend to score higher on physical symptoms compared to participants with fewer hours of training per week.

School level was a statistically significant positive predictor for the factor depression and vigor, indicating that student-athletes in first grade tend to score lower on depression and vigor, compared to student-athletes in second- and third grade. Previous research has indicated that freshmen (first year) and sophomores (second year) have higher training distress scores compared to juniors (third year) and seniors (fourth year), and for this reason, year in school has been identified as a possible variable that could serve as an indicator of training distress [32]. A study by Gustafsson, et al. [112] that used the Profile of Mood States (POMS) [113] discussed that vigor might be an important indicator of maladaptation and NFOR. For example, fatigue is more sensitive and captures general training fatigue, whereas a decrease in vigor might indicate a more severe state. According to Meeusen, Duclos,

Gleeson, Rietjens, Steinacker and Urhausen [9], when the balance between training and recovery is not sufficiently respected, symptoms of prolonged training distress, including decreased vigor, will occur, leading to NFOR. However, a possible explanation of the results of vigor in this study could be attributed to the fact that the student-athletes in the first grade are fresh comers and not adapted to the increased training load, suggesting that school coaches and club coaches should pay attention to the total training load for fresh student-athletes. Another potential explanation for decreased vigor among student athletes in first grade might be due to biological reasons. Boolani, et al. [114] found that feelings of vigor are associated with mitochondrial function, which is usually lower in people who are not as well trained and those who are younger and do not have as much muscle mass. Further, their findings suggest that vigor is associated with normalized resting metabolic rate, which is usually higher in those who are not well trained [114].

4.3. Estimating Group Differences in Factor Indicators

The extended MIMIC model was conducted to investigate if there existed DIF in the responses of MTDS-N by examining the effect of covariates on factor indicators (i.e., items) and to assess if DIF would have an effect on the factor structure and goodness of fit. Such analysis can be considered as an extended method of construct validity, taking variables outside the questionnaire into account [115]. The main findings indicated that the estimated factor structure remained unchanged and the model fit remained within acceptable values (χ^2 = 414.661, p-value of χ^2 < 0.001, RMSEA = 0.043 (90% CI: 0.038–0.049), CFI = 0.958, TLI = 0.925, and SRMR = 0.036). However, the results indicated that 13 of 22 items exhibited statistically significant DIF. Responses to scale items were mostly affected by gender (seven DIF) and school program (eight DIF). However, the impacts of gender and school program on item responses were not systematic across the item set (i.e., four of seven items exhibited positive DIF for gender and five of eight items exhibited positive DIF for school program). The effect of the school program on item response was notable because two of the items (str2 and str3) were very large in magnitude (β > 0.50). The results of DIF in the present study indicate that the MTDS-N items functions differently for different groups; that is, they have a different probability of giving a certain response to the corresponding item given the same underlying factor score [116]. However, investigating the CFA factor loadings indicates that DIFs have been canceled out at the total test score. This means that while males and females have seven DIF and participants attending the school program specialization in general studies and participants attending the school program sport and physical education have eight DIF, differences were small in magnitude and their effect on the sociability dimension were negligible (Table 11). What are the practical consequences of the DIF in MTDS-N? Whether bias matters depends not just on the amount of bias, but also the purposes of the researcher [117]. Hence, one could shift the question from "is the test biased?" to "does the amount of bias in the test matter?". This shifting is especially vital because DIF would be detected in all items of all scales with sufficiently large samples [117]. In the present study, most of the statistically significant DIF was small in magnitude (Table 11). Borsboom [117] considers three possible uses of the test score. Firstly, if a researcher is interested in comparing means, biasing effects may be negligible if they are small in magnitude. Thus, violations of measurement invariance do not need to be a serious threat to validity. Secondly, if a researcher is interested in comparing within-group relations, bias may be entirely irrelevant. Finally, if the purpose is to select specific individuals (e.g., selection of diseases), then measurement invariance is a necessary condition for fair selection. However, further investigations are recommended to produce a more nuanced picture of the presence of DIF in the MTDS-N. If the scale is to be modified, different authors have proposed solutions to handle the presence of DIF in practice [118]. According to the authors of the review, researchers have recommended to split items exhibiting DIF to calibrate them in each group separately when the scale is used in a study; to remove items exhibiting DIF from the scale; or reformulate items exhibiting DIF [118].

The results from the present study must be considered in light of some limitations. First, data are based on self-report, which can result in response bias [20,119]. Additionally, the purpose of this study was to investigate the psychometric properties of the Norwegian version of MTDS, and therefore the data was collected at a single time point. Hence, a longitudinal approach would be ideal for investigating the perceptions captured by the MTDS-N over time. Regarding the choice of statistical analysis, the MIMIC model can only test non-invariances in factor means and item intercepts. To test non-invariance in factor loadings, factor variances, and measurement error variances, a multigroup CFA would be preferable. However, the MIMIC model has some advantages compared to the multigroup CFA. First, it does not require a large sample size. Further, it is possible to include continuous measures for the covariates in the MIMIC model, which is not appropriate for multigroup CFA [52].

5. Conclusions

The main objective of the present study was to examine the validity and reliability of the translated English version of MTDS into the Norwegian language to be able to assess the psychometric properties among Norwegian student-athletes. The alternative CFA model reported in this study yielded acceptable fit indices and strong scale reliability, indicating the suitability of the MTDS-N to be used in a Norwegian population to assess student-athletes training distress. There were indications of group effects, suggesting that different groups could score differently on the MTDS-N. Thus, caution is required if group comparison is the intended purpose when using the MTDS-N among student-athletes.

Supplementary Materials: The following are available online at http://www.mdpi.com/1660-4601/17/20/7603/s1. Table S1: Score values of on the factors for the different groups; Table S2: Score values of the factor predictors for the different groups; results of the preliminary pilot testing; results of the preliminary pilot testing with new model with "BY" statement; Mplus Code; source data.

Author Contributions: Conceptualization, C.N.H. and S.A.I.S.; methodology, C.N.H. and S.A.I.S.; validation, C.N.H. and S.A.I.S.; formal analysis, C.N.H.; investigation, C.N.H. and S.A.I.S.; resources, C.N.H. and S.A.I.S.; data curation, C.N.H. and S.A.I.S.; writing—original draft preparation, C.N.H.; writing—review and editing, C.N.H. and S.A.I.S.; supervision, S.A.I.S.; project administration, S.A.I.S.; funding acquisition, S.A.I.S. All authors have read and agreed to the published version of the manuscript.

Funding: This research received no external funding.

Acknowledgments: The authors would like to acknowledge the following persons for their contribution: Translation: Deborah Lynn Sorton Larssen (Senior Lecturer of English linguistics); Rebecca Anne Charboneau Stuvland (Associate Professors of English linguistics); Silje Henriette Amalia Normand (Associate Professors of English linguistics), Anders Otterbech Jølbo Myrset (Ph.D. Candidate of English linguistics). Expert committee: Rune Giske (Professor in Sport Psychology), Milica Savic (Associate Professors of English linguistics), Silje Henriette Amalia Normand (Associate Professors of English linguistics). Coordination in the pilot data collection (distribution): Espen Tønnessen (Professor in sport Sciences), Sigbjørn Bø (Physical Education student), Gerd Lise Midtgaard Nilsen Nordbotten (Senior Lecturer of sport and exercise), Håvard Myklebust (Professor in sport Sciences), Halvard Øen Grova (Manager at Viking soccer club), Tore Arne Jakobsen (Team manager at Rana soccer club).

Conflicts of Interest: The authors declare no conflict of interest.

References

1. Stambulova, N.B.; Engström, C.; Franck, A.; Linnér, L.; Lindahl, K. Searching for an optimal balance: Dual career experiences of Swedish adolescent athletes. *Psychol. Sport Exerc.* **2015**, *21*, 4–14. [CrossRef]
2. Kristiansen, E. Walking the line: How young athletes balance academic studies and sport in international competition. *Sport Soc.* **2017**, *20*, 47–65. [CrossRef]
3. Christensen, M.K.; Sørensen, J.K. Sport or school? Dreams and dilemmas for talented young Danish football players. *Eur. Phys. Educ. Rev.* **2009**, *15*, 115–133. [CrossRef]
4. Hamlin, M.J.; Wilkes, D.; Elliot, C.A.; Lizamore, C.A.; Kathiravel, Y. Monitoring training loads and perceived stress in young elite university athletes. *Front. Physiol.* **2019**, *10*, 34. [CrossRef] [PubMed]
5. McKay, C.D.; Cumming, S.P.; Blake, T.J.B.P.; Rheumatology, R.C. Youth sport: Friend or Foe? *Best Pract. Res. Clin. Rheumatol.* **2019**, *33*, 141–157. [CrossRef] [PubMed]
6. Jones, C.M.; Griffiths, P.C.; Mellalieu, S.D. Training load and fatigue marker associations with injury and illness: A systematic review of longitudinal studies. *Sports Med.* **2017**, *47*, 943–974. [CrossRef]

7. Eckard, T.G.; Padua, D.A.; Hearn, D.W.; Pexa, B.S.; Frank, B.S. The relationship between training load and injury in athletes: A systematic review. *Sports Med.* **2018**, *48*, 1929–1961. [CrossRef]
8. Kellmann, M.; Bertollo, M.; Bosquet, L.; Brink, M.; Coutts, A.J.; Duffield, R.; Erlacher, D.; Halson, S.L.; Hecksteden, A.; Heidari, J.; et al. Recovery and Performance in Sport: Consensus Statement. *Int. J. Sports Physiol. Perform.* **2018**, *13*, 240–245. [CrossRef]
9. Meeusen, R.; Duclos, M.; Gleeson, M.; Rietjens, G.; Steinacker, J.; Urhausen, A. Prevention, diagnosis and treatment of the overtraining syndrome: ECSS position statement 'task force'. *Eur. J. Sport Sci.* **2006**, *6*, 1–14. [CrossRef]
10. Takarada, Y. Evaluation of muscle damage after a rugby match with special reference to tackle plays. *Br. J. Sports Med.* **2003**, *37*, 416–419. [CrossRef]
11. McLellan, C.P.; Lovell, D.I.; Gass, G.C. Biochemical and endocrine responses to impact and collision during elite Rugby League match play. *J. Strength Cond. Res.* **2011**, *25*, 1553–1562. [CrossRef] [PubMed]
12. Cunniffe, B.; Hore, A.J.; Whitcombe, D.M.; Jones, K.P.; Baker, J.S.; Davies, B. Time course of changes in immuneoendocrine markers following an international rugby game. *Eur. J. Appl. Physiol.* **2010**, *108*, 113–122. [CrossRef] [PubMed]
13. McLellan, C.P.; Lovell, D.I.; Gass, G.C. Creatine kinase and endocrine responses of elite players pre, during, and post rugby league match play. *J. Strength Cond. Res.* **2010**, *24*, 2908–2919. [CrossRef] [PubMed]
14. West, D.J.; Finn, C.V.; Cunningham, D.J.; Shearer, D.A.; Jones, M.R.; Harrington, B.J.; Crewther, B.T.; Cook, C.J.; Kilduff, L.P. Neuromuscular function, hormonal, and mood responses to a professional rugby union match. *J. Strength Cond. Res.* **2014**, *28*, 194–200. [CrossRef]
15. Gill, N.D.; Beaven, C.M.; Cook, C. Effectiveness of post-match recovery strategies in rugby players. *Br. J. Sports Med.* **2006**, *40*, 260–263. [CrossRef]
16. Soligard, T.; Schwellnus, M.; Alonso, J.-M.; Bahr, R.; Clarsen, B.; Dijkstra, H.P.; Gabbett, T.; Gleeson, M.; Hägglund, M.; Hutchinson, M.R. How much is too much?(Part 1) International Olympic Committee consensus statement on load in sport and risk of injury. *Br. J. Sports Med.* **2016**, *50*, 1030–1041. [CrossRef]
17. Chiu, L.Z.F.; Barnes, J.L. The Fitness-Fatigue Model Revisited: Implications for Planning Short- and Long-Term Training. *Strength Cond. J.* **2003**, *25*, 42–51. [CrossRef]
18. Matos, N.F.; Winsley, R.J.; Williams, C.A. Prevalence of nonfunctional overreaching/overtraining in young English athletes. *Med. Sci. Sports Exerc.* **2011**, *43*, 1287–1294. [CrossRef]
19. Bourdon, P.C.; Cardinale, M.; Murray, A.; Gastin, P.; Kellmann, M.; Varley, M.C.; Gabbett, T.J.; Coutts, A.J.; Burgess, D.J.; Gregson, W. Monitoring athlete training loads: Consensus statement. *Int. J. Sports Physiol. Perform.* **2017**, *12*, S2–S161. [CrossRef]
20. Saw, A.E.; Kellmann, M.; Main, L.C.; Gastin, P.B. Athlete self-report measures in research and practice: Considerations for the discerning reader and fastidious practitioner. *Int. J. Sports Physiol. Perform.* **2017**, *12*, S2–S127. [CrossRef]
21. Borg, G.A. Psychophysical bases of perceived exertion. *Med. Sci. Sports Exerc.* **1982**, *14*, 377–381. [CrossRef] [PubMed]
22. Calvert, T.W.; Banister, E.W.; Savage, M.V.; Bach, T. A systems model of the effects of training on physical performance. *IEEE Trans. Syst. ManCybern.* **1976**, 94–102. [CrossRef]
23. Foster, C. Monitoring training in athletes with reference to overtraining syndrome. *Med. Sci. Sports Exerc.* **1998**, *30*, 1164–1168. [CrossRef] [PubMed]
24. Foster, C.; Florhaug, J.A.; Franklin, J.; Gottschall, L.; Hrovatin, L.A.; Parker, S.; Doleshal, P.; Dodge, C. A new approach to monitoring exercise training. *J. Strength Cond. Res.* **2001**, *15*, 109–115.
25. Taylor, K.; Chapman, D.; Cronin, J.; Newton, M.J.; Gill, N. Fatigue monitoring in high performance sport: A survey of current trends. *J. Aust. Strength. Cond.* **2012**, *20*, 12–23.
26. Windt, J.; Taylor, D.; Nabhan, D.; Zumbo, B.D. What is unified validity theory and how might it contribute to research and practice with athlete self-report measures. *Br. J. Sports Med.* **2019**, *53*, 1203–1204. [CrossRef]
27. Jeffreys, I. A System for Monitoring Training Stress and Recovery in High School Athletes. *Strength Cond. J.* **2004**, *26*, 28–33. [CrossRef]
28. Saw, A.E.; Main, L.C.; Gastin, P.B. Monitoring the athlete training response: Subjective self-reported measures trump commonly used objective measures: A systematic review. *Br. J. Sports Med.* **2016**, *50*, 281–291. [CrossRef]

29. Main, L.; Grove, J.R. A multi-component assessment model for monitoring training distress among athletes. *Eur. J. Sport Sci.* **2009**, *9*, 195–202. [CrossRef]
30. Main, L.C.; Warmington, S.A.; Korn, E.; Gastin, P.B. Utility of the multi-component training distress scale to monitor swimmers during periods of training overload. *Res. Sports Med.* **2016**, *24*, 254–265. [CrossRef]
31. Woods, A.L.; Garvican-Lewis, L.A.; Lundy, B.; Rice, A.J.; Thompson, K.G. New approaches to determine fatigue in elite athletes during intensified training: Resting metabolic rate and pacing profile. *PLoS ONE* **2017**, *12*, e0173807. [CrossRef] [PubMed]
32. Agwuenu, I.C.; Bettencourt, H.A.; Van Ness, J.M.; Jensen, C.D. Multicomponent training distress scale (MTDS) questionnaire to detect training distress in collegiate soccer players. *Med. Sci. Sports Exerc.* **2017**, *49*, 579. [CrossRef]
33. Hofacker, M.L. *Changes in Nutritional Biomarkers, Sleep, Perceived Stress, and Performance in Division I Female Soccer Players throughout a Competitive Season*; Rutgers University-School of Graduate Studies: New Brunswick, NJ, USA, 2019.
34. Woods, A.L.; Rice, A.J.; Garvican-Lewis, L.A.; Wallett, A.M.; Lundy, B.; Rogers, M.A.; Welvaert, M.; Halson, S.; McKune, A.; Thompson, K.G. The effects of intensified training on resting metabolic rate (RMR), body composition and performance in trained cyclists. *PLoS ONE* **2018**, *13*, e0191644. [CrossRef] [PubMed]
35. Davis, P.; Halvarsson, A.; Lundström, W.; Lundqvist, C. Alpine ski coaches' and athletes' perceptions of factors influencing adaptation to stress in the classroom and on the slopes. *Front. Psychol.* **2019**, *10*, 1641. [CrossRef]
36. Gescheit, D.T.; Cormack, S.J.; Reid, M.; Duffield, R. Consecutive days of prolonged tennis match play: Performance, physical, and perceptual responses in trained players. *Int. J. Sports Physiol. Perform.* **2015**, *10*, 913–920. [CrossRef] [PubMed]
37. Nässi, A.; Ferrauti, A.; Meyer, T.; Pfeiffer, M.; Kellmann, M. Psychological tools used for monitoring training responses of athletes. *Perform. Enhanc. Health* **2017**, *5*, 125–133. [CrossRef]
38. Kretzschmar, A.; Gignac, G.E. At what sample size do latent variable correlations stabilize? *J. Res. Personal.* **2019**, *80*, 17–22. [CrossRef]
39. Schönbrodt, F.D.; Perugini, M. At what sample size do correlations stabilize? *J. Res. Personal.* **2013**, *47*, 609–612. [CrossRef]
40. Hirschfeld, G.; Brachel, R.V.; Thielsch, M. Selecting items for Big Five questionnaires: At what sample size do factor loadings stabilize? *J. Res. Personal.* **2014**, *53*, 54–63. [CrossRef]
41. Cohen, J. *Statistical Power Analysis for the Behavioral Sciences*; Routledge: New York, NY, USA, 1988.
42. Cohen, S.; Kamarck, T.; Mermelstein, R. A global measure of perceived stress. *J. Health Soc. Behav.* **1983**, *24*, 385–396. [CrossRef]
43. Terry, P.C.; Lane, A.M.; Fogarty, G.J. Construct validity of the Profile of Mood States—Adolescents for use with adults. *Psychol. Sport Exerc.* **2003**, *4*, 125–139. [CrossRef]
44. Fry, R.; Grove, J.; Morton, A.; Zeroni, P.; Gaudieri, S.; Keast, D. Psychological and immunological correlates of acute overtraining. *Br. J. Sports Med.* **1994**, *28*, 241–246. [CrossRef]
45. Raedeke, T.D.; Smith, A.L. Development and Preliminary Validation of an Athlete Burnout Measure. *J. Sport Exerc. Psychol.* **2001**, *23*, 281–306. [CrossRef]
46. Guillemin, F.; Bombardier, C.; Beaton, D. Cross-cultural adaptation of health-related quality of life measures: Literature review and proposed guidelines. *J. Clin. Epidemiol.* **1993**, *46*, 1417–1432. [CrossRef]
47. International Test Commission. The ITC Guidelines for Translating and Adapting Tests (Second edition). *Int. J. Test.* **2017**, *18*, 101–134.
48. Guillemin, F.; Briancon, S.; Pourel, J. Validity and discriminant ability of a French version of the Health Assessment Questionnaire in early RA. *Disabil Rehabil* **1992**, *14*, 7.
49. Leadingsystem. SurveyXact. Available online: http://www.surveyxact.com/about-us (accessed on 24 September 2020).
50. Muthén, L.K.; Muthén, B. *(1998–2017) Mplus User's Guide*, 8th ed.; Muthén & Muthén: Los Angeles, CA, USA, 2017.
51. George, D.; Mallery, P. *SPSS for Windows Step by Step: A Simple Guide and Reference, 11.0 Update*, 4th ed.; Allyn and Bacon: Boston, MA, USA, 2003.
52. Wang, J.; Wang, X. *Structural Equation Modeling: Applicatins Using Mplus*, 2nd ed.; Wiley & Sons Ltd.: Hoboken, NJ, USA, 2020.

53. Field, A. *Discovering Statistics Using IBM SPSS Statistics: And Sex and Drugs and Rock 'n' Roll*, 4th ed.; SAGE: Los Angeles, CA, USA, 2013.
54. Schumacker, R.E.; Lomax, R.G. *A Beginner's Guide to Structural Equation Modeling*, 2nd ed.; Lawrence Erlbaum Associates: Mahwah, NJ, USA, 2004.
55. Hu, L.-T.; Bentler, P.M. Cutoff criteria for fit indexes in covariance structure analysis: Conventional criteria versus new alternatives. *Struct. Equ. Model.* **1999**, *6*, 1–55. [CrossRef]
56. Steiger, J.H. Understanding the limitations of global fit assessment in structural equation modeling. *Pers. Individ. Differ.* **2007**, *42*, 893–898. [CrossRef]
57. Hooper, D.; Coughlan, J.; Mullen, M.R. Structural equation modelling: Guidelines for determining model fit. *Electron. J. Bus. Res. Methods* **2008**, *6*, 53–60.
58. Yu, C.-Y. *Evaluating Cutoff Criteria of Model Fit Indices for Latent Variable Models with Binary and Continuous Outcomes*; University of California: Los Angeles, CA, USA, 2002; Volume 30.
59. Harrington, D. *Confirmatory Factor Analysis*; Oxford University Press: Oxford, UK, 2009.
60. Brown, T.A. *Confirmatory Factor Analysis for Apllied Research*; The Guildford Press: New York, NY, USA, 2006.
61. Mplus. Chi-Square Difference Testing Using the Satorra-Bentler Scaled Chi-Square. Available online: https://www.statmodel.com/chidiff.shtml (accessed on 14 October 2020).
62. Funder, D.C.; Ozer, D.J. Evaluating effect size in psychological research: Sense and nonsense. *Adv. Methods Pract. Psychol. Sci.* **2019**, *2*, 156–168. [CrossRef]
63. Raykov, T. Bias of coefficient afor fixed congeneric measures with correlated errors. *Appl. Psychol. Meas.* **2001**, *25*, 69–76. [CrossRef]
64. Hayes, A.F.; Coutts, J.J. Use omega rather than Cronbach's alpha for estimating reliability. But . . . . *Commun. Methods Meas.* **2020**, *14*, 1–24. [CrossRef]
65. McNeish, D. Thanks coefficient alpha, we'll take it from here. *Psychol. Methods* **2018**, *23*, 412. [CrossRef]
66. Peters, G.-J.Y. The Alpha and the Omega of Scale Reliability and Validity: Why and how to Abandon Cronbach's alpha and the route towards more comprehensive assessment of scale quality. *Eur. Health Psychol.* **2014**, *16*, 56–69.
67. Dunn, T.J.; Baguley, T.; Brunsden, V. From alpha to omega: A practical solution to the pervasive problem of internal consistency estimation. *Br. J. Psychol.* **2014**, *105*, 399–412. [CrossRef] [PubMed]
68. Lance, C.E.; Butts, M.M.; Michels, L.C. The Sources of Four Commonly Reported Cutoff Criteria:What Did They Really Say? *Organ. Res. Methods* **2006**, *9*, 202–220. [CrossRef]
69. Taber, K.S. The Use of Cronbach's Alpha When Developing and Reporting Research Instruments in Science Education. *Res. Sci. Educ.* **2018**, *48*, 1273–1296. [CrossRef]
70. Streiner, D.L. Starting at the beginning: An introduction to coefficient alpha and internal consistency. *J Pers Assess* **2003**, *80*, 99–103. [CrossRef]
71. Kaplan, D. *Structural Equation Modeling: Foundations and Extensions*, 2nd ed.; SAGE: Los Angeles, CA, USA, 2009; Volume 10.
72. Jöreskog, K.G.; Goldberger, A.S. Estimation of a model with multiple indicators and multiple causes of a single latent variable. *J. Am. Stat. Assoc.* **1975**, *70*, 631–639.
73. Muthén, B.O. Latent variable modeling in heterogeneous populations. *Psychometrika* **1989**, *54*, 557–585. [CrossRef]
74. Woods, C.M. Evaluation of MIMIC-model methods for DIF testing with comparison to two-group analysis. *Multivar. Behav. Res.* **2009**, *44*, 1–27. [CrossRef]
75. Woods, C.M.; Oltmanns, T.F.; Turkheimer, E. Illustration of MIMIC-model DIF testing with the schedule for nonadaptive and adaptive personality. *J. Psychopathol. Behav. Assess.* **2009**, *31*, 320. [CrossRef] [PubMed]
76. Chernoff, H. Large-Sample Theory: Parametric Case. *Ann. Math. Stat.* **1956**, *27*, 1–22. [CrossRef]
77. Lehmann, E.L. *Elements of Large-Sample Theory*; Springer: New York, NY, USA, 1956. [CrossRef]
78. Miles, D.A. Risk Factors and Business Models: Understanding the Five Forces of Entrpreneurial Risk and the Causes of Business Failure. In *Risk Factors and Business Models*; Dissertation.com: Boca Raton, FL, USA, 2010.
79. McQueen, A.; Tiro, J.A.; Vernon, S.W. Construct validity and invariance of four factors associated with colorectal cancer screening across gender, race, and prior screening. *Cancer Epidemiol. Prev. Biomark.* **2008**, *17*, 2231–2237. [CrossRef]
80. Zhang, C.-Q.; Si, G.; Chung, P.-K.; Du, M.; Terry, P.C. Psychometric properties of the Brunel Mood Scale in Chinese adolescents and adults. *J. Sports Sci.* **2014**, *32*, 1465–1476. [CrossRef] [PubMed]

81. Lan, M.F.; Lane, A.M.; Roy, J.; Hanin, N.A. Validity of the Brunel Mood Scale for use with Malaysian athletes. *J. Sports Sci. Med.* **2012**, *11*, 131.
82. Cañadas, E.; García, C.M.; Sanchis, C.; Fargueta, M.; Herráiz, E.B. Spanish Validation of BRUMS in Sporting and Non-Sporting Populations. *Eur. J. Hum. Mov.* **2017**, *38*, 105–117.
83. Puffer, J.C.; McShane, J.M. Depression and chronic fatigue in athletes. *Clin. Sports Med.* **1992**, *11*, 327–338. [CrossRef]
84. Knight, S.; Harvey, A.; Towns, S.; Payne, D.; Lubitz, L.; Rowe, K.; Reveley, C.; Hennel, S.; Hiscock, H.; Scheinberg, A. How is paediatric chronic fatigue syndrome/myalgic encephalomyelitis diagnosed and managed by paediatricians? An Australian Paediatric Research Network Study. *J. Paediatr. Child. Health* **2014**, *50*, 1000–1007. [CrossRef]
85. Boolani, A.; Manierre, M. An exploratory multivariate study examining correlates of trait mental and physical fatigue and energy. *Fatigue Biomed. Health Behav.* **2019**, *7*, 29–40. [CrossRef]
86. Nixdorf, I.; Frank, R.; Hautzinger, M.; Beckmann, J. Prevalence of depressive symptoms and correlating variables among German elite athletes. *J. Clin. Sport Psychol.* **2013**, *7*, 313–326. [CrossRef]
87. Hammen, C.; Kim, E.Y.; Eberhart, N.K.; Brennan, P.A. Chronic and acute stress and the prediction of major depression in women. *Depress Anxiety* **2009**, *26*, 718–723. [CrossRef] [PubMed]
88. De Francisco, C.; Arce, C.; Vílchez, M.d.P.; Vales, Á. Antecedents and consequences of burnout in athletes: Perceived stress and depression. *Int. J. Clin. Health Psychol.* **2016**, *16*, 239–246. [CrossRef] [PubMed]
89. Kask, A.; Svanberg, K. *Mental Health among Swedish Elite Athletes: Depression, Overtraining, Help Seeking, and Stigma*; Umeå Univeristy: Umeå, Sweden, 2017.
90. Bettencourt, H.A. *Does Heart Rate Recovery Detect Training Distress in Collegiate Soccer Players?* University of the Pacific: Stockton, CA, USA, 2016.
91. Gitchel, W.D.; Roessler, R.T.; Turner, R.C. Gender effect according to item directionality on the perceived stress scale for adults with multiple sclerosis. *Rehabil. Couns. Bull.* **2011**, *55*, 20–28. [CrossRef]
92. Gerber, M.; Best, S.; Meerstetter, F.; Walter, M.; Ludyga, S.; Brand, S.; Bianchi, R.; Madigan, D.J.; Isoard-Gautheur, S.; Gustafsson, H. Effects of stress and mental toughness on burnout and depressive symptoms: A prospective study with young elite athletes. *J. Sci. Med. Sport* **2018**, *21*, 1200–1205. [CrossRef] [PubMed]
93. Wu, A.D.; Zhen, L.; Zumbo, B.D. Decoding the meaning of factorial invariance and updating the practice of multi-group confirmatory factor analysis: A demonstration with TIMSS data. *Pract. Assess. Res. Eval.* **2007**, *12*, 3.
94. Carle, A.C.; Millsap, R.E.; Cole, D.A. Measurement bias across gender on the Children's Depression Inventory: Evidence for invariance from two latent variable models. *Educ. Psychol. Meas.* **2008**, *68*, 281–303. [CrossRef]
95. Nolen-Hoeksema, S. Gender differences in depression. *Am. Psychol. Soc.* **2001**, *10*, 173–176. [CrossRef]
96. Thayer, J.F.; Rossy, L.A.; Ruiz-Padial, E.; Johnsen, B.H. Gender differences in the relationship between emotional regulation and depressive symptoms. *Cogn. Ther. Res.* **2003**, *27*, 349–364. [CrossRef]
97. Terry, P.C.; Malekshahi, M.; Delva, H.A. Development and initial validation of the Farsi Mood Scale. *Int. J. Sport Exerc. Psychol.* **2012**, *10*, 112–122. [CrossRef]
98. Sigmon, S.T.; Pells, J.J.; Boulard, N.E.; Whitcomb-Smith, S.; Edenfield, T.M.; Hermann, B.A.; LaMattina, S.M.; Schartel, J.G.; Kubik, E. Gender differences in self-reports of depression: The response bias hypothesis revisited. *Sex Roles* **2005**, *53*, 401–411. [CrossRef]
99. Brody, L.R.; Hall, J.A. Gender, emotion, and expression. In *Handbook of Emotions*, 2nd ed.; Lewis, M., Haviland-Jones, J.M., Eds.; Guilford Press: NewYork, NY, USA, 2000; pp. 338–349.
100. Chevron, E.S.; Quinlan, D.M.; Blatt, S.J. Sex roles and gender differences in the experience of depression. *J. Abnorm. Psychol.* **1978**, *87*, 680–683. [CrossRef] [PubMed]
101. Conway, M. On Sex Roles and Representations of Emotional Experience: Masculinity, Femininity, and Emotional Awareness. *Sex Roles* **2000**, *43*, 687–698. [CrossRef]
102. Pluhar, E.; McCracken, C.; Griffith, K.L.; Christino, M.A.; Sugimoto, D.; Meehan, W.P., III. Team sport athletes may be less likely to suffer anxiety or depression than individual sport athletes. *J. Sports Sci. Med.* **2019**, *18*, 490.
103. Nixdorf, I.; Frank, R.; Beckmann, J. Comparison of athletes' proneness to depressive symptoms in individual and team sports: Research on psychological mediators in junior elite athletes. *Front. Psychol.* **2016**, *7*, 893. [CrossRef]

104. Elbe, A.-M.; Nylandsted Jensen, S. Commentary: Comparison of athletes' proneness to depressive symptoms in individual and team sports: Research on psychological mediators in junior elite athletes. *Front. Psychol.* **2016**, *7*, 1782. [CrossRef] [PubMed]
105. Jewett, R.; Sabiston, C.M.; Ashdown-Franks, G.; Brunet, J.; Bélanger, M.; O'Loughlin, E.K.; O'Loughlin, J.L. Team versus individual sports participation in adolescence and depressive symptoms in early adulthood. *J. Exerc. Mov. Sport Scapps Refereed Abstr. Repos.* **2014**, *46*, 157.
106. Birrer, D.; Lienhard, D.; Williams, C.A.; Röthlin, P.; Morgan, G. Prevalence of non-functional overreaching and the overtraining syndrome in Swiss elite athletes. *Schweiz Z Sportmed. Sporttraumatol* **2013**, *61*, 23–29.
107. Houlihan, B.; Green, M. Comparative elite sport development. In *Comparative Elite Sport Development: Systems, Structures and Public Policy*; Houlihan, B., Green, M., Eds.; Elsevier: Oxford, UK, 2008; pp. 1–21.
108. Houlihan, B. Mechanisms of international influence on domestic elite sport policy. *Int. J. Sport Policy Politics* **2009**, *1*, 51–69. [CrossRef]
109. Skille, E.Å.; Chroni, S.A. Norwegian sports federations' organizational culture and national team success. *Int. J. Sport Policy Politics* **2018**, *10*, 321–333. [CrossRef]
110. Tavares, F.; Healey, P.; Smith, T.B.; Driller, M. The effect of training load on neuromuscular performance, muscle soreness and wellness during an in-season non-competitive week in elite rugby athletes. *J. Sports Med. Phys. Fit.* **2017**, *58*, 1565–1571. [CrossRef] [PubMed]
111. Moalla, W.; Fessi, M.S.; Farhat, F.; Nouira, S.; Wong, D.P.; Dupont, G. Relationship between daily training load and psychometric status of professional soccer players. *Res. Sports Med.* **2016**, *24*, 387–394. [CrossRef]
112. Gustafsson, H.; Holmberg, H.-C.; Hassmen, P. An elite endurance athlete's recovery from underperformance aided by a multidisciplinary sport science support team. *Eur. J. Sport Sci.* **2008**, *8*, 267–276. [CrossRef]
113. Droppleman, L.; Lorr, M.; McNair, D. *Profile of Mood States (POMS)- Revised Manual*; Educational and Industrial Testing Service: San Diego, CA, USA, 1992.
114. Boolani, A.; O'Connor, P.J.; Reid, J.; Ma, S.; Mondal, S. Predictors of feelings of energy differ from predictors of fatigue. *Fatigue: Biomed. Health Behav.* **2019**, *7*, 12–28. [CrossRef]
115. Groenvold, M.; Petersen, M.A. The role and use of differential item functioning (DIF) analysis of quality of life data from clinical trials. In *Assessing Quality of Life in Clinical Trials*, 2nd ed.; Fayers, P., Hays, R., Eds.; Oxford University Press: Oxford, NY, USA, 2005; pp. 195–208.
116. Bartolucci, F.; Bacci, S.; Gnaldi, M. *Statistical Analysis of Questionnaires: A Unified Approach Based on R and Stata*; CRC Press: Broken Sound Parkway, FL, USA, 2016.
117. Borsboom, D. When does measurement invariance matter? *Med Care* **2006**, *44*, S176–S181. [CrossRef] [PubMed]
118. Rouquette, A.; Hardouin, J.B.; Vanhaesebrouck, A.; Sébille, V.; Coste, J. Differential Item Functioning (DIF) in composite health measurement scale. Recommendations for characterizing DIF with meaningful consequences within the Rasch model framework. *PLoS ONE* **2019**, *14*, e0215073. [CrossRef] [PubMed]
119. Caputo, A. Social desirability bias in self-reported well-being measures: Evidence from an online survey. *Univ. Psychol.* **2017**, *16*, 245–255. [CrossRef]

Publisher's Note: MDPI stays neutral with regard to jurisdictional claims in published maps and institutional affiliations.

International Journal of
Environmental Research and Public Health

MDPI

Article

Influences of Differing Menarche Status on Motor Capabilities of Girls, 13 To 16 Years: A Two-Year Follow-Up Study

Barry Gerber [1,*], Anita E. Pienaar [1] and Ankebe Kruger [2]

[1] Physical Activity, Sport and Recreation (PhASRec), School of Human Movement Sciences, Faculty of Health Sciences, Potchefstroom Campus, North-West University, Private Bag X6001, Potchefstroom 2520, South Africa; anita.pienaar@nwu.ac.za

[2] Centre of Health and Human Performance (CHHP), Faculty of Health Sciences, Potchefstroom Campus, Institute for Psychology and Wellbeing (IPW), North-West University, Private Bag X6001, Potchefstroom 2520, South Africa; ankebe.kruger@nwu.ac.za

* Correspondence: barry.gerber@nwu.ac.za; Tel.: +27-018-299-1773 or +27-72-581-9629

Abstract: Puberty and the onset of menarche influences the motor performance of girls. However, the magnitude of these influences during varying maturity status, is not clear. This longitudinal study over two years aimed to investigate differences in motor fitness between early and late developing girls based on pre- and post-menarche status. A convenience sample (n = 58) of girls aged 13.51 ± 3.51, divided by means of the Status Quo method into pre (n = 13) and post-menarche (n = 45) groups, was used. Motor fitness was tested once annually by standardized protocols. Basic statistics, independent t-testing and a repeated measures ANOVA with a post hoc Bonferonni correction were used ($p < 0.05$ = statistical significance). Effect sizes were determined by Cohen's d-values. Only explosive upper body strength differed significantly between groups during baseline, favoring post-menarche girls. Initially, post-menarche girls showed advantages in hand-eye coordination and speed ($p > 0.05$) with pre-menarche girls performing better in agility and explosive leg strength ($p > 0.05$). At 15.51 years, no significant, between-group differences were found. Pre-menarche girls surpassed post-menarche girls in hand-eye coordination and 0–40 m speed and post-menarche girls displayed higher explosive leg and upper body strength scores ($p > 0.05$). Our data show that the potential to excel in sport based on motor capabilities can only be accurately estimated 1–2 years after reaching menarche.

Keywords: growth; longitudinal; menarche; motor capabilities

Citation: Gerber, B.; Pienaar, A.E.; Kruger, A. Influences of Differing Menarche Status on Motor Capabilities of Girls, 13 To 16 Years: A Two-Year Follow-Up Study. *Int. J. Environ. Res. Public Health* **2021**, *18*, 5539. https://doi.org/10.3390/ijerph18115539

Academic Editors: Shaher A.I. Shalfawi and Paul B. Tchounwou

Received: 15 March 2021
Accepted: 10 May 2021
Published: 22 May 2021

1. Introduction

Differential timing of the onset of menarche has various consequences for girls [1–10]. Understanding these effects, especially on the physical and motor abilities of girls, can provide coaches, physical education teachers and others involved in the health and well-being of adolescent girls, with valuable insight into the physiology of young girls, especially the potential effects of early and late exposure to sex hormones on their motor and physical abilities [1,2]. In this regard, researchers [3,4] report that the largest variation in sexual maturity among girls is found between the ages of 12 and 16 years, showing clear associations with anthropometric characteristics and motor fitness [5]. Due to menarche being associated with various physical changes that occur during puberty [6], researchers have described differential age of onset of menarche as a risk factor for a number of adverse health outcomes, including obesity [7], type 2 diabetes [8] and cardio-metabolic traits [9], all mostly associated with girls who reach menarche at a young age (early developing girls). In addition, the timing of the onset of menarche also influences the development of motor and physical fitness capabilities of adolescent girls which has consequences for sport performance [10].

Menarche, which is reached during puberty (11.8 to 13 years), on average at the age of 12.8 years [11,12] is a critical milestone in female's journey to adulthood, from both a socio-cultural and medical perspectives [13]. Age of menarche, which occurs about 6 months to 1 year after reaching the maximum growth spurt or peak height velocity (PHV) [12,14], is not rigid and is influenced by a variety of factors, such as genetic factors, nutrition and health status [15,16]. The menstrual cycle is comprehended as a biofeedback system; therefore, each structure and or gland is affected by the activity of the others [17]. The onset of menarche, in turn, directly affects the physical and motor capabilities of girls which have consequences, specifically, for those who participate in sport [11]. The time period of puberty induces critical morpho-functional transitions across the adolescence period [18]. These changes influence anthropometric characteristics and body composition (height, weight, body fat and muscle mass) which again affects motor performance (speed, agility, explosive power, hand-eye coordination and muscle strength) of girls [11,19] and subsequently, sport performance [11,20–24]. More specifically, speed, agility and explosive power are directly influenced by body dimensions such as sitting height and arm span [11].

The literature, however, indicates that biological maturity is not the only role player in girls' motor development, as biological maturity for example only accounts for approximately 2.8% of variation in girls' coordination. Literature also indicates that anaerobic improvement still occurs after puberty indicating that biological maturity plays a significant role in speed [11]. In this regard, peak development in muscle strength and endurance, which is directly related to speed and agility, commences approximately 0.5–1 years after reaching PHV [11].

Various studies that focused on changes in girl's motor and physical capabilities during adolescence have been conducted globally [25–36] although to a lesser extent in South Africa [22,27,32–40]. Results from the above studies concluded that motor capabilities are influenced by biological maturity, although neurological development and fitness and sport training also showed influences. However, biological maturity differences related to the age of onset of menarche were not the main differential factor in these analyses. Furthermore, contradictory results regarding the influence of menarche on girl's motor capabilities are also found, where some research [11] reports no correlations between peak motor development before, during and after menarche in relation to the onset of menarche, while others found [22] significant differences between early, middle and late developing girls. Results of the studies that were reviewed indicated that physical and motor fitness are influenced in different ways by biological maturation during puberty. Most of these studies are older than 10 years old, which questions the relevance of the findings for modern populations. In addition, limited studies analyzed influences of varying menarche status (or the phenomena of early and late development) on motor fitness longitudinally. This background identifies gaps in the literature regarding the understanding of pathways of change in motor fitness as a result of the interrelatedness of different human systems, more specifically, how the differential timing of menarche status will affect the motor fitness capabilities of early and late developing girls.

Consequently, as it can take up to ten years to reach elite performance in a particular sport [41] and as late menarche occurrence seems to favor athletic performance [22,42] it is important to understand developmental motor fitness pathways in girls of differing maturity status especially during the mid to late adolescence period. Such knowledge can aid the process of identifying girls with true sporting potential during this time period or earlier to ensure optimal development. Furthermore, knowledge in this regard will aid coaches and trainers to address maturational differences to the benefit of all girls of similar chronological ages. This can aid the implementation of physiologically sound long-term athlete development plans that will address the developmental needs of all girls, especially late maturing girls, who will most probably be the sporting stars in the future. The aim of this study is therefore to investigate the extent of developmental differences in speed, agility, explosive power and coordination in pre (or late developing) and post-menarche (or early developing) girls by studying it over a longitudinal period during the mid-adolescence period. Findings from the study will aid in a better understanding of the influence of the phenomena of menarche on girls' explosive upper body strength, hand-eye coordination, explosive leg strength, agility and speed development. This understanding can then contribute to the compilation of sport development programs that are aligned with girls' maturational status. In addition, the results of this study can contribute to a more accurate selection of girls during the mid-adolescent period who have the potential to excel in sport, based on motor specific characteristics.

2. Materials and Methods

2.1. Research Design

This study is a sub-study of the longitudinal project "Growth and sport psychological characteristics of talented adolescents" that was conducted over a two-year follow-up period spanning a 3-year school period (2010–2012). The data were collected using anthropometric and motor tests as well as questionnaires. Anthropometric measurements took place three times a year (four months apart) with the motor tests measured once annually. Baseline measurements were taken in February 2010 and the last measurements took place in November 2012, resulting in nine time-point measures for growth (T1–9) and three-time point follow-up measures for motor fitness skills (T1, T2, T3). This time period includes girls between the ages of 13 and 16 years of age.

2.2. Research Group

The participants were recruited by means of convenience sampling. All grade 8 learners of one quintile 5 school (quintile 1 = low socio-economic quintile, to quintile 5 = high socio-economic quintile) in Potchefstroom in the Northwest Province of South Africa were invited to take part in the study. Since the school had boarding facilities, all grade 8 learners enrolled in 2010 represented 46 different primary schools. In 2010, 95 girls with a mean age of 13.73 + 0.48 years participated in the baseline measurements. The final group, who completed all follow-up measurements in November 2012, consisted of 58 girls with a mean age of 16.27 ± 0.36 years. A power calculation indicated that group sizes of 14 participants are needed to observe medium effects of differences. The loss of subjects to follow-up were 37 girls (38%) due to various reasons including parents of children moving elsewhere, children moving between schools or incomplete datasets.

2.3. Ethical Approval

Ethical approval for the execution of the study based on the Declaration of Helsinki was obtained from the Health Research Ethics Committee of the North-West University's Potchefstroom Campus (NWU 00199-15-A1). Permission for the project was also obtained from the principal of the school involved. Learners who had parental permission and who gave assent themselves were subjected to the testing protocol.

2.4. Measuring Instruments

All measurements were conducted by trained researchers from the North-West University. Post graduate students in Human Movement science, specializing in Sport Science and Kinderkinetics assisted in the data collections. These students were trained intensively beforehand on the standardized processes that had to be followed. All of them also had Level 3 certification in Kinatropometry measurements. The principle investigator of the study oversaw all data aspects of the data collection to ensure valid and accurate data at each time point of the follow up period.

Age of Menarche

The age of menarche was determined by the Status Quo method [37,43] during the baseline measurements of each year in February in 2010, 2011 and 2012 (T1, T2 and T3). The girls had to indicate on a questionnaire by selecting YES or NO whether they have had their first menstrual cycle on or before the date of testing. If they have answered YES, they also had to indicate the month and year when their first menstrual cycle had started.

A high percentage of the final group (77%, $n = 45$) already reached menarche during the baseline measurement in grade 8 (2010) at a mean age of 13.51 years. For the purpose of this study, the group was divided into a pre-menarche group ($n = 13$) and post-menarche group ($n = 45$) according to the menarche status at baseline. All comparisons were done based on this grouping.

2.5. Motor Measurements

The Australian Sport Search Program protocol commonly used in Australia for sports talent identification in children of 12 years and older was used [44]. The test protocol involves six motor tests (beep test, basketball throw, 40 m speed test, 10 m agility test, vertical jump and throw-and-catch-test). All motor tests were conducted according to this protocol. In addition, girls 0–10 m speed were also tested. To obtain more details regarding the methods use, please refer to Gerber et.al [45].

2.6. Body Composition

The protocol as developed by the International Society for the Advancement of Kinanthropometry (ISAK) was used for stature and body weight measurements [46]. Stature was measured by using a standardized calibrated stadiometer and body weight was measured by means of an electronically calibrated scale (Omro BF 511). Body weight in kilograms divided by height in meters squared or, BMI = x KG/[y M (×) y M] (x = bodyweight in KG, y = height in M) were used to calculate BMI. Percentage fat mass and muscle mass were measured with an electronically calibrated bio-impedance, body composition apparatus (Omro BF 511). Accuracy of the Omron models differs from model-to-model (+3.5 and 4.1%) based on the Standard Estimation Error (SEE). The SEE indicates that 68% of all measurements for different users are accurate within 3.5–4.1%, relative to body fat percentage (kg/m^2). (https://www.omron-healthcare.com/en/products/weightmanagement, accessed on 15 March 2021). Unfortunately, no data were available for baseline muscle and fat mass measurements due to the measurements obtained from the body composition analyzer only being available from the second year of the study as a result of unforeseen circumstances (T2). BMI was, however, calculated and reported for T1 from mass and stature measurements.

2.7. Statistical Analysis

The data were analyzed with the "Statistica for Windows 2017" Statsoft computer program [47]. Descriptive characteristics, including means, standard deviations (sd) and minimum and maximum values were calculated. The data were firstly checked for normality. By checking the distributions of the variables, no serious deviations of normality were detected. Independent t-testing were used to determine group differences in motor fitness characteristics at each time point with statistical significance set at $p < 0.05$. Effect sizes of these differences were also calculated to determine practical significance of differences using Cohen's d-values with $d > 0.2$ indicating a small effect size, $d > 0.5$ a medium effect size and $d > 0.8$ a large effect size [48].

Repeated measures ANOVA was used to analyze changes in motor skills and capabilities over time followed by a post hoc Bonferonni adjustment to determine the statistical significance of group differences over time as well as the interaction effect over time, with statistical significance set at $p < 0.05$ ($p < 0.05$).

3. Results

Table 1 reports the group's baseline and follow-up descriptive characteristics.

Fifty-eight girls, that included the pre-menarche ($n = 13$, 23%) and post-menarche group ($n = 45$, 77%) completed all measurements. Although the pre- and post-menarche groups as divided at baseline, were used for all analysis, 91% (T2) and 98% (T3) of the group had reached menarche respectively during follow-up measurements. No significant age differences (0.01 years, $p > 0.05$) were found between the groups during baseline measurements, with a mean group age of 13.51 years at baseline.

Table 1. Descriptive characteristics of the pre- and post-menarche groups.

	Year 1 (T1)		Year 2 (T2)		Year 3 (T3)	
	N	Mean Age ± SD	N	Mean Age ± SD	N	Mean Age ± SD
Group	58	(T1) 13.51 ± 3.5	58	(T2) 14.51 ± 3.51	58	(T3) 15.51 ± 3.51
Pre-menarche	13	(T1) 13.52 ± 3.58	13	(T2) 14.52 ± 3.58	13	(T3) 15.52 ± 3.58
Post-menarche	45	(T1) 13.51 ± 3.53	45	(T2) 14.51 ± 3.53	45	(T3) 15.51 ± 3.53

T1 = Year one (Gr8); T2 = Year 2 (Grade 9); T3 = Year 3 (Grade 10); N = number of subjects.

Table 2 displays the body composition (fat and muscle mass percentage) of the subgroups during the first and second follow-up measurements. Unfortunately, no data were available for baseline muscle and fat mass measurements due to the body composition analyzer only being introduced during T2. A lower BMI at all three time points and higher muscle mass and lower fat mass were found in the pre-menarche group during T2 and T3. Group differences in fat mass decreased from T2 (4.82%; $p < 0.05$, $d = 0.68$) to 2.71% ($p > 0.05$; $d = 0.31$). Differences in muscle mass of the groups stayed unchanged from T2 to T3. Group differences were also only of small to medium practical significance. BMI differences between groups were borderline statistically significant ($p = 0.06$) during baseline, although became insignificant at T2 and T3. These differences in BMI were of medium practical significance during T1 ($d = 0.60$), but declined to small practical significant differences during T2 ($d = 0.35$) and T3 ($d = 0.25$).

Table 2. Body composition differences between pre- and post-menarche groups during T2 and T3.

	Pre	Post	Difference	*p*-Value	*d*-Value
		T1 (Grade 8)			
BMI Δ	19.59 + 3.50	21.79 + 3.73	2.2	0.06 ►	0.60 ##
		T2 (Grade 9)			
Fat %	21.02 ± 7.62	25.84 ± 6.45	4.82	0.02 *	0.68 ##
Muscle %	34.90 ± 2.63	33.38 ± 2.33	1.25	−2.02	0.61 ##
BMI	21.02 ± 4.07	22.36 ± 3.36	1.34	0.23	0.35 #
		T3 (Grade 10)			
Fat %	26.26 ± 10.01	28.97 ± 7.54	2.71	0.29	0.31 #
Muscle %	40.24 ± 5.68	38.98 ± 4.25	1.26	0.39	0.25 #
BMI	21.65 ± 3.78	22.49 ± 2.91	0.84	0.39	0.25 #

T1 = Baseline measurements (Grade 8); T2 = First follow up measurement (Grade 9); T3 = Second follow up measurement (Grade 10); Pre = Pre-menarche; Post = Post menarche; * = Statistical significance ($p < 0.05$); ► = Borderline significant $0.05 < p > 0.07$; # = small effect size ($d > 0.2$); ## = medium effect size ($d > 0.5$); ### = large effect size ($d > 0.8$). Note Δ BMI at T1 was calculated from mass and stature.

Table 3 shows the descriptive characteristics and the statistical and practical significance of group differences in motor fitness capabilities. Post-menarche girls outperformed the pre-menarche girls in four of the six motor tests during baseline (T1), including EUBS, HEC, 0–10 m and 0.40 speed (Table 3). However, only the difference of 0.59 m in EUBS was of statistically significance ($p = 0.01$, $d = 0.80$). All other differences were only of practical significance in HEC (catches = 0.76, $d = 0.17$), 0.10 m speed (0.05 s, $d = 0.27$) and 0–40 m speed (0.17 s, $d = 0.27$) (Table 3).

Table 3. Motor fitness characteristics and differences between the pre- and post-menarche groups at T1, T2 and T3.

	Pre-Menarche (n = 13)			Post-Menarche (n = 45)			Significance of Differences		
TP	**M ± SD**	**Min**	**Max**	**M ± SD**	**Min**	**Max**	**Diff**	***p*-Value**	***d*-Value**
Explosive upper body strength (EUBS) (m) (Maturity group * Time F = 2.65; p = 0.11)									
T1	4.65 ± 0.83	3.1	6.18	5.24 ± 0.63	4.05	6.72	0.59	0.01 *	0.80 ###
T2	5.42 ± 0.97	4.2	7.2	5.58 ± 0.57	4.5	7	0.12	0.58	0.15
T3	5.34 ± 0.80	4.04	6.73	5.60 ± 0.63	4.2	7.1	0.26	0.23	0.36 #
Explosive leg strength (ELS) (cm) (Maturity group * Time F = 0.02; p = 0.87)									
T1	32.57 ± 4.16	26	39	31.23 ± 5.77	18.5	45	1.34	0.43	0.26 #
T2	29.80 ± 8.60	19	42.5	29.13 ± 7.96	16.5	51.5	0.67	0.79	0.08
T3	31.43 ± 6.98	21	41.5	33.97 ± 6.06	22	48.2	2.54	0.2	0.38 #
Agility (s) (Maturity group * Time F = 0.06; p = 0.80)									
T1	20.46 ± 1.22	18.57	22.43	20.72 ± 1.27	18.02	24.88	0.26	0.52	0.20 #
T2	19.23 ± 1.35	17.87	22.91	19.23 ± 1.86	16.37	24.71	0	0.99	0
T3	20.53 ± 1.31	18.24	22.32	20.62 ± 1.28	18.84	24.27	0.09	0.83	0.06
Speed (0–10 m) (s) (Maturity group * Time F = 0.53; p = 0.47)									
T1	2.18 ± 0.15	1.92	2.45	2.13 ± 0.14	1.9	2.54	0.05	0.3	0.34 #
T2	3.67 ± 0.62	1.9	4.28	3.50 ± 0.59	1.78	4.34	0.16	0.42	0.28 #
T3	2.13 ± 0.15	1.88	2.39	2.12 ± 0.11	1.9	2.41	0.01	0.79	0.07
Speed (0–40 m) (s) (Maturity group * Time F = 0.04; p = 0.84)									
T1	7.12 ± 0.61	6.17	8.39	6.95 ± 0.64	5.81	8.9	0.17	0.39	0.27 #
T2	6.88 ± 0.69	5.87	8.04	6.74 ± 0.63	5.67	8.61	0.14	0.5	0.21 #
T3	6.75 ± 0.70	5.84	8.15	6.80 ± 0.63	6	8.59	0.05	0.82	0.07
Hand-eye coordination (HEC) (n) (Maturity group * Time F = 0.41; p = 0.52)									
T1	4.84 ± 4.45	0	14	5.60 ± 4.08	0	15	0.76	0.56	0.17
T2	6.15 ± 4.68	0	14	8.06 ± 5.02	0	20	1.91	0.22	0.39 #
T3	5.61 ± 4.53	0	12	5.46 ± 4.02	0	16	0.15	0.88	0.04

TP = Time points; T1 = Baseline measurements (Grade 8), T2 = First follow up measurement (Grade 9); T3 = Second follow up measurement (Grade 10); Pre = Pre-menarche; Post = Post menarche; M = Mean values; SD = Standard deviation; * = Statistical significance ($p < 0.05$); Practical significance # = small effect size ($d > 0.2$); ## = medium effect size ($d > 0.5$); ### = large effect size ($d > 0.8$).

At T2, the, post-menarche group still displayed slightly higher mean values in EUBS, HEC, 0–10 m and 0–40 m speed ($p > 0.05$) with pre-menarche having a slight advantage in ELS ($p > 0.05$) (Table 3). No difference was evident in the agility scores of the groups (Table 3). Differences between the groups also declined ($p > 0.05$) in EUBS (0.12 m), ELS (0.67 cm), agility (0.00 s) and 0–40 m speed (0.14 s), although it increased in HEC and 0–10 m speed. These differences between the groups at T2 were only of small practical significance for 0.10 m speed ($d = 0.28$), 0–40 m speed ($d = 0.21$) and HEC ($d = 0.39$) (Table 3).

At T3, no statistically significant group differences were evident, although the differences in the strength tests, EUBS ($d = 0.36$) and ELS ($d = 0.36$), showed small practical significance (Table 3). Post-menarche girls caught up and surpassed the pre-menarche group in ELS where the difference of 2.54 cm (T3) between the groups also increased from 0.67 cm during T2 to T3 ($p > 0.05$, $d = 0.38$) (Table 3). The post-menarche group still showed more favorable EUBS where between groups differences increased with 0.26 cm from T2 to T3 ($p > 0.05$, $d = 0.36$) (Table 3). The post-menarche group also showed a slight advantage in 0–10 m speed as the between-group difference of 0.01 s decreased further to similar values from T2 to T3 ($p > 0.05$, Table 3). The pre-menarche group, however, caught up and surpassed the post-menarche group during T3 in HEC (+0.15 catches) and 0–40 m (−0.05 s) speed although these both these differences were insignificant on a practical ($d < 0.2$) and statistical level ($p > 0.05$) insignificant. The pre-menarche group still showed slightly lower agility values although the difference of 0.09 s between groups increased slightly from T2 to T3, although still statistically insignificant (Table 3). Maturity group differences over time were insignificant for all motor skills ($p > 0.05$) (Table 3).

Table 4 reports the significance of changes in motor capabilities between measurements. Although various changes between measurements were of statistical significance, only changes in explosive upper body strength and 0–40 m speed in both groups and explosive leg strength in the post-menarche group were of significance from T1–T3 (Table 4). This contributed to evidence portraying that the pre-menarche group catching up and surpassing the post-menarche group in HEC and 0–40 m speed. Their larger increase in EUBS could not, however, result in them catching up to the post-menarche group (Table 3). Larger changes in ELS of post-menarche girls contributed to them surpassing pre-menarche girls during T3 although they could not catch up with pre-menarche girls in agility after showing a bigger increase as well (Table 4). Overall, the means in the different tests over this follow-up period portray that the pre-menarche groups' motor performance, was lagging that of the post-menarche group with approximately two years. This is evident from the similar values that the pre-menarche group obtained at T3 compared to the values that were obtained by the post-menarche group at T1.

Table 4. Significance of changes in motor fitness characteristics of pre- and post-menarche groups.

	T1–T2		T2–T3		T1–T3	
	Pre	Post	Pre	Post	Pre	Post
Explosive upper body strength	0.81 *	0.34 *	−0.12	0.02	0.69 *	0.36 *
Explosive leg strength	−2.77	−1.9	1.63	4.75 *	−1.14	2.85 *
Agility	−1.23 *	−1.38 *	1.30 *	1.24 *	0.07	−0.14
Speed (1–10 m)	1.42 *	1.36 *	−1.45 *	−1.38 *	−0.03	−0.02
Speed (0–40 m)	−0.23 *	−0.17 *	−0.04	0	−0.27 *	−0.17 *
Hand-eye coordination	1.31	2.46 *	−0.54	−2.64 *	0.77	−0.18

* = Statistical significance ($p < 0.05$); T1 = Baseline measurements (Grade 8), T2 = First follow-up measurement (Grade 9); T3 = Second follow-up measurement (Grade 10); Pre = Pre-menarche; Post = Post-menarche.

Table 5 presents the results of interaction effect between the groups over the three time points (T1–T3) derived from a repeated measures ANOVA. Interaction effects over time points were only significant for explosive upper body strength [F (2.112) = 5.9670, $p = 0.00345$], although marginally significant for explosive leg strength [F (2.108) = 2.7179, $p = 0.06986$] (Table 5).

Table 5. Interaction effects between pre- and post-menarche groups over time of.

Variable	Interaction Effect
Explosive upper body strength	F (2.112) = 5.9670, $p = 0.00345$
Hand-eye coordination	F (2.112) = 2.2069, $p = 0.11480$
Vertical jump	F (2.108) = 2.7179, $p = 0.06986$
Agility	F (2.98) = 0.12702, $p = 0.88086$
Speed 0–10 m	F (2.92) = 0.10077, $p = 0.90424$
Speed 0– 40 m	F (2.100) = 0.54467, $p = 0.58174$

p = statistical significance set at $p < 0.05$.

4. Discussion

The objective of this study was to determine if differences exist in explosive power, speed, agility and hand-eye coordination of girls with differing menarcheal status over a two-year follow-up period. This aim was investigated by comparing pre (or late developing) and post-menarche (or early developing) girls longitudinally over time, based on their menarche status at baseline (February of Grade 8) when they had a mean age of 13.51 years.

Developmental differences between the pre- and post-menarche groups was found to be relatively small and mostly insignificant in speed, agility and hand-eye coordination. This finding agrees with most other studies, as reviewed by Malina et al. [11], that also reported similar findings. This finding is most probably attributable to the groups being already late in their pubertal phase with most of the participants (n = 45, 77%) having already reached menarche at baseline (T1) (Table 1). A large percentage (<38%) of the post-menarche group were also in their menarche phase for a considerable time as 4.4%

reached menarche at 10 years, 2.2% at 11 years, 31.1% at 12 years and 60% at 13 years and only 2.2% at 14 years. Of the pre-menarche group, 9 (93%) reached menarche during Grade 9 (T2) at 14.51 years and all but one (98%) of this group before (T3) in their grade 10 year at the mean age of 15.51 years.

The post-menarche girls showed slightly more favorable results in the 10 m and 40 m speed although differences between the groups were insignificant. These differences were of small practical significance at 13.51 years (10 m and 20 m speed) and at 14.51 years for 40 m speed. The largest, although also insignificant differences ($p > 0.05$) were found in 10 m speed during T2 at a mean age of 14.51 years and in 40 m speed during T1 at a mean age of 13.51 years. These results coincide with the findings of Van den Berg et al. [22] who also found insignificant differences between 14-year-old girl tennis players of differing maturity levels in 10 m speed. Our study also showed similar non-significant differences in agility with the largest, mean differences ($p > 0.05$) found during T1, favoring the pre-menarche group. This could also be ascribed to pre-menarche girls having a higher percentage muscle mass (34.9%) and lower percentage fat mass (21.02%) compared to the post-menarche group (33.8%) as well as fat mass (25.84%) at T2 ($p < 0.05$), although differences in body composition became insignificant at T3 (Table 2). Hand-eye co-ordination showed insignificant differences of 1.91 catches at T2, favoring the post-menarche group. These small insignificant differences that were found and also mostly during the baseline measurements, could in some way be ascribed to the explained small differences in the time of reaching maturational status during baseline measurements in the groups. As most of the group have reached menarche in grade 9 at age 14.51 years, it can be assumed that almost all have already experienced PHV at the baseline measurements, as this event occurs on average one year before reaching menarche. The adolescent growth spurt in muscle strength and muscle endurance, which is directly linked to speed and agility, takes an onset approximately 0.5–1 year after reaching PHV where after a plateau is reached at around 14 years of age [11,49]. Therefore, due to the current maturational status of our group, where most of the participants have already reached menarche, which occurs on average two years after PHV, most participants, including participants from the pre-menarche group would have reached peak development in speed and agility. This might explain the small difference between the groups in speed and agility. Furthermore, with regard to body composition influences, Aberberga-Augskalne and Kemper [50] state that the biggest increase in mass occurs between 12 and 14 years, congruent to the average age of menarche. From the onset of menarche, estrogen plays an important role in the lipogenic profile of girls during the puberty phase [51]. Consequently, higher levels of estrogen results in a higher percentage body-fat and also the distribution of fat within the body changes to where a large percentage of fat is being distributed among the hips and surrounding areas. Increased fat distribution will have an effect on girls' BMI and according to Kaplowitz et al. [52], girls with a higher BMI and fat percentage tend to be more advanced in their maturation status compared to girls with a lower BMI and fat percentage. As peak mass increases are concurrent with the onset of menarche, the BMI of pre-menarche girls' (who are still to reach peak mass increases) were not affected as much compared to the post-menarche groups' BMI. These changes could, therefore, be suggestive as possible explanations for the insignificant differences that were found in the speed and agility of girls of differing maturity levels where pre-menarche girls are still to be affected by mass increases, while post-menarche girls most probably have already adapted to peak mass increases.

Our results also showed signified interaction effects of differences in muscle strength between the pre- and post-menarche groups. A significant interaction effect was found in upper body strength (EUBS) ($p = 0.003$) with a marginally significant interaction effect in explosive leg strength (ELS) ($p = 0.069$) (Table 5), although group differences over time were insignificant for EUBS (F = 2.65; $p = 0.11$) and ELS (F = 0.02; $p = 0.87$). Differences in upper body strength during baseline measurements were also of statistical ($p = 0.01$) and large practical significance ($d = 0.80$), favoring post-menarche girls (Table 3). Post-menarche girls, furthermore, outperformed the pre-menarche group throughout the study, although the differences declined from T1 to T3, but remained practically significant (Table 3). With regard to explosive leg strength, post-menarche group also outperformed ($p > 0.05$, $d = 0.38$) the pre-menarche group although the pre-menarche group initially had an advantage in ELS ($p > 0.05$, $d = 0.26$). The results that still showed an increase in strength of post-menarche girls between 14.51 and 15.51 years in EUBS ($p > 0.05$) and ELS ($p < 0.05$), can possibly be ascribed to peak development of submaximal power output in girls that occurs more than a year after peak height velocity [11]. Therefore, due to a large percentage of our group who had already surpassed menarche and PHV, as PHV occurs approximately 12–24 months before menarche, the post-menarche group still had a slight strength advantage due to their advanced maturation. Furthermore, post-menarche girls, usually have broader shoulders because of earlier growth in body dimensions such as shoulder width [11], which may have aided them in producing more power to perform upper-body strength tests. To the contrary, peak mass increases take place between 12 and 14 years, congruent to the average age of menarche and, consequently, the pre-menarche group was most probably still affected by significant mass changes that result in fat deposits such as around the hips, which again moves the center of gravity point lower. As a result, they will have to displace more weight during upward jumping which in turn can affect performance in activities performed against gravitation negatively. The post-menarche girls might in turn, have most probably, already adapted to these body compositional changes.

Our results, furthermore, showed that the performance of the pre-menarche girls, in the different tests, based on the means that are reported during each year of measurement, was approximately two years behind that of the post-menarche group. In this regard, only small differences of 0.10 m (EUBS), 0.20 cm (ELS), 0.19 s (agility), 0.20 s (0–40 m speed) and 0.01 catches (HEC) were seen in the mean values of the pre-menarche group at T3 compared to the post-menarche girls' performance during T1 (Table 3). This coincides with findings reported by Malina and co-workers [11] that showed a two-year difference in the mean onset of menarche between early (11.8 years) and late (>13.8 years) maturing girls. Furthermore, the adolescent acceleration in muscle strength and muscle endurance, that are directly linked to motor abilities, takes an onset approximately 0.5–1 year after reaching PHV [6]. This link between the last-mentioned factor is the result of similar accelerations in morphological and biochemical determinants (the proportion of various muscle vessel types) [53]. Furthermore, in the course of maturation, a variety of biological and physiological structures in the body functions at a higher level [24] and consequently, individuals of the same chronological age, but differing maturity status, will differ in terms of physical- and motor performance [22,54]. In this regard, Freitas et al. [26] report that factors including neuromuscular maturation, specific instruction, practice and sport participation will also affect motor capabilities between the ages of 11 and 14 years and that skeletal maturity (skeletal age according to chronological age) explains only a maximum of 2.8% variance in motor capabilities in girls, after corrections for stature and body mass. The hand–eye coordination that was tested in the study is based on a skill, which might be affected by experience and training which might explain the inconsistent results that were found in this test.

Due to growth and maturation differences that were leveled-out by the end of the follow-up period at a mean age of 15.51 years, where no significant differences were evident between the groups, it can be concluded that the speed, agility and coordination and also strength of pre- and post-menarche girls can be considered to be nearly alike in girls of the same chronological age at 16 years. Differences between pre- and post-menarche groups decreased to almost similar values in 5 of the 6 motor fitness capabilities that were tested. Explosive leg strength differences, however, increased from T1–T3 (13.51–15.51 years) in favor of the post-menarche group although the difference was still insignificant. This could be due to a larger muscle mass in relation to total body mass. Furthermore, although it was not analyzed and reported, the post-menarche girls could have had a better, well-established ratio between sitting height and leg-length, possibly resulting in a more efficient weight distribution/center of gravity. Lastly, because of earlier maturation, post-menarche girls could have a higher functioning neurological system that contributes to improved coordination, which pre-menarche girls have not yet reached.

This study had limitations that need to be acknowledged. All participants were recruited from one school, which make the results mainly relevant to the study population and thereby limits the generalization of the findings. However, the school had hostel facilities which represented children enrolling from various different primary schools from the surrounding area. Our final sample size was small and also did not evenly represent different racial groups and results are mostly based on data of white (Caucasian) girls. A power calculation of the group sizes did show that medium effects can be observed from the results. The late developing group was, however, already limited in numbers at baseline that would have constrained the power and thereby limited us in dividing this group any further at later time points because some changed to full menarcheal status at T2 and T3 which might have added further understanding of differences. Changes in environmental conditions such as weather conditions (rain, hot conditions) over the 3-year period were out of the researchers' control and could have influenced the results. Although the data were collected over a longitudinal period of two years, which strengthens the results of the study, it has to be kept in mind that the study only incorporated secondary school learners and could subsequently only focused on a late age period in the development of girls which was between 13 and 16 years of age. It is acknowledged that a larger age period is needed to fully investigate the influences that are associated with changes in pubertal status. Although groups would have become too small for comparison purposes in the current study, it can be considered in future studies to only include girls who are the furthest in the menarche phase (post-menarche) group and those who are the furthest away from reaching menarche (pre-menarche), to make a more realistic comparison of early and late development differences. It is also advisable that influences of sport participation should also be taken into consideration in future analyses of this nature.

5. Conclusions

The findings of this study add to existing knowledge and provided more insight into the effect of biological and physiological changes that occur in girls before and after the onset of menarche, more specifically how these changes influence their motor fitness capabilities. The results confirm that, although there were differences in the motor capabilities of girls of differing maturity status, based on their menarche status during mid to late adolescence, these differences were only of statistical and practical significance in strength. Differences were, however, of small practical significance in agility and speed at the mean age of 13.51 years. Differences were also larger at a younger age (13.51 years) but declined with increased age. Performance in the motor tests of pre-menarche girls, were approximately two years behind that of the post-menarche girls. Based on these findings, it is concluded that the motor capabilities of girls, once they have reached menarche, will only be comparable with other girls of the same chronological age who have reached menarche earlier, 1–2 years later when the influences of puberty on their fitness performance can be considered to have been levelled-out. This knowledge can be incorporated by coaches into designing well-planned training programs, which again can aid in optimal skill development and reduce the risk of injury and drop-out. It can also contribute to improved sports development and talent identification processes, by providing more understanding of the temporary weaknesses in speed, agility and hand-eye coordination and gains in strength associated with early or late development and by applying this knowledge in appropriate short and long-term motor performance goals. Further research is, however, recommended that includes a longer developmental period, especially from a younger age. This will aid in obtaining a deeper and more complete understanding of growth differences between early and late developing girls and, consequently, the effect of differential growth on girls of different maturation's motor capability profiles. Our study should be seen as a pilot study that can serve as a reference study and it is suggested that the findings can be used for direction and new topics when studies of this nature is planned and conducted in the future.

Author Contributions: Conceptualization A.E.P. and A.K.; methodology A.E.P.; software, B.G., A.E.P. and A.K.; validation A.E.P. and A.K.; formal analysis B.G. and A.E.P.; investigation B.G., A.E.P. and A.K.; resources, B.G., A.E.P. and A.K.; data curation, B.G., A.E.P. and A.K.; writing—original draft preparation B.G.; writing—review and editing A.E.P. and A.K.; visualization B.G., A.E.P. and A.K.; supervision A.E.P. and A.K.; project administration A.E.P.; funding acquisition A.E.P. All authors have read and agreed to the published version of the manuscript.

Funding: This research was funded by The Department of Sport and Recreation in South-Africa (SRSA).

Institutional Review Board Statement: Based on approval by Health Research Ethics Committee (HREC), the North-West University Institutional Research Ethics Regulatory Committee (NWU-IRERC) hereby approves your project as indicated below. This implies that the NWU-IRERC grants its permission that, provided the special conditions specified below are met and pending any other authorization that may be necessary, the project may be initiated, using the ethics number NWU-00199-15-A1.

Informed Consent Statement: Informed consent was obtained from all subjects involved in the study.

Data Availability Statement: The dataset is the property of the North-West University under supervision of Prof Anita E Pienaar. In this regard, Prof. AE Pienaar should be contacted if, for any reason, the data included in this paper needs to be shared.

Acknowledgments: All post-graduate students specializing in Kinderkinetics and Sport Science are also thanked for their assistance during the collection of the data.

Conflicts of Interest: The authors declare no conflict of interest. The funders had no role in the design of the study; in the collection, analyses, or interpretation of data; in the writing of the manuscript, or in the decision to publish the results.

References

1. Global Burden of Disease Study 2013 Collaborators. Global, regional, and national incidence, prevalence, and years lived with disability for 301 acute and chronic diseases and injuries in 188 countries, 1990–2013: A systematic analysis for the Global Burden of Disease Study, 2013. *Lancet* **2015**, *386*, 743–800.
2. Mendelsohn, M.E.; Karas, R.H. Molecular and cellular basis of cardiovascular gender differences. *Science* **2005**, *308*, 1583–1587. [CrossRef]
3. Osiński, W. Relation between motor abilities and body features and components in children and adolescents from metropolitan populations. *Phys. Educ. Sport* **1988**, *4*, 11–27.
4. Saczuk, J.; Popławska, H.; Wilczewski, A. Biological age and the physical fitness of girls and boys. *Phys. Educ. Sport* **1999**, *1*, 3–18.
5. Gill, D.; Sheehan, N.A.; Wielscher, M.; Shrine, N.; Amaral, A.F.S.; Thompson, J.R.; Granell, R.; Leynaert, B.; Real, F.G.; Hall, I.P.; et al. Age at menarche and lung function: A Mendelian randomization study. *Eur. J. Epidemiol.* **2017**, *32*, 701–710. [CrossRef] [PubMed]
6. Gill, D.; Brewer, C.F.; Del Greco, M.F.; Sivakumaran, P.; Bowden, J.; Sheehan, N.A.; Minelli, C. Age at menarche and adult body mass index: A Mendelian randomization study. *Int. J. Obes.* **2018**, *42*, 1574–1581. [CrossRef] [PubMed]
7. Pierce, M.B.; Leon, D.A. Age at menarche and adult BMI in the Aberdeen children of the 1950s cohort study. *Am. J. Clin. Nutr.* **2005**, *82*, 733–739. [CrossRef]
8. He, C.; Zhang, C.; Hunter, D.J.; Hankinson, S.E.; Louis, G.M.B.; Hediger, M.L.; Hu, F.B. Age at Menarche and Risk of Type 2 Diabetes: Results From 2 Large Prospective Cohort Studies. *Am. J. Epidemiol.* **2009**, *171*, 334–344. [CrossRef]
9. Remsberg, K.E.; Demerath, E.W.; Schubert, C.M.; Chumlea, W.C.; Sun, S.S.; Siervogel, R.M. Early menarche and the development of cardiovascular disease risk factors in adolescent girls: The fels longitudinal study. *J. Clin. Endocrinol. Metab.* **2005**, *90*, 2718–2724. [CrossRef] [PubMed]
10. Balyi, I.; Way, R. *Canadian Sports for Life: The Role of Monitoring Growth in Long-Term Athlete Development*; Canadian Sports Centre: Calgary, AB, Canada, 2010.
11. Malina, R.M.; Bouchard, C.; Bar-Or, O. *Growth, Maturation and Physical Activity*; Human Kinetics: Champaign, IL, USA, 2004; 712p.
12. Gluckman, P.D.; Handson, M.A. Evolution, development and timing of puberty. *Trends Endocr. Meta* **2006**, *17*, 7–12. [CrossRef] [PubMed]
13. Biro, F.M.; Pajak, A.; Wolff, M.S.; Pinney, S.M.; Windham, G.C.; Galvez, M.P.; Greenspan, L.C.; Kushi, L.H.; Teitelbaum, S. Age of menarche in a longitudinal US cohort. *J. Pediatr. Adolesc. Gynecol.* **2018**, *31*, 339–345. [CrossRef] [PubMed]
14. Karapanou, O.; Papadimitriou, A. Determinants of menarche. *Reprod. Biol. Endocrinol.* **2010**, *8*, 115–122. [CrossRef]

15. Kaprio, J.; Rimpelä, A.; Winter, T.; Viken, R.J.; Rimpelä, M.; Rose, M.J. Common genetic influences on BMI and age at menarche. *Hum. Biol.* **1995**, *67*, 739–753. [PubMed]
16. Salces, I.; Rebato, E.M.; Susanne, C.; San Martin, L.; Rosique, J. Familial resemblance for the age at menarche in Basque population. *An. Hum. Biol.* **2001**, *28*, 143–156.
17. Reka, S.; Samraj, P. Differences between menstrual cycle phases on selected motor fitness components among college women kho-kho players. *IJPESH* **2018**, *5*, 76–77.
18. Do Bonfim, B.M.A.; Bonuzzi, G.M.G.; Domingues, V.L.; Reiser, F.C. The influence of maturational and morphological status pre- and post-menarche on the 100-m freestyle swimming performance of competitive teenagers. *Motriz Rio Claro* **2020**, *26*, 1–6.
19. Erlandson, M.C.; Sherar, L.B.; Mirwald, R.L.; Maffulli, N.; Baxter-Jones, A.D.G. Growth and Maturation of Adolescent Female Gymnasts, Swimmers, and Tennis Players. *Med. Sci. Sport Exerc.* **2008**, *40*, 34–42. [CrossRef] [PubMed]
20. Bronikowski, M.; Bronikowska, M. Motor fitness in relation to the maturational process of pubertal boys and girls. *Pap. Anthropol.* **2008**, *7*, 28–37.
21. Baquet, C.; Twisk, J.W.R.; Kemper, E.; van Praagh, E.; Berthoin, S. Longitudinal follow-up of fitness during childhood: Interaction with physical activity. *Am. J. Hum. Biol.* **2006**, *18*, 51–58. [CrossRef]
22. Van Den Berg, L.; Coetzee, B.; Pienaar, A.E. The influence of biological maturity on physical and motor performance talent identification determinants of u-14 provincial girl tennis players. *Afr. J. Phys. Health Educ. Recreat. Dance* **2006**, *18*, 510–515.
23. Des te Croix, M. Advances in paediatric strength assessment: Changing our perspective on strength development. *J. Sports Sci. Med.* **2007**, *6*, 292–304.
24. Pienaar, A.E. *Motor Development, Growth, Motor Assessment and the Intervention Thereof: A Textbook for Students in Kinderkinetics*, 10th ed.; Ivyline Printers: Potchefstroom, South Africa, 2018; 682p.
25. Anderson, S. *Collins English Dictionary: Complete & Unabridged*, 10th ed.; Harper Collins: London, UK, 2009; 2336p.
26. Freitas, D.L.; Lausen, B.; Maia, J.A.; Lefevre, J.; Gouveia, E.R.; Thomis, M.; Malina, R.M. Skeletal maturation, fundamental motor capabilities and motor coordination in children 7–10 years. *J. Sports Sci.* **2015**, *33*, 924–934. [CrossRef]
27. Van Gent, M.M. Anthropometrical, Physical and Motor Fitness Characteristics of 10- to 15-Year Old Girls in the Northwest Province. Master's Thesis, NWU, Potchefstroom, South Africa, 2001.
28. Rodrıguez, G.; Moreno, L.A.; Blay, M.G.; Blay, V.A.; Garagorri, J.M.; Sarrı, A.; Bueno, M. Body composition in adolescents: Measurements and metabolic aspects. *Int. J. Obes.* **2004**, *28*, S54–S58. [CrossRef]
29. Garnier, D.; Simondon, K.B.; Benefice, E. Longitudinal estimates of pubertal timing in Senegalese adolescent girls. *Am. J. Hum. Biol.* **2005**, *17*, 718–730. [CrossRef]
30. Fredriks, A.M.; van Buuren, S.; van Heel, W.J.M.; Dijkman-Neerincx, R.H.M.; Verloove, S.P.; Wit, J.M. Nationwide age reference for sitting height, leg length, and sitting height/height ratio, and their diagnostic value for disproportionate growth disorders. *Arch. Dis. Child.* **2005**, *90*, 807–812. [CrossRef]
31. Deborah, C.; Russel, V. ABC of adolescence: Adolescent development. *BMJ* **2005**, *330*, 301–304.
32. Beunen, G.P.; Ostyn, M.; Simons, J.; Renson, R.; Claessens, A.; Eynde, V.; Van't Hof, M.A. Development and tracking in fitness components: Leuven longtudinal study on lifestyle, fitness and health. *Int. J. Sport Med.* **1997**, *18*, S171–S178. [CrossRef]
33. Prahl-Anderson, B.; Kowalski, C.J.; Heydendael, P. *A Mix Longitudinal Interdisciplinary Study of Growth and Development*; Academic Press: New York, NY, USA, 1994.
34. Kemper, H.C.G.; Snel, J.; van Mechelen, W. Amsterdam growth and health longitudinal study. *J. Sci. Med. Sport* **2004**, *47*, 1–198.
35. Lee, T.S.; Chao, T.; Tang, R.B.; Hsieh, C.C.; Chen, S.J.; Ho, L.T. A longitudinal study of growth in schoolchildren in one Taipei district II: Sitting height, arm span, body mass index and skinfold thickness. *Chin. Med. J.* **2005**, *68*, 16–20. [CrossRef]
36. Volver, A.; Viru, A.; Viru, M. A two-year longitudinal study of sexual maturation effects on motor abilities of girls. *Med. Della Sport.* **2007**, *60*, 57–63.
37. Henneberg, M.; Louw, G.J. Average menarcheal age of higher socioeconomic status urban Cape coloured girls assessed by means of status quo and recall methods. *Am. J. Phys. Anthropol.* **1995**, *96*, 1–5. [CrossRef] [PubMed]
38. Travill, A.L. Growth and physical fitness of socially disadvantage boys and girls aged 8–17 years living in the Western Cape, South Africa. *Afr. J. Phys. Health Educ. Recreat. Dance* **2007**, *13*, 279–293.
39. Monyeki, K.D.; Koppes, L.L.J.; Kemper, H.C.G.; Monyeki, K.D.; Toriola, A.L.; E Pienaar, A.; Twisk, J.W.R. Body composition and physical fitness of undernourished South African rural primary school children. *Eur. J. Clin. Nutr.* **2006**, *59*, 877–883. [CrossRef]
40. Richter, L.; Norris, S.; Yack, D.; Cameron, N. Cohort profile: Mandela's children. The 1990 birth to twenty study in South Africa. *Int. J. Epidemiol.* **2007**, *36*, 504–511. [CrossRef] [PubMed]
41. Durand-Bush, N.; Salmela, J.H. The development and maintenance of expert athletic performance: Perceptions of world and Olympic champions. *J. Appl. Sport Psychol.* **2002**, *14*, 154–171. [CrossRef]
42. Little, N.G.; Day, J.A.P.; Steinke, L. Relationship of physical performance to maturation in perimenarchal girls. *Am. J. Hum. Biol.* **1997**, *9*, 163–171. [CrossRef]
43. Wang, Z.; Dang, S.; Yuan, X.; Li, Q.; Hong, Y. Correlation of body mass index levels with menarche in adolescent girls in Shaanxi, China: A cross sectional study. *BMC Women's Health* **2016**, *16*, 61. [CrossRef]
44. Australian Sport Commission. *Sport Search Program*; ASC: Canberra, NSW, Australia, 1996.
45. Gerber, B.P.; Pienaar, A.E.; Kruger, A. Interrelations between anthropometric and fitness changes during mid-adolescence in boys: A 2-year longitudinal study. *Am. J. Hum. Biol.* **2014**, *26*, 617–626. [CrossRef]

46. Steward, A.D.; Marfell-Jones, M.; Olds, T.; de Ridder, H. *International Standards for Anthropometric Assessment*; International Society for Advancement of Kinanthropometry (ISAK): Potchefstroom, South Africa, 2011.
47. Statsoft. *Statistica for Windows: General Conventions and Statistics*; Statsoft: Tulsa, OK, USA, 2017.
48. Cohen, J.A. Power primer. *Psychol. Bull.* **1992**, *112*, 155–159. [CrossRef]
49. Pauole, K.; Madole, K.; Garhammer, J.; Lacourse, M.; Rozenek, R. Reliability and validity of the t-test as a measure of agility, leg power, and leg speed in college-aged men and women. *J. Strength Cond. Res.* **2000**, *14*, 443–450.
50. Aberberga-Augskalne, L.; Kemper, H.C.G. Longitudinal relationship between cardiovascular functioning and peak height velocity during exercise in 7- to 16-year-old boys and girls. *Hum. Mov. Sci.* **2007**, *8*, 5–11.
51. Rogol, D.R.; Roemmich, J.N.; Clark, P.A. Growth at Puberty. *J. Adolesc. Health* **2002**, *31*, 192–200. [CrossRef]
52. Kaplowitz, P.B.; Slora, E.J.; Wasserman, R.C.; Pedlow, S.E.; Herman-Giddens, M.E. Earlier onset of puberty in girls: Relation to increased body mass index and race. *Paediatrics* **2001**, *108*, 347–353. [CrossRef] [PubMed]
53. Little, T.; Williams, A.G. Specificity of acceleration, maximum speed, and agility in professional soccer players. *J. Strength Cond. Res.* **2005**, *19*, 76–78.
54. Davis, B.; Bull, R.; Roscoe, J.; Roscoe, D. *Physical Education and the Study of Sport*, 3rd ed.; Mosby: London, UK, 1997.

International Journal of
Environmental Research and Public Health

MDPI

Article

Moderate Exercise Combined with Enriched Environment Enhances Learning and Memory through BDNF/TrkB Signaling Pathway in Rats

Liyuan Xu, Linna Zhu, Lina Zhu, Dandan Chen, Kelong Cai, Zhimei Liu and Aiguo Chen *

College of Physical Education, Yangzhou University, Yangzhou 225127, China; MX120180363@yzu.edu.cn (L.X.); MX120180361@yzu.edu.cn (L.Z.); zhulina827@mail.bnu.edu.cn (L.Z.); DX120200078@yzu.edu.cn (D.C.); MX120170353@yzu.edu.cn (K.C.); DX120200076@yzu.edu.cn (Z.L.)
* Correspondence: agchen@yzu.edu.cn; Tel.: +86-139-5272-5968

Abstract: This study aimed to investigate the effects and potential mechanisms of exercise combined with an enriched environment on learning and memory in rats. Forty healthy male Wistar rats (7 weeks old) were randomly assigned into 4 groups ($N = 10$ in each group): control (C) group, treadmill exercise (TE) group, enriched environment (EE) group and the TE + EE group. The Morris water maze (MWM) test was used to evaluate the learning and memory ability in all rats after eight weeks of exposure in the different conditions. Moreover, we employed enzyme-linked immunosorbent assay (ELISA) to determine the expression of brain-derived neurotrophic factor (BDNF) and receptor tyrosine kinase B (TrkB) in the rats. The data showed that the escape latency and the number of platform crossings were significantly better in the TE + EE group compared to the TE, EE or C groups ($p < 0.05$). In addition, there was upregulation of BDNF and TrkB in rats in the TE + EE group compared to those in the TE, EE or C groups ($p < 0.05$). Taken together, the data robustly demonstrate that the combination of TE + EE enhances learning and memory ability and upregulates the expression of both BDNF and TrkB in rats. Thus, the BDNF/TrkB signaling pathway might be modulating the effect of exercise and enriched environment in improving learning and memory ability in rats.

Keywords: combined intervention; exercise; enriched environment; learning and memory ability; BDNF/TrkB signaling pathway

Citation: Xu, L.; Zhu, L.; Zhu, L.; Chen, D.; Cai, K.; Liu, Z.; Chen, A. Moderate Exercise Combined with Enriched Environment Enhances Learning and Memory through BDNF/TrkB Signaling Pathway in Rats. *Int. J. Environ. Res. Public Health* **2021**, *18*, 8283. https://doi.org/10.3390/ijerph18168283

Academic Editor: Shaher A. I. Shalfawi

Received: 28 May 2021
Accepted: 28 July 2021
Published: 5 August 2021

1. Introduction

Learning and memory are fundamental features in the development and survival of humans and animals. Besides being critical for higher-order brain functions, they are intimately associated with behavioral and psychological consequences. Previous studies have associated the brain-derived neurotrophic factor (BDNF) signaling pathway with learning and memory [1]. BDNF exerts widespread effects throughout the central nervous system, thus mediating critical processes in learning and memory [2]. Furthermore, other reports have demonstrated a correlation between central and peripheral BDNF in rats and other animals as well as its ability to cross the blood–brain barrier [3–5]. Therefore, the peripheral BDNF might be a biomarker for learning and memory functions. BDNF binds to its specific receptor tyrosine kinase B (TrkB) to promote learning and memory performance and participates in the growth, differentiation and repair of neurons [6]. For instance, exogenous introduction of BDNF and its receptor TrkB agonist was shown to prevent stress-induced spatial memory deficits [7,8]. Understanding the role of the BDNF/TrkB signaling pathway in mediating learning and memory development remains of immense research interest. An increasing body of evidence from in vivo experiments has shown that enriched environment, physical exercise, learning experiences or social interactions induce changes in the BDNF/TrkB signaling pathway, resulting in learning and memory shifts.

The effects of physical exercise on memory retention and learning have been demonstrated both in animal models and humans [9–11]. Other studies have demonstrated the neuroprotective effect of regular physical exercise in improving learning and memory in healthy individuals [12,13]. Moreover, recent studies have associated exercise with an increased release of BDNF and TrkB, which are delivered to the brain and might play a role in learning and memory [14,15]. On the other hand, whereas regular physical activity benefits learning and memory over the whole life course, the benefits are dependent on aspects of physical exercise plans such as speed, time or slope [16–18]. For instance, moderate treadmill exercise was shown to positively modulate the concentrations of BDNF and its TrkB receptor in experimental animals [19,20]. Therefore, the different exercise intensities have different effects on learning and memory as well as BDNF/TrkB signaling activities. Thus, exercise dosage appears to be an important factor in the achievement of enhanced cognitive capabilities.

On the other hand, an enriched environment entails a combination of complex inanimate and social stimulations [21]. An enriched environment consists of physical exercise, novel stimulants and social interactions [22]. Previous findings showed that learning and memory impairment can be attenuated by a relatively short (a few weeks) exposure to environmental conditions; provision of sensory, exercise or cognitive stimulations; as well as sustained social interactions in rodents [23]. In addition, BDNF and TrkB have been shown to be upregulated in the brain in animals maintained in an enriched environment compared to those in impoverished conditions (isolation, no stimulation for physical or learning experiences) [24]. Moreover, an enriched environment could improve learning and memory, and the up-regulation of BDNF/TrkB is considered to be an important pathway in the improved features. One clear difference between treadmill exercise and voluntary exercise in the enriched environment is the ability to quantify the exercise plans for animals undergoing treadmill exercise. On the contrary, the amount of voluntary exercise in the enriched environment cannot be controlled [25].

Previous studies have demonstrated that either the enriched environment or exercise could be promising strategies in enhancing learning and memory as well as upregulation of the BDNF/TrkB signaling pathway, thus highlighting their therapeutic potential [26–28]. It has been shown that, compared to a single intervention, combined exercise and enriched environment interventions yield better effects in healthy animals [29–32]. However, data on the effect of forced exercise combined with voluntary exercise in an enriched environment remains scant. Besides, previous research on learning and memory and the BDNF/TrkB signaling pathway has focused on the effectiveness of a single intervention. Here, we evaluated the effect of a combination of exercise and enriched environment interventions on learning and memory ability, as well profiling the expression of the BDNF/TrkB signaling pathway in healthy Wistar rats. Based on the above research, we put forward the following hypothesis that the combination of treadmill exercise and enriched environment enhances the learning and memory ability by upregulating the concentrations of BDNF/TrkB in rats.

2. Experimental Procedures

2.1. Animals

Male Wistar rats (6 weeks old), purchased from Laboratory Animal Center (Yangzhou University) [certificate: SCXK (SU) 2017-0007], were used in this study. The study was approved by the Institutional Animal Care and Use Committee and Ethical Committee of Yangzhou University. Initially, the rats were housed in standard cages 46 × 30 × 16 cm (L × W × H), 5 per cage for 7 days. On day 8, 40 healthy rats were pulled together and then placed in the same environment, to allow random grouping. Then, all rats were randomly selected and assigned by an independent technician as follows: each rat was randomly picked up from the cage and assigned to the control (C) group, the treadmill exercise (TE) group, the enriched environment (EE) group and the treadmill exercise combined with enriched environment (TE + EE) group in sequence, and the assignment was repeated until all groups reached the designated number of animals ($N = 10$ in each group). In order to reduce the treadmill exercise stress, the rats in TE and TE + EE groups were allowed to adapt to treadmill exercise for one week period prior to the commencement of the experiments. The experimental protocol consisted of 40 min of daily exercise for 6 days and rest for 1 day. The rats were housed in groups in a controlled room (temperature 23 ± 2 °C; 12 h light/12 h dark cycle, light on at 6 PM and off at 6 AM). Except for the C and the TE groups, food and water were delivered from both sides of the cage. Sawdust bedding (SPF) was provided at approximately 2 cm depth. The rats were 8 weeks of age at the onset of the experiments.

2.2. Groups

2.2.1. Control Group

Five animals per cage were housed in standard cages as a control group. The cages had bedding, regular rate chow and plain boiled water (Figure 1).

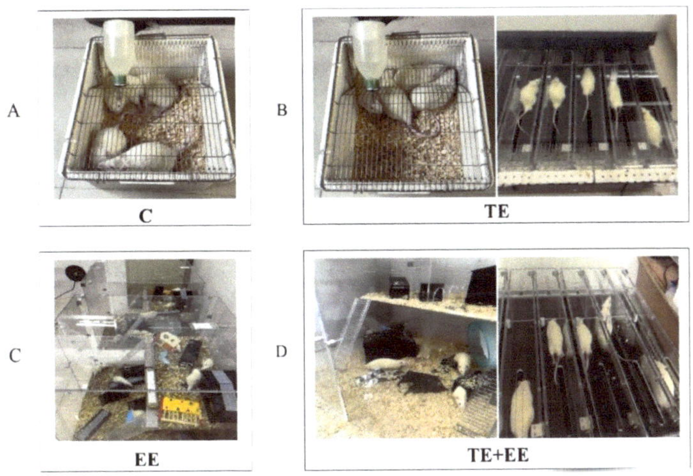

Figure 1. Study groups: (**A**) Control (C); (**B**) Treadmill Exercise (TE); (**C**) Enriched Environment (EE); (**D**) Treadmill Exercise Combined with Enriched Environment (TE + EE).

2.2.2. Treadmill Exercise

The rats were familiarized with the treadmill to eliminate any exercise-related stress. The rats were adapted to a running treadmill for 40 min daily for 6 days (running at a speed of 5 m/min for the 1st and 2nd days, 10 m/min for the 3rd and 4th days, and 20 m/min for the 5th and 6th days, with 0° inclination.).

As indicated, exercise-induced benefits are dependent on various quantifiable plans of physical exercise such speed, time and slope. We performed regular moderate exercise with newfangled dynamics and exercise load standards as previously described (Bedford et al.).

Eight-week-old rats were then forced to run on a treadmill, with the 0° inclination, at a speed of 20 m/min for 40 min daily, 6 days a week, for 8 consecutive weeks [33].

2.2.3. Enriched Environment

The rats in the EE group were housed for a whole day and then divided into 2 cages (83 × 83 × 83 cm) in order to promote social interaction. Each cage had two floors connected by ramps to promote physical exercise and movement. Various elements of different shapes and textures such as balls, stairs, cubes, tunnels, swings and wheels were placed in the cages and were available to the animals for the 8 weeks of the experiment. The objects in each cage were rotated once a week to stimulate sensory, motor and cognitive functions.

2.2.4. Treadmill Exercise Combined with Enriched Environment

Like in the TE or EE group, one dimension of the intervention contained the treadmill while the other contained toys and food treats. Prior to the intervention, the rats underwent the same adaptive exercise as described in the TE group for 1 week. After 40 min on the treadmill exercise, the rats were kept in the enriched environment for the rest of the day.

2.3. Experimental Design

The rats in each group underwent the experimental protocols for 8 weeks (N = 10 per group). Thereafter, the animals were allowed to acclimatize to the laboratory environment for one day. 6-day Morris water maze (MWM) tests were employed to assess the learning and memory functions in the rats. Testing took place during the light phase of the light/dark cycle and the animals were immediately returned to cages after the tests. To prevent the 6-day MWM test from affecting the intervention effects, all rats were given the intervention for four extra days [34]. On the fifth day, the rats were anaesthetized with urethane and then blood was collected from the abdominal aorta and snap frozen (−80 °C) for further biochemical analysis.

2.4. Morris Water Maze

The Morris water maze (MWM) consisted of a circular galvanized steel pool (diameter = 120 cm; wall height = 50 cm), filled with water at 23 ± 1 °C. A small round escape platform (12 cm diameter) was fixed at the center of one quadrant, 2 cm beneath the water surface. The learning phase consisted of five training days, which randomly started at four different positions. We conducted four trials daily. The rats were placed into the pool facing the maze wall at fixed entry points. In case a rat could not find the platform within 120 s, the experimenter guided the rat to the platform [35]. The rat was then allowed to stay on the platform for 10s to memorize the location [36]. The water maze was surrounded by fixed clues. Moreover, the experimental room was kept invariable during the MWM testing [37]. We recorded the duration the rats spent searching for the platform in each quadrant, with an average of escape latency in the four quadrants as the final escape latency. On the sixth day, the platform was removed, and rats were placed in water to swim with a limitation of 60 s. We then recorded the number of times the rats crossed the exact place containing the submerged platform in each quadrant, with the average number of platform crossings in the four quadrants considered the probe trial of the day. Images of swimming rats were captured by a video camera placed above the center of the pool, which was connected to a computer system running specialized tracking software (ANY-maze, Stoelting Co., Wood Dale, IL, USA).

2.5. ELISA for Plasma BDNF and TrkB

Using the enzyme-linked immunosorbent assay (ELISA), we quantified the concentrations of BDNF and TrkB in the plasma of the rats, following the manufacturer's instructions (Shanghai Enzyme-linked Biotechnology Co., Ltd, Shanghai, China). Dispensed antigen standards and samples were added to each well in the 96-well plates, precoated with primary antibodies. After the addition of biotin and enzyme conjugate reagents into the wells, the plates were incubated at 37 °C for 60 min. We then washed the plates five times in distilled water. Within 15 min of chromogenic reaction, the absorbance was read at 450 nm using a microplate reader (Nano Drop ND-1000, Waltham, MA, USA).

2.6. Statistical Analysis

Data were analyzed using JAMOVI (version 1.6.1) statistical software. A $p < 0.05$ was considered statistically significant. For the MWM test acquisition, the average escape latency time(s) to reach the platform per day was analyzed by repeated measure analysis with days as the within-subjects factor and treatment (C, TE, EE, TE + EE) as the between-subjects factor. The Tukey post-hoc tests were used to evaluate pair-wise differences between the group means. For the probe trial, the number of platform crossings was analyzed using a two-way ANOVA with exercise factors (running versus not running) and enrichment (enriched versus not enriched); data were not corrected. In addition, we used the post-hoc tests to evaluate pair-wise differences between the group means. The BDNF and TrkB concentrations were analyzed using a two-way ANOVA using exercise factors (exercise versus not exercise) and enriched environment (enriched versus non enriched environment); data were not corrected. Furthermore, we used post-hoc tests to evaluate pair-wise differences between the group means.

3. Results

3.1. Behavioral Performance: The Morris Water Maze (MWM)

The escape latency data showed that the time effect [F (4,144) = 68.77, $p < 0.001$, partial $\eta^2 = 0.66$] and the group effect [F (3,36) = 103, $p < 0.001$, partial $\eta^2 = 0.90$] were statistically significant, but the time × group interaction effect [F (12,144) = 1.69, $p > 0.05$, partial $\eta^2 = 0.12$] was not statistically significant. In addition, the escape latency of each group decreased with the increase in days. Further analysis showed that the TE, EE and TE + EE groups' escape latency were better compared to that of the C group ($p < 0.001$) while that of the TE + EE group was better than that of the EE or C groups ($p < 0.001$) (Figure 2).

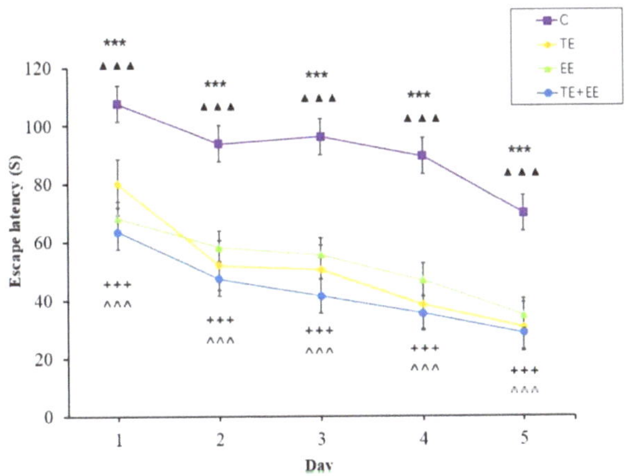

Figure 2. Average escape latency in the Control (C), Treadmill Exercise (TE), Enriched Environment (EE) and Treadmill Exercise Combined with Enriched Environment (TE + EE) groups ($N = 10$, $\overline{x} \pm s$). Note: EE group versus C group, *** $p < 0.001$; TE group versus C group, ▲▲▲ $p < 0.001$; TE + EE group versus C group, + + + $p < 0.001$; TE + EE group versus EE group, ^^^ $p < 0.001$.

Data from the number of platform crossings showed a statistically significant difference between the exercise effect [F (1,36) = 56.90, $p < 0.001$, partial $\eta^2 = 0.61$], the enriched environment effect [F (1,36) = 47.80, $p < 0.001$, partial $\eta^2 = 0.57$] and the interaction effect of the exercise × enriched environment [F (1,36) = 11.20, $p < 0.01$, partial $\eta^2 = 0.24$] in the probe trail of the rats. Further post-hoc analysis showed that the rats in the TE + EE, TE, or EE groups had a significantly increased number of platform crossings compared with those in the C group ($p < 0.001$). Unlike between the TE and EE groups, the number of platform crossings of the rats in the TE + EE group was significantly higher than those in the TE or EE groups ($p < 0.05$) (Figure 3).

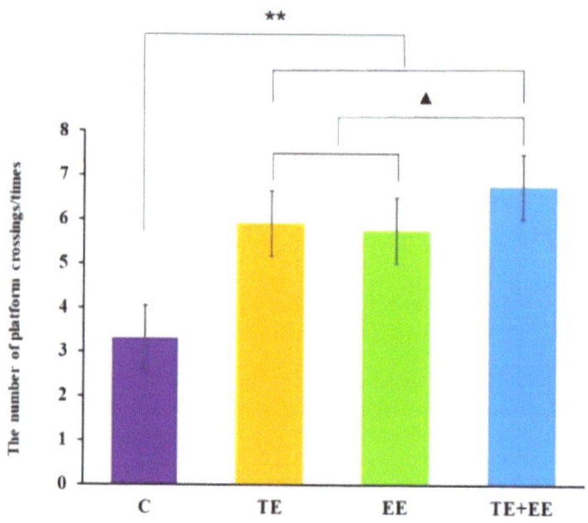

Figure 3. Average number of platform crossings in the Control (C), Treadmill Exercise (TE), Enriched Environment (EE) and Treadmill Exercise Combined with Enriched Environment (TE + EE) groups ($N = 10$, $\bar{x} \pm s$). Note: compared with the C group, ** $p < 0.01$; compared with TE + EE group, ▲ $p < 0.05$.

3.2. BDNF and TrkB in Plasma

To define the mechanism of learning and memory in rats exposed to the combination of exercise and an enriched environment, we interrogated the expression profile of the BDNF and TrkB in the rats' plasma.

Our data demonstrated that there was a significant difference between the exercise effect [F (1,36) = 28.95, $p < 0.01$, partial $\eta^2 = 0.45$] and the enriched environment effect [F (1,36) = 27.02, $p < 0.01$, partial $\eta^2 = 0.43$] as well as the interaction effect [F (1,36) = 5.03, $p < 0.05$, partial $\eta^2 = 0.12$] in the expression of BDNF in the rats. Post-hoc analysis showed that the BDNF concentration was significantly increased in the TE + EE, TE or EE groups compared with those in the C group ($p < 0.01$). In addition, the BDNF concentration in the TE + EE group was significantly higher than that in the TE or EE groups ($p < 0.05$). On the contrary, there was no statistically significant difference in the BDNF concentration between the TE and EE groups ($p > 0.05$).

Similarly, the data showed a significant difference between the exercise effect [F (1,36) = 53.44, $p < 0.01$, partial $\eta^2 = 0.60$] and the enriched environment effect [F (1,36) = 27.88, $p < 0.01$, partial $\eta^2 = 0.44$] as well as the interaction effect [F (1,36) = 4.99, $p < 0.05$, partial $\eta^2 = 0.12$] in the expression of TrkB in the rats. Post-hoc analysis showed that the TrkB concentration was significantly upregulated in the TE + EE, TE or EE groups compared with those in the C group ($p < 0.01$). Moreover, the TrkB concentration in the TE + EE group was significantly higher than that in the TE or EE groups ($p < 0.05$). There was, however, no statistically significant difference in the TrkB concentration between the TE and EE groups ($p > 0.05$) (Table 1).

Table 1. Comparison of the plasma concentrations of BDNF and TrkB in the groups ($\bar{x} \pm s$).

Group	N	BDNF	TrkB
C	10	492.22 ± 77.03	1538.34 ± 133.86
TE	10	707.19 ± 63.63 **▲	2049.94 ± 122.38 **▲
EE	10	702.05 ± 106.30 **▲	1941.09 ± 239.68 **▲
TE + EE	10	790.49 ± 102.57 **	2213.22 ± 156.81 **

Note: compared with the C group, ** $p < 0.01$; compared with TE + EE group, ▲ $p < 0.05$. Study groups: Control (C); Treadmill Exercise (TE); Enriched Environment (EE); Treadmill Exercise Combined with Enriched Environment (TE + EE).

4. Discussion

This study investigated the effects and mechanisms of moderate exercise combined with an enriched environment on learning and memory in rats. We further interrogated the role of the BDNF/TrkB signaling pathway in mediating learning and memory effects in rats. Our data demonstrate that exercise, enriched environment or exercise combined with an enriched environment intervention improves the learning and memory ability in rats and the effect is mediated by BDNF/TrkB. Interestingly, exercise combined with the enriched environment conferred the best effect.

Our study showed that exercise could improve learning and memory ability and increase the expression of BDNF and TrkB in rats. Our findings are consistent with previous data which used exercise intervention methods alone in rats. Many studies have shown that moderate treadmill exercise has a positive effect on learning and memory. However, the intensity of the exercise determines the optimal learning and memory effects [38,39]. Control of the frequency, duration and intensity of exercise, which are essential aspects in evaluating the beneficial effects of exercise, is more feasible with treadmill exercise, while moderate-intensity running (speed up to 21 m/min) positively affects information acquisition, learning and memory [40,41]. In our study, we used treadmill workouts with defined parameters (such as intensity, duration and cycle). This would explain the fact that the escape latency of the rats in the TE group was lower than that of the C group. In addition, recent data have demonstrated a positive correlation between BDNF expression and different types of physical exercises [42–46]. Similarly, exercise-induced elevation of brain BDNF was reported to be intensity-dependent [47,48]. Moreover, the upregulation of BDNF expression might also be dependent on the duration and frequency of exercise [49–51]. This phenomenon has been shown to not only be beneficial to the peripheral nervous system, but also to the central nervous system [52].

We demonstrated that the rats in the EE group exhibited significantly improved learning and memory as well as upregulation in the BDNF/TrkB pathway. Novel stimulants, social interactions and physical exercise are components of the enriched environment. Our study used novel objects, and their rearrangement triggered fresh exploration of the enriched environment by the EE and TE + EE rats. Furthermore, compared with the standard squirrel cage, the enriched environment box had more companions and doorways for communication. Thus, it is possible that the effects of an enriched environment are a function of interaction with the cage mates [53]. In addition, physical exercise has been proposed as a critical component of an enriched environment. However, there is a difference between voluntary exercise in an enriched environment and treadmill exercise. Unlike in a previous study, our findings showed that there was no difference in the learning and memory of rats in the TE and EE groups [54]. This was probably because there was no autonomous runner in the enriched environment. In our study, the two layers of rats in the enriched environment were connected by ramps and contained autonomous runners, which obviously promoted their exercise. In addition, the enriched environment has been shown to increase brain and blood BDNF concentration [55–57]. Previous studies reported that BDNF signaling is closely associated with learning and memory functions. The acquisition of learning and memory is accompanied by an increase in the BDNF gene expression in specific brain regions. Blocking the effect of BDNF would lead to declined learning and memory abilities. An appealing feature in the use of BDNF as an indicator for effective enrichment is the correlation between the blood and brain BDNF concentrations, as BDNF can cross the blood–brain barrier [58,59]. Hence, blood-based measures of BDNF have been used as a proxy for brain BDNF [60], allowing for a less invasive assessment of brain changes. BDNF through TrkB receptors contributes to the proliferation, survival and differentiation of neurons in the hippocampus and other brain regions closely related to learning and memory, as well as promoting the induction of long-term potentiation and improving the ability of learning and memory in experimental animals [61]. Long-term potentiation in the hippocampus is an activity-dependent modification of synaptic strength and is considered a potential cellular mechanism underlying learning and memory. Our study demonstrated that the rats housed in total exercise and enriched environment conditions had changes in behavioral and physiological outcomes.

To improve the effectiveness of a single intervention method, the combination of two effective behavioral strategies, such as exercise combined with an enriched environment, presents a feasible alternative. Our analysis showed that exercise combined with an enriched environment intervention has a significant effect in improving the learning and memory ability as well as the expression of the BDNF/TrkB signaling pathway in rats. Compared with a single intervention method, exercise combined with a rich environment confers superior effects on improving the learning and memory of rats. In agreement, Wang Chaolei et al. showed that an enriched environment intervention was slightly better than a swimming intervention, while swimming combined with rich environmental intervention was slightly better than enriched environment or swimming interventions [62]. On the other hand, previous studies have assessed the molecular mechanisms involved in the regulation of the BDNF/TrkB signaling pathway. For instance, Du Mingyang et al. showed that memantine and enriched environment therapy could effectively improve the learning and memory abilities in rapidly aging mice. Moreover, it increases the expression of BDNF and TrkB in the hippocampus [63]. Nasroallah Moradi Kor showed that combined enrichment of spirulina or combined exercise of spirulina has a synergistic effect on the hippocampal BDNF levels and dendritic morphology [64].

A number of limitations need to be noted regarding the present study. Firstly, our study only included male rats and could not be duplicated in female rats. It is reported that estrogen might affect the behavior of female rats [65,66]. Secondly, we only included healthy rats. It is possible that these results might not be applicable to other groups with cognitive dysfunctional model rats. Future studies need to assess cognitive ability after intervention in impaired models to provide early treatment strategies. Lastly, although our data robustly demonstrates that 8-week treadmill exercise can improve the learning and memory ability and upregulated expression of BDNF/TrkB in rats, previous literature proposed that a longer intervention period may stabilize the intervention effect on learning and memory [67,68]. Future studies need to investigate the effects of longer intervention cycles on learning and memory, as well as related mechanisms. In short, these limitations mean that the study findings need to be interpreted cautiously.

5. Conclusions

Taken together, our data robustly demonstrates that exercise combined with an enriched environment can improve the learning and memory ability in rats. The improve learning and memory ability might be mediated by the upregulated expression of BDNF/TrkB.

Author Contributions: A.C. designed and performed the study. L.Z. (Lina Zhu) oversaw the data collection. L.X. and L.Z. (Linna Zhu) analyzed the data and wrote the initial manuscript. D.C., K.C. and Z.L. monitored the data quality. All authors have read and agreed to the published version of the manuscript.

Funding: This study was partly funded by grants received by Aiguo Chen from the National Natural Science Foundation of China (31771243) and the Fok Ying Tung Education Foundation (141113).

Institutional Review Board Statement: The Institutional Animal Care and Use Committee of Yangzhou University following the Ethical Committee approved this study (ethical code: YZU-TYXY-32 and date of approval: 1 April 2019).

Informed Consent Statement: Not applicable.

Data Availability Statement: The raw data supporting the conclusions of this article will be made available by the authors, without undue reservation.

Conflicts of Interest: The authors declare that the research was conducted in the absence of any commercial or financial relationships that could be construed as a potential conflict of interest.

References

1. Huang, E.J.; Reichardt, L.F. Neurotrophins: Roles in neuronal development and function. *Annu. Rev. Neurosci.* **2001**, *24*, 677–736. [CrossRef]
2. McAllister, A.K.; Katz, L.C.; Lo, D.C. Neurotrophins and synaptic plasticity. *Annu. Rev. Neurosci.* **1999**, *22*, 295–318. [CrossRef]
3. Sartorius, A.; Hellweg, R.; Litzke, J.; Vogt, M.; Dormann, C.; Vollmayr, B.; Danker-Hopfe, H.; Gass, P. Correlations and discrepancies between serum and brain tissue levels of neurotrophins after electroconvulsive treatment in rats. *Pharmacopsychiatry* **2009**, *42*, 270–276. [CrossRef]
4. Karege, F.; Schwald, M.; Cisse, M. Postnatal developmental profile of brain-derived neurotrophic factor in rat brain and platelets. *Neurosci. Lett.* **2002**, *328*, 261–264. [CrossRef]
5. Lang, U.E.; Hellweg, R.; Seifert, F.; Schubert, F.; Gallinat, J. Correlation between serum brain-derived neurotrophic factor level and an in vivo marker of cortical integrity. *Biol. Psychiatry* **2007**, *62*, 530–535. [CrossRef]
6. Tyler, W.J. From acquisition to consolidation: On the role of brain-derived neurotrophic factor signaling in hippocampal-dependent learning. *Learn. Mem.* **2002**, *9*, 224–237. [CrossRef]
7. Kim, D.M.; Leem, Y.H. Chronic stress-induced memory deficits are reversed by regular exercise via ampk-mediated BDNF induction. *Neuroscience* **2016**, *324*, 271–285. [CrossRef]
8. Sanz-García, A.; Knafo, S.; Pereda-Pérez, I.; Esteban, J.A.; Venero, C.; Armario, A. Administration of the TrkB receptor agonist 7,8-dihydroxyflavone prevents traumatic stress-induced spatial memory deficits and changes in synaptic plasticity. *Hippocampus* **2016**, *26*, 1179–1188. [CrossRef]
9. Sabouri, M.; Kordi, M.; Shabkhiz, F.; Taghibeikzadehbadr, P.; Geramian, Z.S. Moderate treadmill exercise improves spatial learning and memory deficits possibly via changing PDE-5, IL-1 beta and pCREB expression. *Exp. Gerontol.* **2020**, *139*, 111056. [CrossRef] [PubMed]
10. Erickson, K.I.; Voss, M.W.; Prakash, R.S.; Basak, C.; Szabo, A.; Chaddock, L.; Kim, J.S.; Heo, S.; Alves, H.; White, S.M.; et al. Exercise training increases size of hippocampus and improves memory. *Proc. Natl. Acad. Sci. USA* **2011**, *108*, 3017–3022. [CrossRef]
11. van Dongen, E.V.; Kersten, I.H.P.; Wagner, I.C.; Morris, R.G.M.; Fernández, G. Physical exercise performed four hours after learning improves memory retention and increases hippocampal pattern similarity during retrieval. *Curr. Biol.* **2016**, *26*, 1722–1727. [CrossRef] [PubMed]
12. Joubert, C.; Chainay, H. Aging brain: The effect of combined cognitive and physical training on cognition as compared to cognitive and physical training alone—A systematic review. *Clin. Interv. Aging* **2018**, *13*, 1267–1301. [CrossRef]
13. Lago, T.R.; Hsiung, A.; Leitner, B.P.; Duckworth, C.J.; Balderston, N.L.; Chen, K.Y.; Grillon, C.; Ernst, M. Exercise modulates the interaction between cognition and anxiety in humans. *Cogn. Emot.* **2019**, *33*, 863–870. [CrossRef]
14. Vaynman, S.; Ying, Z.; Gómez-Pinilla, F. Exercise induces BDNF and synapsin I to specific hippocampal subfields. *J. Neurosci. Res.* **2004**, *76*, 356–362. [CrossRef] [PubMed]
15. Aguiar, A.J.; Tuon, T.; Pinho, C.A.; Silva, L.A.; Andreazza, A.C.; Kapczinski, F.; Quevedo, J.; Streck, E.L.; Pinho, R.A. Intense exercise induces mitochondrial dysfunction in mice brain. *Neurochem. Res.* **2008**, *33*, 51–58. [CrossRef] [PubMed]
16. Azimi, M.; Gharakhanlou, R.; Naghdi, N.; Khodadadi, D.; Heysieattalab, S. Moderate treadmill exercise ameliorates amyloid-beta-induced learning and memory impairment, possibly via increasing AMPK activity and up-regulation of the PGC-1alpha/FNDC5/BDNF pathway. *Peptides* **2018**, *102*, 78–88. [CrossRef]
17. Tsai, S.F.; Ku, N.W.; Wang, T.F.; Yang, Y.H.; Shih, Y.H.; Wu, S.Y.; Lee, C.W.; Yu, M.; Yang, T.T.; Kuo, Y.M. Long-Term Moderate Exercise Rescues Age-Related Decline in Hippocampal Neuronal Complexity and Memory. *Gerontology* **2018**, *64*, 551–561. [CrossRef]
18. Shafia, S.; Vafaei, A.A.; Samaei, S.A.; Bandegi, A.R.; Rafiei, A.; Valadan, R.; Hosseini-Khah, Z.; Mohammadkhani, R.; Rashidy-Pour, A. Effects of moderate treadmill exercise and fluoxetine on behavioural and cognitive deficits, hypothalamic-pituitary-adrenal axis dysfunction and alternations in hippocampal BDNF and mRNA expression of apoptosis-related proteins in a rat model of post-traumatic stress disorder. *Neurobiol. Learn. Mem.* **2017**, *139*, 165–178. [CrossRef]
19. Just-Borras, L.; Hurtado, E.; Cilleros-Mane, V.; Biondi, O.; Charbonnier, F.; Tomas, M.; Garcia, N.; Tomas, J.; Lanuza, M.A. Running and swimming prevent the deregulation of the BDNF/TrkB neurotrophic signalling at the neuromuscular junction in mice with amyotrophic lateral sclerosis. *Cell Mol. Life Sci.* **2020**, *77*, 3027–3040. [CrossRef]
20. Almeida, M.F.; Chaves, R.S.; Silva, C.M.; Chaves, J.C.S.; Melo, K.P.; Ferrari, M.F.R. BDNF trafficking and signaling impairment during early neurodegeneration is prevented by moderate physical activity. *IBRO Rep.* **2016**, *1*, 19–31. [CrossRef]
21. Rosenzweig, M.R.; Bennett, E.L.; Hebert, M.; Morimoto, H. Social grouping cannot account for cerebral effects of enriched environments. *Brain Res.* **1978**, *153*, 563–576. [CrossRef]
22. Robison, L.S.; Francis, N.; Popescu, D.L.; Anderson, M.E.; Hatfield, J.; Xu, F.; Anderson, B.J.; Van Nostrand, W.E.; Robinson, J.K. Environmental enrichment: Disentangling the influence of novelty, social, and physical activity on cerebral amyloid angiopathy in a transgenic mouse model. *Int. J. Mol. Sci.* **2020**, *21*, 843. [CrossRef]
23. Mora-Gallegos, A.; Rojas-Carvajal, M.; Salas, S.; Saborio-Arce, A.; Fornaguera-Trias, J.; Brenes, J.C. Age-dependent effects of environmental enrichment on spatial memory and neurochemistry. *Neurobiol. Learn. Mem.* **2015**, *118*, 96–104. [CrossRef]

24. Stratta, P.; Sanità, P.; Bonanni, R.L.; de Cataldo, S.; Angelucci, A.; Rossi, R.; Origlia, N.; Domenici, L.; Carmassi, C.; Piccinni, A.; et al. Clinical correlates of plasma brain-derived neurotrophic factor in post-traumatic stress disorder spectrum after a natural disaster. *Psychiatry Res.* **2016**, *244*, 165–170. [CrossRef]
25. Solinas, M.; Thiriet, N.; El, R.R.; Lardeux, V.; Jaber, M. Environmental enrichment during early stages of life reduces the behavioral, neurochemical, and molecular effects of cocaine. *Neuropsychopharmacology* **2009**, *34*, 1102–1111. [CrossRef] [PubMed]
26. Austin, M.W.; Ploughman, M.; Glynn, L.; Corbett, D. Aerobic exercise effects on neuroprotection and brain repair following stroke: A systematic review and perspective. *Neurosci. Res.* **2014**, *87*, 8–15. [CrossRef] [PubMed]
27. Bondi, C.O.; Klitsch, K.C.; Leary, J.B.; Kline, A.E. Environmental enrichment as a viable neurorehabilitation strategy for experimental traumatic brain injury. *J. Neurotraum.* **2014**, *31*, 873–888. [CrossRef]
28. Gajhede Gram, M.; Gade, L.; Wogensen, E.; Mogensen, J.; Malá, H. Equal effects of typical environmental and specific social enrichment on posttraumatic cognitive functioning after fimbria-fornix transection in rats. *Brain Res.* **2015**, *1629*, 182–195. [CrossRef]
29. Ahmadalipour, A.; Ghodrati-Jaldbakhan, S.; Samaei, S.A.; Rashidy-Pour, A. Deleterious effects of prenatal exposure to morphine on the spatial learning and hippocampal BDNF and long-term potentiation in juvenile rats: Beneficial influences of postnatal treadmill exercise and enriched environment. *Neurobiol. Learn. Mem.* **2018**, *147*, 54–64. [CrossRef]
30. Xie, H.; Wu, Y.; Jia, J.; Liu, G.; Zhang, Q.; Yu, K.; Guo, Z.; Shen, L.; Hu, R. Enrichment-induced exercise to quantify the effect of different housing conditions: A tool to standardize enriched environment protocols. *Behav. Brain Res.* **2013**, *249*, 81–89. [CrossRef] [PubMed]
31. Fabel, K.; Wolf, S.A.; Ehninger, D.; Babu, H.; Leal-Galicia, P.; Kempermann, G. Additive effects of physical exercise and environmental enrichment on adult hippocampal neurogenesis in mice. *Front. Neurosci.* **2009**, *3*, 50. [CrossRef] [PubMed]
32. Kapgal, V.; Prem, N.; Hegde, P.; Laxmi, T.R.; Kutty, B.M. Long term exposure to combination paradigm of environmental enrichment, physical exercise and diet reverses the spatial memory deficits and restores hippocampal neurogenesis in ventral subicular lesioned rats. *Neurobiol. Learn. Mem.* **2016**, *130*, 61–70. [CrossRef] [PubMed]
33. Bedford, T.G.; Tipton, C.M.; Wilson, N.C.; Oppliger, R.A.; Gisolfi, C.V. Maximum oxygen consumption of rats and its changes with various experimental procedures. *J. Appl. Physiol.* **1979**, *47*, 1278–1283. [CrossRef] [PubMed]
34. Jing, L.; Zhongming, L.; Haijun, L.; Yan, Z.; Yongliang, W. Effects of different exercise loads on cognitive ability and expression of VEGF/VEGI in hippocampus of aged rats. *Chin. J. Neuroanat.* **2018**, *34*, 572–578.
35. Frye, C.A. Estrus-associated decrements in a water maze task are limited to acquisition. *Physiol. Behav.* **1995**, *57*, 5–14. [CrossRef]
36. Sakata, A.; Mogi, M.; Iwanami, J.; Tsukuda, K.; Min, L.J.; Jing, F.; Iwai, M.; Ito, M.; Horiuchi, M. Female exhibited severe cognitive impairment in type 2 diabetes mellitus mice. *Life Sci.* **2010**, *86*, 638–645. [CrossRef]
37. Chen, W.Q.; Zhao, X.L.; Hou, Y.; Li, S.T.; Hong, Y.; Wang, D.L.; Cheng, Y.Y. Protective effects of green tea polyphenols on cognitive impairments induced by psychological stress in rats. *Behav. Brain Res.* **2009**, *202*, 71–76. [CrossRef]
38. Pietrelli, A.; Matkovic, L.; Vacotto, M.; Lopez-Costa, J.J.; Basso, N.; Brusco, A. Aerobic exercise upregulates the BDNF-Serotonin systems and improves the cognitive function in rats. *Neurobiol. Learn. Mem.* **2018**, *155*, 528–542. [CrossRef] [PubMed]
39. Pietrelli, A.; López-Costa, J.J.; Goñi, R.; López, E.M.; Brusco, A.; Basso, N. Effects of moderate and chronic exercise on the nitrergic system and behavioral parameters in rats. *Brain Res.* **2011**, *1389*, 71–82. [CrossRef]
40. Wang, X.Q.; Wang, G.W. Effects of treadmill exercise intensity on spatial working memory and long-term memory in rats. *Life Sci.* **2016**, *149*, 96–103. [CrossRef]
41. Okudan, N.; Belviranlı, M. Long-term voluntary exercise prevents post-weaning social isolation-induced cognitive impairment in rats. *Neuroscience* **2017**, *360*, 1–8. [CrossRef]
42. Berchtold, N.C.; Castello, N.; Cotman, C.W. Exercise and time-dependent benefits to learning and memory. *Neuroscience* **2010**, *167*, 588–597. [CrossRef]
43. Gradari, S.; Palle, A.; McGreevy, K.R.; Fontan-Lozano, A.; Trejo, J.L. Can Exercise Make You Smarter, Happier, and Have More Neurons? A Hormetic Perspective. *Front. Neurosci.* **2016**, *10*, 93. [CrossRef]
44. Gómez-Pinilla, F.; Ying, Z.; Roy, R.R.; Molteni, R.; Edgerton, V.R. Voluntary exercise induces a bdnf-mediated mechanism that promotes neuroplasticity. *J. Neurophysiol.* **2002**, *88*, 2187–2195. [CrossRef] [PubMed]
45. Gomez-Pinilla, F.; Ying, Z.; Opazo, P.; Roy, R.R.; Edgerton, V.R. Differential regulation by exercise of BDNF and NT-3 in rat spinal cord and skeletal muscle. *Eur. J. Neurosci.* **2001**, *13*, 1078–1084. [CrossRef]
46. Hauser, S.L.; Johnston, S.C. Of ghosts and sirens: The subtlest lures of industry. *Ann. Neurol.* **2007**, *61*, A11–A12. [CrossRef]
47. Lou, S.J.; Liu, J.Y.; Chang, H.; Chen, P.J. Hippocampal neurogenesis and gene expression depend on exercise intensity in juvenile rats. *Brain Res.* **2008**, *1210*, 48–55. [CrossRef]
48. Shih, P.; Yang, Y.; Wang, R. Effects of exercise intensity on spatial memory performance and hippocampal synaptic plasticity in transient brain ischemic rats. *PLoS ONE* **2013**, *8*, e78163. [CrossRef]
49. Sheikhzadeh, F.; Etemad, A.; Khoshghadam, S.; Asl, N.A.; Zare, P. Hippocampal BDNF content in response to short- and long-term exercise. *Neurol. Sci.* **2015**, *36*, 1163–1166. [CrossRef] [PubMed]
50. Costa, M.S.; Ardais, A.P.; Fioreze, G.T.; Mioranzza, S.; Botton, P.H.S.; Souza, D.O.; Rocha, J.B.T.; Porciúncula, L.O. The impact of the frequency of moderate exercise on memory and brain-derived neurotrophic factor signaling in young adult and middle-aged rats. *Neuroscience* **2012**, *222*, 100–109. [CrossRef]

51. Dalise, S.; Cavalli, L.; Ghuman, H.; Wahlberg, B.; Gerwig, M.; Chisari, C.; Ambrosio, F.; Modo, M. Biological effects of dosing aerobic exercise and neuromuscular electrical stimulation in rats. *Sci. Rep.* **2017**, *7*, 10830. [CrossRef]
52. Li, X.; Wu, Q.; Xie, C.; Wang, C.; Wang, Q.; Dong, C.; Fang, L.; Ding, J.; Wang, T. Blocking of BDNF-TrkB signaling inhibits the promotion effect of neurological function recovery after treadmill training in rats with spinal cord injury. *Spinal Cord* **2019**, *57*, 65–74. [CrossRef]
53. Schapiro, S.J. Effects of social manipulations and environmental enrichment on behavior and cell-mediated immune responses in rhesus macaques. *Pharm. Biochem. Behav.* **2002**, *73*, 271–278. [CrossRef]
54. Ambrogini, P.; Lattanzi, D.; Ciuffoli, S.; Betti, M.; Fanelli, M.; Cuppini, R. Physical exercise and environment exploration affect synaptogenesis in adult-generated neurons in the rat dentate gyrus: Possible role of BDNF. *Brain Res.* **2013**, *1534*, 1–12. [CrossRef] [PubMed]
55. Rasmussen, P.; Brassard, P.; Adser, H.; Pedersen, M.V.; Leick, L.; Hart, E.; Secher, N.H.; Pedersen, B.K.; Pilegaard, H. Evidence for a release of brain-derived neurotrophic factor from the brain during exercise. *Exp. Physiol.* **2009**, *94*, 1062–1069. [CrossRef] [PubMed]
56. Branchi, I.; D Andrea, I.; Fiore, M.; Di Fausto, V.; Aloe, L.; Alleva, E. Early social enrichment shapes social behavior and nerve growth factor and brain-derived neurotrophic factor levels in the adult mouse brain. *Biol. Psychiatry* **2006**, *60*, 690–696. [CrossRef]
57. Zhu, S.; Yee, B.K.; Nyffeler, M.; Winblad, B.; Feldon, J.; Mohammed, A.H. Influence of differential housing on emotional behaviour and neurotrophin levels in mice. *Behav. Brain Res.* **2006**, *169*, 10–20. [CrossRef] [PubMed]
58. Lu, B. BDNF and activity-dependent synaptic modulation. *Learn. Mem.* **2003**, *10*, 86–98. [CrossRef]
59. Klein, A.B.; Williamson, R.; Santini, M.A.; Clemmensen, C.; Ettrup, A.; Rios, M.; Knudsen, G.M.; Aznar, S. Blood BDNF concentrations reflect brain-tissue BDNF levels across species. *Int. J. Neuropsychopharmacol.* **2011**, *14*, 347–353. [CrossRef]
60. Pan, W.; Banks, W.A.; Fasold, M.B.; Bluth, J.; Kastin, A.J. Transport of brain-derived neurotrophic factor across the blood-brain barrier. *Neuropharmacology* **1998**, *37*, 1553–1561. [CrossRef]
61. Bliss, T.V.; Collingridge, G.L. A synaptic model of memory: Long-term potentiation in the hippocampus. *Nature* **1993**, *361*, 31–39. [CrossRef] [PubMed]
62. Wang, C.L. The Effects of Swimming Movement and Rich Environment on Autism Rats' Learning and Memory Ability and Mechanism Research. Master's Thesis, Jilin University, Changchun, China, 2016.
63. Du, M.; Guan, Q.; Wang, X. Effects of Memantine combined with enriched environment on the expression of brain derived neurophic factor and tyrosine kinase receptor B in hippocampus and the learning and memory ability of senescence accelerated mouse prone 8. *J. Clin. Neurol.* **2013**, *26*, 278–281.
64. Moradi-Kor, N.; Ghanbari, A.; Rashidipour, H.; Yousefi, B.; Bandegi, A.R.; Rashidy-Pour, A. Beneficial effects of Spirulina platensis, voluntary exercise and environmental enrichment against adolescent stress induced deficits in cognitive functions, hippocampal BDNF and morphological remolding in adult female rats. *Horm. Behav.* **2019**, *112*, 20–31. [CrossRef] [PubMed]
65. Warren, S.G.; Juraska, J.M. Spatial and nonspatial learning across the rat estrous cycle. *Behav. Neurosci.* **1997**, *111*, 259–266. [CrossRef]
66. Galea, L.A.; Kavaliers, M.; Ossenkopp, K.P.; Hampson, E. Gonadal hormone levels and spatial learning performance in the Morris water maze in male and female meadow voles, Microtus pennsylvanicus. *Horm. Behav.* **1995**, *29*, 106–125. [CrossRef]
67. Kennard, J.; Woodruff-Pak, D.S. Aging and exercise effects on motor learning and spatial memory. *Ageing Res.* **2011**, *2*, 2. [CrossRef]
68. Qingwei, Y.; Bo, X.; Qing, T. Treadmill exercise improves hippocampal mitochondrial function and learning and memory ability of APP/PS1 mice. *Chin. J. Biochem. Mol. Biol.* **2019**, *35*, 669–677. [CrossRef]

International Journal of
Environmental Research and Public Health

MDPI

Article

Absolute Accelerometer-Based Intensity Prescription Compared to Physiological Variables in Pregnant and Nonpregnant Women

Philipp Birnbaumer [1], Pavel Dietz [2], Estelle Dorothy Watson [3], Gudani Mukoma [3,4], Alexander Müller [1], Matteo Christian Sattler [1], Johannes Jaunig [1], Mireille Nicoline Maria van Poppel [1] and Peter Hofmann [1,*]

1 Institute of Human Movement Science, Sport and Health, University of Graz, 8010 Graz, Austria; philipp.birnbaumer@uni-graz.at (P.B.); alexander.mueller@uni-graz.at (A.M.); matteo.sattler@uni-graz.at (M.C.S.); jaunig.johannes@uni-graz.at (J.J.); mireille.van-poppel@uni-graz.at (M.N.M.v.P.)
2 Institute of Occupational, Social and Environmental Medicine, University Medical Center of the University of Mainz, 55131 Mainz, Germany; pdietz@uni-mainz.de
3 School of Therapeutic Sciences, Faculty of Health Sciences, University of the Witwatersrand, Johannesburg 2000, South Africa; estelle.owen@googlemail.com (E.D.W.); mukomagudani@gmail.com (G.M.)
4 South African MRC/Wits Developmental Pathways for Health Research Unit, Faculty of Health Sciences, University of the Witwatersrand, Johannesburg 2000, South Africa
* Correspondence: peter.hofmann@uni-graz.at

Received: 3 June 2020; Accepted: 3 August 2020; Published: 5 August 2020

Abstract: Estimation of the intensity of physical activity (PA) based on absolute accelerometer cut points (Cp) likely over- or underestimates intensity for a specific individual. The purpose of this study was to investigate the relationship between absolute moderate intensity Cp and the first ventilatory threshold (VT_1). A group of 24 pregnant and 15 nonpregnant women who performed a submaximal incremental walking test with measures of ventilatory parameters and accelerations from three different accelerometers on the wrist (ActiGraph wGT3X-BT, GENEActiv, Axivity AX3) and one on the hip (Actigraph wGT3X-BT) were analyzed. Cp were determined corresponding to 3 metabolic equivalents of task (MET), using the conventional MET definition ($Cp_{3.5}$) (3.5 mL/kg×min) and individual resting metabolic rate (Cp_{ind}). The ventilatory equivalent (VE/VO_2) was used to determine VT_1. Accelerations at VT_1 were significantly higher ($p < 0.01$) compared to $Cp_{3.5}$ and Cp_{ind} in both groups. $Cp_{3.5}$ and Cp_{ind} were significantly different in nonpregnant ($p < 0.01$) but not in pregnant women. Walking speed at VT_1 (5.7 ± 0.5/6.2 ± 0.8 km/h) was significantly lower ($p < 0.01$) in pregnant compared to nonpregnant women and correspondent to 3.8 ± 0.7/4.9 ± 1.4 conventional METs. Intensity at absolute Cp was lower compared to the intensity at VT_1 independent of the device or placement in pregnant and nonpregnant women. Therefore, we recommend individually tailored cut points such as the VT_1 to better assess the effect of the intensity of PA.

Keywords: ventilatory threshold; walking test; ENMO; raw accelerations; accelerometer cut point

1. Introduction

Accelerometers are often used as a measure of free-living physical activity (PA) to estimate frequency, duration, and intensity [1]. In order to estimate the intensity of PA, calibration of accelerometers based on physiological responses to various activities is required. Calibration studies use oxygen consumption as the criterion measure and specific statistical methods, such as regression models or machine learning-based modeling, to determine the corresponding accelerometer cut point at a certain intensity threshold [2,3]. Usually, these intensity thresholds are used to define activity classes based on the average energy expenditure, expressed in multiples of the conventional metabolic equivalent of task (MET) ratio. The 1 MET value is defined as the energy expended by a subject at rest, which equals an oxygen consumption of 3.5 mL/kg×min for a 70 kg person [4]. Common classifications of PA intensity classes are light (< 3 METs), moderate (3–5.9 METs), and vigorous (≥ 6 METs) [5–7]. However, using the conventional 1 MET to classify PA intensity classes already causes misclassifications, compared to approaches where the individual resting metabolic rate would have been used [8,9]. Moreover, it must be considered that accelerometer cut points, which are based on the same absolute approach, are independent of individual performance capacity which leads to different physiological and metabolic strain (internal load) at the same absolute intensity [10]. To counteract that, relative accelerometer cut points based on the individual maximum performance capacity can be used. Several studies showed that the estimation of the duration of moderate-to-vigorous physical activity (MVPA) was shorter when relative comparisons to absolute cut points were applied, independent of body mass index (BMI). Therefore, absolute cut points overestimate MVPA compared to relative cut points [2,11]. When applying relative cut points, activity counts at a fixed relative intensity (e.g., 60% heart rate reserve (HRR)) increase with increasing fitness level [12]. On the contrary, low-fit persons had significantly higher percentage of maximum oxygen uptake (%VO_{2max}) at absolute cut points (e.g., 2020 cpm) compared to fit persons [11]. The use of absolute accelerometer cut points is therefore likely to over- or underestimate PA intensity and volume in a certain PA intensity class for a specific individual. Individualized activity measurements (i.e., relative accelerometer cut points), which take into account the performance capacity of each individual, will allow us to draw more valid conclusions about the internal loads due to different intensities of PA.

Relative accelerometer cut points are usually derived using fixed percentages of an individual's maximum heart rate (HR_{max}), maximum oxygen uptake (VO_{2max}), or HRR [13]. Such an individualized approach improves validity, but will still lead to some inaccuracy in the prescription of exercise intensity, because exercising at a calculated and fixed relative intensity such as 85% HR_{max} causes different metabolic and cardiorespiratory responses across individuals [14,15]. To overcome these problems, exercise can be prescribed based on submaximal markers such as the first and second ventilatory or lactate thresholds (VT_1 and VT_2; LTP_1 and LTP_2) which rely on the detection of physiological thresholds dependent on exercise intensity [16,17]. Hence, less variability in interindividual metabolic responses is expected when being active at a certain intensity relative to these thresholds. Indeed, Moser et al. [18] recently showed consistent metabolic responses during continuous cycle ergometer exercise five percent above and below LTP_1 and LTP_2. Furthermore, lactate thresholds as well as their physiological equivalents VT_1 and VT_2 allow conclusions about the fitness level and adaptations to exercise, and are very sensitive in reflecting differences in endurance performance [16,17].

Two studies by Gil-Rey et al. [19,20] estimated the intensity of PA from individually tailored accelerometer cut points derived from lactate thresholds in postmenopausal women. Individually tailored cut points revealed similar time for MVPA in high- and low-fit groups. In contrast, MVPA was overestimated in low-fit and more strongly in the high-fit group when absolute accelerometer cut points at moderate intensity (3–5.9 METs) were applied. They showed that individually tailored rather than traditional absolute accelerometer cut points estimate an individual's activity level (i.e., time spent in different intensities of PA) more accurately. Thus, using individually tailored cut points from physiological thresholds may provoke greater adaptions to exercise and reduced interindividual variability of metabolic responses, as well as less overestimation of PA intensity. To date, it is unknown how well absolute accelerometer cut points are related to a physiological threshold such as the VT_1 in pregnant as well as in young nonpregnant women. We hypothesized that the two absolute accelerometer cut points, derived from the 3 MET moderate intensity definition using either the conventional 3.5 mL/kg×min or the individual resting metabolic rate, will be lower compared to the individual threshold derived from VT_1.Therefore, the aim of this study was to compare accelerometer cut points from different devices and placements, derived from the 3-MET absolute moderate intensity definition with the first ventilatory threshold (VT_1) determined in a short submaximal incremental walking test (IWT) in a sample of pregnant and younger nonpregnant women.

2. Materials and Methods

2.1. Subjects

In total, a group of 30 pregnant (second and third trimester) and 17 nonpregnant women were tested at the University of Graz, Austria and the University of the Witwatersrand, Johannesburg, South Africa (22 pregnant, 9 nonpregnant). Subjects in Graz were active pregnant women and a mix of highly active and well-trained nonpregnant women (mainly students). In South Africa, subjects were sedentary and low-active pregnant women and a mix of sedentary, low-active, and well-trained nonpregnant women. Before any study procedures were undertaken, the participants completed informed consent forms and were familiarized with the testing protocol. The study protocol was approved by the local ethics committees (SA clearance certificate no. M160532; GZ. 39/42/63 ex 2015/16).

2.2. Test Protocol

Participants performed one IWT while wearing a portable gas analyzer and four different accelerometers. Before the IWT, resting metabolic rate was measured during 15 min of supine resting. IWT was conducted on a 400 m outdoor running track and started at 3 km/h. Walking speed was paced by audio signals given in 10 m intervals and increased by 0.5 km/h every 50 m up to the maximum individual walking speed. Maximum walking speed was defined as the speed where participants were unable to walk the given pacer speed.

2.3. Measurements

Gas exchange data were continuously measured breath by breath by a portable gas analyzer in Graz (CORTEX METAMAX 3B, Cortex Biophysik GmbH, Germany) and Johannesburg (OXYCON Mobile, CareFusion GmbH, Hoechberg, Germany). Calibration of volume, O_2, and CO_2 gas sensors was performed prior to every test according to the manufacturer's guidelines. For activity measurements, all participants were equipped with four accelerometers in total. Three different types of accelerometers were attached on the nondominant wrist, placed in a random order: ActiGraph wGT3X-BT (ActiGraph, Pensacola, FL), GENEActive (Activeinsights, Kimbolton, UK), Axivity AX3 (Axivity Ltd., Newcastle upon Tyne, UK). In addition, one accelerometer (ActiGraph wGT3X-BT) was placed on the left hip. Prior to the measurements, all accelerometers were initialized with a data sampling frequency of 100 Hz and a sampling range of ± 8 g.

2.4. Determination of Physiological Thresholds and Accelerometer Cut Points

Gas exchange data were exported into Microsoft Excel files (Microsoft Corporation, Redmond, WA, USA) in 15 s epochs using the manufacturer's software. Oxygen uptake (VO_2) was converted to $MET_{3.5}$ by using the conventional conversion factor (1 MET = 3.5 mL/kg×min) and to MET_{ind} by using the individual resting metabolic equivalent (1 MET_{ind}) defined as mean oxygen uptake from the last 10 min of the 15 min supine resting position. Based on the raw triaxial accelerations, the vector magnitude (expressed in milligravity (mg) units) was calculated using the Euclidian norm minus one (ENMO = $\sqrt{(a_x^2+a_y^2+a_z^2)}$-1g) [21]. Therefore, the raw files from all devices were imported into R statistical software V3.1.2 (R Foundation for Statistical Computing, Vienna, Austria) by which the metric ENMO was calculated in 15 s epoch using the package GGIR V1.2-0. Processed files were then exported into Microsoft Excel. To determine the absolute accelerometer cut points at moderate intensity (3 METs), we performed an individual linear regression analysis between the ENMO and the oxygen uptake during the IWT, based on $MET_{3.5}$ ($Cp_{3.5}$) and MET_{ind} (Cp_{ind}). Individual physiological threshold was defined as the first ventilatory threshold (VT_1), using the ventilatory equivalent (VE/VO_2) to determine VT_1 as the minimum of VE/VO_2 without an increase in VE/VCO_2. The evaluation was carried out by two independent examiners using computer-supported linear regression analysis to increase objectivity. In case of disagreement, the results were discussed with a further examiner.

2.5. Statistical Analysis

Data analysis was performed using GraphPad Prism 7 (GraphPad Software, San Diego, CA, USA). The Shapiro–Wilk test was used for confirmation of normality. For normally distributed data, independent t tests were used to assess differences between pregnant and nonpregnant women. If data were not normally distributed, Mann–Whitney U tests were applied. To determine the effect of different cut points ($Cp_{3.5}$, Cp_{ind}, and VT_1) and devices/placement (GENEActiv, Axivity, ActiGraph wrist and hip) on acceleration (ENMO), we applied a two-way repeated measures ANOVA (two within subject factors) with post hoc Tukey multiple comparison test in pregnant and nonpregnant women. If sphericity was violated, the Geisser–Greenhouse correction was used. Spearman correlation coefficient was applied to evaluate the relationship between walking speed and accelerations at VT_1. Data are presented as means ± standard deviation (M ± SD). Statistical significance was set at $p < 0.05$.

3. Results

We analyzed 39 data sets of healthy pregnant ($n = 24$; 27.7 ± 4.6 yrs) and nonpregnant ($n = 15$; 24.3 ± 2.2 yrs) women. In total, eight tests were excluded from the analysis because of incomplete data sets (six in the pregnant and two in the nonpregnant group). The mean age, weight, and BMI were significantly higher in pregnant women (gestational age: 26 ± 7 weeks), but maximum walking speed (v_{max}), VO_{2max}, speed at VT_1 (v_{VT1}), and MET_{ind} were significantly lower compared to nonpregnant women. Absolute oxygen uptake at VT_1 (VO_{2VT1}) was not different ($p = 0.07$) between pregnant (0.9 ± 0.2 L/min) and nonpregnant (1.0 ± 0.2 L/min) women, but calculated conventional MET values at VT_1 were significantly lower in pregnant compared to nonpregnant women (3.8 ± 0.7 vs. 4.9 ± 1.4 METs, $p < 0.01$). Determined 1 MET_{ind} was significantly higher compared to the conventional 1 MET value (3.5 mL/kg×min) in pregnant and nonpregnant women (Table 1). Bland–Altman interobserver comparison of VT_1 determination (VO_{2VT1} bias: 0.01 ± 0.08 L/min) revealed a high level of agreement for the analysis.

Table 1. Comparison of anthropometrics, performance of the incremental walking test (IWT), and the individual resting metabolic equivalent between pregnant and nonpregnant women.

Variables	Pregnant ($n = 24$)	Nonpregnant ($n = 15$)
Age (yrs)	27.7 ± 4.6 [1]	24.3 ± 2.2
Weight (kg)	69.1 ± 10.6 [1]	61.2 ± 7.8
BMI (kg/m)	26.5 ± 4.9 [1]	22.5 ± 3.4
VO_{2max} (mL/kg×min)	18.2 ± 4.4	26.5 ± 8.0 [1]
VO_{2VT1} (METs/L/min)	3.8 ± 0.7/0.9 ± 0.2	4.9 ± 1.4 [1] / 1.0 ± 0.2
v_{max} (km/h)	7.8 ± 0.5	8.3 ± 0.5 [1]
v_{VT1} (km/h)	5.7 ± 0.5	6.2 ± 0.8 [1]
MET_{ind} (mL/kg×min)	3.7 ± 0.5 [2]	4.2 ± 0.6 [1,2]

BMI = Body Mass Index, VO_{2max} = maximum oxygen uptake, VO_{2VT1} = oxygen uptake at the first ventilatory threshold, v_{max} maximum walking speed, v_{VT1} = walking speed at the first ventilatory threshold, MET_{ind} = calculated individual resting metabolic equivalent, METs = rates of energy expenditure (1 MET is equivalent to 3.5 $mL \cdot kg^{-1} \cdot min^{-1}$, results are shown as $M \pm SD$. [1] significantly higher than the comparison group ($p < 0.05$). [2] significantly higher compared to conversion 1 MET = 3.5 mL/kg×min ($p < 0.05$).

In general, accelerometer cut points (ENMO) showed higher values and higher interindividual variability in pregnant compared to nonpregnant women (e.g., SD = 136 vs. SD = 50 for Cp3.5). In both groups, interindividual variability was less for the hip worn device (Table 2). Two-way repeated measures ANOVA in pregnant woman showed a significant effect for the determination of cut points ($F(1.76, 141.30) = 51.27$, $p < 0.01$) and a significant effect for devices/placement ($F(3, 80) = 3.16$, $p < 0.05$)

and no significant effect of interaction (F (6, 160) = 0.35, p = 0.91). Post hoc multiple comparison revealed no difference between $Cp_{3.5}$ and Cp_{ind}, but ENMO was significantly lower for $Cp_{3.5}$ and Cp_{ind} compared to the ENMO at VT_1 in pregnant women. Comparison of devices in pregnant women showed significantly higher ENMOs for wrist-worn GENEActiv compared to hip-worn ActiGraph ($p < 0.05$) and for wrist-worn ActiGraph compared to hip-worn ActiGraph and wrist-worn Axivity ($p < 0.05$). In nonpregnant women, there was a significant effect for the determination of cut points (F (1.28, 69.36) = 56.19, $p < 0.01$) and no significant effect for devices/placement and interaction (F (3, 54) = 0.42, p = 0.74; F (6, 108) = 0.38, p = 0.88). ENMO was significantly different for $Cp_{3.5}$ and Cp_{ind} compared to the ENMO at VT_1 and between $Cp_{3.5}$ and Cp_{ind} ($p < 0.01$).

Table 2. Metric Euclidian norm minus one (ENMO) of the determined accelerometer cut points of the different devices for pregnant and nonpregnant women.

	Pregnant (n = 24)			Nonpregnant (n = 15)		
Devices	$Cp_{3.5}$ (mg)	Cp_{ind} (mg)	VT_1 (mg)	$Cp_{3.5}$ (mg)	Cp_{ind} (mg)	VT_1 (mg)
GENEActiv (wrist)	190 ± 136 [2]	204 ± 109 [2]	290 ± 120 [1]	106 ± 50 [2]	156 ± 50 [1,2]	240 ± 85 [1]
Axivity (wrist)	165 ± 118 [2]	178 ± 94 [2]	271 ± 154 [1]	95 ± 43 [2]	145 ± 68 [1,2]	268 ± 204 [1]
ActiGraph (wrist)	238 ± 171 [2]	245 ± 142 [2]	350 ± 166 [1]	108 ± 58 [2]	169 ± 58 [1,2]	276 ± 129 [1]
ActiGraph (hip)	139 ± 93 [2]	145 ± 50 [2]	215 ± 129 [1]	106 ± 36 [2]	152 ± 37 [1,2]	236 ± 85 [1]

$Cp_{3.5}$ = absolute accelerometer cut point at moderate intensity (3 MET) calculated using the conventional 1 MET = 3.5 m/kg×min value, Cp_{ind} = absolute accelerometer cut point at moderate intensity (3 MET) calculated using the individual resting metabolic equivalent, VT_1 = first ventilatory threshold, mg = milligravity. [1] significantly different compared to $Cp_{3.5}$ ($p < 0.05$). [2] significantly different compared to VT_1 ($p < 0.0001$).

Figure 1 shows the oxygen uptake expressed in $MET_{3.5}$ and MET_{ind} as well as the ENMO of all devices at comparable walking speeds of the IWT for pregnant and nonpregnant women. Walking speed and accelerations at VT_1 were not significantly correlated in pregnant (r_{preg}) but significantly correlated in nonpregnant (r_{non}) women for GENEActiv (r_{preg} = 0.13/r_{non} = 0.57) and Axivity (r_{preg} = 0.30/r_{non} = 0.69). Both groups showed no significant correlation between v_{VT1} and ENMO at VT_1 for wrist-worn ActiGraph (r_{preg} = 0.10/r_{non} = 0.41), but for hip-worn ActiGraph, values were significantly correlated (r_{preg} = 0.62/r_{non} = 0.69). Comparing ENMOs within all wrist-worn devices, GENEActiv and Axivity were similar in their measurements while wrist-worn ActiGraph showed higher mean accelerations with increasing speed. This difference was stronger in pregnant compared to nonpregnant women and at higher speeds above VT_1. Walking speed at VT_1 corresponded to 3.8 ± 0.7 and 4.9 ± 1.4 conventional METs in pregnant and nonpregnant women, respectively. Values ranged between 2.48 and 7.73 conventional METs and were lower at VT_1 compared to the 3-MET absolute moderate intensity definition in three cases in pregnant and in one case in nonpregnant women.

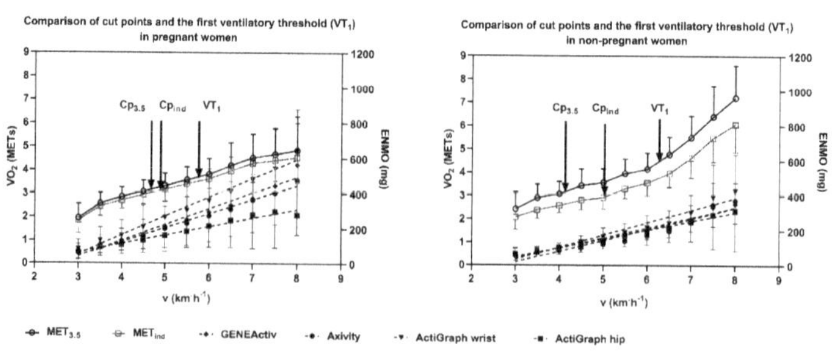

Figure 1. Mean ± SD oxygen uptake (VO_2) expressed in $MET_{3.5}$ (1 MET = 3.5 mL/kg×min) and MET_{ind} (1 MET = 3.7 ± 0.5/4.2 ± 0.6 mL/kg×min in pregnant/nonpregnant women) as well as the Euclidian norm minus one (ENMO=$\sqrt{(a_x^2+a_y^2+a_z^2)}$-1g) from GENEActiv, Axivity, ActiGraph wrist and hip for each single load step of the incremental walking test (IWT). Arrows mark cut point values determined from $MET_{3.5}$ ($Cp_{3.5}$), MET_{ind} (Cp_{ind}), and the first ventilatory threshold (VT_1).

4. Discussion

Accelerometer cut points at absolute moderate intensity definition (3 METs) were significantly lower compared to the intensity at VT_1 in a short maximal incremental walking test. The underestimation of intensity compared to VT_1 was independent of the accelerometer device or placement and the applied 1 MET value in pregnant and nonpregnant women. Walking speed at VT_1 was 5.7 ± 0.5 and 6.2 ± 0.8 km/h, which corresponded to an oxygen uptake of 3.8 ± 0.7 and 4.9 ± 1.4 conventional METs in pregnant and nonpregnant women, respectively. Whether during pregnancy or not, a certain duration of moderate-intensity physical activity (MPA), vigorous-intensity physical activity (VPA), or a combination of them (MVPA) is recommended in order to gain specific health benefits. Application of PA recommendations using fixed absolute intensities (e.g., MPA: 3–6 METs) [22] may lead to insufficient health benefits in our group of pregnant and nonpregnant women. In our sample, activity according to fixed absolute moderate intensity may be not intense enough to provoke larger adaptions of the cardiorespiratory system since 3 METs were lower compared to the intensity at VT_1 in all women except four. On the contrary, in individuals with lower fitness level, overloading or discouragement due to unattainable recommendations could be the result of recommendations based on absolute intensities [10]. Individually tailored metabolic or physiological accelerometer cut points were already shown to reduce this methodological error and to provide more meaningful results [19,20]. To determine individualized accelerometer cut points, a three-phase model [16] can be applied which allows one to detect the transition from phase 1 to phase 2 of energy supply, independent of the individual performance level, by using an individual threshold like VT_1. Phase 1 is characterized by a metabolically inter- and intramuscular balanced situation. Activities within this phase can be maintained for several hours without becoming fatigued [23]. The metabolic situation in phase 2 is systemically balanced but activity duration is limited [16]. Deliberate activity in phase 1 or 2 will therefore cause specific adaptions on a local and systemic level and the exact definition of these phases enables precise prescription and interpretation of intensity [14,24]. Therefore, optimized health benefits are suspected when recommendations are based on individual metabolic thresholds (i.e., VT_1 = lower limit for MPA), which are standard in performance development in structured training processes [25]. Furthermore, a more accurate assessment of the intensity of PA would enable better associations with health outcomes, dose–response relationships, and behavior surveillance [19,26].

The accelerations at absolute cut points ($Cp_{3.5}$, Cp_{ind}) were significantly lower compared to VT_1. Mean values for $Cp_{3.5}$ were higher in pregnant compared to nonpregnant women (e.g., Axivity: 165 ± 118 vs. 95 ± 43 mg). This difference of accelerations between groups was smaller for Cp_{ind} and VT_1 values as well as for the hip-worn device (Table 2). Such interindividual variability has already been shown for intensity cut points relative to heart rate reserve in a group with heterogeneous cardiorespiratory fitness. A high-fit group had higher accelerometer counts at the same relative intensity compared to a low-fit group [12]. Clear influence on varying accelerometer cut points was also shown for age and overweight/obesity [27,28]. However, age and weight affect cardiorespiratory fitness, which tends to decrease with both age [29] and obesity [30]. In our study, pregnant women had significantly higher body mass and maximum performance capacity was significantly lower compared to nonpregnant women. However, accelerometer cut points were higher (for wrist-worn devices) within pregnant women but showed no correlation with the walking speed at VT_1. Therefore, accelerometer values from wrist-worn devices could not be attributed to intensity in pregnant women. As walking economics were shown to change in pregnancy [31], higher accelerations in pregnant woman might more likely show differences in walking style. In nonpregnant women, high interindividual variability at the single cut points can be explained by differences in performance capacity, due to walking speeds at VT_1 (higher speed implicates a higher performance capacity) being significantly correlated to cut points, except for the wrist-worn ActiGraph. Accelerations in wrist-worn devices generally varied between the constant speed increments of IWT and were in some cases generally higher from the start of IWT compared to average values. In contrast, the hip-worn device showed less variability and significant correlations between walking speed and accelerations at VT_1 (r_{preg} = 0.62/r_{non} = 0.69) in pregnant and nonpregnant women, which is in line with a study by Ozemek et al. [12]. The hip-worn device seems to be less affected by the walking style and may therefore provide more meaningful results, especially in pregnant women. Mean ENMO accelerometer values in nonpregnant women for $Cp_{3.5}$ were in line with recent findings from the literature, presenting similar values for wrist-worn GENEActive (93.2 mg) and ActiGraph (100.6 mg) and hip-worn ActiGraph (69.1 mg) devices [5].

Mean speed at VT_1 in our study (pregnant: 5.7 km·h^{-1} and nonpregnant: 6.2 km·h^{-1}) is comparable to other studies, which determined a walking speed of ≈ 5 km·h^{-1} in older healthy men and women (56 ± 16 yrs) [32] and of 5.1 and 5.5 km/h in postmenopausal women [19,20]. Determination of VT_1 in a walking test seems to be applicable in a wide range of populations. Furthermore, walking tests are highly practicable due to the short duration of the test (average duration 6.5 min) and the fact that VT_1 can also be assessed using heart rate variability measurement of a simple heart rate monitor [32]. This enables testing several subjects at once in a short period of time requiring only heart rate monitors and pacing.

In both groups, 1 MET_{ind} was significantly higher compared to the conventional 1 MET value (3.5 mL/kg×min). Higher resting metabolic rates in pregnant women compared to the conventional 1 MET value are different compared to the literature, where no difference to the conventional 1 MET value was found [9]. This might be due to no acclimatization period and the relatively short measurement period of the resting state in our study. Higher resting metabolic rates of our sample of mainly active and well-trained women are in line with the recent literature, where energy expenditure of active healthy women was found to be underestimated by the conventional 1 MET [33]. Determination of the absolute accelerometer cut points at moderate intensity (3 METs) by the MET_{ind} resulted in higher values compared to the conventional equivalent ($MET_{3.5}$), but in significantly different values compared to VT_1. Therefore, using the MET_{ind} can partly compensate for the error made by using the fixed 1 MET definition, but not for the differences in performance capacity.

However, this study is not without limitations. The protocol of the IWT, with 50 m speed increases, allows a time-efficient determination of the first threshold (average duration 6.5 min). Although small increases of 0.5 km/h per increment favor a fast adaption, 50 m is a relatively short distance to adjust to the pacing speed. However, with increasing speed, walking time of the single increments decreases, which might have increased variance at higher speeds. For the definition of accelerations at a constant speed, increments with longer and equal duration would provide more precise results. Prior to IWT, individual resting metabolic rates were defined from a 15 min supine rest position without any guidance regarding the fasting state. This is not according to the general practice, as usually subjects have to be overnight fasted, run through an acclimating period and a longer measurement period [9,33], which would not have been feasible in pregnant women. Because of this, the determined resting metabolic equivalent needs to be considered with caution. Nevertheless, our resting metabolic equivalent determination was sufficient to get performance parameters related to the subject's actual metabolic status, considering their actual weight, age, and performance capacity. Furthermore, one could criticize that the tests were conducted by two research groups in different countries. Between groups, we used different gas analyzer devices, possibly influencing the results, although appropriate calibration was performed and devices were shown to provide reliable measurements with adequate validity for field-based measurements [34]. Furthermore, the majority of women in South Africa were black Africans, compared to Caucasian in the Austrian population, which was not considered in the analysis even though African Americans were shown to have lower accelerometer cut points compared to Caucasians in a maximal graded exercise treadmill test [2]. Assessing differences in thresholds, the role of race was considered negligible due to individual analysis. Nevertheless, this approach might have increased interindividual variability of accelerometer data. However, the generalizability of these findings is limited due to the small number of subjects. Future research should take these limitations into consideration and validate the findings in a larger, more representative sample.

5. Conclusions

Intensity at absolute 3 MET accelerometer cut points was lower compared to the intensity at VT_1 independent of the device or placement in pregnant and nonpregnant women. The application of the individual resting metabolic equivalent results in an approximation to the first ventilatory threshold but does not provide an alternative for individually tailored activity cut points. Using absolute accelerometer cut points, which are independent of the individual performance capacity, can lead to different physiological and metabolic strain at the same absolute intensity, possibly causing under- or overloading for a particular person. Therefore, individual thresholds based on physiological parameters, such as the VT_1, are recommended to quantify the intensity of PA. A short incremental walking test can be a time-efficient method to define these thresholds and, thus, can be used for tailoring accelerometer cut points to individual differences in performance capacity.

Author Contributions: Conceptualization, M.N.M.v.P., P.D., and P.H.; Methodology, P.D., A.M., M.N.M.v.P., and P.H.; Software, M.C.S., J.J., and P.B.; Validation, P.B.; Formal analysis, M.C.S., J.J., and P.B.; investigation, P.D., A.M., E.D.W., G.M., and P.B.; Resources, P.H.; Data curation, G.M. and P.B.; writing—original draft preparation, P.B.; Writing—Review and editing, M.N.M.v.P., P.D., E.D.W., M.C.S., J.J., G.M., and P.H. All authors have read and agreed to the published version of the manuscript.

Funding: This research received no external funding.

Acknowledgments: "Open Access Funding by the University of Graz".

Conflicts of Interest: The authors declare no conflict of interest.

References

1. Sanders, S.G.; Jimenez, E.Y.; Cole, N.H.; Kuhlemeier, A.; McCauley, G.L.; Van Horn, M.L.; Kong, A.S. Estimated Physical Activity in Adolescents by Wrist-Worn GENEActiv Accelerometers. *J. Phys. Act. Health* **2019**, *16*, 792–798. [CrossRef] [PubMed]
2. Siddique, J.; Aaby, D.; Montag, S.E.; Sidney, S.; Sternfeld, B.; Welch, W.A.; Carnethon, M.R.; Liu, K.; Craft, L.L.; Pettee, G.K.; et al. Individualized Relative-Intensity Physical Activity Accelerometer Cut Points. *Med. Sci. Sports Exerc.* **2020**, *52*, 398–407. [CrossRef] [PubMed]
3. De Almeida Mendes, M.; Da Silva, I.C.M.; Ramires, V.V.; Reichert, F.F.; Martins, R.C.; Tomasi, E. Calibration of raw accelerometer data to measure physical activity: A systematic review. *Gait Posture* **2018**, *61*, 98–110. [CrossRef] [PubMed]
4. Jetté, M.; Sidney, K.; Blümchen, G. Metabolic equivalents (METS) in exercise testing, exercise prescription, and evaluation of functional capacity. *Clin. Cardiol.* **1990**, *13*, 555–565. [CrossRef] [PubMed]
5. Hildebrand, M.; VAN Hees, V.T.; Hansen, B.H.; Ekelund, U. Age group comparability of raw accelerometer output from wrist- and hip-worn monitors. *Med. Sci. Sports Exerc.* **2014**, *46*, 1816–1824. [CrossRef] [PubMed]
6. Arvidsson, D.; Fridolfsson, J.; Börjesson, M.; Andersen, L.B.; Ekblom, Ö.; Dencker, M.; Brønd, J.C. Re-examination of accelerometer data processing and calibration for the assessment of physical activity intensity. *Scand. J. Med. Sci. Sports* **2019**, *29*, 1442–1452. [CrossRef]
7. Vähä-Ypyä, H.; Vasankari, T.; Husu, P.; Mänttäri, A.; Vuorimaa, T.; Suni, J.; Sievänen, H. Validation of Cut-Points for Evaluating the Intensity of Physical Activity with Accelerometry-Based Mean Amplitude Deviation (MAD). *PLoS ONE* **2015**, *10*, e0134813. [CrossRef]
8. Kozey, S.; Lyden, K.; Staudenmayer, J.; Freedson, P. Errors in MET estimates of physical activities using 3.5 $ml{\cdot}kg^{-1}{\cdot}min^{-1}$ as the baseline oxygen consumption. *J. Phys. Act. Health* **2010**, *7*, 508–516. [CrossRef]
9. Melzer, K.; Heydenreich, J.; Schutz, Y.; Renaud, A.; Kayser, B.; Mäder, U. Metabolic equivalent in adolescents, active adults and pregnant women. *Nutrients* **2016**, *8*, 438. [CrossRef]
10. Kujala, U.M.; Pietilä, J.; Myllymäki, T.; Mutikainen, S.; Föhr, T.; Korhonen, I.; Helander, E. Physical Activity: Absolute Intensity versus Relative-to-Fitness-Level Volumes. *Med. Sci. Sports Exerc.* **2017**, *49*, 474–481. [CrossRef]
11. Raiber, L.; Christensen, R.A.G.; Randhawa, A.K.; Jamnik, V.K.; Kuk, J.L. Do moderate- to vigorous-intensity accelerometer count thresholds correspond to relative moderate- to vigorous-intensity physical activity? *Appl. Physiol. Nutr. Metab.* **2019**, *44*, 407–413. [CrossRef] [PubMed]

12. Ozemek, C.; Cochran, H.L.; Strath, S.J.; Byun, W.; Kaminsky, L.A. Estimating relative intensity using individualized accelerometer cutpoints: The importance of fitness level. *BMC Med. Res. Methodol.* **2013**, *13*, 53. [CrossRef] [PubMed]
13. ACSM. *ACSM's Guidelines for Exercise Testing and Prescription*, 10th ed.; Lippincot Williams & Wilkins: Philadelphia, PA, USA, 2016; 472p.
14. Hofmann, P.; Tschakert, G. Special needs to prescribe exercise intensity for scientific studies. *Cardiol. Res. Pract.* **2010**, *2011*, 209302. [CrossRef] [PubMed]
15. Scharhag-Rosenberger, F.; Meyer, T.; Gässler, N.; Faude, O.; Kindermann, W. Exercise at given percentages of VO2max: Heterogeneous metabolic responses between individuals. *J. Sci Med. Sport.* **2010**, *13*, 74–79. [CrossRef] [PubMed]
16. Binder, R.K.; Wonisch, M.; Corra, U.; Cohen-Solal, A.; Vanhees, L.; Saner, H.; Schmid, J.-P. Methodological approach to the first and second lactate threshold in incremental cardiopulmonary exercise testing. *Eur. J. Cardiovasc. Prev. Rehabil.* **2008**, *15*, 726–734. [CrossRef]
17. Mezzani, A. Cardiopulmonary exercise testing: Basics of methodology and measurements. *Ann. Am. Thorac. Soc.* **2017**, *14*, 3–11. [CrossRef]
18. Moser, O.; Tschakert, G.; Mueller, A.; Groeschl, W.; Hofmann, P.; Pieber, T.; Lawrence, J.; Koehler, G. Short-Acting Insulin Reduction Strategies for Continuous Cycle Ergometer Exercises in Patients with Type 1 Diabetes Mellitus. *Asian J. Sports Med.* **2017**, *8*, e42160. [CrossRef]
19. Gil-Rey, E.; Maldonado-Martín, S.; Palacios-Samper, N.; Gorostiaga, E.M. Objectively measured absolute and relative physical activity intensity levels in postmenopausal women. *Eur. J. Sport Sci.* **2019**, *19*, 539–548. [CrossRef]
20. Gil-Rey, E.; Maldonado-Martín, S.; Gorostiaga, E.M. Individualized Accelerometer Activity Cut-Points for the Measurement of Relative Physical Activity Intensity Levels. *Res. Q. Exerc. Sport* **2019**, *90*, 327–335. [CrossRef]
21. Bakrania, K.; Yates, T.; Rowlands, A.V.; Esliger, D.W.; Bunnewell, S.; Sanders, J.; Davies, M.; Khunti, K.; Edwardson, C.L. Intensity thresholds on raw acceleration data: Euclidean norm minus one (ENMO) and mean amplitude deviation (MAD) approaches. *PLoS ONE* **2016**, *11*, e0164045. [CrossRef]
22. Garber, C.E.; Blissmer, B.; Deschenes, M.R.; Franklin, B.A.; Lamonte, M.J.; Lee, I.-M.; Nieman, D.C.; Swain, D.P. American College of Sports Medicine position stand. Quantity and quality of exercise for developing and maintaining cardiorespiratory, musculoskeletal, and neuromotor fitness in apparently healthy adults: Guidance for prescribing exercise. *Med. Sci. Sports Exerc.* **2011**, *43*, 1334–1359. [CrossRef] [PubMed]
23. Pokan, R.; Ocenasek, H.; Hochgatterer, R.; Miehl, M.; Vonbank, K.; Von Duvillard, S.P.; Franklin, B.; Würth, S.; Volf, I.; Wonisch, M.; et al. Myocardial dimensions and hemodynamics during 24-h ultraendurance ergometry. *Med. Sci. Sports Exerc.* **2014**, *46*, 268–275. [CrossRef] [PubMed]
24. Tschakert, G.; Hofmann, P. High-Intensity Intermittent Exercise: Methodological and Physiological Aspects. *Int. J. Sports Physiol. Perform.* **2013**, *8*, 600–610. [CrossRef] [PubMed]
25. Sellés Pérez, S.; Fernández-Sáez, J.; Cejuela, R. Polarized and pyramidal training intensity distribution: Relationship with a half-ironman distance triathlon competition. *J. Sport Sci. Med.* **2019**, *18*, 708–715.
26. Rennie, K.L.; Wareham, N.J. The validation of physical activity instruments for measuring energy expenditure: Problems and pitfalls. *Public Health Nutr.* **1998**, *1*, 265–271. [CrossRef]
27. Miller, N.E.; Strath, S.J.; Swartz, A.M.; Cashin, S.E. Estimating absolute and relative physical activity intensity across age via accelerometry in adults. *J. Aging Phys. Act.* **2010**, *18*, 158–170. [CrossRef]
28. Lopes, V.; Magalhães, P.; Bragada, J.; Vasques, C. Actigraph calibration in obese/overweight and type 2 diabetes mellitus middle-aged to old adult patients. *J. Phys. Act. Health* **2009**, *6* (Suppl. 1), S133–S140. [CrossRef]
29. Dishman, R.K.; Sui, X.; Church, T.S.; Kline, C.E.; Youngstedt, S.D.; Blair, S.N. Decline in cardiorespiratory fitness and odds of incident sleep complaints. *Med. Sci. Sports Exerc.* **2015**, *47*, 960–966. [CrossRef]
30. McEligot, A.J.; Mitra, S.; Beam, W. The association between fitness and obesity in diverse multi-ethnic college students. *J. Am. Coll Health* **2020**. Epub ahead of print. [CrossRef]
31. Forczek, W.; Ivanenko, Y.; Salamaga, M.; Sylos-Labini, F.; Frączek, B.; Masłoń, A.; Curylo, M.; Suder, A. Pelvic movements during walking throughout gestation—the relationship between morphology and kinematic parameters. *Clin. Biomech.* **2019**, *71*, 146–151. [CrossRef]
32. Dourado, V.Z.; Banov, M.C.; Marino, M.C.; de Souza, V.L.; Antunes, L.D.O.; McBurnie, M.A. A simple approach to assess VT during a field walk test. *Int. J. Sports Med.* **2010**, *31*, 698–703. [CrossRef] [PubMed]

33. Heydenreich, J.; Schutz, Y.; Melzer, K.; Kayser, B. Comparison of Conventional and Individualized 1-MET Values for Expressing Maximum Aerobic Metabolic Rate and Habitual Activity Related Energy Expenditure. *Nutrients* **2019**, *11*, 458. [CrossRef] [PubMed]
34. Overstreet, B.S.; Bassett, D.R.; Crouter, S.E.; Rider, B.C.; Parr, B.B. Portable open-circuit spirometry systems. *J. Sport Med. Phys. Fit.* **2017**, *57*, 227–237.

International Journal of
Environmental Research and Public Health

MDPI

Article

Soft Tissue Mobilization and Stretching for Shoulder in CrossFitters: A Randomized Pilot Study

Marcos Jusdado-García and Rubén Cuesta-Barriuso *

Department of Physiotherapy, Faculty of Sport Sciences, European University of Madrid, 28670 Madrid, Spain; marcosgarjus@gmail.com
* Correspondence: ruben.cuesta@um.es; Tel.: +34-8688-87286

Abstract: Background. The shoulder in CrossFit should have a balance between mobility and stability. Glenohumeral internal rotation deficit and posterior shoulder stiffness are risk factors for overhead shoulder injury. Objective. To determine the effectiveness of instrument-assisted soft tissue mobilization and horizontal adduction stretch in CrossFit practitioners' shoulders. Methods: Twenty-one regular CrossFitters were allocated to experimental (stretching with isometric contraction and instrument-assisted soft tissue mobilization) or control groups (instrument-assisted soft tissue mobilization). Each session lasted 5 min, 2 days a week, over a period of 4 weeks. Shoulder internal rotation and horizontal adduction (digital inclinometer), as well as posterior shoulder stretch perception (Park scale), were evaluated. Shapiro–Wilk test was used to analyze the distribution of the sample. Parametric Student's *t*-test was used to obtain the intragroup differences. The inter- and intra-rater differences were calculated using a repeated measures analysis of variance (ANOVA). Results. Average age was 30.81 years (SD: 5.35), with an average height of 178 (SD: 7.93) cm and average weight of 82.69 (SD: 10.82) kg. Changes were found in the experimental group following intervention ($p < 0.05$), and when comparing baseline and follow-up assessments ($p < 0.05$) in all variables. Significant differences were found in the control group following intervention ($p < 0.05$), in right horizontal adduction and left internal rotation. When comparing the perception of internal rotation and horizontal adduction in both groups, significant differences were found. Conclusions. Instrument-assisted soft tissue mobilization can improve shoulder horizontal adduction and internal rotation. An instrument-assisted soft tissue mobilization technique yields the same results alone as those achieved in combination with post-isometric stretch with shoulder adduction.

Keywords: instrument-assisted soft tissue mobilization; muscle stretching exercises; range of motion; manual therapy

Citation: Jusdado-García, M.; Cuesta-Barriuso, R. Soft Tissue Mobilization and Stretching for Shoulder in CrossFitters: A Randomized Pilot Study. *Int. J. Environ. Res. Public Health* **2021**, *18*, 575. https://doi.org/10.3390/ijerph18020575

Received: 10 December 2020
Accepted: 8 January 2021
Published: 12 January 2021

1. Introduction

CrossFit is a physical fitness system featuring the performance of a wide variety of exercises covering sports disciplines (weightlifting, powerlifting, and gymnastics) in addition to activities such as running, rowing, or cycling. Workouts are combined with little or no rest, involving high-intensity training [1].

With regard to the incidence of injuries in the practice of CrossFit, there is a scarce amount of data published in the literature [2], with an estimated rate of 3.1 injuries per 1000 h of training. This prevalence is similar to that found in sports such as weightlifting, gymnastics, and rugby (3–3.3/1000 h). The prevalence of musculoskeletal injury was 24.0%, and the most affected regions of the body were the lumbar spine, shoulders, and knees [3].

CrossFit is an overhead sport, in which many of the movements are performed above the head, as in other sports such as baseball, volleyball, or tennis. However, unlike these, the burden does not rest exclusively on the dominant upper limb, but is shared between the two extremities [3]. This sport requires a sufficiently lax shoulder to be able to reach extreme positions of movement above the head, but with enough stability to prevent luxation.

CrossFit performance is thus associated with different power-, strength-, and aerobic-related markers [4]. In most CrossFit exercises, athletes not only have to lift or throw an external load, but also their own body mass. For this reason—as in other sports—trying to reach a balance between maximum strength and body mass will be of paramount importance [5].

Training more than four days a week and not receiving regular physiotherapeutic care were associated with CrossFit-related musculoskeletal injuries [3]. The high incidence of injury in the shoulder joint is due to various etiological factors. In Olympic lifting (typically in weightlifting) and gymnastics movements, the shoulders need to reach extreme positions of flexion, adduction, external rotation, and internal shoulder and elbow extension is required. These movements occur when the head is placed under the bar in Olympic lifts and kipping pull-ups in gymnastics, in this case, using the moment of inertia below the bar in the performance of chin-ups or similar exercises [1]. These movements are performed through a series with long reps and using large weights at high intensity, which can lead to muscle fatigue, poor technique, and an alteration in shoulder joint alignment [6].

The stability of the glenohumeral joint depends, to a great extent, on its active stability. Muscle fatigue, caused by repetitive high-intensity exercises in CrossFit, can have a detrimental effect on the activity and muscle response in these athletes. This muscle alteration caused by fatigue produces a decrease of the dynamic joint stability; a poorer technique; and, as a result, a greater likelihood of injury [1].

Most injuries in CrossFit occur as a result of repetitive strain, implying an extended process in time, which can lead to a higher prevalence of injury. Athletes acquire adaptations from the sport itself, including alterations in strength, flexibility, and posture, which induce changes in the biomechanics and movement patterns [7]. Therefore, overhead athletes are participant to the risk of injury in the shoulder joint due to overuse, such as deficient glenohumeral internal rotation and total rotation, deficit of strength in the rotator cuff, and scapular dyskinesia. The most common biomechanics adaptation is posterior stiffness of the shoulder, causing a decreased horizontal adduction of the shoulder and reduced mobility in internal rotation, causing capsular tightness, and muscle spasm. In the same way, posterior shoulder stiffness, therefore, has been suggested to be a causative or perpetuating factor in shoulder impingement and labral pathology [7].

Soft tissue mobilization techniques [8] can increase internal rotation and horizontal adduction movements of the shoulder [9] and the range of knee and hip motion affecting quadriceps and hamstrings [10,11]. It has been reported [12] that these techniques can reduce rotator cuff stiffness to improve the range of motion, as well as reduce the pain threshold of an active and musculoskeletal movement [9,13]. In the same way, soft tissue mobilization techniques may have an inhibitory effect on hyperactive muscles, thus favoring intermuscular balance [14].

The current literature provides support for instrument-assisted soft tissue mobilization (IASTM) in improving the range of motion (ROM) in uninjured individuals as well as pain and patient-reported function (or both) in injured patients [15]. Horizontal adduction shoulder stretch or post-isometric cross-body stretch can improve the range of motion in horizontal adduction and the glenohumeral internal rotation [16], by decreasing the posterior stiffness of the shoulder [17]. Moreover, IASTM appeared to be effective in yielding short-term improvements in shoulder horizontal adduction and internal rotation among uninjured participants [12]. It is recommended to perform stretching by stabilizing the scapula to decrease infraspinatus stiffness and avoid subacromial impingement [18].

The hypothesis of this study was that an intervention using instrument-assisted soft tissue mobilization and horizontal adduction shoulder produces improvements in the mobility of internal rotation and horizontal adduction of the shoulder, as well as the perception of stretching of the back of the shoulder in CrossFitters.

The aim of this study is to evaluate the effectiveness of a physical therapy intervention through instrument-assisted soft tissue mobilization and horizontal adduction shoulder stretches in CrossFitters aged from 18 to 40 years.

2. Materials and Methods

2.1. Study Design and Approvals

Randomized, single-blind pilot study was conducted with CrossFit athletes from the gym Acero CrossFit, located in the city of Toledo (Spain). The study compared clinical outcome after instrument-assisted soft tissue mobilization techniques and post-isometric horizontal adduction stretches or underwent soft tissue mobilization with 21 athletes randomised to each intervention type.

The study was registered at www.clinicaltrials.gov (NCT03830346.). This study has been approved by the Research Committee of the European University of Madrid (registration no.: CIPI/18/033). Prior to the commencement of the study, all the participants selected signed an informed consent document, as defined by the Helsinki Rules.

2.2. Study Population

We calculated the sample size needed for this study (effect size = 0.25 (medium), α error = 0.05, power = 0.8) using the G*power software (Version 3.1., Heinrich Heine University, Duesseldorf, Germany). The effect size used herein was in accordance with a previous study [19]. The results showed that 18 participants were required. Given the likelihood of dropouts during the study, a total of 24 participants were recruited, of which 21 met the selection criteria and were included in the study. The athletes were invited (in February) to participate in the study. The study period was from January to June 2018.

The inclusion criteria to participate in the study were as follows: participants of both sexes, being regular CrossFitters (workouts at least two days a week), and in the age range of 18 to 40 years. On the other hand, participants excluded were those who had suffered a shoulder injury in the 3 months prior to the study, had undergone shoulder surgery in the previous six months, had a non-attendance rate of over 15% of the intervention sessions (2 sessions), and had not signed the informed consent document.

2.3. Randomisation

Participants who met the selection criteria, and after signing the informed consent document, were randomly assigned by the opaque envelope system to each study group: experimental group (n = 11) and control (n = 10). Participants were randomly allocated by a person not involved in the study.

2.4. Outcome Evaluation

Three dependent variables were evaluated: mobility of internal rotation and horizontal adduction of the shoulder, and the perception of stretching of the back of the shoulder in each movement.

The assessment of the internal rotation and horizontal adduction of the shoulder was performed according to the protocol described by Laudner et al. [20]. In order to measure the internal rotation of the shoulder, the patient was placed in the supine position on the stretcher with the arm to be assessed at 90 degrees shoulder adduction, 90 degrees elbow flexion, and with the elbow at the height of the acromion with a towel. By stabilizing the scapula at the acromion, the shoulder was taken at a maximum range of internal rotation. The range of motion was measured with a digital inclinometer, model Tacklife MDP01. The angle of the edge of the ulna coincided with a line perpendicular to the stretcher. For horizontal adduction, the arm was placed in the same initial position in neutral rotation and, while stabilizing the lateral edge of the scapula, the arm was adducted to its maximum range of motion. The angle between the line of the ventral edge of the humerus and a line perpendicular to the stretcher was measured with the inclinometer. Intraclass correlation coefficient and standard error of measurement values were 0.93 and 1.6° for passive Glenohumeral (GH) horizontal adduction ROM and 0.98 and 2.0° for internal rotation ROM, respectively.

To assess the perception of stretch, the scale described by Park et al. [21] was used. This 11-point scale evaluates the discomfort from least to most, asking each participant to define the level of discomfort in the back of the shoulder in the maximum range of motion of internal rotation and horizontal adduction of the shoulder. Intraclass correlation coefficient for this scale was 0.97 (95% confidence interval (CI) = 0.96 to 0.98).

The main anthropometric independent variables were collected (height, weight, and body mass index), as well as sociodemographic variables (sex, age, profession, experience, weekly training sessions, duration of training, competition, and so on).

Three assessments were carried out in this study: prior to intervention (T0), following intervention (T1), and after a 4-week follow-up period (T2). Another physical therapist oversaw conducting the three study assessments, blinded with respect to participant allocation to each study group. All assessments were carried out following the same protocol and under the same conditions.

2.5. Intervention

Each session lasted 2 to 5 min, 2 days a week, over a period of 4 weeks, prior to each workout. In the experimental group, instrument-assisted soft tissue mobilization techniques and post-isometric horizontal adduction stretches were performed, while the control group only underwent soft tissue mobilization.

The soft tissue mobilization techniques were applied with the participant in prone position, as described by Laudner et al. [20]. The technique lasted 20 s in a parallel direction and 20 s in a perpendicular direction on the posterior shoulder and scapula muscles. While the dominant hand was used to hold the instrument, the other hand was used to tighten the skin medially to ensure an even area of treatment (Figure 1).

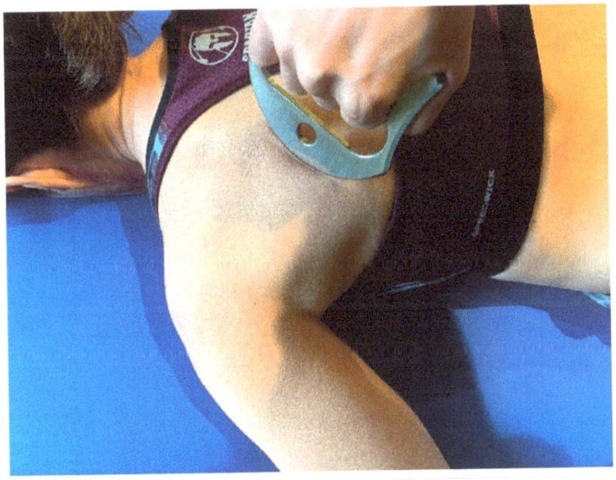

Figure 1. Soft tissue mobilization techniques in prone position.

The post-isometric horizontal adduction stretch was carried out according to the protocol by Moore et al. [22] in the movement evaluation position described by Laudner et al. [20] with the participant in the supine position, passively adducting the arm horizontally until the first motion barrier and performing active horizontal adduction for 5 s at 25% of force. The arm was then taken to the new motion barrier, repeating this process three times.

2.6. Statistics

Sample distribution analysis was performed using the Shapiro–Wilk test. The differences between the three assessments were analyzed, in each group, for the different variables using the non-parametric Wilcoxon test. An analysis of variance (ANOVA) of repeated measures was carried out to compare the experimental and control groups at the three assessment times: baseline (T0), posttreatment (T1), and follow-up (T2). The results of the F test depend on whether the Mauchly spherical test was significant or not. If significant, the Greenhouse–Geisser correction was used. Bonferroni correction has been applied to control the error rate of the significance level. When the interaction was significant, pairwise comparison tests were performed on the group. The partial eta-squared value was calculated as an indicator of effect size (classified as small 0.01, medium 0.06, and large 0.14) [23]. An analysis by intention to treat was conducted. The level of significance of the study was estimated at 95%.

3. Results

During the study and follow-up, none of the participants included in the experimental group (n = 11) or control group (n = 10) dropped out. Figure 2 shows the flowchart of the research study.

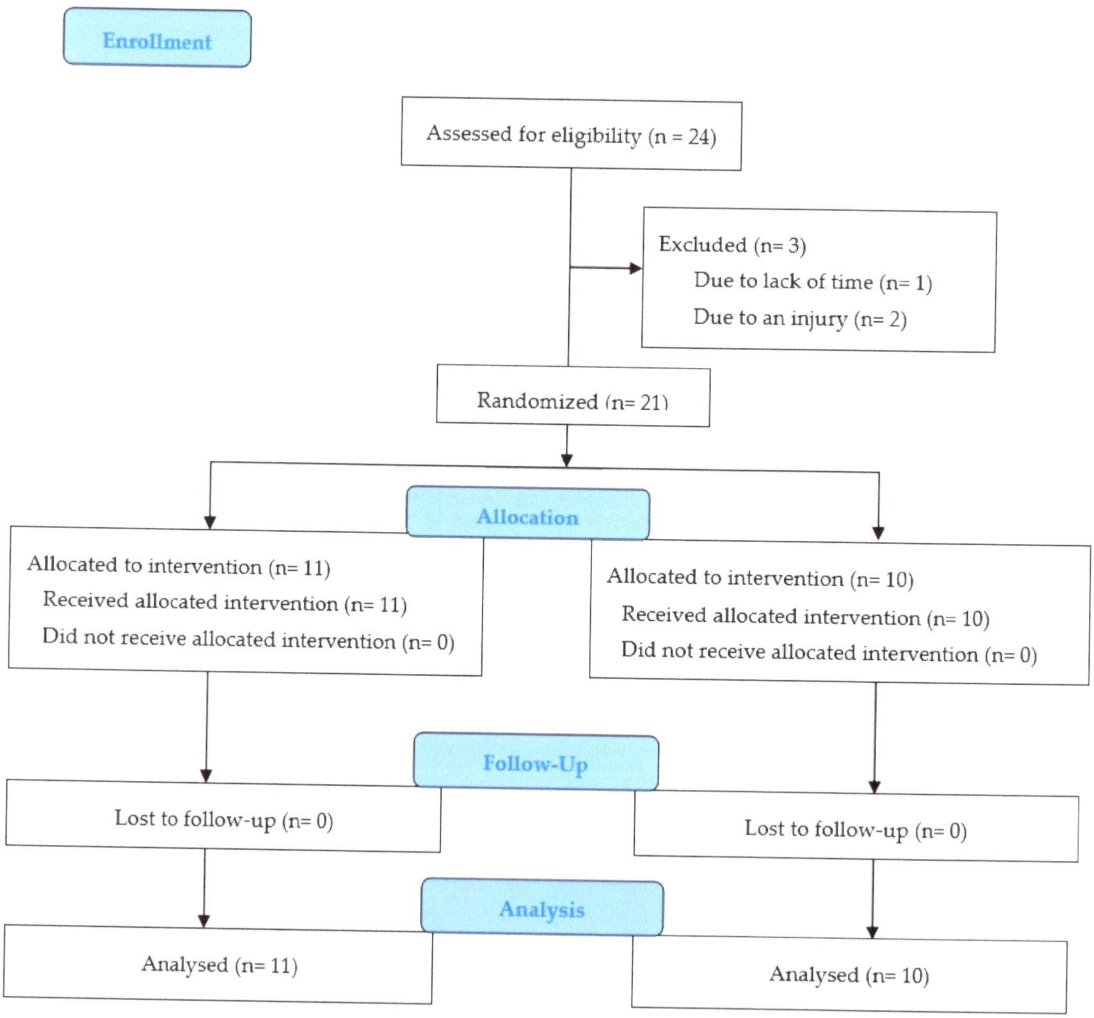

Figure 2. CONSORT 2010 flow diagram.

The average age of the 21 participants included in the study was 30.81 years (SD: 5.35), with an average height of 178 (SD: 7.93) cm, an average weight of 82.69 (SD: 10.82) kg, and a mean body mass index of 25.98 (SD: 3.04) kg/m^2. The mean of weekly training sessions was 4.1, with an average session duration of 82 min, and the length of time since initiating in the practice of CrossFit being 29.38 months on average. Furthermore, 90.5% of participants were males, and only 28.6% of the participants had ever competed. Although the pretreatment assessment revealed no differences ($p > 0.05$) in anthropometric variables and internal rotation and horizontal adduction movements, all other independent variables and the measurements of perception of stretching of all movements showed differences ($p < 0.05$) between the two groups. The description of the whole sample, and according to the group, is shown in Table 1.

Table 1. Descriptive characteristics of all patients mean (and standard deviation) at baseline and in each group of the study.

Psychometric Variables	All Sample		Experimental Group		Control Group		Sig.
Age (years)	30.81 (5.35)		31.45 (6.02)		30.10 (4.72)		0.16 [a]
Height (cm)	178.33 (7.93)		178.27 (9.07)		175.36 (7.68)		0.14 [a]
Weight (kg)	82.69 (10.82)		81.82 (12.18)		70.93 (11.81)		0.48 [a]
Body mass index (kg/m^2)	25.98 (3.04)		25.60 (2.29)		22.92 (2.44)		0.06 [a]
Clinical variables							
Time practicing CrossFit (months) *	29.38 (20.69)		41 (19.32)		16.6 (13.81)		0.02 [a]
Training per week (days) *	4.1 (1.22)		4.73 (0.90)		3.40 (1.17)		0.03 [a]
Time per training (minutes) *	82.14 (28.31)		91.36 (28.81)		72 (25.29)		0.00 [a]
Sociodemographic variables	*n*	%	*n*	%	*n*	%	
Gender (Male/Female)	19/2	90.5/9.5	10/1	90.9/9.1	9/1	90/10	0.78 [b]
Participation in competition (Yes/No) *	6/15	28.6/71.4	4/7	36.4/63.6	2/8	20/80	0.04 [b]

M: mean; SD: standard deviation; *n*: number of participants; %: percentage; Sig.: significance. [a] Shapiro–Wilks test. [b] Fisher exact test. * Significant difference ($p < 0.05$).

Table 2 shows the statistical analysis of the dependent variables of the study at baseline, post-treatment, and follow-up assessment. The experimental group revealed changes in all variables ($p < 0.001$) after the intervention. When comparing T0 and T2 assessments, we found improvements in all variables ($p < 0.01$) The calculation of the effect size in the post-treatment results produced high values (d > 0.80) in all variables, except perception of left internal rotation (d = −0.58) and perception of left horizontal adduction (d = −0.80). Similarly, the effect size obtained after follow-up period was high (d > 0.80) in range of motion variables, and moderate (range: −0.58 to −0.75) in the other variables.

Table 2. Statistical analysis and median (and interquartile range) of the dependent variables of the study at baseline, post-treatment, and follow-up assessment.

Variables	Experimental Group			Control Group		
	T0	T1	T2	T0	T1	T2
Right internal rotation	36.4 (18.0)	51.1 (11.8)	48.5 (12.0)	38.65 (15.8)	44.00 (16.4)	55.90 (10.8)
Perception of right internal rotation	3.00 (2.0)	2.00 (1.0)	2.00 (1.0)	1.00 (1.5)	2.00 (2.2)	3.00 (2.7)
Right horizontal adduction	12.2 (12.0)	19.2 (4.0)	19.1 (5.0)	12.9 (10.2)	16.85 (7.1)	16.80 (17.1)
Perception of right horizontal adduction	3.00 (2.0)	2.00 (2.0)	2.00 (1.0)	2.00 (3.0)	2.00 (0.25)	3.00 (1.0)
Left internal rotation	38.5 (13.1)	43.9 (15.8)	54.8 (5.5)	44.15 (23.4)	50.45 (10.1)	58.35 (12.0)
Perception of left internal rotation	3.00 (4.0)	2.00 (3.0)	2.00 (4.0)	2.00 (2.25)	3.00 (1.5)	2.50 (2.2)
Left horizontal adduction	15.7 (6.9)	20.30 (4.8)	21.5 (9.3)	11.90 (5.9)	16.05 (9.1)	22.45 (13.4)
Perception of left horizontal adduction	4.00 (1.0)	2.00 (2.0)	2.00 (2.0)	2.50 (3.0)	2.50 (3.0)	2.50 (3.0)

Outcome measures at the baseline (T0), after the four-week period of soft tissue mobilization and control interventions (T1), and after a further four weeks as follow-up (T2).

Differences were found ($p < 0.01$) in the control group between T0 and T1 assessments in right horizontal adduction and left internal rotation. When comparing T0 and T2 assessments, we found improvements in five variables: right internal rotation, perception of right internal rotation, right horizontal adduction left internal rotation, and left horizontal adduction ($p < 0.01$). The effect size obtained after the follow-up period was high (d > 0.80) in range of motion variables and perception of right internal rotation (d = 1.67). Table 3 shows the main statistics of the three assessments performed in the two groups.

Table 3. Mean difference and changes (and effect size) after post-treatment and follow-up period of the dependent variables of the study with non-parametric Wilcoxon test.

Variables	Experimental Group		Control Group	
	T0–T1	T0–T2	T0–T1	T0–T2
Right internal rotation	−13.87 (1.07) *	−16.58 (1.28) *	−3.88 (0.33)	−14.90 (1.29) *
Perception of right internal rotation	1.27 (−0.81) **	1.00 (−0.64) *	−0.90 (0.83)	−1.80 (1.67) *
Right horizontal adduction	−6.79 (1.21) **	−6.93 (1.23) **	−3.16 (0.46) *	−6.13 (0.89) *
Perception of right horizontal adduction	2.00 (−0.86) **	1.45 (−0.62) **	0.10 (−0.06)	−0.20 (0.12)
Left internal rotation	−12.05 (1.47) **	−18.25 (−6.56) **	−8.77 (0.54) *	−13.48 (0.83) *
Perception of left internal rotation	1.36 (−0.58) **	1.36 (−0.58) **	−0.800 (0.38)	−0.900 (0.42)
Left horizontal adduction	−4.40 (1.20) **	−6.03 (1.64) **	−4.01 (0.65)	−9.27 (1.51) *
Perception of left horizontal adduction	1.63 (−0.80) **	1.54 (−0.75) **	0.10 (−0.04)	−0.30 (0.14)

Outcome measures at the baseline (T0), after the four-week period of treatment and control interventions (T1), and after a further four weeks as follow-up (T2). * Significant difference between improvements of the study groups ($p < 0.01$). ** Significant difference between improvements of the study groups ($p < 0.001$).

There were differences between the three evaluations in the perception of stretch in all motions; however, no differences were found in the group interaction in terms of range of motion. No significant difference was reported in dependent variables, upon comparing the three assessments (T0, T1, and T2). Table 4 shows the results of the repeated measures analysis including baseline (T0), T1, and T2 assessments.

Table 4. Statistical analysis of repeated measures of the dependent variables in the three study assessments.

Variables	Intra-Group Effect			Inter-Group Effect		
	F	Sig.	η^2_p	F	Sig.	η^2_p
Right internal rotation [a]	0.53	0.59	0.02	0.87	0.36	0.04
Perception of right internal rotation [a]	8.38	0.00 *	0.30	0.08	0.77	0.01
Right horizontal adduction [a]	2.02	0.15	0.09	0.20	0.65	0.01
Perception of right horizontal adduction [a]	8.49	0.01 *	0.30	0.13	0.71	0.01
Left internal rotation [a]	1.46	0.24	0.07	0.68	0.41	0.03
Perception of left internal rotation [a]	3.70	0.04 *	0.16	0.02	0.86	0.01
Left horizontal adduction [a]	1.56	0.22	0.07	0.01	0.89	0.00
Perception of left horizontal adduction	4.98	0.01 *	0.20	1.11	0.30	0.05

Sig.: significance; η^2_p: partial Eta-squared. [a] the df corresponds to Greenhouse–Geisser test. * Interaction with the group ($p < 0.05$).

4. Discussion

The study examined the effectiveness of instrument-assisted soft tissue mobilization and post-isometric horizontal adduction stretches in CrossFitters. The results of this study support the assumption that this intervention may have a positive effect on range of motion and perception of stretch. The high effect size found after post-treatment and follow-up assessments indicates a high power of the results. These data suggest that the application of instrument-assisted soft tissue mobilization techniques and post-isometric horizontal adduction stretches can generate improvements after 4 weeks of intervention that are maintained after 4 weeks of follow-up.

CrossFit is a highly popular conditioning program combining elements of strength, coordination, balance, and mobility. It represents one of the most common examples of high-intensity interval training [24] However, there are no clinical studies on CrossFitters comparable to our study. This absence of scientific evidence complicates the possibility of comparing results in similar samples, although the techniques used have already been used in other studies. Laudner et al. [20] observed improvements in baseball players in range of motion in horizontal adduction and internal rotation of the dominant shoulder, through a single application of instrument-assisted mobilization, without assessing whether the improvements were maintained over time. Despite involving different populations and not being comparable, our study included 39 shoulders, observing an improvement that is maintained even after 4 weeks.

The literature suggests that IASTM is effective in increasing acute shoulder ROM in overhead athletes with asymptomatic ROM deficiency. The lack of a standardized IASTM treatment protocol in the current research presents a limitation to utilize it in clinical practice [12]. McMurray et al. [25] reported that treatment sessions usually last approximately 5–6 min per treatment region.

McClure et al. [26] noted, after 4 weeks of intervention, how cross-body stretches in asymptomatic participants were more effective than sleeper stretches commonly used in the improvement of horizontal adduction and internal rotation of the shoulder. Similarly, Manske et al. [27] showed how cross-body stretches with joint mobilization were more effective than stretching alone in the improvement of range of motion in internal rotation in asymptomatic participants. Our study includes this technique, where the interventions were carried out before the training session, with the goal of providing CrossFitters with that range of motion for their exercises, and thus be able to perpetuate the effect of the intervention. Moreover, the improvement observed in the study prior [27] is maintained in our results in terms of shoulder ROM.

Bailey et al. [28] evaluated the effectiveness of cross-body and sleeper self-stretches both alone and combined with instrument-assisted soft tissue mobilization, with each intervention lasting 4 min, noting how the group treated with soft tissue mobilization improved internal rotation and horizontal adduction of the shoulder. Our study found improvements in both movements, with special significance for horizontal adduction. However, our intervention protocol included shorter application times. Thus, it can be established that shorter treatment times, as shown in our study, produce improvements after 4 weeks of intervention, and that these are maintained over time.

The study findings show that the time needed for treatment in shoulder movement restriction can be reduced. By applying a soft tissue mobilization technique for 40 s, instead of over a minute and a half stretch per shoulder, the time of treatment is reduced by almost three quarters. The use of this protocol as a preventive measure of shoulder injuries would be desirable in CrossFit participants favoring an improved mobility.

Study limitations include the low sample size, although no participant dropped out of the study. To address this limitation, the values of effect size were calculated to observe the statistical power of the results in our sample. A larger team of researchers would have been desirable to facilitate the process of intervention and evaluation. Finally, the completion of the three assessments on the same day of the week and at the same time could provide different results to those found in this study.

The current review highlights three important factors associated with injury incidence and incidence rates in CrossFit: training frequency, duration of CrossFit experience, and individuals that compete in CrossFit competitions [29]. Future research should include a larger sample size, with the sample being homogeneous. In addition, more dependent variables such as muscle strength of the shoulder should be assessed.

5. Conclusions

The instrument-assisted soft tissue mobilization technique with post-isometric horizontal adduction stretches may improve the range of motion of the shoulder. These improvements can be maintained for up to four weeks. A protocol that includes an instrument-assisted soft tissue mobilization technique can improve horizontal adduction and internal rotation. Better results would potentially be attainable by adding the horizontal adduction shoulder stretch technique. Instrument-assisted soft tissue mobilization has no adverse effects or complications in asymptomatic participants.

Author Contributions: Conceptualization, M.J.-G. and R.C.-B.; methodology, M.J.-G. and R.C.-B.; software, R.C.-B.; validation, M.J.-G.; formal analysis, M.J.-G. and R.C.-B.; investigation, M.J.-G. and R.C.-B.; resources, M.J.-G.; data curation, M.J.-G.; writing—original draft preparation, M.J.-G. and R.C.-B.; writing—review and editing, R.C.-B.; visualization, M.J.-G. and R.C.-B.; supervision, M.J.-G. and R.C.-B.; project administration, M.J.-G. and R.C.-B. All authors have read and agreed to the published version of the manuscript.

Funding: This research received no external funding.

Institutional Review Board Statement: The study was conducted according to the guidelines of the Declaration of Helsinki and approved by the Institutional Ethics Committee of European University of Madrid (protocol code CIPI/18/033 on 9 February 2018).

Informed Consent Statement: Informed consent was obtained from all subjects involved in the study.

Acknowledgments: The author thanks the owners of AceroCrossFit Toledo for putting their facilities and customers at our full disposal for the study. Further, many thanks to Manuel Garcia for his essential collaboration as rater.

Conflicts of Interest: The authors declare no conflict of interest.

References

1. Durkalec-Michalski, K.; Nowaczyk, P.; Siedzik, K. Effect of a four-week ketogenic diet on exercise metabolism in CrossFit-trained athletes. *J. Int. Soc. Sports Nutr.* **2019**, *16*, 16. [CrossRef] [PubMed]
2. Klimek, C.; Ashbeck, C.; Brook, A.J.; Durall, C. Are Injuries More Common with Crossfit Training than other Forms of Exercise? *J. Sport Rehabil.* **2018**, *27*, 295–299. [CrossRef] [PubMed]
3. Lima, P.O.; Souza, M.B.; Sampaio, T.V.; Almeida, G.P.; Oliveira, R.R. Epidemiology and associated factors for CrossFit-related musculoskeletal injuries: A cross-sectional study. *J. Sports Med. Phys. Fitness* **2020**, *60*, 889–894. [CrossRef] [PubMed]
4. Martínez-Gómez, R.; Valenzuela, P.L.; Alejo, L.B.; Gil-Cabrera, J.; Montalvo-Pérez, A.; Talavera, E.; Lucia, A.; Moral-González, S.; Barranco-Gil, D. Physiological Predictors of Competition Performance in CrossFit Athletes. *Int. J. Environ. Res. Public Health* **2020**, *17*, 3699. [CrossRef]
5. Andersen, E.; Lockie, R.; Dawes, J.J. Relationship of Absolute and Relative Lower-Body Strength to Predictors of Athletic Performance in Collegiate Women Soccer Players. *Sports* **2018**, *6*, 106. [CrossRef]
6. Hak, P.; Hodzovic, E.; Hickey, B. The nature and prevalence of injury during CrossFit training. *J. Strength Cond. Res.* **2013**. [CrossRef]
7. Cools, A.M.; Johansson, F.R.; Borms, D.; Maenhout, A. Prevention of shoulder injuries in overhead athletes: A science-based approach. *Braz. J. Phys. Ther.* **2015**, *19*, 331–339. [CrossRef]
8. Cheatham, S.W.; Lee, M.; Cain, M.; Baker, R. The efficacy of instrument assisted soft tissue mobilization: A systematic review. *J. Can. Chiropr. Assoc.* **2016**, *60*, 200–211.
9. Coviello, J.P.; Kakar, R.S.; Reynolds, T.J. Short-term effects of instrument-assisted soft tissue mobilization on pain free range of motion in a weightlifter with subacromial pain syndrome. *Int. J. Sports Phys. Ther.* **2017**, *12*, 144–154.
10. Baker, R.T.; Hansberger, B.L.; Warren, L.; Nasypany, A. A novel approach for the reversal of chronic apparent hamstring tightness: A case report. *Int. J. Sports Phys. Ther.* **2015**, *10*, 723–733.
11. Markovic, G. Acute effects of instrument assisted soft tissue mobilization vs. foam rolling on knee and hip range of motion in soccer players. *J. Bodyw. Mov. Ther.* **2015**, *19*, 690–696. [CrossRef] [PubMed]
12. Bailey, L.B.; Shanley, E.; Hawkins, R.; Beattie, P.F.; Fritz, S.; Kwartowitz, D.; Thigpen, C.A. Mechanisms of Shoulder Range of Motion Deficits in Asymptomatic Baseball Players. *Am. J. Sports Med.* **2015**, *43*, 2783–2793. [CrossRef] [PubMed]
13. Kim, J.; Sung, D.J.; Lee, J. Therapeutic effectiveness of instrument-assisted soft tissue mobilization for soft tissue injury: Mechanisms and practical application. *J. Exerc. Rehabil.* **2017**, *13*, 12–22. [CrossRef] [PubMed]
14. Lee, J.J.; Lee, J.J.; Kim, D.H.; Hyun You, S.J. Inhibitory effects of instrument-assisted neuromobilization on hyperactive gastrocnemius in a hemiparetic stroke patient. *Bio. Med. Mater. Eng.* **2014**, *24*, 2389–2394. [CrossRef]
15. Seffrin, C.B.; Cattano, N.M.; Reed, M.A.; Gardiner-Shires, A.M. Instrument-Assisted Soft Tissue Mobilization: A Systematic Review and Effect-Size Analysis. *J. Athl. Train.* **2019**, *54*, 808–821. [CrossRef]
16. Yamauchi, T.; Hasegawa, S.; Nakamura, M.; Ishishita, S.; Yanase, K.; Fujita, K.; Umehara, J.; Ji, X.; Ibuki, S.; Ichihashi, N. Effects of two stretching methods on shoulder range of motion and muscle stiffness in baseball players with posterior shoulder tightness: A randomized controlled trial. *J. Shoulder Elbow Surg.* **2016**, *25*, 1395–1403. [CrossRef]
17. Mine, K.; Nakayama, T.; Milanese, S.; Grimmer, K. Effectiveness of Stretching on Posterior Shoulder Tightness and Glenohumeral Internal-Rotation Deficit: A Systematic Review of Randomized Controlled Trials. *J. Sport Rehabil.* **2017**, *26*, 294–305. [CrossRef]
18. Umehara, J.; Hasegawa, S.; Nakamura, M.; Nishishita, S.; Umegaki, H.; Tanaka, H.; Fujita, K.; Kusano, K.; Ichihashi, N. Effect of scapular stabilization during cross-body stretch on the hardness of infraspinatus, teres minor, and deltoid muscles: An ultrasonic shear wave elastography study. *Musculoskelet. Sci. Pract.* **2017**, *27*, 91–96. [CrossRef]

19. Umehara, J.; Ikezoe, T.; Nishishita, S.; Nakamura, M.; Umegaki, H.; Kobayashi, T.; Fujita, K.; Ichihashi, N. Effect of hip and knee position on tensor fasciae latae elongation during stretching: An ultrasonic shear wave elastography study. *Clin. Biomech.* **2015**, *30*, 1056–1059. [CrossRef]
20. Laudner, K.; Compton, B.D.; McLoda, T.A.; Walters, C.M. Acute effects of instrument assisted soft tissue mobilization for improving posterior shoulder range of motion in collegiate baseball players. *Int. J. Sports Phys. Ther.* **2014**, *9*, 1–7.
21. Park, K.N.; Kwon, O.Y.; Weon, J.H.; Choung, S.S.; Kim, S.H. Comparison of the effects of local cryotherapy and passive cross-body stretch on extensibility in subjects with posterior shoulder tightness. *J. Sports Sci. Med.* **2014**, *13*, 84–90. [PubMed]
22. Moore, S.D.; Laudner, K.G.; McLoda, T.A.; Shaffer, M.A. The immediate effects of muscle energy technique on posterior shoulder tightness: A randomized controlled trial. *J. Orthop. Sports Phys. Ther.* **2011**, *41*, 400–407. [CrossRef]
23. Pallant, J. *SPSS Survival Manual*, 6th ed.; McGraw-Hill Education: New York, NY, USA, 2016.
24. Meyer, J.; Morrison, J.; Zuniga, J. The benefits and risks of CrossFit: A systematic review. *Workplace Health Saf.* **2017**, *65*, 612–618. [CrossRef]
25. McMurray, J.; Landis, S.; Lininger, K.; Baker, R.T.; Nasypany, A.; Seegmiller, J. A comparison and review of indirect myofascial release therapy, instrument assisted soft tissue mobilization, and active release techniques to inform clinical decision making. *Int. J. Athl. Ther. Train.* **2015**, *20*, 29–34. [CrossRef]
26. McClure, P.; Balaicuis, J.; Heiland, D.; Broersma, M.E.; Thorndike, C.K.; Wood, A. A randomized controlled comparison of stretching procedures for posterior shoulder tightness. *J. Orthop. Sports Phys. Ther.* **2007**, *37*, 108–114. [CrossRef]
27. Manske, R.C.; Meschke, M.; Porter, A.; Smith, B.; Reiman, M. A randomized controlled single-blinded comparison of stretching versus stretching and joint mobilization for posterior shoulder tightness measured by internal rotation motion loss. *Sports Health* **2010**, *2*, 94–100. [CrossRef] [PubMed]
28. Bailey, L.B.; Thigpen, C.A.; Hawkins, R.J.; Beattie, P.F.; Shanley, E. Effectiveness of Manual Therapy and Stretching for Baseball Players With Shoulder Range of Motion Deficits. *Sports Health* **2017**, *9*, 230–237. [CrossRef]
29. Gardiner, B.; Devereux, G.; Beato, M. Injury risk and injury incidence rates in CrossFit. *J. Sports Med. Phys. Fitness* **2020**, *60*, 1005–1013. [CrossRef]

International Journal of *Environmental Research and Public Health*

MDPI

Article

The Validation of Direct and Meta Versions of the Coach–Athlete Relationship Questionnaire (ArCART-Q) in the Arabic Language: Their Relationship to Athlete's Satisfaction with Individual Performance

Hasan Ahmad [1,*], Elif Nilay Ada [2], Sophia Jowett [3], Kholoud Alabduljader [1] and Zişan Kazak [4]

1 The College of Basic Education, The Public Authority for Applied Education and Training, Al Adiliya Area, Kuwait City 13092, Kuwait; Kholoud911@gmail.com
2 Faculty of Sport Sciences, Mersin University, Mersin 33343, Turkey; elifnilayada@gmail.com
3 School of Sport, Exercise and Health Sciences, Loughborough University, Loughborough LE11 3TT, UK; S.Jowett@lboro.ac.uk
4 Faculty of Sport Sciences, Ege University, Bornova, Izmir 35040, Turkey; f.zisan.kazak@gmail.com
* Correspondence: dr.hasanattiya@gmail.com

Abstract: Background: The first aim of this study is to achieve validation of the direct and meta-perspective versions of the Coach–Athlete Relationship Questionnaire in the Arabic language, and the second aim of this study is to determine the quality of the coach-athlete relationship to athlete' satisfaction with individual performance according to sport participation type, sport duration, and sport achievement. **Methods**: A total of 259 athletes with a mean age of 22 years were recruited from various athletic clubs in Kuwait. Participants completed The Coach–Athlete Relationship Questionnaire and The Athlete Satisfaction Questionnaire. For this study, the factorial structure of the Arabic version of the Coach–Athlete Relationship Questionnaire (CART-Q) was used in Kuwait and was prepared with both direct and meta perspectives. **Results**: The results of this study show evidence of the validity of the direct and meta-perspective Arabic versions of the CART-Q. The fit indices of the data collected by direct-method were as follows ($x^2/df = 2.21$; RMSEA = 0.06; CFI = 0.98; GFI = 0.95; AGFI = 0.91); data for the meta-method were as follows ($x^2/df = 2.32$; RMSEA = 0.08; CFI = 0.99; GFI = 0.93; AGFI = 0.87). Female participants have obtained higher means than males from all questionnaires. **Conclusions**: The results of the present study could help coaches and athletes from the Middle East to understand the reasons and methods that lead to a quality coach–athlete relationship.

Keywords: coach–athlete relationship; validation; satisfaction

Citation: Ahmad, H.; Ada, E.N.; Jowett, S.; Alabduljader, K.; Kazak, Z. The Validation of Direct and Meta Versions of the Coach–Athlete Relationship Questionnaire (ArCART-Q) in the Arabic Language: Their Relationship to Athlete's Satisfaction with Individual Performance. *Int. J. Environ. Res. Public Health* **2021**, *18*, 1998. https://doi.org/10.3390/ijerph18041998

Academic Editors: Fraser Carson and Shaher A. I. Shalfawi

Received: 27 December 2020
Accepted: 13 February 2021
Published: 19 February 2021

1. Introduction

There are different social (e.g., coach–administrator, athlete–athlete) and personal relationships (e.g., athlete–parent, athlete–partner) that can be found in the sport context, however, the coach–athlete relationship is the most important for both performance accomplishments and psychological well-being [1,2]. While coaches need to ensure that they are creating an environment that allows athletes to feel open, accessible, and available (as opposed to withdrawn, hostile, and distant) [3], athletes find it difficult to produce top-level performances without the support of their coaches [4]. Moreover, coaches are unlikely to be successful without athletes' talent, passion, and enthusiasm [5]. In many cases, neither the coach nor the athlete can do it alone [6]. Coaches may have to deliberately create situations that provide opportunities to connect with the athlete and create an environment that is genuinely and constantly nurturing, supportive, and caring [7]. Athletes reach out to their coaches for their expertise and knowledge, and as a result often have to set aside the sort of insecurities that are likely to prevent them from building a close, trustworthy, and committed relationship if they are to develop and succeed in sport [8].

Sports coaches encourage new skills and challenges, even in the face of adversity, and provide a platform for growth and development [9]. Through a series of studies [10,11], it was found that coaches were viewed by their athletes as persons who are likely to provide a source of comfort and security during times of need and who provide a sound platform from which athletes can explore autonomously. A high-quality interdependent coach–athlete relationship is central to effective coaching and is a fundamental precursor of athletes' optimal functioning [9,12,13]. The benefit of investigating relationships is not for the coaches and athletes exclusively. The need for more research in this area is prompted by the requirements of a systematic, comprehensive, and empirical knowledge, which contains practical implications for coaches, athletes, as well as parents, practitioners, and sport administrators [13]. Jowett et al.'s [14] qualitative case studies and relevant literature were used to generate items for an instrument that measures affective, cognitive, and behavioral aspects of the coach–athlete relationship [15].

Through the Coach–Athlete Relationship Questionnaire (CART-Q), the relationship between coach and athlete has been identified as an important research area for sport psychology [16]. The CART-Q provides an opportunity to pursue research questions that would promote knowledge and understanding of the complex dynamics involved between athletes and coaches from a relationship perspective. It could also contribute to the development of interventions for enhancing the quality of this athletic relationship and its associated outcomes (e.g., motivation, performance, well-being) [17]. The CART-Q [17] includes two versions, namely, direct and meta perspectives, and the investigations and studies that have been conducted focused on both versions; how one person perceives how the other person views him/her (meta-perspective) can dictate/change one's perception (direct-perspective). The results obtained with the CART-Q can provide relevant information to help professionals in the sport psychology area, and help coaches to develop experiences that promote a positive relationship between coaches and athletes [18]. The relationship between coaches and athletes is crucial for sports performance and individual well-being [19].

The 3Cs model was utilized to understand and investigate the impact of the coach–athlete relationship, namely the constructs of closeness, commitment, and complementarity on the outcomes of the interpersonal relationships. Various studies found associations between the coach–athlete relationship and the outcomes of its interpersonal relationship (e.g., satisfaction, dissatisfaction, anxiety). A study by Jowett and Nezlek [20] aimed to investigate the association between coach–athlete relationship interdependence and satisfaction level as a function of competition level, relationship length, and gender has found that the association between interdependence and satisfaction with training, instruction, and personal treatment are higher within higher-level competitors (e.g., regional, national, and international) rather than lower-level (e.g., club) competitors. The coach–athlete relationship is defined and operationalized as a situation in which both coaches' and athletes' feelings of closeness, thoughts of commitment, and behaviors of complementarity (3Cs) are interconnected. Closeness refers to the affective bonds developed between coaches and athletes and includes relational interpersonal properties such as mutual trust and respect. Commitment is defined as an athlete's and a coach's intention to maintain a close athletic partnership and long-term relationship that aims to maximize its outcomes. Complementarity refers to the type of interaction that the coach and the athlete engage in that reflects corresponding actions and interactions that are co-operative and affiliative [20].

The Coach–Athlete Relationship Questionnaire (CART-Q) has been validated widely during the last decade. The validation's attempts crossed the European borders and reached the Far East (China) [21]. Validating the CART-Q began with a study by Jowett and Ntoumanis [15] that consisted of two separate studies. The study aimed to develop an instrument that could be used to assess the nature of the coach–athlete relationship, validate the instrument, and examine the relationships between interpersonal satisfaction and the 3Cs within coaches and athletes. Consequently, the validation studies of the Coach–Athlete Relationship Questionnaire continued targeting different regions, cultures, and countries. Balduck and Jowett [22] examined the psychometric properties of the CART-Q utilizing 144 Belgian coaches. The result supported previous studies that validated this specific instrument, and the psychometric properties of the Belgian version were verified. On the other hand, Yang and Jowett [23] attempted to universalize the CART-Q by conducting a study that recruited participants from seven different countries (United States, Britain, China, Greece, Belgium, Sweden, and Spain). As the results of this study showed a variation within the intensity of the athletes' perceptions towards the quality of the relationships with their coaches, the validity of the CART-Q was proved using a three-first-order factor model across the seven countries.

Since this important measurement tool was validated in many countries across the world, it is also still unheard of in many other countries. There is still a gap when it comes to investigating the coach–athlete relationship in the Middle East. Therefore, the first aim of this study was to fill that gap and add to the literature by validating this measurement tool; the translated direct and meta-perspective Arabic versions of the CART-Q in the Middle East. Validating the Arabic version of the CART-Q is beneficial to most countries in the Middle East, as most of the countries are Arabic speaking. The CART-Q is highly beneficial to Middle Eastern countries as the sport field in that area is rapidly growing and developing. Many sports events and tournaments take place in the Middle East, as well as the World Cup scheduled to take place in Qatar in 2022, the first-ever World Cup to be held in an Arabic country. Needless to say, many athletes want to pursue professional sport careers in the Middle East, making the coach–athlete relationship a very important relationship to investigate. This leads to emphasizing once again the importance of utilizing and validating the Arabic versions of the CART-Q and helping coaches and athletes to perform at an optimum level. While sport psychology in the Middle East region is underutilized in theoretical, empirical, and practical terms, its various applications may be critical in facilitating harmony and stability in the ways coaches and athletes, as well as other significant individuals, including sport administrators and officials, could operate and interact. The interrelation of both the coach and the athlete makes effective and successful coaching. The wide and various interests from all around the world in exploring the coach–athlete relationship has motivated several sport psychologists to adopt the Coach–Athlete Relationship Questionnaire (CART-Q). It is especially necessary for those who are aiming to develop the sports field in their country. Reaching an optimum level for an athlete can depend on the relationship with her/his coach. As stated, the nature of this relationship includes three important constructs. When these constructs can operationalize well in the relationship of the coach and athlete, the satisfaction level can increase for the athlete. The second aim of this study was to determine the quality of the coach–athlete relationship in relation to athlete's satisfaction with individual performance. The Athlete Satisfaction Questionnaire (ASQ) is a measure of the experiences of sport participants based on Riemer and Chelladurai's [24] classification of the facets of athlete satisfaction [25]. Even though research on athlete satisfaction remains limited [26], findings from various studies highlight the importance of satisfaction within the coach–athlete relationship, such as a study by Davis et al. [27], which found that the coach–athlete relationship quality positively predicted athlete satisfaction. Since athlete satisfaction was not fully explored in the Middle East, and since it is highly linked to the coach–athlete relationship, it is very important to discover the facets of athlete satisfaction to predict the quality of the coach–athlete relationship.

This study was conducted in Kuwait, one of the Middle Eastern countries. Satisfaction is very important amongst the Kuwaiti coach–athlete relationships, as satisfaction is a fulfillment of one's expectations and needs. Once an athlete is fulfilled, it will lead to successful performances and sport results.

2. Materials and Methods

2.1. Participants

A total of 259 athletes (male and female) were recruited from various athletic clubs in Kuwait. The sample was comprised of 187 male and 72 female athletes, with a mean age of 22 years old (M_{age} = 22.33, SD = 4.61). The athletes participated in either team or individual sports. Any sport where individuals are organized into opposing teams that compete to win and involves competition between teams of players has been accepted as a team sport. Sport participation type ($n_{individual}$ = 71; n_{team} = 186), sport duration (experience in sport participation) (M_{year} = 6.68), and sport achievement (n_{yes} = 123; n_{no} = 134) variables were collected from participants. The participants had to answer a question about their achievements with their current coach. Sport achievement criteria were classified by athletes who won trophies or medals with their current coach and athletes who did not, at the time the questionnaires were conducted. The subjects were extracted randomly. All the participants completed at senior level, and they were members of local clubs.

2.2. Measures

2.2.1. The Coach–Athlete Relationship Questionnaire (CART-Q)

CART-Q [17] was used to assess how athletes believe the coach perceives the athletic relationship with them. The questionnaire consists of 11-item meta-perspective items and 3 sub-dimensions: meta-closeness (4 items; e.g., "My coach likes me"), meta-commitment (3 items; e.g., "My coach is committed to me"), and meta-complementarity (4 items; e.g., "My coach is responsive to my efforts during training"). The direct version of the questionnaire also includes 11 direct-perspective items (3 items for direct-closeness; e.g., "I like my coach"; 3 items for direct commitment; e.g., "I am committed to my coach"; 3 items for direct complementarity; e.g., "When I am coached by my coach, I am responsive to his/her efforts"). For this study, the factorial structure of the Arabic version of the CART-Q was used in Kuwait and was prepared with both direct and meta perspectives. The items were assigned a score ranging from 1 (strongly agree) to 7 (strongly disagree) with a mid-point of 4 (half-way). The Cronbach's internal consistency coefficients for these 3 sub-scales for direct and meta versions were 0.82 and 0.85 for closeness, 0.70 and 0.82 for commitment, 0.65 and 0.82 for complementarity, respectively.

2.2.2. Athlete Satisfaction Questionnaire (ASQ)

ASQ [25] measure the facets of athlete satisfaction. The questionnaire contains 56-items and 15 subscales. These subscales include individual performance, team integration, personal dedication, team performance, ability utilization, strategy, personal treatment, training and instruction, team task contribution, team social contribution, ethics, budget, medical personnel, academic support services, and external agents. In this study, only 3 items were employed to measure athletes' satisfaction with individual performance (e.g., "I am satisfied with the improvement in my performance over the previous season"). The response scale of these measures ranged from 1 (strongly disagree) to 7 (strongly agree). Cronbach's alpha reliability estimates ranged from 0.78 to 0.95 [25]. In this study, the internal consistency coefficient for the individual performance subscale was 0.81.

2.3. Translation Procedures

The translation and cultural adaptation of the CART-Q was done by six Arabic professionals (three English teachers and three Ph.D. graduates in Physical Education and Sport Science) in Kuwait. Subsequently, the translated items were independently translated back into English. The back-translated version was then compared with the original British version and any inconsistencies, and ways of eliminating them were discussed. This process was repeated until the final versions were accurate and comprehensive translations of the original CART-Q were developed.

2.4. Procedures

The approval of the institutional ethics board was not required as per the institution's guidelines and applicable regulations in the city where the study was conducted. That is, why we cannot provide formal approval by the institutional ethics committee. However, we verified that the study is in accordance with established ethical guidelines. Participation was voluntary, it was not obligatory. All the participants were informed about the anonymity, confidentiality, and the voluntary nature of the study. Before athletes completed forms, written informed consent forms were received from them and from the parents of the athletes who were under the age of 18. Thereby, all potential participants were well-informed about the study. The information stated in the informed consent form was not exceeded. In Kuwait, female athletes are not easy to target since there are very few females participating in sport, and those who do participate are difficult to contact due to their cultural restrictions. An information sheet that explained the aims of the study was also given to the participants. The questionnaires were handed out to the participants and collected at different times. Necessary explanations on how to fill out the questionnaires were given by the first researcher. The questionnaire contained three pages in addition to the demographics section and took 10–15 min to complete.

2.5. Data Analysis

The study has two aims. The first aim was to achieve validation of the direct and meta-perspective versions of the CART-Q in the Arabic language, and the second aim was to discover the differentiations of the CART-Q with other variables (e.g., gender, sport participation type, and achievement) using independent sample *t*-tests and to discover the relationships with the variables of age, satisfaction, and sport duration using Pearson correlation coefficients. First of all, all preconditions, which are missing values, normal distribution, and multi-collinearity situations, were checked. A series of descriptive statistics for all variables and sub-dimensions of both meta and direct data were controlled. Mean (*M*), standard deviation (*SD*), skewness, and kurtosis values were obtained to determine whether the data set has a normal distribution. It was seen that skewness and kurtosis values ranged between −0.09 to −2.01. There were no missing values or outliers in the data. Descriptive statistics were calculated for all variables of the study including means, and standard deviations. Multi-collinearity was checked and results showed that tolerance and the variance inflation factor (VIF) value ranges were as they should be. According to Hair, Black, Babin, Anderson, and Tatham [28], the VIF value range is less than 5 and tolerance is more than 0.2.

As the main aim of this study was to examine the psychometric properties of the CART-Q, the first-order confirmatory factor analysis (CFA) was used to confirm the factor structure of the scale. Lisrel 8.1. software package was used to perform the CFA. The covariance matrix was created by using the maximum likelihood calculation method. Furthermore, Pearson correlation was used to examine the relationship of the coach–athlete relationship quality (both direct and meta, separately) with other variables. Independent sample *t*-tests were used to determine the differentiation between gender, sport type, and achievement situation, with direct-meta coach–athlete relationship and satisfaction.

3. Results

According to the results obtained from the path analysis with the parameter values for the first level confirmatory factor analysis results (CFA), fit indices (RMSEA: root Mean square error of approximation; CFI: comparative fit index; GFI: goodness of fit index; and AGFI: adjusted goodness of fit index) of the data collected by direct-method were as follows ($x^2/df = 2.21$; RMSEA = 0.06; CFI = 0.98; GFI = 0.95; AGFI = 0.91); data for the meta-method were as follows ($x^2/df = 2.32$; RMSEA = 0.08; CFI = 0.99; GFI = 0.93; AGFI = 0.87). According to acceptable criteria, fit index values should be between <2–3 for x^2/df; <0.05–0.10 for RMSEA; <0.95–0.97 for CFI; <0.90–0.95 for GFI; and <0.90–0.95 for AGFI [29]. Results show that the results obtained for both scales are compatible with the model data and are acceptable. These results show that the data obtained from the research corresponds to the predicted theoretical structure of the CART-Q versions for Kuwait. On the other hand, when interpreting the CFA, Lambda (factor loading), t, and R^2 values of the substances are also important (Tables 1 and 2).

Table 1. According to The Coach–Athlete Relationship Questionnaire (CART-Q)'s confirmatory factor analysis (CFA) results, standardized Lambda (λ), t, and R^2 values for the direct method.

Subscales and Items	λ	t	R^2
Closeness 1	0.87	17.17 *	0.74
Closeness 2	0.80	15.42 *	0.67
Closeness 3	0.58	9.62 *	0.33
Closeness 4	0.74	13.71 *	0.54
Commitment 1	0.69	12.43 *	0.47
Commitment 2	0.48	7.79 *	0.23
Commitment 3	0.83	15.93 *	0.70
Complementarity 1	0.88	16.97 *	0.74
Complementarity 2	0.32	5.31 *	0.11
Complementarity 3	0.46	7.68 *	0.23
Complementarity 4	0.52	8.95 *	0.28

Note. * $p < 0.05$.

Table 2. According to CART-Q's CFA results, standardized Lambda (λ), t, and R^2 values for the meta-method.

Subscales and Items	λ	t	R^2
Meta-Closeness 1	0.82	15.98 *	0.67
Meta-Closeness 2	0.78	14.87 *	0.60
Meta-Closeness 3	0.67	11.97 *	0.45
Meta-Closeness 4	0.88	18.13 *	0.78
Meta-Commitment 1	0.82	15.95 *	0.67
Meta-Commitment 2	0.78	14.94 *	0.61
Meta-Commitment 3	0.74	13.83 *	0.55
Meta-Complementarity 1	0.74	13.98 *	0.55
Meta-Complementarity 2	0.67	12.08 *	0.44
Meta-Complementarity 3	0.82	16.08 *	0.67
Meta-Complementarity 4	0.72	13.26 *	0.51

Note. * $p < 0.05$.

As seen in Table 1, Lambda (λ), t, and R^2 values obtained as significant at 0.05 level. When lambda values showing factor loads are examined, it is seen that factor loads vary between 0.32 and 0.87. These values show that the factor loadings of the items are acceptable. In addition, t values of the observed variables (items) regarding the explanation of latent variables (dimensions) were found to be significant at the 0.05 level. On the other hand, when R^2 values are analyzed, it is seen that the variance amount explained by the sub-factors in the items varies between 0.11 and 0.74. All these findings can be considered as evidence that the scale has satisfactory construct validity.

Lambda (λ), t, and R^2 values obtained in Table 2 are significant at the 0.05 level. When lambda values showing factor loads are examined, it is seen that factor loads vary between 0.67 and 0.88. These values show that the factor loadings of the items are acceptable. Besides, t values of the observed variables (items) regarding the explanation of latent variables (dimensions) were found to be significant at 0.05 level. On the other hand, when R^2 values are analyzed, it is seen that the variance amount, explained by the sub-factors in the items, varies between 0.44 and 0.78. All these findings can be considered as evidence that the scale has satisfactory construct validity.

Means and standard deviations of all subscales in the study concerning gender, sports participation type, and achievement situation are presented in Table 3.

Table 3. Means and standard deviations of all sub-scales concerning gender, sport participation type (SPT), and achievement situation.

Gender	SPT	Achievement	$M \pm SD$	Closeness	Commitment	Complementarity	Meta-Closeness	Meta-Commitment	Meta-Complementarity	Satisfaction
Female	Individual	No	*M*	6.15	6.03	6.27	6.35	5.93	6.15	5.51
			SD	0.96	1.23	0.84	0.88	1.11	1.26	2.10
		Yes	*M*	6.76	6.44	6.56	6.80	6.28	6.62	6.13
			SD	0.30	0.46	0.46	0.30	0.64	0.47	0.75
		Total	*M*	6.52	6.28	6.44	6.62	6.14	6.43	5.88
			SD	0.70	0.85	0.64	0.62	0.86	0.88	1.44
	Team	No	*M*	6.10	5.41	6.37	5.43	5.16	5.96	5.77
			SD	0.84	0.93	0.47	1.15	1.24	0.80	1.23
		Yes	*M*	6.49	6.13	6.45	6.45	6.24	6.38	6.00
			SD	0.64	.88	0.67	0.73	0.93	0.73	1.07
		Total	*M*	6.36	5.89	6.43	6.11	5.87	6.24	5.92
			SD	0.73	0.95	0.61	1.01	1.15	0.77	1.12
	Total	No	*M*	6.12	5.65	6.33	5.78	5.46	6.03	5.67
			SD	0.87	1.08	0.63	1.13	1.23	0.98	1.59
		Yes	*M*	6.58	6.23	6.49	6.56	6.26	6.46	6.04
			SD	0.56	0.78	0.61	0.64	0.84	0.66	0.97
		Total	*M*	6.41	6.02	6.43	6.28	5.97	6.31	5.91
			SD	0.72	0.93	0.61	0.92	1.06	0.814	1.23
Male	Individual	No	*M*	5.50	5.11	5.75	5.36	4.88	5.19	5.11
			SD	1.29	1.09	0.99	1.21	1.13	1.13	1.77
		Yes	*M*	6.35	6.00	6.28	6.34	6.05	6.30	5.55
			SD	0.80	0.95	0.64	0.63	0.96	0.77	1.32
		Total	*M*	6.18	5.83	6.17	6.15	5.82	6.08	5.46
			SD	0.96	1.03	0.74	.858	1.08	0.953	1.41
	Team	No	*M*	5.88	5.46	5.95	5.60	5.04	5.49	5.20
			SD	1.22	1.31	0.941	1.38	1.49	1.33	1.30
		Yes	*M*	6.25	5.74	6.08	6.10	5.72	5.94	5.35
			SD	1.01	1.01	0.82	0.87	1.05	1.00	1.37
		Total	*M*	6.06	5.63	6.04	5.87	5.42	5.76	5.31
			SD	1.11	1.17	0.864	1.16	1.33	1.18	1.34
	Total	No	*M*	5.85	5.43	5.93	5.57	5.02	5.47	5.19
			SD	1.23	1.29	0.94	1.36	1.46	1.31	1.34
		Yes	*M*	6.29	5.85	6.16	6.20	5.86	6.09	5.43
			SD	0.92	0.98	0.75	0.78	1.02	0.92	1.35
		Total	*M*	6.06	5.63	6.04	5.87	5.42	5.76	5.31
			SD	1.11	1.17	0.86	1.16	1.33	1.18	1.34

Note. *M*: Mean; *SD*: Standard deviation.

Table 3 shows the means and standard deviations of all sub-scales concerning gender, sports participation type, and achievement situation. According to this, both females and males with achievement had higher means than participants without achievement. Furthermore, individual sports participants for both female and male, with achievement, had higher means than team sport participants without achievement.

As seen in Table 4, there was a positive correlation between age and sport duration (r = 0.41, $p < 0.01$). Commitment (r = 0.16, $p < 0.05$) and complementarity (r = 0.17, $p < 0.01$) were positively associated with age; while any subscale was significantly associated with sport duration. Furthermore, satisfaction was positively correlated with closeness (r = 0.24, $p < 0.01$), commitment (r = 0.33, $p < 0.01$), and complementarity (r = 0.28, $p < 0.01$). Additionally, all subscales were positively associated with itself. According to these findings, commitment and complementarity scores increased with increasing age; however, it was found that there was no difference between the duration of sports and any sub-dimension.

Table 4. Correlation coefficients among age, sport duration, satisfaction, and direct data.

Variables	1	2	3	4	5	6
1. Age	1					
2. Sport Duration	0.41 **	1				
3. Satisfaction	0.03	0.01	1			
4. Closeness	0.07	0.02	0.24 **	1		
5. Commitment	0.16 *	0.07	0.33 **	0.72 **	1	
6. Complementarity	0.17 **	0.03	0.28 **	0.70 **	0.77 **	1

Note. * $p < 0.05$, ** $p < 0.01$.

As seen in Table 5, there was a positive correlation between age and sport duration (r = 0.41, $p < 0.01$). Meta-commitment (r = 0.14, $p < 0.05$) and meta-complementarity (r = 0.14, $p < 0.05$) were positively associated with age; while sport duration was significantly associated with meta-closeness (r = 0.16, $p < 0.05$) and meta-commitment (r = 0.14, $p < 0.05$). Furthermore, satisfaction was positively correlated again with meta-closeness (r = 0.29, $p < 0.01$), meta-commitment (r = 0.33, $p < 0.01$), and meta-complementarity (r = 0.30, $p < 0.01$). Additionally, all subscales were positively associated with itself. According to these results, meta-commitment and meta-complementarity scores increased with increasing age; it was also found that as the duration of sports increased, meta-closeness and meta-commitment scores increased. The scores of the athletes on satisfaction and the CART-Q (both meta and direct) scales were examined according to gender.

Table 5. Correlation coefficients among age, sport duration, satisfaction, and metadata.

Variables	1	2	3	4	5	6
1. Age	1					
2. Sport Duration	0.41 **	1				
3. Satisfaction	0.03	0.01	1			
4. Meta-closeness	0.09	0.16 *	0.29 **	1		
5. Meta-commitment	0.14 *	0.14 *	0.33 **	0.84 **	1	
6.Meta-complementarity	0.14 *	0.09	0.30 **	0.85 **	0.87 **	1

Note. * $p < 0.05$, ** $p < 0.01$.

The independent sample *t*-test results were presented in Table 6. According to the findings, significant differences were found in terms of satisfaction and CART-Q scores according to gender. In all sub-dimensions, the means of female athletes were significantly higher than the means of male athletes.

Table 6. Independent sample *t*-test results for gender and each scale.

	Gender	*n*	*M*	*SD*	df	t	*p*
Satisfaction	Female Male	72 185	5.91 5.31	1.23 1.34	255	3.26 ***	0.001
Closeness	Female Male	72 185	6.41 6.06	0.72 1.11	255	2.97 **	0.003
Commitment	Female Male	72 185	6.02 5.63	0.94 1.17	255	2.79 **	0.006
Complementarity	Female Male	72 185	6.43 6.04	0.62 0.86	255	4.05 ***	0.000
Meta-Closeness	Female Male	72 185	6.28 5.87	0.93 1.16	255	2.68 **	0.008
Meta-Commitment	Female Male	72 185	5.97 5.42	1.06 1.33	255	3.11 **	0.002
Meta-Complementarity	Female Male	72 185	6.31 5.76	0.81 1.18	255	3.58 ***	0.000

Note. ** $p < 0.01$; *** $p < 0.001$; *M*: Mean; *SD*: Standard deviation; df: Degrees of freedom.

According to the findings in Table 7, significant differences were found in favor of individual participants in some dimensions according to the sport participation type. Accordingly, the means obtained were commitment ($M_{individual} = 5.99$; $SD = 0.99$; t (255) = 2.33; $p < 0.05$), meta-closeness ($M_{individual} = 6.31$; $SD = 0.81$; t (255) = 3.45 $p < 0.01$), meta-commitment ($M_{individual} = 5.94$; $SD = 1.02$; t (255) = 3.20; $p < 0.01$), and meta-complementarity ($M_{individual} = 6.20$; $SD = 0.94$; t (255) = 2.84; $p < 0.01$). In all of the dimensions where there is a significant difference, the means of athletes who participated in individual sports were higher than the means of athletes who participated in team sports. These results showed that the perceived relationship levels of the athletes who participated in individual sports with their coaches were higher than the athletes who participated in team sports.

Table 7. Independent sample *t*-test results for sport participation type (SPT) and each scale.

	SPT	*n*	*M*	*SD*	df	t	*p*
Satisfaction	Individual Team	71 186	5.61 5.42	1.42 1.30	255	0.99	0.325
Closeness	Individual Team	71 186	6.30 6.11	0.89 1.07	255	1.46	0.182
Commitment	Individual Team	71 186	5.99 5.65	0.99 1.16	255	2.33 *	0.021
Complementarity	Individual Team	71 186	6.27 6.10	0.72 0.86	255	1.54	0.156
Meta-Closeness	Individual Team	71 186	6.31 5.86	0.81 1.19	255	3.45 **	0.004
Meta-Commitment	Individual Team	71 186	5.94 5.44	1.02 1.35	255	3.20 **	0.005
Meta-Complementarity	Individual Team	71 186	6.20 5.80	0.94 1.16	255	2.84 **	0.010

Note. * $p < 0.05$, ** $p < 0.01$; *M*: Mean; *SD*: Standard deviation; df: Degrees of freedom.

Regarding the findings that represented in Table 8, significant differences were obtained in all satisfaction and CART-Q scores according to the achievement status of the athletes. The means of the athletes having success in all sub-dimensions were higher than the athletes who did not. These results showed that the coach–athlete relationship quality scores of the athletes with achievement are higher than the athletes without achievement.

Table 8. Independent sample *t*-test results for achievement and each scale.

	Achievement	*n*	*M*	*SD*	df	t	*p*
Satisfaction	No	123	5.29	1.40	255	−2.09 *	0.038
	Yes	134	5.64	1.26			
Closeness	No	123	5.91	1.16	255	−3.80 ***	0.000
	Yes	134	6.39	0.83			
Commitment	No	123	5.48	1.25	255	−3.64 ***	0.000
	Yes	134	5.98	0.94			
Complementarity	No	123	6.01	0.89	255	−2.53 **	0.012
	Yes	134	6.27	0.72			
Meta-Closeness	No	123	5.62	1.31	255	−5.24 ***	0.000
	Yes	134	6.33	0.76			
Meta-Commitment	No	123	5.11	1.42	255	−5.74 ***	0.000
	Yes	134	6.00	0.98			
Meta-Complementarity	No	123	5.59	1.26	255	−4.63 ***	0.000
	Yes	134	6.22	0.86			

Note. * $p < 0.05$; ** $p < 0.01$; *** $p < 0.001$; *M*: Mean; *SD*: Standard deviation; df: Degrees of freedom.

4. Discussion

The development of the Coach–Athlete Relationship Questionnaire (CART-Q) was guided by the findings of previous qualitative studies, and the development of the British [15], the Greek [30], and the Chinese [21] versions of the CART-Q. The CART-Q is expanding around the world and its validation is evidenced across the globe, despite its linguistic differences, such as in Brazil [18], China [21], and Belgium [22]. The CART-Q has become an important measurement tool and it is time to develop and utilize the CART-Q in new regions, such as the Middle East. New versions of a translated CART-Q to Arabic, Persian, and other languages are needed. These areas have different cultures, traditions, and beliefs, which make it necessary and encouraging to explore the coach–athlete relationship in such regions. The results of the CART-Q could help researchers and practitioners who aim to investigate the nature of the coach–athlete relationship in the Middle East or among the Arab nations. This study shows robust evidence of the validity of the direct and meta-perspectives of the Arabic version of the CART-Q. Moreover, the CART-Q could help coaches and athletes from the Middle East to understand the reasons and methods that lead to a quality coach–athlete relationship.

The first aim of this present study was to examine the validity of the direct and meta-perspective versions of the Coach–Athlete Relationship Questionnaire (CART-Q) in the Middle East area (Kuwait) and to discover the differentiations of the CART-Q with other variables. An understanding of the nature and content of the coach–athlete relationship, as well as its functions, is important because such knowledge could contribute toward the development of strategies that help to establish and maintain effective and successful coach–athlete relationships [13,31]. Confirmatory factor analysis (CFA) was used to examine the validity of the Arabic CART-Q version, which is consistent with a study by Vieira et al., [18] which confirmed the construct validity of the Brazilian coach–athlete questionnaire by using CFA. The methodological procedures that were used in this study to examine the factorial validity of the direct and meta-perspective versions of the Arabic CART-Q are coupled with the procedures in previous studies [15,17,23]. When the factorial construct was examined for Arabic culture, the factor loadings of direct complementarity were seen lower than other dimensions. This result can be caused by Arabic culture than itself because complementarity reflects the members' reciprocal and corresponding cooperation [32]. In Arabic culture, considering the lower number of female participants in the sport field, this result may make sense more. Furthermore, complementarity has been studied as an issue [33] across cultures, because the nature of the attitude of friendly and relaxed can be differentiated in a different culture. To avoid incomplete implications, measurement invariance analyses are recommended for the future.

The second aim of this present study was to determine the quality of the coach–athlete relationship to athlete satisfaction. Other researchers such as Jowett et al. [34], approached this relationship similarly and it showed that athletes who feel that their relationship with the coach is underlined by trust, respect, and co-operation, are more likely to be satisfied. High satisfaction leads to a high-quality coach–athlete relationship, and the coach–athlete relationship quality positively predicts athlete satisfaction [27].

The scores of the athletes on satisfaction and the CART-Q (both meta and direct) scales were examined according to gender. According to the findings, significant differences were found in terms of satisfaction and CART-Q scores according to gender. In all sub-dimensions, the means of female athletes were significantly higher than the means of male athletes. It can be presumed that these results are because in Kuwait, the cultural norm is for female athletes to have female coaches. This gives the female athletes a sense of satisfaction within their sport environment. Every culture has its unique norms, values, and beliefs, however, less attention has been given to how culture affects the coach–athlete relationship. Within the sport psychology literature, it has been noted that there is less attention paid to the cultural impact and the cultural background effect [35].

Females are more emotional, caring, understanding of one another, and they structurally have more intense connectedness and trust needs than men [36], therefore, the female athletes tend to be committed to their coaches. However, in Kuwait, the media is a male-dominated setting where women's sport is rarely broadcasted and female athletes do not get the attention they deserve. Therefore, once females become athletes, they try to prove that they deserve the same attention as men, giving importance to their sports career, showing their athletic abilities, and committing to their coaches. This level of commitment makes the sport environment a safe and satisfactory place for female athletes. Females have a very strong ability to connect, and the female coaches have the right strategies to create a comfort zone for their female athletes. These findings were similar to what was found in the study by Jowett and Nezlek [20], where it was mentioned that "all-female dyads were more satisfied with training and instruction than the other gender combinations considered together" [20]. The findings of this study show that the same gender coach–athlete dyads make a successful combination, and are consistent with a study by Jowett [37], where it was found that the same gender coach–athlete dyads may feel they have something in common that connects them.

This reflects a high degree of commitment between dyads and a desire to maintain a long-term sport relationship. The dyads invest in each other and are committed to each other. These results are consistent with the study by Jowett and Nezlek [20], as it was found that coaches invest their knowledge, skills, and expertise, while athletes invest their raw talent, long and hard hours of training, passion, determination, and motivation to achieve.

The results also showed that the perceived relationship levels of the athletes who participated in individual sports with their coaches were higher than the athletes who participated in team sports. The coach–athlete relationship is important in individual sports, as the leadership and orientation of the coach are very important for the athletes who are in direct contact with them [36]. Baker et al., [38] found that team sport athletes require greater coach control, and when those needs were not met, it created less satisfaction in both the athlete and the coach in team sports. Significant differences were obtained in all satisfaction and CART-Q scores according to the achievement status of the athletes. The means of the athletes having success in all sub-dimensions were higher than the athletes who did not. These results showed that the coach–athlete relationship quality scores of the athletes with achievement are higher than the athletes without achievement. Moreover, coaches' satisfaction is likely to be linked to their own and their athletes' perspectives of the coach–athlete relationship quality, while athletes' satisfaction is likely to be associated with their meta-perspectives and their coaches' meta-perspectives of the relationship quality [39].

The findings of this study revealed that there was a positive correlation between age and sport duration and no difference between the duration of sports and any sub-dimension. According to the results, older athletes had higher commitment and complementarity. It was observed that as the sport duration increased, meta-closeness and meta-commitment increased. This study shows evidence of the validity of the direct and meta-perspective Arabic versions of the CART-Q. These results could help researchers and practitioners who aim to investigate the nature of the coach–athlete relationship in the Arabic speaking nations in the Middle East. Moreover, the results of the present study could help coaches and athletes from the Middle East to understand the reasons and methods that lead to a quality coach-athlete relationship.

The present study includes also some limitations that needed to be explained. Firstly, the sample was taken for this study only targeted athletes and therefore did not include a full dyad. It would have been more beneficial to target coaches in the study, however, in Kuwait, there is a very large number of foreign coaches. Getting the foreign, non-Arabic speaking coaches involved in this study would require the coaches to use the original (English) version of the CART-Q, and that would go against the purpose of this study, as this study requires the use of the Arabic version of the CART-Q. Secondly, there are very few female athletes in the sample as it is not popular to find female athletes in Kuwait due to the cultural differences that discourage the existence of women in the sports field. That is why the results should be interpreted with caution as the sample sizes are significantly different (gender and sport type). Thirdly, at the time this study was conducted, Kuwait was banned from international sport competitions. As a result, athletes in Kuwait were significantly affected in terms of their commitment, and motivation. Most of the athletes lacked ambition, had fewer training hours, and had less desire to improve or prepare for a sports career. In turn, they were frustrated and disappointed. This situation could have greatly affected the results of this study. In the future, it would be highly beneficial to investigate such issues and the impact they have on the coach–athlete relationship.

5. Conclusions

The results of the Arabic version of the CART-Q could help researchers and practitioners investigate the nature of the coach–athlete relationship in the Middle East or among the Arab nations. Furthermore, the CART-Q could help coaches and athletes understand the steps that lead to a quality coach–athlete relationship while investigating the obstacles that stand in the way of achieving a harmonious relationship. Once coaches and athletes understand what builds up their relationship, they can achieve their goals together and reach a state of overall well-being. The constructs of the CART-Q have shown that high satisfaction is strongly associated with a high quality, successful, harmonious, and supportive coach–athlete relationship [17]. The CART-Q is highly beneficial to Middle Eastern countries as the sports field in that area is rapidly growing and developing.

Author Contributions: Conceptualization, H.A.; methodology, H.A., E.N.A., Z.K. and K.A.; software, E.N.A. and Z.K.; validation, E.N.A., Z.K., H.A., K.A. and S.J.; formal analysis, E.N.A. and Z.K.; investigation, H.A., E.N.A., Z.K. and K.A.; resources, H.A. and K.A.; writing—original draft preparation, H.A., E.N.A. and Z.K.; writing—review and editing, Z.K. and H.A.; visualization, H.A., Z.K. and E.N.A.; supervision, Z.K. and S.J.; project administration, H.A. All authors have read and agreed to the published version of the manuscript.

Funding: This research received no external funding.

Institutional Review Board Statement: Ethical review and approval were waived for this study, as the First author's College does not require Ethical approval.

Informed Consent Statement: Informed consent was obtained from all subjects involved in the study.

Data Availability Statement: The data presented in this study are available on request from the corresponding author.

Conflicts of Interest: The author declares no conflict of interest.

References

1. Jowett, S. On enhancing and repairing the coach-athlete relationship. In *The Psychology of Coaching*; Jowett, S., Jones, M., Eds.; The British Psychological Society, Sport and Exercise Psychology Division: Leicester, UK, 2005; pp. 14–26.
2. Lyle, J. The coaching process: An overview. In *The Coaching Process: Principles and Practice for Sports*; Cross, N., Lyle, J., Eds.; Butterworth-Heinman: Oxford, UK, 1999; pp. 3–24.
3. Felton, L.; Jowett, S.; Begg, C.; Zhong, X. A multi-study examination of the complementarity dimension of the coach-athlete relationship. *J. Sport Exerc. Perform. Psychol.* **2020**. [CrossRef]
4. Hemery, D. *The Pursuit of Sporting Excellence: A Study of Sport's Highest Achievers*; Willow Books Collins: London, UK, 1986.
5. Philippe, R.A.; Seiler, R. Closeness, co-orientation and complementarity in coach-athlete relationships: What male swimmers say about their male coaches? *Psychol. Sport Exerc.* **2006**, *7*, 159–171. [CrossRef]
6. Jowett, S.; Chaundy, V. An investigation into the impact of coach leadership and coach-athlete relationship on group cohesion. *Group Dyn. Theory Res. Pract.* **2004**, *8*, 302–311. [CrossRef]
7. Davis, L.; Jowett, S. Coach-Athlete attachment and the quality of the coach-athlete relationship: Implications for athlete's well-being. *J. Sport Sci.* **2014**, *32*, 1454–1464. [CrossRef] [PubMed]
8. Davis, L.; Jowett, S. Attachment styles within the coach-athlete dyad: Prelimenary investigation and assessment development. *J. Clin. Sport Psychol.* **2013**, *7*, 120–145. [CrossRef]
9. Lyle, J. *Sports Coaching Concepts: A Framework for Coaches' Behaviour*; Routledge: London, UK, 2002.
10. Davis, L.; Jowett, S. Investigating the interpersonal dynamics between coaches and athletes based on fundamental principles of attachment. *J. Clin. Sport Psychol.* **2010**, *4*, 112–132. [CrossRef]
11. Davis, L.; Jowett, S.; Lafreniere, M.K. An attachment theory perspective in the examination of relational processes associated with coach-athlete dyads. *J. Sport Exerc. Psychol.* **2013**, *35*, 156–167. [CrossRef]
12. Gould, D.; Collins, K.; Lauer, L.; Chung, Y. Coaching life skills through football: A study of award winning high school coaches. *Int. J. Sport Psychol.* **2007**, *19*, 16–37. [CrossRef]
13. Jowett, S. (Ed.) Interdependence analysis and the 3 + 1 Cs in the coach-athlete relationship. In *Social Psychology in Sport*; Human Kinetics: Champaign, IL, USA, 2007; pp. 15–27.
14. Jowett, S.; Meek, G.A. The coach-athlete relationship in married couples: An exploratory content analysis. *Sport Psychol.* **2000**, *14*, 157–175. [CrossRef]
15. Jowett, S.; Ntoumanis, N. The Coach-Athlete Relationship Questionnaire (CART–Q): Development and initial validation. *Scand. J. Med. Sci. Sports* **2004**, *14*, 245–257. [CrossRef]
16. Auweele, Y.V.; Rzewnicki, R. Putting relationship issues in sport in perspective. *Int. J. Sport Psychol.* **2000**, *31*, 573–577.
17. Jowett, S. Validating coach-athlete relationship measures with the nomological network. *Meas. Phys. Educ. Exerc. Sci.* **2009**, *13*, 34–51. [CrossRef]
18. Vieira, L.F.; Nascimento, J.; Puials, C.; Jowett, S. Cross-cultural adaptation and psychometric properties of the Brazilian coach-athlete relationship questionnaire (CART-Q)-Athlete version. *Braz. J. Kinanthropometry Hum. Perform.* **2015**, *17*, 635–649. [CrossRef]
19. Wachsmuth, S.; Jowett, S.; Harwood, C. Third party interventions in coach-athlete conflict: Can sport psychology practitioners offer the necessary support? *J. Appl. Sport Psychol.* **2020**, 1–26. [CrossRef]
20. Jowett, S.; Nezlek, J. Relationship interdependence and satisfaction with important outcomes in coach–athlete dyads. *J. Soc. Pers. Relatsh.* **2012**, *29*, 287–330. [CrossRef]
21. Yang, S.X.; Jowett, S. An examination of the psychometric properties of the Chinese coach-athlete relationship questionnaire (CART-Q). *Int. J. Coach. Sci.* **2010**, *4*, 73–89. [CrossRef]
22. Balduck, A.L.; Jowett, S. Psychometric properties of the Belgian coach version of the coach-athlete relationship questionnaire (CART-Q). *Scand. J. Med. Sci. Sports* **2010**, *20*, 779–786. [CrossRef]
23. Yang, S.X.; Jowett, S. Psychometric properties of the Coach–Athlete Relationship Questionnaire (CART-Q) in seven countries. *Psychol. Sport Exerc.* **2012**, *13*, 36–43. [CrossRef]
24. Riemer, H.A.; Chelladurai, P. A classification of facets of athlete satisfaction. *J. Sport Manag.* **1997**, *11*, 133–159. [CrossRef]
25. Riemer, H.A.; Chelladurai, P. Development of the Athlete Satisfaction Questionnaire (ASQ). *J. Sport Exerc. Psychol.* **1998**, *20*, 127–156. [CrossRef]
26. Burns, G.; Jasinski, D.; Dunn, S.; Fletcher, D. Athlete identity and athlete satisfaction: The nonconformity of exclusivity. *Personal. Individ. Differ.* **2012**, *52*, 280–284. [CrossRef]
27. Davis, L.; Jowett, S.; Tafvelin, S. Communication strategies: The fuel for quality coach-athlete relationships and athlete satisfaction. *Front. Psychol.* **2019**, *10*, 2156. [CrossRef]
28. Hair, J.; Black, W.; Babin, B.; Anderson, R.; Tatham, R. *Multivariate Data Analysis*; Prentice Hall: Englewood Cliffs, NJ, USA, 2010.
29. Çelik, H.E.; Yılmaz, V. Chapter II: Evaluation of Model and Fit Indices. In *Structural Equation Modelling with Lisrel 9.1*; Anı Publishing: Ankara, Turkey, 2016; ISBN 978-605-5213-48-0.
30. Jowett, S.; Ntoumanis, N. The Greek Coach-Athlete Relationship Questionnaire (GrCART-Q): Scale development and validation. *Int. J. Sport Psychol.* **2003**, *34*, 101–124. [CrossRef]
31. Jowett, S. Coach-athlete relationships ignite groupness. In *Group Dynamics Advances in Sport and Exercise Psychology*; Beauchamp, M., Eys, M., Eds.; Routledge: New York, NY, USA, 2007; pp. 63–77.

32. Jowett, S.; Kanakoglou, K.; Passmore, J. The application of the 3+1Cs relationship model in executive coaching. *Consult. Psychol. J. Pract. Res.* **2012**, *64*, 183–197. [CrossRef]
33. Yang, S.X.; Jowett, S. Conceptual and measurement issues of the complementarity dimension of the coach–athlete relationship across cultures. *Psychol. Sport Exerc.* **2013**, *14*, 830–841. [CrossRef]
34. Jowett, S.; Yang, X.; Lorimer, R. The role of personality, empathy, and satisfaction with instruction within the context of the coach-athlete relationship. *Int. J. Coach. Sci.* **2012**, *6*, 3–20.
35. Peters, H.J.; Williams, J.M. Rationale for developing a cultural sport psychology. In *Cultural Sport Psychology*; Schinke, R.J., Hanraham, S.J., Eds.; Human Kinetics: Champaign, IL, USA, 2009; pp. 13–21.
36. Gullu, S.; Keskin, B.; Ates, O.; Hanbay, E. Coach-athlete relationship and sport passion in individual sports. *Acta Kinesiol.* **2020**, *14*, 9–15.
37. Jowett, S. Coaching Effectiveness: The coach-athlete relationship at its heart. *Curr. Opin. Psychol.* **2017**, *16*, 154–158. [CrossRef]
38. Baker, J.; Cote, J.; Abernethy, B. Sport-specific practice and the development of expert decision-making in team ball sports. *J. Appl. Sport Psychol.* **2003**, *15*, 12–25. [CrossRef]
39. Yang, S.X.; Jowett, S.; Chan, D.K.C. Effects of big-five personality traits on the quality of relationship and satisfaction in Chinese coach-athlete dyads. *Scand. J. Med. Sci. Sports* **2015**, *25*, 568–580. [CrossRef] [PubMed]

International Journal of
Environmental Research and Public Health

MDPI

Article

Too Much of a Good Thing? Exercise Dependence in Endurance Athletes: Relationships with Personal and Social Resources

Zsuzsanna Zimanyi [1], Wanja Wolff [1,2] and Julia Schüler [1,*]

[1] Department of Sport Science, Sport Psychology, University of Konstanz, 78464 Konstanz, Germany; zimanyizsuzsanna@gmail.com (Z.Z.); wanja.wolff@uni-konstanz.de (W.W.)
[2] Institute of Educational Science, Educational Psychology, University of Bern, 3012 Bern, Switzerland
* Correspondence: julia.schueler@uni-konstanz.de

Abstract: (1) Background: A large body of research has examined the positive effects of physical activity on physical and mental health. However, for some, excessive exercise can develop into an addiction that is detrimental to their health. In the present study, we examine potential personal (self-control, self-concordance) and social (social support) resources that we assume to be related to exercise dependence. (2) Methods: One hundred and forty athletes from different endurance sports participated in an online survey. Exercise dependence, self-control, self-concordance, and social support were assessed using questionnaires that are well-established in health and sport psychology. Additionally, further sport-relevant and demographic variables were assessed. (3) Results: Correlational analyses supported our hypotheses that exercise dependence is negatively correlated with the personal resources trait, state self-control, and self-concordance. Social support, however, was not significantly correlated with exercise dependence. Furthermore, the results of a mediation analysis revealed that the relationship between both personal traits (self-control, self-concordance) and exercise dependence was mediated by state self-control. (4) Conclusions: Our results indicate that trait self-control and self-concordance might be important personal resources that protect against exercise dependence by making state self-control available.

Keywords: exercise dependence; endurance sports; self-control; self-concordance; social support

Citation: Zimanyi, Z.; Wolff, W.; Schüler, J. Too Much of a Good Thing? Exercise Dependence in Endurance Athletes: Relationships with Personal and Social Resources. *Int. J. Environ. Res. Public Health* **2021**, *18*, 2966. https://doi.org/10.3390/ijerph18062966

Academic Editor: Shaher A.I. Shalfawi

Received: 31 January 2021
Accepted: 11 March 2021
Published: 14 March 2021

Publisher's Note: MDPI stays neutral with regard to jurisdictional claims in published maps and institutional affiliations.

1. Introduction

A large body of research has shown that physical activity has a positive effect on physical and mental health [1]. Recommendations for the minimum level of physical activity that is needed for beneficial health effects are given by the World Health Organization (WHO) [2]. For adults aged 18–64 years, the WHO recommends 150 min at moderate intensity, or 75 min at vigorous intensity. Moreover, the health benefits increase with increased physical activity [2,3]. However, the WHO provides no recommendations for upper limits in terms of intensity, frequency and duration of physical activity exist. Upper limits would help to address a health-related problem: while most people exercise too little, some exercise too much and even display addiction-like behavior [4]. Excessive exercising can have harmful effects on physical (e.g., injury) and mental health (e.g., withdrawal symptoms during absence). Szabo and colleagues defined exercise addiction as "a morbid pattern of behavior in which the habitually exercising individual loses control over his or her exercise habits and acts compulsively, exhibits dependence, and experiences negative consequences to health as well as in his or her social and professional life" [5]. According to the components model by Griffiths, addictions, in general, are characterized by a number of common symptoms, among them withdrawal symptoms, tolerance, mood modification, salience, personal conflict and relapse [6–8].

Various studies in previous decades have attempted to clarify the psychological and physiological etiology of exercise dependence [9–11]. Synthesizing this research in their review, Berczik and colleagues [4] addressed the necessity of future research into the personal and environmental factors sustaining, maintaining or developing exercise addiction. Susceptibility to addictive behavior in exercise [4] and in other domains has already been associated with factors within a person's personality, referred to as "personal factors" [12,13], as well as the social environment [14]. Researchers found self-control [13], self-concordant goal setting [12] and social support [14] to be predictive of addictive behavior in other life domains. In the present study, we aim to examine the relationship of self-control, self-concordance (personal factors) and social support (social factor) with exercise dependence.

By suggesting self-concordance as a potential predictor of exercise dependence, we refer to motivation psychology [15]. Sheldon and Elliott (1999) described self-concordance as "the extent to which a goal reflects personal interests and values versus something one feels compelled to do by external or internal pressures [16]. Engaging in self-concordant goals leads to optimal functioning and well-being [15]. Deeper insights to the underlying assumptions can be found in the self-determination theory [17,18]. Attesting to the importance of self-concordance in regard to addictive behaviors, self-concordance is associated with less excessive alcohol consumption [12]. In the same vein, dysfunctional goal characteristics lead to a higher risk of substance abuse and alcoholism [19]. Based on these studies, we assume that self-concordance might also be negatively related to exercise dependence.

Besides the self-concordance of goals [15], self-control is needed to translate goals into action [20]. Self-control is defined as the ability to suppress or control impulses and thereby control one's own behavior [13,21]. Therefore, persons with stronger self-control can better pursue and succeed in their long-term goals, because they are better at resisting distractions and temptations that might derail goal pursuit. Accordingly, self-control is important for effective self-regulation [22]. Besides the inhibition facet of self-control (e.g., to suppress the urge to eat chocolate in front of the TV), Hoyle and Davisson postulate that the initiation of behavior (e.g., starting to go for a run instead of watching TV), and the continuation of this behavior (e.g., staying with jogging, even when it becomes strenuous) are all facets of the ability of self-control [23].

Studies show that people who can control themselves well have more career success, more stable social relationships and enjoy better physical and mental health [22]. Low self-control, on the other hand, is linked with various individual problems or even social issues, like unhealthy eating, less exercising, impulsive buying, academic failure or underachievement, procrastination, substance abuse or even criminal activities [24–31]. In this study, we examine trait self-control (the relatively stable tendency to exert self-control successfully) as well as state self-control (perception of momentary ability/willingness to apply self-control) as correlates of exercise dependence.

The third variable we assume to be related to exercise dependence is social support. Social support can be provided by a peer group, by friends, or by the family, for example. Social support is defined as "social interactions or relationships that provide individuals with actual assistance or with a feeling of attachment to a person or group that is perceived as loving or caring [32]. Social support is differentiated into perceived social support (perception of the availability of social support) [33] and received social support (the retrospective perception of having been supported) [34].

A large body of evidence shows that social support can contribute to health [35–38]. Lower mortality rates [39,40], better recovery from surgery [41] and sport injuries [42], conveyance of healthy behavior [43,44], and the enhancement of well-being and motivation [45,46] are just a few examples of these positive effects. Most importantly, in the present research, social support acted as a protective factor for the use of substances or alcohol [47], the frequency of gambling [48] and social media addiction [14]. However, studies analyzing the effects of social support on exercise dependence are scarce. The findings of Lukács and colleagues showed that feelings of not being socially integrated can increase an exerciser's volume of sport activity [49]. Furthermore, a study with Australian elite athletes from various sports revealed that athletes who are at risk of exercise dependence report lower social support scores compared to their non-at-risk peers [50].

The present research aims to examine personal and social resources simultaneously in order to determine the strength of their potential relationship with exercise dependence. Specifically, we test the hypothesis that athletes with high self-control (trait and state), high exercise-related self-concordance and high levels of social support are less likely to be exercise dependent. Because endurance sports athletes show the greatest risk of exercise dependence [51], we focused on endurance athletes from all types of endurance sports, without any age restrictions except the age of majority in order to increase sample heterogeneity, and therefore the generalizability of our findings. Thus, we extend previous research that focused on specific types of endurance sports [49,52–54].

2. Materials and Methods

2.1. Participants

Two hundred and eleven athletes from different endurance sports took part in an online survey. The subjects were recruited by social media and mailing lists, as well as by written advertisements in sports medicine centers. The inclusion criteria were that athletes had to engage in regular exercise in an endurance sport and had to be a minimum of 18 years old. Due to incomplete data (premature cancellation of the questionnaire), 58 subjects had to be excluded from the study. A further 13 athletes were excluded because they did not meet the inclusion criteria. Finally, the data of 82 male and 58 female ($N = 140$) endurance athletes aged between 18 and 76 years ($M = 36.35$, $SD = 14.66$) were analyzed. Most of the athletes were runners ($n = 67$), triathletes ($n = 29$), and mixed ($n = 24$, for example, running and swimming). Swimming ($n = 9$), cycling ($n = 10$) and rowing ($n = 1$) were less represented in the sample. More detailed descriptions of the sample are presented in the results section.

2.2. Procedure

Participants completed a web survey that contained informed consent questions with regard to their sporting activity, as well as the frequency and intensity of the sport, and questionnaires assessing the relevant variables for this research (exercise dependence, self-control, self-concordance, and social support; see below). Participants filled in further questionnaires, which will not be discussed in this paper as they do not relate to the present research question. The web survey ended with a detailed debrief and the information that participants could receive feedback about their scores, as well as some additional information. If they were interested in receiving feedback, they subscribed with their email address, which was saved using a web survey separate from the data provided by the participants. The study was carried out in accordance with the guidelines that were laid out in the Declaration of Helsinki in 1975. Moreover, according to the guidelines of the ethics committee of the first author's university, no separate Institutional Review Board statement was required for this study. Participants who entered the online study were informed about the purpose of the study, delivered informed consent and confirmed that they voluntarily agreed to participate. In data collection and data processing we followed the compliance of the Health Insurance Portability and Accountability Act (HIPAA).

2.3. Measures

Participants indicated their sex, age, occupational status, the frequency and duration of their training sessions, and whether they participate in competitions or not.

In order to assess addictive behavior, the Exercise Dependence Scale (EDS) was used [55]. The scale is based on the Diagnostic and Statistical Manual of Mental Disorders-IV criteria for substance dependence [56]. Hausenblas and Downs used these criteria to operationalize their multidimensional questionnaire for maladaptive behavior in exercising. The athletes were asked to rate their exercise beliefs and behaviors that have occurred in the past three months. Each of the seven dimensions, tolerance ("I continually increase my exercise duration to achieve the desired effects/benefits."), withdrawal ("I exercise to avoid feeling tense."), intention effects ("I exercise longer than I intend."), lack of control

("I am unable to reduce how often I exercise."), time ("I spend most of my free time exercising."), reduction in other activities ("I would rather exercise than spend time with family/friends.") and continuance ("I exercise when injured.") each had three items with a rating scale from 1 (never) to 6 (always). Average scores for each dimension as well as an overall score were calculated. The EDS allows us to categorize responses in the following manner: (1) at risk—this category includes individuals whose responses are in the "at risk" range, which corresponds to a Likert-scale score of five or six for at least three of the seven criteria; (2) nondependent-symptomatic—this category includes people for whom at least three of the seven criteria are in the "nondependent-symptomatic" range (on the Likert scale, these are the values three and four); and (3) nondependent-asymptomatic—people who are neither addicted nor show symptoms of a sports addiction (on the Likert scale, values of one or two can be found here). Cronbach´s alpha for the overall scale showed an internal consistency of $\alpha = 0.88$.

Perceived and received social support were measured with the Berlin Social Support Scale [57]. While the perceived scale with eight items measures a prospective ("When everything becomes too much for me to handle, others are there to help me."), the received scale with 15 items measures a retrospective perspective ("This person made me feel valued and important.") of social support. Participants rated each statement using a four-point scale ranging from 1 (not at all) to 4 (exactly true). In the present study, the scales showed a high internal consistency (perceived $\alpha = 0.94$, received $\alpha = 0.90$).

The Capacity for Self-Control Scale (CSCS) was used to measure the trait dimension of self-control [23]. The scale consists of 20 items that have to be answered on a five-point Likert-scale from 1 (hardly ever) to 5 (nearly always). Examples for items are "I have trouble resisting my cravings." and "I get started on new projects right away". Cronbach´s alpha was $\alpha = 0.86$.

Momentary available self-control was measured using the 25-item State Self-Control Capacity Scale ($\alpha = 0.94$) [58]. Participants indicated their agreement with statements (e.g., "Example") using a seven-point rating scale ranging from 1 (not correct at all) to 7 (fully correct). In both questionnaires for self-control the athletes were made aware that the statements did not only refer to sport, but more to life in general.

To measure the self-concordance of participants´ sport- and exercise-related goals, the Self-Concordance in Sport Scale was used [59]. The scale is based on Deci and Ryan´s self-determination theory as well on Sheldon and Elliot´s self-concordance model [15,17]. Participants were asked to rate their intention to exercise in the next few weeks on a six-point Likert scale ranging from 1 (does not apply at all) to 6 (fully applies). Therefore, they had to complete the sentence "In the next few weeks and months, I intend to exercise ... ". Intrinsic ("...because I enjoy exercising"), identified (" ... by personal decision"), introjected (" ... I feel guilty, when I don´t exercise") and extrinsic (" ... I exercise because other people say I should") forms of regulation were assessed with three items for each subscale. An overall self-concordance score was created by summing the identified and intrinsic scores and then subtracting the introjected and external scores. The internal consistency for the four subscales ranged from $\alpha = 0.60$ to $\alpha = 0.73$.

2.4. Data Analysis

In all analyses, the assumption of normal distribution was tested with the Shapiro–Wilk test and variance homogeneity was tested with the Levene test. In case of significant main effects, Bonferroni-corrected post hoc tests were calculated to compare differences between specific factor levels. For all tests, statistical significance was set at $p < 0.05$. Cohen´s ds were calculated as effect size estimates, where d > 0.20 represents a small, d > 0.50, moderate, and d > 0.80 a large effect respectively $r > 0.10$ represents a small, $r > 0.30$, moderate, and $r > 0.50$ a large effect at the correlation analyses [60].

In order to test for differences between risk groups in workload and state self-control, one-way analyses of variance (ANOVA) were run. We used T-Tests or Mann–Whitney-U-tests (if normal distribution was violated) to analyze whether men and women differ in the measured variables.

Assessing our hypotheses, correlations between variables were calculated via Pearson correlation coefficients, if the data in the investigated parameters were normal distributed. Otherwise, Spearman correlations were computed. Subsequently, a hierarchical multiple regression with exercise dependence as dependent variable was calculated. At first, the trait factors, self-concordance and trait self-control, were included in the regression equation. As a second step, state self-control was added. For the supplemental analyses, we also conducted a mediation analysis according to the procedure suggested by Baron and Kenny [61]. All analyses were run with JASP, Version 0.14.1, [62] and the statistical software environment R [63]. The plots were created with GGPLOT 2 [64].

3. Results

3.1. Characteristics of the Sample

Besides the overall score for exercise dependence, we classified athletes into three different risk groups (at risk, nondependent symptomatic, and nondependent asymptomatic) according to a classification system proposed by Hausenblas and Downs [55]. Eight athletes were identified as "at risk" for exercise dependence while 93 athletes could be classified as "nondependent symptomatic" and 39 athletes as "nondependent asymptomatic".

On average, the athletes had been involved with their sports for 12.77 years (SD = 9.25) and reported that they exercise M = 6.01 (SD = 3.18) times per week for M = 85.46 min (SD = 33.45) per session. This results in an average workload of M = 512.23 min (SD = 305.88) per week. Eleven participants reported that they do not take part in competitions. Furthermore, seven athletes train with a coach, while 83 exercise alone and 50 practice in a group. Related to the classification of exercise dependence, the "at risk" group exercises for 110 min (SD = 58.80) per training session and exercises more often (M_{units} = 8.31, SD = 3.72) than the nondependent symptomatic ($M_{minutes}$ = 86.71, SD = 30.59; M_{units} = 6.37, SD = 3.42) and the nondependent asymptomatic groups ($M_{minutes}$ = 77.42, SD = 31.52; M_{units} = 4.69, SD = 1.70). In order to test the differences between workload, a one-way ANOVA was run. Levene´s test showed a significant result, so the analysis was corrected with the Welch test. The analysis revealed a significant main effect, $F(2, 18.54) = 14.26$, $p < 0.001$, $\eta^2 = 0.15$. Post hoc tests with Bonferroni correction showed that athletes in the "at risk" group showed a significantly higher workload (M = 840.00 min per week, SD = 353.42) compared to athletes in the "nondependent symptomatic" group (M = 548.89 min per week, SD = 312.95), $t = -2.77$, $p = 0.019$, $d = -0.92$, and the athletes in the nondependent asymptomatic group (M = 357.58 min per week, SD = 177.95), $t = -4.37$, $p < 0.001$, $d = -2.25$. Furthermore, athletes in the "nondependent symptomatic" group have a significantly higher workload than persons with no symptoms, $t = -3.53$, $p = 0.002$, $d = -0.68$. The different workloads are illustrated in Figure 1.

3.2. Preliminary Analysis

In their review, Dumitru and colleagues [65] examined gender differences in the prevalence of exercise dependence and concluded that men are more at risk for exercise addiction than women. Therefore, we tested for gender differences in exercise dependence and in the other dependent variables. Table 1 shows the results of t-tests (for normally distributed variables) and Mann–Whitney U-tests (for non-normally distributed variables). The analyses revealed a significant difference for state self-control with higher scores for men (M = 5.27, SD = 1.00) compared to women (M = 4.92, SD = 1.04), W = 2842, p = 0.050, d = 0.20.

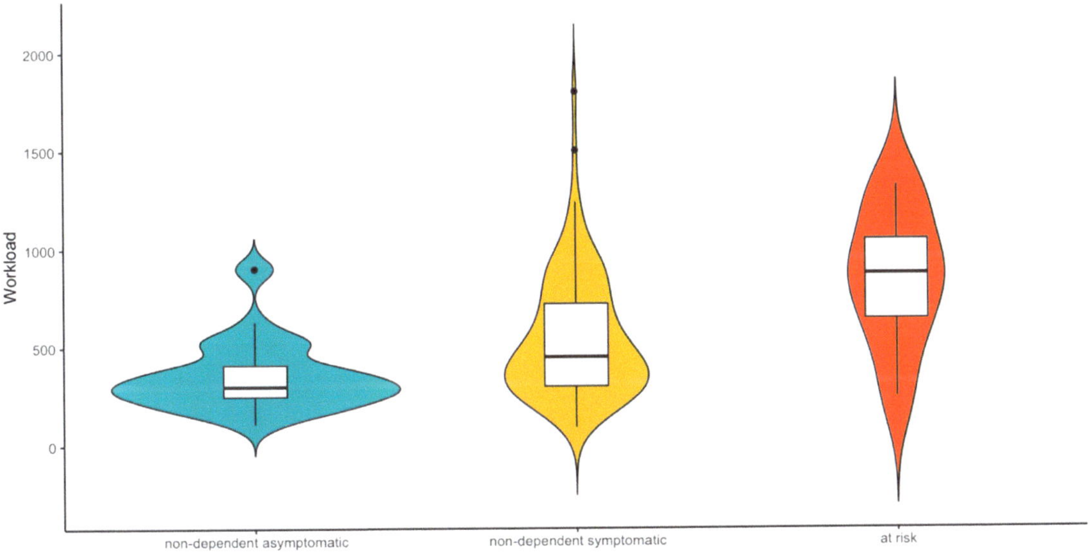

Figure 1. Workload per week (minutes × unit) illustrated for the three classifications of exercise dependence.

Table 1. Descriptive statistics and tests for differences between male and female athletes.

	Total (N = 140)	Male (n = 82)	Female (n = 58)	t/U	p
	M (SD)	M (SD)	M (SD)		
Exercise dependence	2.98 (0.70)	2.94 (0.73)	3.04 (0.65)	−0.85	0.395
Self-control (trait)	3.52 (0.54)	3.49 (0.58)	3.56 (0.47)	−0.76	0.446
Self-concordance *	3.16 (0.98)	3.15 (0.92)	3.17 (1.08)	2311.50	0.780
Self-control (state) *	5.13 (1.03)	5.27 (1.00)	4.92 (1.04)	2842.00	0.050
Perceived support *	3.61 (0.51)	3.56 (0.55)	3.69 (0.45)	1986.00	0.087
Received support *	3.33 (0.54)	3.28 (0.57)	3.39 (0.50)	2117.50	0.271
Workload *	512.16 (305.88)	549.54 (320.39)	459.48 (278.30)	2814.50	0.065

Note. * Assumption of normal distribution was violated. Therefore, a non-parametric test was used.

3.3. Descriptive Statistics and Correlation Analyses

Pearson correlations and Spearman correlations (if nonparametric test is required) were computed between trait and state self-control, self-concordance, perceived and received social support and exercise dependence (see Table 2). Small to moderate negative correlations were observed between exercise dependence and self-concordance ($r = -0.23$, $p = 0.006$), trait self-control ($r = -0.26$, $p = 0.002$) and state self-control ($r = -0.39$, $p < 0.001$). In contrast, exercise dependence was not significantly related to social support.

Moderate to large positive correlations were found between self-concordance and trait self-control ($r = 0.36$, $p < 0.001$) and self-concordance and state self-control ($r = 0.53$, $p < 0.001$). Furthermore, a large positive correlation of trait and state self-control was observed ($r = 0.49$, $p < 0.001$). Self-concordance and social support were positively correlated (perceived: $r = 0.21$, $p = 0.002$; received: $r = 0.18$, $p = 0.038$). State and trait self-control were positively correlated to perceived social support (trait: $r = 0.21$, $p = 0.008$; state: $r = 0.29$, $p < 0.001$).

Table 2. Correlations and descriptive statistics for the dependent variables.

Variables	EDS	SCT	SSC	SCS	PER	REC	WKL
Exercise dependence—EDS	1						
Self-control (trait)—SCT	−0.26 **	1					
Self-concordance—SSC	−0.23 **	0.36 ***	1				
Self-control (state)—SCS	−0.39 ***	0.49 ***	0.53 ***	1			
Perceived support—PER	−0.10	0.21 *	0.21 *	0.29 ***	1		
Received support—REC	0.01	0.18 *	0.18 *	0.14	0.52 ***	1	
Workload—WKL	0.31 ***	0.10	0.05	0.06	−0.01	0.12	1
Mean	3.01	3.50	3.08	5.09	3.59	3.32	526.28
SD	0.70	0.55	1.04	1.03	0.54	0.54	334.11
Range	1–7	1–5	−6–6	1–7	1–4	1–4	90–1800

Note 2. The Pearson correlation was run for the Exercise Dependence Scale (EDS) and self-concordance (SSC), for EDS and self-control (state) (SCS) and for SSC and SCS. For all other analyses, Spearman's Rho was calculated. * $p < 0.05$, ** $p < 0.01$, *** $p < 0.001$.

3.4. Regression Analyses

The correlation analyses showed that social support (social factor) is not related to exercise dependence, whereas all three personal factors revealed a negative relationship with exercise dependence. To further explore the strength of the effects and disentangle the effects of trait and state effects, a hierarchical multiple regression was computed. At first, the trait factors, self-concordance and trait self-control, were included in the regression equation (Model 1). Then, as a second step, state self-control was added in Model 2.

The results of these regression analyses are summarized in Table 3. Model 1 was significant, $F(2, 137) = 5.84$, $p = 0.004$, but neither self-concordance, nor trait self-control were revealed as significant predictors. However, their effects were marginally significant at $p < 0.10$, explaining why Model 1 was significant. When accounting for state self-control (Model 2), the trait factors became nonsignificant (see Table 3) and state self-control was the only significant statistical predictor of exercise dependence. Overall, Model 2 was significant, $F(3, 136) = 8.54$, $p = 0.001$.

Table 3. Regression analyses predicting exercise dependence.

Variable	Model 1					Model 2				
	b	*SE b*	*β*	*p*	95% CI	*b*	*SE b*	*β*	*p*	95% CI
Intercept	4.14	0.38		0.001		4.52	0.38		0.001	
Self-concordance	−0.12	0.06	−0.16	0.066	[−0.241, 0.008]	−0.02	0.07	−0.03	0.751	[−0.151, 0.109]
Trait self-control	−0.23	0.12	−0.18	0.052	[−0.453, 0.002]	−0.07	0.12	−0.05	0.556	[−0.305, 0.165]
State self-control						−0.24	0.07	−0.35	0.001	[−0.371, −0.108]
R^2	0.08					0.16				
Adj. R^2	0.07					0.14				

Note. SE: standard error. CI = Confidence interval.

3.5. Mediation Analyses—Self-Control, Self-Concordance and Exercise Dependence

The results of the correlational pattern between variables suggest that the effects of self-concordance and trait self-control on exercise dependence could be mediated by state self-control. A mediation analysis including both predictors (see Figure 2) showed that the relationship between self-concordance and exercise dependence (indirect effect: $z = -2.99$, $se = 0.05$, $p = 0.003$, 95% CI [−0.227, −0.047], total effect: $z = -1.88$, $se = 0.09$, $p = 0.061$, 95% CI [−0.342, 0.007]) as well as the relationship between trait self-control and dependence (indirect effect: $z = -2.87$, $se = 0.08$, $p = 0.004$, 95% CI [−0.375, −0.070], total effect: $z = -1.98$, $se = 0.16$, $p = 0.048$, 95% CI [−0.643, −0.003]), were fully mediated by state self-control. An overview of the unstandardized model parameters is given in Figure 2.

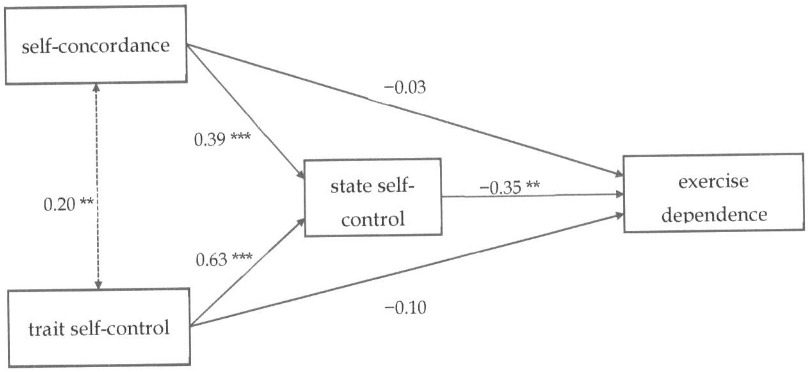

Figure 2. The pathways of the mediation model. Coefficients are unstandardized. ** $p < 0.01$, *** $p < 0.001$.

3.6. Supplemental Analysis—Risk Factor Groups

The linear regression analyses revealed that momentary available self-control predicts exercise dependence. A one-way ANOVA testing whether risk factor groups differed in state self-control was significant $F(2, 18.65) = 7.60$, $p = 0.004$, $\eta^2 = 0.10$. A Bonferroni-corrected post hoc test revealed that the nondependent asymptomatic group ($M = 5.58$, $SD = 0.96$) scored significantly higher score on state self-control than the nondependent symptomatic ($M = 5.01$, $SD = 0.99$; $t = 3.06$, $p = 0.008$, $d = 0.59$), and the at-risk groups ($M = 4.26$, $SD = 1.03$; $t = 3.47$, $p = 0.002$, $d = 1.36$). There was no significant difference between the nondependent symptomatic and at-risk groups ($t = 2.07$, $p = 0.122$, $d = 0.76$).

4. Discussion

The aim of this study was to promote research in exercise dependence by taking personal factors from motivational research (self-concordance) and volitional research (self-control), as well as social support, into account simultaneously. In support for our hypotheses, self-control and self-concordance were negatively related to exercise dependence. Further unpacking this relationship, we found that state self-control mediated the link between trait self-control, self-concordance and exercise dependence. Trait self-control and self-concordance of exercise goals seem to activate high momentary available self-control, which, in turn, was associated with a reduced risk of exercise dependence. This is in line with prior work by Sheldon and Elliot [15], which found that self-concordant goals lead to sustained effort, which, in turn, led to better goal attainment and well-being. In the context of the present study, high self-concordance might facilitate heightened perceptions of momentary self-control (triggering higher effort), which might protect against detrimental behavioral tendencies (e.g., excessive exercise). The perception of higher momentary self-control might result from the fact that striving for goals that are *not* self-concordant requires additional effort, while current theorizing on self-control indicates that the exertion of self-control reduces the willingness to invest further effort [66]. In contrast, self-concordant goals themselves require less effort, which could, in turn, be invested into successful task execution.

The findings from this study reveal that trait and state self-control are linked to each other in predicting the risk of addictive behavior in exercising. Several approaches regarding how trait self-control might elucidate state self-control can be found in the literature (for an overview, see de Ridder, 2018) [67]. First, besides the assumption that successfully dealing with self-control dilemmas can be traced back to successful inhibition, a meta-analysis from de Ridder and colleagues [22] emphasizes that individuals with high trait self-control reported stronger automatized adaptive behavior like habits or routines that can be performed without effort. Second, they organize themselves and their environment in a way that means they need to deal with effortful inhibitions to a lesser extent in everyday life because this structure prevents them from being constantly confronted with problematic temptations [68]. This is also in line with Duckworth´s considerations on situational self-control [69].

According to Ent et al., 2015, self-control could be interpreted as a proactive trait that is helpful avoiding harmful behaviors [70]. In terms of our study context, it is likely that athletes with high trait self-control structure their lives in a more adaptive way, and that maintenance of their lives is less demanding in terms of the application of constant self-control. Nevertheless, once a self-control dilemma occurs, these individuals are able to deal with this dilemma more efficiently [71]. In relation to the expression of the exercise dependence scale in terms of continuance, for example, a dilemma could be that an athlete striving for an improvement in their personal best in a half marathon is interrupted by an injury. In order to reach this goal, regular exercising is necessary. Therefore, the athlete's aim to improve is in conflict with the need to recover from the injury. Thus, an athlete with high state self-control would be able to make a better choice when an injury occurred, as further exercising would be harmful to their health.

Furthermore, the supplemental analysis on the group level supports our findings from the linear analysis. Athletes in the "nondependent asymptomatic" group showed significantly higher momentary self-control than the "nondependent symptomatic and at risk" group.

In our sample, 7% of endurance sport athletes belonging to the "at risk" group, 66% to the "nondependent symptomatic" group and 28% to the "nondependent asymptomatic" group. Previous studies display similar distributions for the risk of exercise dependence in their samples [49,51,72–74]. Moreover, comparing the three groups "at risk", "non-dependent symptomatic", and "nondependent asymptomatic" shows that the different workloads in the groups can be traced back to the fact that athletes in these groups attend more training sessions per week rather than to the duration of a session. This finding is supported by studies that revealed a positive relationship between the total duration spent training and the risk of exercise dependence [75,76].

Contrary to our assumptions, neither perceived nor received support is directly related to exercise dependence in this study. Moreover, unexpectedly, social support was positively related to self-concordance and self-control, and is therefore associated with facets of self-regulation. Why social support does not affect a specific domain of self-regulation (exercise dependence) remains an unanswered question. We can only speculate that the different levels of abstraction of the concepts (general: self-control, self-concordance; sport-specific: dependence) might provide a rationale that should be tested empirically.

There are some limitations to this study that should be acknowledged. Our study is cross-sectional. Therefore, the line of reasoning in mediation analysis is based on theoretical deliberations and cannot take temporal sequencing of variables into account. Furthermore, estimated mediation effects are based on correlational relations between the variables, which does not allow for any specifications about directionality. Deeper insights and advanced interpretations of directions and causality of effects would be enabled by longitudinal data, especially since developing an exercise dependence is likely to develop gradually and over time. In consideration of the fluctuation of personal state factors in contrast to stable personal trait factors (e.g., self-control) [66], a longitudinal design could further lead to a better understanding of the observed relation between state and trait factors predicting the risk of harmful exercising.

Although our study extends the current research on exercise dependence by simultaneously taking motivational and volitional factors into account, our study is limited in its design. We used a self-report questionnaire (EDS), which is based on a risk score and risk categorization (at risk, nondependent symptomatic and nondependent asymptomatic) and is not a clinical diagnosis instrument for addiction. However, it should be mentioned that exercise dependence is not classified within any medical or psychological diagnostic frameworks [4]. Moreover, the interpretation of self-reported data is complicated because of possible bias due to the nature of the studied sample (e.g., demographics, gender and race/ethnicity). Szabo and colleagues suggested that future research in the field of exercise dependence should be extended with in-depth interviews with athletes suspected to be at risk of exercise dependence by those instruments [5]. This kind of mixed-methods approach, using quantitative as well as qualitative data, could lead to a better understanding and characterization of exercise dependence and its symptoms, as well as its promoting and preventing factors (like self-control and self-concordance). Once these mechanisms become clearer, it will be easier to explore possible prevention strategies and recommend appropriate interventions.

Practical implications can be derived from our findings that address the three components in our mediation model (see Figure 2). According to self-concordance, athletes and coaches were recommend spending effort to choose goals that fit the values, interests, and personality of the athlete. As reported by Sheldon, knowing one's implicit motivations and potentials are important for setting more self-concordant goals. This can be reached by interpersonal contexts (e.g., coach–athlete relationships) that promote accurate self-insights and provide autonomy support [77]. Moreover, Weinberg and Gould provide a good overview of implementation strategies of goal setting and explain the underlying key processes [78].

Self-control, as the second component of our mediation model, can be improved by specific self-control training (for a review of self-control training effects see Friese and colleagues) [79]. These trainings are theoretically based on the assumption of the strength model of self-control that self-control can be trained as a muscle [80]. Repeated exposure to self-control (for example by pressing a hand-grip device regularly or simply brushing one´s teeth with the non-dominant hand) build up self-control [81].

The third component, state self-control, can be modified by reducing other tasks that require self-control (see ego depletion effect) [21,80,82]. A simple example would be to reduce stress at work or to better structure daily life and environment.

5. Conclusions

Our results showed that self-control and self-concordance play a key role in predicting exercise dependence in endurance athletes, whereas, unexpectedly, social support did not explain the variance in exercise dependence. Additionally, the present study suggests that both trait factors decrease the risk of exercise dependence by increasing perceptions of momentary self-control. These findings can help to enhance awareness when dealing with high training volumes and the development of addictive exercising behavior in endurance sports at recreational and elite levels. Mixed-methods procedures (e.g., also including lab experiments, in that self-concordance of an exercise goal is experimentally manipulated) and longitudinal studies are recommended to shed further light on the assumed mechanism.

Author Contributions: J.S. and Z.Z. conceptualized the experimental design. Z.Z. carried out the data collection. Data analysis was performed by Z.Z., W.W., J.S. The first draft was written by Z.Z.; W.W. and J.S. revised and edited the manuscript which was then finalized by Z.Z. All authors have read and agreed to the published version of the manuscript.

Funding: This research received no external funding.

Institutional Review Board Statement: Ethical review and approval were waived for this study, due to the fact that research in the field of sports science that is non-invasive and mainly addresses sport-scientific questions is not supervised by the Ethics Committee of the University of Konstanz.

Informed Consent Statement: Informed consent was obtained from all subjects involved in the study.

Data Availability Statement: Data will be provided by the authors upon request.

Acknowledgments: The authors thank all participants for their contribution. Furthermore, we thank the students from our project seminar for their assistance in data collection.

Conflicts of Interest: The authors declare no conflict of interest.

References

1. Reiner, M.; Niermann, C.; Jekauc, D.; Woll, A. Long-term health benefits of physical activity—A systematic review of longitudinal studies. *BMC Public Health* **2013**, *13*, 813. [CrossRef]
2. WHO. Guidelines on Physical Activity and Sedentary Behaviour. Available online: https://www.who.int/publications/i/item/9789240015111 (accessed on 1 December 2020).
3. O'Donovan, G.; Blazevich, A.J.; Boreham, C.; Cooper, A.R.; Crank, H.; Ekelund, U.; Fox, K.R.; Gately, P.; Giles-Corti, B.; Gill, J.M.R.; et al. The ABC of Physical Activity for Health: A consensus statement from the British Association of Sport and Exercise Sciences. *J. Sports Sci.* **2010**, *28*, 573–591. [CrossRef] [PubMed]
4. Berczik, K.; Szabó, A.; Griffiths, M.D.; Kurimay, T.; Kun, B.; Urbán, R.; Demetrovics, Z. Exercise addiction: Symptoms, diagnosis, epidemiology, and etiology. *Subst. Use Misuse* **2012**, *47*, 403–417. [CrossRef] [PubMed]
5. Szabo, A.; Griffiths, M.D.; Marcos, R.D.L.V.; Mervó, B.; Demetrovics, Z. Methodological and conceptual limitations in exercise addiction research. *Yale J. Biol. Med.* **2015**, *88*, 303. [PubMed]
6. Brown, R.I.F. Some contributions of the study of gambling to the study of other addictions. In *Gambling Behavior and Problem Gambling*; Eadington, W.R., Cornelius, J.A., Eds.; University of Nevada Press: Reno, NV, USA, 1993; pp. 241–272.
7. Griffiths, M. A 'components' model of addiction within a biopsychosocial framework. *J. Subst. Use* **2005**, *10*, 191–197. [CrossRef]
8. Szabo, A. *Addiction to Exercise: A Symptom or a Disorder?* Nova Science Publishers: New York, NY, USA, 2010.
9. Adams, J.; Kirkby, R.J. Excessive exercise as an addiction: A review. *Addict. Res. Theory* **2002**, *10*, 415–437. [CrossRef]
10. Landolfi, E. Exercise addiction. *Sports Med.* **2013**, *43*, 111–119. [CrossRef]
11. Nogueira, A.; Molinero, O.; Salguero, A.; Márquez, S. Exercise addiction in practitioners of endurance sports: A literature review. *Front. Psychol.* **2018**, *9*, 1484. [CrossRef] [PubMed]
12. Caudwell, K.M.; Mullan, B.A.; Hagger, M.S. Combining motivational and volitional approaches to reducing excessive alcohol consumption in pre-drinkers: A theory-based intervention protocol. *BMC Public Health* **2016**, *16*, 45. [CrossRef] [PubMed]
13. Tangney, J.P.; Baumeister, R.F.; Boone, A.L. High self-control predicts good adjustment, less pathology, better grades, and interpersonal success. *J. Pers.* **2004**, *72*, 271–324. [CrossRef]
14. Brailovskaia, J.; Rohmann, E.; Bierhoff, H.W.; Schillack, H.; Margraf, J. The relationship between daily stress, social support and Facebook Addiction Disorder. *Psychiatry Res.* **2019**, *276*, 167–174. [CrossRef]
15. Sheldon, K.M.; Elliot, A.J. Goal striving, need satisfaction, and longitudinal well-being: The self-concordance model. *J. Pers. Soc. Psychol.* **1999**, *76*, 482. [CrossRef] [PubMed]
16. Koestner, R.; Lekes, N.; Powers, T.A.; Chicoine, E. Attaining personal goals: Self-concordance plus implementation intentions equals success. *J. Pers. Soc. Psychol.* **2002**, *83*, 231. [CrossRef]
17. Deci, E.L.; Ryan, R.M. The "what" and "why" of goal pursuits: Human needs and the self-determination of behavior. *Psychol. Inq.* **2000**, *11*, 227–268. [CrossRef]
18. Deci, E.L.; Ryan, R.M. Overview of self-determination theory: An organismic dialectical perspective. In *Handbook of Self-Determination Research*; Deci, E.L., Ryan, R.M., Eds.; University of Rochester: Rochester, NY, USA, 2002; pp. 3–33.
19. Cox, W.M.; Klinger, E. Motivational structure: Relationships with substance use and processes of change. *Addict. Behav.* **2002**, *27*, 925–940. [CrossRef]
20. Heckhausen, J.; Heckhausen, H. *Motivation and Action*; Cambridge University Press: New York, NY, USA, 2008; Volume 2.
21. Baumeister, R.F.; Bratslavsky, E.; Muraven, M.; Tice, D.M. Ego depletion: Is the active self a limited resource? *J. Pers. Soc. Psychol.* **1998**, *74*, 1252. [CrossRef]
22. De Ridder, D.T.D.; Lensvelt-Mulders, G.; Finkenauer, C.; Stok, F.M.; Baumeister, R.F. Taking stock of self-control: A meta-analysis of how trait self-control relates to a wide range of behaviors. *Pers. Soc. Psychol. Rev.* **2012**, *16*, 76–99. [CrossRef]
23. Hoyle, R.H.; Davisson, E.K. Varieties of self-control and their personality correlates. In *Handbook of Self-Regulation: Research, Theory, and Applications*; Vohs, K.D., Baumeister, R.F., Eds.; The Guilford Press: New York, NY, USA, 2016; pp. 396–413.
24. Duckworth, A.L.; Seligman, M.E.P. Self-discipline outdoes IQ in predicting academic performance of adolescents. *Psychol. Sci.* **2005**, *16*, 939–944. [CrossRef] [PubMed]
25. Gottfredson, M.R.; Hirschi, T. *A General Theory of Crime*; Stanford University Press: Redwood City, CA, USA, 1990.
26. Hagger, M.S.; Wood, C.W.; Stiff, C.; Chatzisarantis, N.L. Self-regulation and self-control in exercise: The strength-energy model. *Int. Rev. Sport Exerc. Psychol.* **2010**, *3*, 62–86. [CrossRef]
27. Hofmann, W.; Friese, M.; Roefs, A. Three ways to resist temptation: The independent contributions of executive attention, inhibitory control, and affect regulation to the impulse control of eating behavior. *J. Exp. Soc. Psychol.* **2009**, *45*, 431–435. [CrossRef]
28. Moffitt, T.E.; Arseneault, L.; Belsky, D.; Dickson, N.; Hancox, R.J.; Harrington, H.L.; Houts, R.; Poulton, R.; Roberts, B.W.; Ross, S.; et al. A gradient of childhood self-control predicts health, wealth, and public safety. *Proc. Natl. Acad. Sci. USA* **2011**, *108*, 2693–2698. [CrossRef]
29. Zhao, J.; Meng, G.; Sun, Y.; Xu, Y.; Geng, J.; Han, L. The relationship between self-control and procrastination based on the self-regulation theory perspective: The moderated mediation model. *Curr. Psychol.* **2019**, 1–11. [CrossRef]
30. Wills, T.A.; DuHamel, K.; Vaccaro, D. Activity and mood temperament as predictors of adolescent substance abuse; Test of a self-regulation mediational model. *J. Pers. Soc. Psycol.* **1995**, *68*, 901–916. [CrossRef]

31. Vohs, K.D.; Faber, R.J. Spent resources: Self-regulatory resource availability affects impulse buying. *J. Consum. Res.* **2007**, *3*, 537–547. [CrossRef]
32. Hobfoll, S.E.; Stokes, J.P. The process and mechanism of social support. In *The Handbook of Research in Personal Relationships*; Duck, S.W., Ed.; Wiley: London, UK, 1998; pp. 497–517.
33. Holt, N.L.; Hoar, S.D. The multidimensional construct of social support. In *Literature Reviews in Sport Psychology*; Hanton, S., Mellalieu, S.D., Eds.; Nova: New York, NY, USA, 2006; pp. 199–225.
34. Sarason, I.G.; Sarason, B.R.; Shearin, E.N. Social support as an individual difference variable: Its stability, origins, and relational aspects. *J. Pers. Soc. Psychol.* **1986**, *50*, 845. [CrossRef]
35. Berkman, L.F.; Glass, T. Social integration, social networks, social support, and health. *Soc. Epidemiol.* **2000**, *1*, 137–173.
36. Ditzen, B.; Heinrichs, M. Psychobiology of social support: The social dimension of stress buffering. *Restor. Neurol. Neurosci.* **2014**, *32*, 149–162. [CrossRef]
37. Pressman, S.D.; Cohen, S. Does positive affect influence health? *Psychol. Bull.* **2005**, *131*, 925. [CrossRef]
38. Uchino, B.N. *Social Support and Physical Health: Understanding the Health Consequences of Relationships*; Yale University Press: New Haven, CT, USA, 2004.
39. Brummett, B.H.; Barefoot, J.C.; Siegler, I.C.; Clapp-Channing, N.E.; Lytle, B.L.; Bosworth, H.B.; Williams, R.B., Jr.; Mark, D.B. Characteristics of socially isolated patients with coronary artery disease who are at elevated risk for mortality. *Psychosom. Med.* **2001**, *63*, 267–272. [CrossRef]
40. Rutledge, T.; Reis, S.E.; Olson, M.; Owens, J.; Kelsey, S.F.; Pepine, C.J.; Mankad, S.; Rogers, W.J.; Merz, C.N.B.; Sopko, G.; et al. Social networks are associated with lower mortality rates among women with suspected coronary disease: The National Heart, Lung, and Blood Institute-Sponsored Women's Ischemia Syndrome Evaluation study. *Psychosom. Med.* **2004**, *66*, 882–888. [CrossRef]
41. Kulik, J.A.; Mahler, H.I. Social support and recovery from surgery. *Health Psychol.* **1989**, *8*, 221. [CrossRef]
42. Bianco, T.; Eklund, R.C. Conceptual considerations for social support research in sport and exercise settings: The case of sport injury. *J. Sport Exerc. Psychol.* **2001**, *23*, 85–107. [CrossRef]
43. DiMatteo, M.R. Social support and patient adherence to medical treatment: A meta-analysis. *Health Psychol.* **2004**, *23*, 207. [CrossRef]
44. Martire, L.M.; Schulz, R. Involving family in psychosocial interventions for chronic illness. *Curr. Dir. Psychol. Sci.* **2007**, *16*, 90–94. [CrossRef]
45. DeFreese, J.D.; Smith, A.L. Athlete social support, negative social interactions and psychological health across a competitive sport season. *J. Sport Exerc. Psychol.* **2014**, *36*, 619–630. [CrossRef] [PubMed]
46. Wang, H.H. A meta-analysis of the relationship between social support and well-being. *Kaohsiung J. Med. Sci.* **1998**, *14*, 717–726.
47. Havassy, B.E.; Hall, S.M.; Wasserman, D.A. Social support and relapse: Commonalities among alcoholics, opiate users, and cigarette smokers. *Addict. Behav.* **1991**, *16*, 235–246. [CrossRef]
48. Thomas, A.C.; Allen, F.L.; Phillips, J.; Karantzas, G. Gaming machine addiction: The role of avoidance, accessibility and social support. *Psychol. Addict. Behav.* **2011**, *25*, 738. [CrossRef] [PubMed]
49. Lukacs, A.; Sasvári, P.; Varga, B.; Mayer, K. Exercise addiction and its related factors in amateur runners. *J. Behav. Addict.* **2019**, *8*, 343–349. [CrossRef] [PubMed]
50. McNamara, J.; McCabe, M.P. Striving for success or addiction? Exercise dependence among elite Australian athletes. *J. Sports Sci.* **2012**, *30*, 755–766. [CrossRef]
51. Di Lodovico, L.; Poulnais, S.; Gorwood, P. Which sports are more at risk of physical exercise addiction: A systematic review. *Addict. Behav.* **2019**, *93*, 257–262. [CrossRef] [PubMed]
52. Mayolas-Pi, C.; Simon-Grima, J.; Peñarrubia-Lozano, C.; Munguía-Izquierdo, D.; Moliner-Urdiales, D.; Legaz-Arrese, A. Exercise addiction risk and health in male and female amateur endurance cyclists. *J. Behav. Addict.* **2016**, *6*, 74–83. [CrossRef] [PubMed]
53. Schüler, J.; Knechtle, B.; Wegner, M. Antecedents of exercise dependence in ultra-endurance sports: Reduced basic need satisfaction and avoidance-motivated self-control. *Front. Psychol.* **2018**, *9*, 1275. [CrossRef] [PubMed]
54. Schipfer, M.; Cook, B.; Stoll, O. OR-95: Examination of changes in exercise dependece symptoms in endurance athletes throughout a competition season. *J. Behav. Addict.* **2016**, *5*, 39.
55. Hausenblas, H.A.; Downs, D.S. How much is too much? The development and validation of the exercise dependence scale. *Psychol. Health* **2002**, *17*, 387–404. [CrossRef]
56. De Coverley Veale, D.M.E. Exercise dependence. *Brit. J. Addict.* **1987**, *82*, 735–740. [CrossRef]
57. Schultz, U.; Schwarzer, R. Social support by coping with illness: The Berlin Social Support Scale (BSSS). *Diagnostica* **2003**, *40*, 73–82.
58. Bertrams, A.; Unger, A.; Dickhäuser, O. Momentan verfügbare Selbstkontrollkraft—Vorstellung eines Messinstruments und erste Befunde aus pädagogisch-psychologischen Kontexten. [Momentarily available self-control strength—Introduction of a measure and first findings from educational-psychological contexts]. *Z. Für Pädagogische Psychol.* **2011**, *25*, 185–196.
59. Seelig, H.; Fuchs, R. Messung der sport-und bewegungsbezogenen Selbstkonkordanz [Measurement of exercise-related self-concordance]. *Z. Für Sportpsychol.* **2006**, *13*, 121–139. [CrossRef]
60. Cohen, J. *Statistical Power Analysis for the Behavioral Sciences*, 2nd ed.; Erlbaum Associates: Hillsdale, NJ, USA, 1988.
61. Baron, R.M.; Kenny, D.A. The moderator–mediator variable distinction in social psychological research: Conceptual, strategic, and statistical considerations. *J. Pers. Soc. Psychol.* **1986**, *51*, 1173. [CrossRef]

62. JASP Team. *JASP (Version 0.14.1) [Computer Software]*; Department of Psychological Methods, University of Amsterdam: Amsterdam, The Netherlands, 2020.
63. R Core Team. *R: A Language and Environment for Statistical Computing*; R Foundation for Statistical Computing: Vienna, Austria, 2018.
64. Wickham, H. *Ggplot2*; Springer: New York, NY, USA, 2009.
65. Dumitru, D.C.; Dumitru, T.; Maher, A.J. A systematic review of exercise addiction: Examining gender differences. *J. Phys. Educ. Sport* **2018**, *18*, 1738–1747.
66. Wolff, W.; Martarelli, C.S. Bored into Depletion? Toward a Tentative Integration of Perceived Self-Control Exertion and Boredom as Guiding Signals for Goal-Directed Behavior. *Perspect. Psychol. Sci.* **2020**, *15*, 1272–1283. [CrossRef] [PubMed]
67. De Ridder, D.T.D.; Kroese, F.; Gillebaart, M. Whatever happened to self-control? A proposal for integrating notions from trait self-control studies into state self-control research. *Motiv. Sci.* **2018**, *4*, 39. [CrossRef]
68. Hofmann, W.; Baumeister, R.F.; Förster, G.; Vohs, K.D. Everyday temptations: An experience sampling study of desire, conflict, and self-control. *J. Pers. Soc. Psychol.* **2012**, *102*, 1318. [CrossRef]
69. Duckworth, A.L.; Gendler, T.S.; Gross, J.J. Situational Strategies for Self-Control. *Perspect. Psychol. Sci.* **2016**, *11*, 35–55. [CrossRef] [PubMed]
70. Ent, M.R.; Baumeister, R.F.; Tice, D.M. Trait self-control and the avoidance of temptation. *Pers. Individ. Differ.* **2015**, *74*, 12–15. [CrossRef]
71. Gillebaart, M.; de Ridder, D.T.D. Effortless self-control: A novel perspective on response conflict strategies in trait self-control. *Soc. Personal. Psychol. Compass* **2015**, *9*, 88–99. [CrossRef]
72. Hale, B.D.; Diehl, D.; Weaver, K.; Briggs, M. Exercise dependence and muscle dysmorphia in novice and experienced female bodybuilders. *J. Behav. Addict.* **2013**, *2*, 244–248. [CrossRef] [PubMed]
73. Miller, K.J.; Mesagno, C. Personality traits and exercise dependence: Exploring the role of narcissism and perfectionism. *Int. J. Sport Exerc. Psychol.* **2014**, *12*, 368–381. [CrossRef]
74. Weik, M.; Hale, B.D. Contrasting gender differences on two measures of exercise dependence. *Br. J. Sports Med.* **2009**, *43*, 204–207. [CrossRef] [PubMed]
75. Karr, T.M.; Zunker, C.; Thompson, R.A.; Sherman, R.T.; Erickson, A.; Cao, L.; Crosby, R.D.; Mitchell, J.E. Moderators of the association between exercise identity and obligatory exercise among participants of an athletic event. *Body Image* **2013**, *10*, 70–77. [CrossRef] [PubMed]
76. Zarauz-Sancho, A.; Ruiz-Juan, F.; Flores-Allende, G.; Arufe Giráldez, V. Predictor variables of the perception of success: Differential aspects in route runners. *Rev. Int. Med. Cienc. Act. Física Del Deporte* **2016**, *16*, 601–615.
77. Sheldon, K.M. Becoming Oneself: The Central Role of Self-Concordant Goal Selection. *Pers. Soc. Psychol. Rev.* **2014**, *18*, 349–365. [CrossRef]
78. Weinberg, R.S.; Gould, D. *Foundations of Sport and Exercise Psychology*; Human Kinetics: Champaign, IL, USA, 2014.
79. Friese, M.; Frankenbach, J.; Job, V.; Loschelder, D.D. Does Self-Control Training Improve Self-Control? A Meta-Analysis. *Perspect. Psychol. Sci.* **2017**, *12*, 1077–1099. [CrossRef]
80. Baumeister, R.F.; Vohs, K.D.; Tice, D.M. The strength model of self-control. *Curr. Dir. Psychol. Sci.* **2007**, *16*, 351–355. [CrossRef]
81. Miles, E.; Sheeran, P.; Baird, H.; Macdonald, I.; Webb, T.L.; Harris, P.R. Does self-control improve with practice? Evidence from a six-week training program. *J. Exp. Psychol. Gen.* **2016**, *145*, 1075–1091. [CrossRef] [PubMed]
82. Muraven, M.; Baumeister, R.F. Self-regulation and depletion of limited resources: Does self-control resemble a muscle? *Psychol. Bull.* **2000**, *126*, 247–259. [CrossRef]

International Journal of
Environmental Research and Public Health

MDPI

Article

Effects of Double-Taped Kinesio Taping on Pain and Functional Performance due to Muscle Fatigue in Young Males: A Randomized Controlled Trial

Haneul Lee [1] and Hyoungwon Lim [2,*]

1 Department of Physical Therapy, Gachon University, Inchon 21936, Korea; leehaneul84@gachon.ac.kr
2 Department of Physical Therapy, Dankook University, Cheonan 31116, Korea
* Correspondence: 11954690@dankook.ac.kr; Tel.: +82-41-550-1641

Received: 11 March 2020; Accepted: 29 March 2020; Published: 31 March 2020

Abstract: Kinesio taping (KT) is widely applied for pain control and rehabilitation in clinical settings. Tape tension is a key factor in the taping method. However, limited evidence exists regarding the reinforced tension effects of KT on functional performance and pain in healthy individuals. This study aimed to investigate the immediate effects of double-taped Kinesio taping (DTKT) on functional performance and pain caused by muscle fatigue after exercise. A total of 44 healthy male students (mean age, 23.3 ± 2.2 years) were randomly assigned to the following three groups: DTKT, normal-tape Kinesio taping (NTKT), and placebo. The single-hopping (SH) distance, vertical jump height (VJH), and power (VJP) were assessed at baseline. The muscle fatigue protocol was then applied to induce muscle soreness. Outcome measures including subjective pain, SH distance, VJH and VJP were evaluated immediately after the muscle fatigue protocol, and KT was then applied; the measures were then again evaluated immediately and 24 h after KT application. No significant interactions between pain and functional performance were observed ($p > 0.05$), and there were no significant differences in SH, VJH, and VJP among the groups ($p > 0.05$). Notably, the DTKT had an immediate effect on the alleviation of pain caused by muscle fatigue. The present findings indicate that DTKT is not superior to NTKT or placebo in terms of pain relief and enhancing functional performance after tape application in healthy male students.

Keywords: functional performance; kinesio taping; muscle fatigue; pain; tension

1. Introduction

Kinesio taping (KT) is one of the most common adhesive therapeutic taping technique and has been shown to be clinically effective for improving the range of motion [1–3] and muscle activities [4,5], shortening of an earlier occurrence of muscle peak torque generation [6,7], and enhancing functional performance [8–10].

In various sports and exercise activities, vertical jumping is a well-known movement [11,12]. Quick extension of the lower limb joints, including the hip, knee, and ankle, occurs before beginning the push-off movement. The vertical jump height (VJH) is an essential factor for sports performance that is often considered an indicator of an individual's ability to participate in exercise or sports activities. [13]. Vertical jumping can be used as exercise training to gain strength and increase power of the lower extremities. Vertical jumping-associated movements comprise actions at multiple joints, including the hip, knee, and ankle, with active contraction of the major muscles such as hamstrings, quadriceps, triceps surae, and muscles of the lower back [14].

In athletes, especially those who perform jumping, vertical jumping movements exhibit relatively normalized patterns in terms of complex movements of multiple joints requiring explosive muscle contraction, which results in maximal muscle performance of the lower joints [15]. Therefore, jumping can be performed to improve muscle strength and endurance of the lower extremities [16]. Several researchers claimed that functional performance can be enhanced by applying KT [2,3]. KT reduces inflammation and promotes joint movement by improving blood flow and lymph circulation [17]. It also helps relieve pain by decreasing pressure on subcutaneous nociceptors and facilitates joint and muscle function by improving sensory feedback and muscle activation for prevention of injuries, rehabilitation, and enhancement of functional performance [2,3,18]. Huang et al. observed significantly better improvements in high-jump performance during the single-leg hop (SH) test and in vertical ground reaction force and enhanced muscle activity of the medial gastrocnemius during vertical jump test with KT than with placebo tape in healthy inactive men [13].

However, the effects of KT on functional performance, especially on muscular strength and endurance, remain controversial because of limited clinical and scientific evidence [2,3,18]; therefore, no clear scientific agreement has yet been reached regarding the effect of KT on athletes' performance in terms of muscular strength and endurance. Nevertheless, many Olympic athletes use KT to improve their performance, and the trend is becoming increasingly popular [19,20].

Some studies have demonstrated that KT application does not immediately enhance functional performance of healthy individuals without pain due to muscle fatigue, regardless of subject deception and changes in tape tension [14,21–23]. This might be because these participants are pain-free and their functional performance is good. However, in individuals with pain caused by muscle fatigue, the functional performance is affected by KT, and KT might help reduce pain.

Neuromuscular activation and proprioception play a key role in maintaining joint function and stability [24]. A previous study suggested that the tension provided by the tape can improve proprioceptive feedback and facilitate correct posture and movement, even after the removal of the tape, which can improve muscle activities for functional performance [25]. Joint proprioception can be enhanced with external supports such as elastic band or taping [24,26].

However, Long et al. showed that KT on the foot and ankle may amplify sensory input, which enhances proprioception of poor ankle performers, but produces an input overload that impairs proprioception in those who were originally good performers [27].

Thus, tape tension is a critical element of the KT method [14]; however, previous studies applied only the stretched tape to increase tension but not the double-taped technique to reinforce tension [28].

Therefore, the present study aimed to compare the effects of double-taped KT (DTKT), normal-tape KT (NTKT), and placebo taping on functional performances such as SH distance, VJH and vertical jump power (VJP), and on subjective pain of the lower extremities in individuals with muscle fatigue. We hypothesized that KT with double tension would reduce pain, which would improve functional performance.

2. Materials and Methods

2.1. Ethical Approval

This study was approved by the institutional review board of Gachon University, registered on the clinicaltrials.gov website (KCT 0003522) and conducted in accordance with the Consolidated Standards of Reporting Trial recommendations. All participants signed a statement of informed consent prior to participation in the study.

2.2. Participants

A total of 50 male students were recruited in this study; among these, 2 declined to participate in the study and 4 did not meet the inclusion criteria; finally, 44 participants (mean age, 23.3 ± 2.2 years) were included. All participants were physically active and healthy, with a body mass index (BMI) of <25 kg/m^2 (mean BMI, 23.3 ± 2.7 kg/m^2) and practice time of >150 min of moderate or intense physical activity per week (mean physical activity time, 262.6 ± 48.5 min per week). Participants who had not received pharmacological therapy or undergone surgery of the lower extremities were eligible for the study, whereas those who had orthopedic, musculoskeletal, or neurological limitations of the lower extremities, and those who presented with signs of allergy or any inconvenience to KT were excluded.

The sample size was calculated using G power 3.0.1. software (Heinrich Heine University Dusseldorf, Dusseldorf, Germany). A sample size of 39 participants (13 participants per group and a 0% attrition rate) was estimated using a moderate effect size of f = 0.25, significance level of 0.05, and power of 0.85. Thirty-nine participants were required to show statistical significance when a clinically significant interaction was observed between the time points and groups. An additional five participants were recruited to provide for unanticipated attrition.

2.3. Procedure

Simple randomization was independently conducted by one of the researchers, and concealed allocation was performed using a computer-generated randomized table of numbers created before data collection. Participants were randomly divided into the following three groups: DTKT (n = 15), NTKT (n = 14), and placebo (n = 15) groups (PG; Figure 1). This study was double-blinded, and different researchers performed randomization (researcher 1), assessment (researcher 2), intervention (researcher 3), and data analysis (researcher 4) to minimize potential bias.

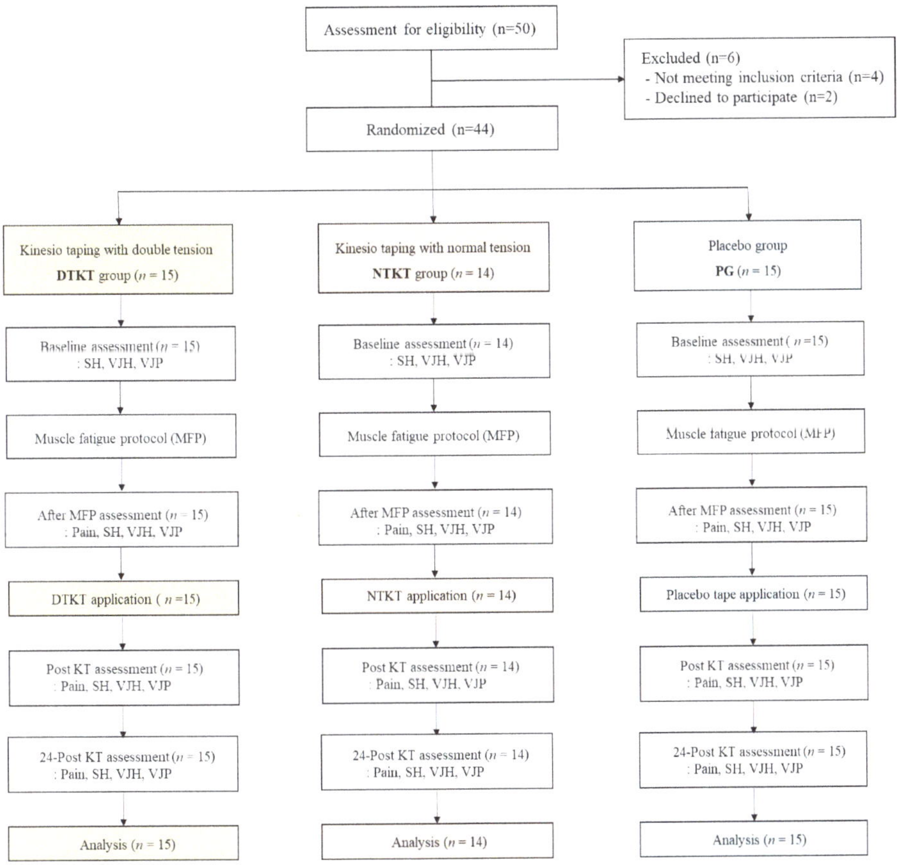

Figure 1. Flowchart diagram of the study. Abbreviations: SH, single hopping; VJH, vertical jump height; VJP, vertical jump power.

Once participants arrived at the research laboratory, they were asked to sit comfortably for 10 min to stabilize their body condition at ambient room temperature. General characteristics (height, weight, and BMI) were measured before the beginning of the test. All participants were asked to perform static stretching of their lower extremities (calf muscles and quadriceps) for 5 min to warm up while they watched an exercise video that demonstrated countermovement jumps and SH for familiarization. Subsequently, the baseline SH distance and maximum VJH and VJP were measured. To induce muscle soreness, participants underwent the muscle fatigue protocol (MFP) under the supervision of researchers. The SH distance, VJH, and VJP were again measured after the MFP, and KT was applied. Outcome measurements were taken immediately (post-KT) and 24 h (24-post KT) after KT application. Subjective pain was also measured, except at baseline. Participants were asked not to perform more than moderate physical activities during 24 h between measurements, and if they did so, they were asked to report them.

2.4. Muscle Fatigue Protocol

The MFP basically included 20 bilateral squats (90° knee flexion) for 5 sets and 20 eccentric contractions of the ipsilateral calf muscles for 5 sets; however, if the participants reached the criteria of muscle fatigue, they would complete the MFP. For eccentric contractions of the ipsilateral calf muscles, participants were asked to stand on a step with the dominant leg and lower the heel over 3 s until they could not lower the heel any further. This MFP was modified based on previous studies [29,30] and determined according to the pilot study findings.

Prior to the MFP, participants were informed about the modified Borg's scale of perceived exertion (scale: 0–10) [31], which was used between the protocol sets to quantify the perceived exertion [29,32]. Participants performed the MFP until they reached the perceived exertion scale of 8 out of 10, and they were then asked to continue the MFP until they were fully exhausted [32,33].

2.5. Intervention (Applying Kinesio Taping)

The ATEX Kinesio sports tape (Atex Medical Co., Seoul, Korea) was applied on clean and dry skin of participants. The length of the KT applied was calculated using anthropometric dimensions and was defined by a change in length of the tape between the origin and insertion points of the rectus femoris and gastrocnemius before and after stretching [18,28].

KT has muscle facilitation effects when it is applied from the direction of origin to insertion points with 75% of the maximum length tension [6,21,34]. However, in the present study, KT was applied from the direction of insertion to origin points with 75% of the maximum length tension to investigate its muscle inhibition effect [18].

In the DTKT group, double-layer KT was applied to the participants while they were in a relaxed prone position, from the surface of the calcaneus bone on the sole of the foot to the end of origin of the medial and lateral gastrocnemius muscles below the knee joint using the Y-shaped taping technique (Figure 2A). The I-shaped taping technique was applied from the tibial tuberosity to the anterior superior iliac spine for the rectus femoris (Figure 2B). Participants in the NTKT group underwent the same procedures as those in the DTKT group, except that the KT was applied only in a single layer. In addition, participants in the PG underwent the same procedures as those in the NTKT group, except that they were asked to stay in a neutral position without tension to the CaduMedi non-woven adhesive sham tape (T&C Healthcare Co. Ltd., Guangzhou, China). All participants were instructed not to remove the applied tapes for 24 h until reassessment. If the tape was removed in 24 h, participants were asked to contact the researchers; indeed, no one had removed the tape within this time period.

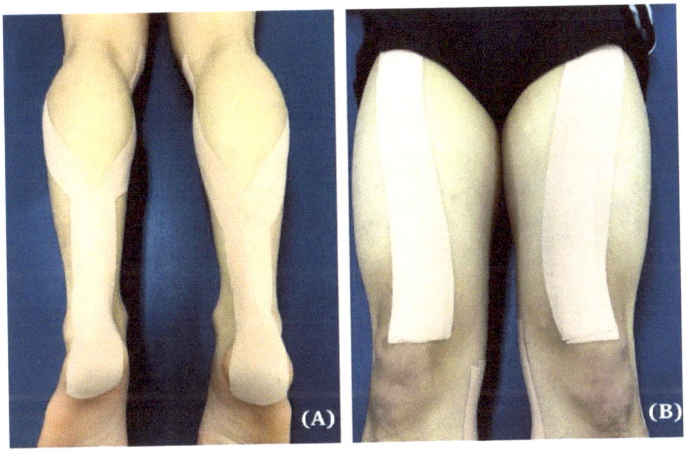

Figure 2. (**A**) Kinesio taping with double-taped application to the calf muscle; (**B**) Kinesio taping with double-taped application to the rectus femoris.

2.6. Outcome Measures

Subjective pain was measured using the visual analog scale for pain [35,36]. Participants were asked to place a vertical mark across a 10-point horizontal line, with the 10-point level indicating the greatest pain [17]. Only 1 scale was marked on each piece of paper so that any bias from previous measures could be eliminated.

The SH and vertical jump tests have been used as reliable methods to assess functional performance [15,37,38]. All measurements were taken with the dominant leg. In the SH test, participants started with single-leg standing with their hands on their waists behind a line on the floor and the knees slightly flexed for a while; then, they were asked to jump forward as quickly as possible and land with the same leg [37]. In the vertical jump test, participants were asked to stand at hip's width, with their hands on their waists, and then asked to jump up from the ground as fast and high as possible with a verbal cue; the body was to remain stretched while jumping [39]. The VJH and VJP were calculated in this test.

The mean value of three attempts was calculated. The SH distance and VJH, and VJP in the SH and vertical jump tests, respectively, were assessed using the OptoGait system (Microgate Srl, Bolzano, Italy). The OptoGait system is a floor-based photocell system for movement analysis and functional assessment consisting of two 1-m transmitting and receiving bars, including a 96-light emitting diode (LED) that communicates via an infrared frequency and a web camera. The OptoGait system was placed 1.5 m apart on a flat surface, and the system calculated the time when the participants touched the floor or stayed in the air and communicated this information by sending and receiving 1000 signals per second, generating accurate data. The OptoGait software (Microgate Srl, Bolzano, Italy) was then used to calculate the precise VJH (cm) and VJP (w/kg) with the acquired data using the following [40,41]:

$$h = \frac{T_V{}^2 \cdot g}{8} \quad p = g^2 \cdot T_V \cdot \frac{(T_V + T_c)}{4 \cdot T_c} \tag{1}$$

h = height (cm), p = power (W/kg), g = gravity acceleration, T_V = flight time, and T_c = contract time.

2.7. Statistical Analysis

The SPSS 23.0 software for Windows 10 was used for data analysis (IBM, Armonk, NY, USA). All data are presented as mean and standard deviation. Normality of the continuous variables was examined using the Shapiro–Wilk test, and all outcome variables were normally distributed. One-way analysis of variance (ANOVA) was conducted to compare general characteristics and baseline SH distance, VJH, and VJP among the three groups. A 3 (group) × 3 (time) two-factor mixed ANOVA was conducted to determine whether any interaction existed between the groups and time points. As no interaction was observed between the groups and time points in all outcome variables, one-way repeated-measures ANOVA was conducted to determine any differences in outcome variables among the time points in each group. Post hoc comparisons using the least significant difference (LSD) test were performed when significant group main effects were detected. The level of significance was set at $\alpha = 0.05$.

3. Result

All 44 participants completed the study (15 in the DTKT group, 14 in the NTKT group, and 15 in the PG). General characteristics of the participants and baseline functional performance, including SH, VJH, and VJP, were not significantly different among the three groups (Table 1).

Table 1. General characteristics of participants ($N = 44$).

	DTKT ($n = 15$)	NTKT ($n = 14$)	PG ($n = 15$)	p Values
Age (years)	23.2 ± 2.0	23.2 ± 2.7	23.4 ± 2.1	0.98
Height (cm)	172.9 ± 4.3	171.6 ± 7.6	174.3 ± 4.5	0.45
Weight (kg)	69.6 ± 8.4	69.6 ± 12.7	69.5 ± 8.2	0.99
BMI (kg/m^2)	23.2 ± 2.4	23.6 ± 3.2	22.9 ± 2.4	0.80
Baseline SH distance (cm)	173.1 ± 16.1	178.6 ± 13.3	180.5 ± 15.0	0.40
Baseline VJH (cm)	31.5 ± 4.7	30.3 ± 5.4	33.7 ± 6.1	0.30
Baseline VJP (w/kg)	15.4 ± 2.5	15.9 ± 3.6	15.7 ± 2.5	0.97

Abbreviations: SH, single hopping; VJH, vertical jump height; VJP, vertical jump power; DTKT, double-taped Kinesio taping; NTKT, normal-taped Kinesio taping; PG, placebo group; BMI, body mass index.

No significant difference was found in subjective pain after the MFP among the groups ($F_{[2,43]} = 1.26$, $p = 0.30$). No significant interaction in subjective pain was observed between the three time points (after MFP, post-KT, and 24-post KT) and groups ($F_{[3.1,41]} = 0.54$, $p = 0.67$, $\eta^2 = 0.03$). Only a significant change in the mean subjective pain was found in the DTKT group from immediately after the MFP to post-KT (3.5 ± 1.9 to 2.5 ± 1.6, $p = 0.004$; Table 2).

Table 2. Subjective pain changes after intervention in the three groups ($N = 44$).

		DTKT ($n = 15$)	NTKT ($n = 14$)	PG ($n = 15$)	F [1]	P [1]	η^2 [1]
Pain	After MFP	3.5 ± 1.9	3.5 ± 2.9	2.3 ± 1.8	0.54	0.67	0.03
	Post	2.5 ± 1.6 *	2.9 ± 1.8	2.1 ± 1.9			
	24-post	3.3 ± 2.4	3.0 ± 2.3	2.2 ± 2.2			

[1] F, P, and η^2: interaction between time and group. * significant decrease after MFP. Abbreviations: DTKT, double-taped Kinesio taping; NTKT, normal-taped Kinesio taping; PG, placebo group; MFP, muscle fatigue protocol.

The post-MFP SH distance was not significantly different among the groups ($F_{[2,43]} = 0.40, p = 0.68$), and a significant decrease in the mean SH distance after the MFP compared to baseline was observed in all three groups ($p < 0.01$). No significant interaction was observed between the three time points (after the MFP, post-KT, and 24-post KT) and groups ($F_{[13.14,41]} = 0.32$, $p = 0.86$, $\eta^2 = 0.02$; Table 3). There was no significant difference in the mean VJH after the MFP among the groups ($F_{[2,43]} = 1.52$, $p = 0.23$). In addition, the mean VJH was lower after the MFP than at baseline in each group ($p < 0.01$). No significant interaction was observed between the time points and groups ($F_{[3.4,41]} = 1.55$, $p = 0.20$, $\eta^2 = 0.07$; Table 3). The VJP results were similar to the SH distance and VJH results. No significant difference in the mean VJP after the MFP was found among the groups ($F_{[2,43]} = 0.70$, $p = 0.50$). A significant decrease in the mean VJP after the MFP was found in all three groups ($p < 0.05$). In addition, no significant interaction in the mean VJP was found between the time points and groups ($F_{[2.4,41]}$ = 0.86, p = 0.45, η^2 = 0.04; Table 3).

Table 3. Functional performance changes after intervention in the three groups (N = 44).

		DTKT (n = 15)	NTKT (n = 14)	PG (n = 15)	F [1]	P [1]	η^2 [1]
SH distance (cm)	Baseline	173.1 ± 16.1	178.6 ± 13.3	180.5 ± 15.0			
	After MFP	163.9 ± 20.0 *	165.0 ± 20.7 *	170.3 ± 22.3 *	0.32	0.86	0.02
	Post KT	168.2 ± 15.6	165.9 ± 21.4	170.8 ± 23.9			
	24-post KT	168.6 ± 14.1	166.3 ± 20.7	172.2 ± 23.1			
VJH (cm)	Baseline	31.5 ± 4.7	30.3 ± 5.4	33.7 ± 6.1			
	After MFP	29.1 ± 4.6 *	26.2 ± 5.5 *	29.8 ± 7.3 *	1.55	0.20	0.07
	Post KT	28.6 ± 3.7	26.9 ± 6.7	30.9 ± 6.8			
	24-post KT	29.8 ± 4.2	27.3 ± 6.3	29.4 ± 8.5			
VJP (w/kg)	Baseline	15.4 ± 2.5	15.9 ± 3.6	15.7 ± 2.5			
	After MFP	14.4 ± 1.0 *	13.8 ± 2.8 *	14.7 ± 2.3 *	0.86	0.45	0.04
	Post KT	14.3 ± 1.0	14.2 ± 3.7	14.8 ± 2.4			
	24-post KT	15.9 ± 1.2	14.9 ± 4.2	14.7 ± 3.5			

[1] F, P, and η^2: interaction between time (After MFP, Post, and 24-Post; 3 time points) and group. Abbreviations: SH, single hopping; VJH, vertical jump height; VJP, vertical jump power; DTKT, double-taped Kinesio taping; NTKT, normal-taped Kinesio taping; PG, placebo group; BMI, body mass index; MFP, muscle fatigue protocol.

4. Discussion

Tape tension is a key factor of the KT method [14]. One study showed that tape tension can improve proprioceptive feedback and facilitate correct posture and movement, even after removal of the tape [25]. However, another study found that the tension might have reversal effects on functional performance [27].

To our knowledge, the present study is the first to investigate the immediate effects of the DTKT technique, which provides more tension, on functional performance including the SH distance, VJH, and VJP of the lower extremities with pain due to muscle fatigue.

Our results indicate that there were no significant interactions in pain, SH distance, VJH, and VJP between the groups and time points (after the MFP, post-KT, and 24-post KT). This finding is consistent with that of previous studies that reported that KT application did not immediately enhance functional performance in healthy individuals, regardless of subject deception and changes in tape tension [14,21,22]. On the other hand, Mendez-Rebolledo et al. found that KT increased VJH and ground reaction force only 72 h, but not 24 h, after KT application on the gluteus maximus, biceps femoris, longissimus, rectus femoris, and gastrocnemius muscles in male athletes [22].

One potential mechanism of KT is that motor neuron threshold reductions can be induced by skin irritation, resulting in easier recruitment of motor units and improved functional performance [42]. In addition, KT is effective in pain control management by inhibiting muscle activities [1,3,19].

Functional performance was more related to muscle strength in the Konishi's study and they showed that the tactile input from KT could inhibit muscle weakness and decrease muscle activities owing to decreased Ia afferents; however, tactile stimulation from KT was not enough to increase muscle strength in individuals without any injuries [43]. Our results indicate that KT, even with double layers, does not increase muscle performance or suppress pain caused by muscle fatigue because it might not be still enough to stimulate the non-nociceptive fibers. Our results support those of a previous study that reported that the tactile input from KT was not strong enough to improve muscle power, which influences VJH [14].

It is difficult to conclude that the effect of KT application is simply due to the placebo effect because its effects on pain, disability, and functional performance have been controversial over a decade [1,3,4,13,18,19,21,23,25,44–46].

The present study has several limitations. First, although tension is a key factor of KT according to a previous study [14], the tension of KT could not be quantified. Second, participants in this study were healthy individuals; therefore, our findings may not be applicable in clinical practice of athletic training and sports medicine. Third, KT was applied only on the rectus femoris and calf muscles to investigate functional performance of the lower extremities; however, more muscles of the lower extremities, such as the gluteus maximus, biceps femoris, tibialis anterior, multifidus, and peroneus are involved in high-speed jumping. Thus, data obtained might not provide accurate evidence on the effect of KT on functional performance. Fourth, this study did not include a control group without any taping. Therefore, further studies should include a control group without any taping to confirm our findings.

Despite these limitations, this study has several strengths: it is the first study to investigate the immediate effects of the KT technique reinforced with tape tension on the functional performance of the lower limbs and pain due to muscle fatigue in healthy individuals, and our study may provide the basis for further research on KT with reinforced tension.

5. Conclusions

In conclusion, the DTKT technique has immediate effects on the alleviation of pain caused by muscle fatigue. However, this technique is not superior to NTKT or placebo in terms of pain relief and functional performance within 24 h after tape application in healthy male students.

Author Contributions: Conceptualization, H.L. (Hyoungwon Lim); methodology, H.L. (Hyoungwon Lim) and H.L. (Haneul Lee); formal analysis, H.L. (Haneul Lee); investigation, H.L. (Hyoungwon Lim) and H.L. (Haneul Lee); data curation, H.L. (Hyoungwon Lim) and H.L. (Haneul Lee); writing—original draft preparation, H.L. (Hyoungwon Lim) and H.L. (Haneul Lee); writing—review and editing, H.L. (Hyoungwon Lim) and H.L. (Haneul Lee); funding acquisition, H.L. (Hyoungwon Lim). All authors have read and agreed to the published version of the manuscript.

Funding: The present research was conducted with research funding from Dankook University (R201800123) in 2018.

Conflicts of Interest: The authors declare no conflict of interest.

References

1. Gonzalez-Iglesias, J.; Fernandez-de-Las-Penas, C.; Cleland, J.A.; Huijbregts, P.; Del Rosario Gutierrez-Vega, M. Short-term effects of cervical kinesio taping on pain and cervical range of motion in patients with acute whiplash injury: A randomized clinical trial. *J. Orthop. Sports Phys. Ther.* **2009**, *39*, 515–521. [CrossRef]
2. Yoshida, A.; Kahanov, L. The effect of kinesio taping on lower trunk range of motions. *Res. Sports Med.* **2007**, *15*, 103–112. [CrossRef]
3. Thelen, M.D.; Dauber, J.A.; Stoneman, P.D. The clinical efficacy of kinesio tape for shoulder pain: A randomized, double-blinded, clinical trial. *J. Orthop. Sports Phys. Ther.* **2008**, *38*, 389–395. [CrossRef] [PubMed]
4. Hsu, Y.H.; Chen, W.Y.; Lin, H.C.; Wang, W.T.; Shih, Y.F. The effects of taping on scapular kinematics and muscle performance in baseball players with shoulder impingement syndrome. *J. Electromyogr. Kinesiol.* **2009**, *19*, 1092–1099. [CrossRef] [PubMed]
5. Slupik, A.; Dwornik, M.; Bialoszewski, D.; Zych, E. Effect of Kinesio Taping on bioelectrical activity of vastus medialis muscle. Preliminary report. *Ortop. Traumatol. Rehabil.* **2007**, *9*, 644–651. [PubMed]
6. Wong, O.M.; Cheung, R.T.; Li, R.C. Isokinetic knee function in healthy subjects with and without Kinesio taping. *Phys. Ther. Sport* **2012**, *13*, 255–258. [CrossRef]
7. Simon, J.; Garcia, W.; Docherty, C.L. The effect of kinesio tape on force sense in people with functional ankle instability. *Clin. J. Sport Med.* **2014**, *24*, 289–294. [CrossRef]
8. Jaraczewska, E.; Long, C. Kinesio taping in stroke: Improving functional use of the upper extremity in hemiplegia. *Top. Stroke Rehabilit.* **2006**, *13*, 31–42. [CrossRef]
9. Yasukawa, A.; Patel, P.; Sisung, C. Pilot study: Investigating the effects of Kinesio Taping in an acute pediatric rehabilitation setting. *Am. Occup. Ther.* **2006**, *60*, 104–110. [CrossRef]

10. Chang, H.Y.; Chou, K.Y.; Lin, J.J.; Lin, C.F.; Wang, C.H. Immediate effect of forearm Kinesio taping on maximal grip strength and force sense in healthy collegiate athletes. *Phys. Ther. Sport* **2010**, *11*, 122–127. [CrossRef]
11. Vanezis, A.; Lees, A. A biomechanical analysis of good and poor performers of the vertical jump. *Ergonomics* **2005**, *48*, 1594–1603. [CrossRef] [PubMed]
12. Bobbert, M.F.; Gerritsen, K.G.; Litjens, M.C.; Van Soest, A.J. Why is countermovement jump height greater than squat jump height? *Med. Sci. Sports Exerc.* **1996**, *28*, 1402–1412. [CrossRef]
13. Huang, C.Y.; Hsieh, T.H.; Lu, S.C.; Su, F.C. Effect of the Kinesio tape to muscle activity and vertical jump performance in healthy inactive people. *Biomed. Eng. Online* **2011**, *10*, 70. [CrossRef]
14. Magalhaes, I.; Bottaro, M.; Freitas, J.R.; Carmo, J.; Matheus, J.P.; Carregaro, R.L. Prolonged use of Kinesiotaping does not enhance functional performance and joint proprioception in healthy young males: Randomized controlled trial. *Braz. J. Phys. Ther.* **2016**, *20*, 213–222. [CrossRef]
15. Lees, A.; Vanrenterghem, J.; De Clercq, D. The maximal and submaximal vertical jump: Implications for strength and conditioning. *J. Strength Cond. Res.* **2004**, *18*, 787–791. [CrossRef]
16. AragonVargas, L.F.; Gross, M.M. Kinesiological factors in vertical jump performance: Differences among individuals. *J. Appl. Biomech.* **1997**, *13*, 24–44. [CrossRef]
17. Stedge, H.L.; Kroskie, R.M.; Docherty, C.L. Kinesio taping and the circulation and endurance ratio of the gastrocnemius muscle. *J. Athl. Train.* **2012**, *47*, 635–642. [CrossRef]
18. Cai, C.; Au, I.P.; An, W.; Cheung, R.T. Facilitatory and inhibitory effects of Kinesio tape: Fact or fad? *J. Sci. Med. Sport* **2016**, *19*, 109–112. [CrossRef]
19. Martinez-Gramage, J.; Merino-Ramirez, M.A.; Amer-Cuenca, J.J.; Lison, J.F. Effect of Kinesio Taping on gastrocnemius activity and ankle range of movement during gait in healthy adults: A randomized controlled trial. *Phys. Ther. Sport* **2016**, *18*, 56–61. [CrossRef]
20. Williams, S.; Whatman, C.; Hume, P.A.; Sheerin, K. Kinesio taping in treatment and prevention of sports injuries: A meta-analysis of the evidence for its effectiveness. *Sports Med.* **2012**, *42*, 153–164. [CrossRef] [PubMed]
21. Cheung, R.T.; Yau, Q.K.; Wong, K.; Lau, P.; So, A.; Chan, N.; Kwok, C.; Poon, K.Y.; Yung, P.S. Kinesiology tape does not promote vertical jumping performance: A deceptive crossover trial. *Man Ther.* **2016**, *21*, 89–93. [CrossRef] [PubMed]
22. Mendez-Rebolledo, G.; Ramirez-Campillo, R.; Guzman-Munoz, E.; Gatica-Rojas, V.; Dabanch-Santis, A.; Diaz-Valenzuela, F. Short-term effects of Kinesio Taping on muscle recruitment order during a vertical jump: A pilot study. *J. Sport Rehabil.* **2018**, *27*, 319–326. [CrossRef] [PubMed]
23. Nakajima, M.A.; Baldridge, C. The effect of Kinesio(R) Tape on vertical jump and dynamic postural control. *Int. J. Sports Phys. Ther.* **2013**, *8*, 393–406. [PubMed]
24. Callaghan, M.J.; Selfe, J.; McHenry, A.; Oldham, J.A. Effects of patellar taping on knee joint proprioception in patients with patellofemoral pain syndrome. *Man Ther.* **2008**, *13*, 192–199. [CrossRef]
25. Macedo, L.B.; Richards, J.; Borges, D.T.; Melo, S.A.; Brasileiro, J.S. Kinesio Taping reduces pain and improves disability in low back pain patients: A randomised controlled trial. *Physiotherapy* **2018**. [CrossRef]
26. Perlau, R.; Frank, C.; Fick, G. The effect of elastic bandages on human knee proprioception in the uninjured population. *Am. J. Sports Med.* **1995**, *23*, 251–255. [CrossRef]
27. Long, Z.; Wang, R.W.; Han, J.; Waddington, G.; Adams, R.; Anson, J. Optimizing ankle performance when taped: Effects of kinesiology and athletic taping on proprioception in full weight-bearing stance. *J. Sci. Med. Sport* **2017**, *20*, 236–240. [CrossRef]
28. De Jesus, J.F.; Franco, Y.R.; Nannini, S.B.; Nakaoka, G.B.; Dos Reis, A.C.; Bryk, F.F. The effects of varied tensions of kinesiology taping on quadriceps strength and lower limb function. *Int. J. Sports Phys. Ther.* **2017**, *12*, 85–93.
29. Lessi, G.C.; Dos Santos, A.F.; Batista, L.F.; de Oliveira, G.C.; Serrao, F.V. Effects of fatigue on lower limb, pelvis and trunk kinematics and muscle activation: Gender differences. *J. Electromyogr. Kinesiol.* **2017**, *32*, 9–14. [CrossRef]
30. Gervasio, S.; Finocchietti, S.; Stevenson, A.J.T.; Mrachacz-Kersting, N. Delayed muscle onset soreness in the gastrocnemius muscle attenuates the spinal contribution to interlimb communication. *Eur. J. Appl. Physiol.* **2018**, *118*, 2393–2402. [CrossRef]

31. Borg, G. Psychophysical scaling with applications in physical work and the perception of exertion. *Scand. J. Work Environ. Health* **1990**, *16* (Suppl. 1), 55–58. [CrossRef] [PubMed]
32. Zanca, G.G.; Gruninger, B.; Mattiello, S.M. Effects of Kinesio taping on scapular kinematics of overhead athletes following muscle fatigue. *J. Electromyogr. Kinesiol.* **2016**, *29*, 113–120. [CrossRef] [PubMed]
33. Fuller, J.R.; Lomond, K.V.; Fung, J.; Cote, J.N. Posture-movement changes following repetitive motion-induced shoulder muscle fatigue. *J. Electromyogr. Kinesiol.* **2009**, *19*, 1043–1052. [CrossRef] [PubMed]
34. Kase, K.; Wallis, J.; Kase, T. *Clinical therapeutic applications of the Kinesio Taping Method*, 3rd ed.; Kinesio Taping Association: Tokyo, Japan, 2003; p. 249.
35. Jensen, M.P.; Karoly, P.; Braver, S. The measurement of clinical pain intensity: A comparison of six methods. *Pain* **1986**, *27*, 117–126. [CrossRef]
36. Carlsson, A.M. Assessment of chronic pain. I. Aspects of the reliability and validity of the visual analogue scale. *Pain* **1983**, *16*, 87–101. [CrossRef]
37. Ross, M.D.; Langford, B.; Whelan, P.J. Test-retest reliability of 4 single-leg horizontal hop tests. *J. Strength Cond. Res.* **2002**, *16*, 617–622.
38. Petschnig, R.; Baron, R.; Albrecht, M. The relationship between isokinetic quadriceps strength test and hop tests for distance and one-legged vertical jump test following anterior cruciate ligament reconstruction. *J. Orthop. Sports Phys. Ther.* **1998**, *28*, 23–31. [CrossRef]
39. Tenelsen, F.; Brueckner, D.; Muehlbauer, T.; Hagen, M. Validity and reliability of an electronic contact mat for drop jump assessment in physically active adults. *Sports* **2019**, *7*, 114. [CrossRef]
40. Alvarez, D.S.A.; Pellitero, L.; Ferrer-Roca, V. Validation of the photoelectric optogait system to measure racewalking biomechanical parameters on a treadmill. *ISBS Proc.* **2017**, *35*, 253.
41. *OPTOGAIT User Manual*. 2010. Available online: http://www.optogait.com/OptoGaitPortal/Media/Manuals/Manual-EN.PDF (accessed on 26 March 2020).
42. Maratou, E.; Theophilidis, G. An axon pacemaker: Diversity in the mechanism of generation and conduction of action potentials in snail neurons. *Neuroscience* **2000**, *96*, 1–2. [CrossRef]
43. Konishi, Y. Tactile stimulation with kinesiology tape alleviates muscle weakness attributable to attenuation of Ia afferents. *J. Sci. Med. Sport* **2013**, *16*, 45–48. [CrossRef] [PubMed]
44. Zhang, S.; Fu, W.; Pan, J.; Wang, L.; Xia, R.; Liu, Y. Acute effects of Kinesio taping on muscle strength and fatigue in the forearm of tennis players. *J. Sci. Med. Sport* **2016**, *19*, 459–464. [CrossRef] [PubMed]
45. Fernandes de Jesus, J.; de Almeida Novello, A.; Bezerra Nakaoka, G.; Curcio Dos Reis, A.; Fukuda, T.Y.; Fernandes Bryk, F. Kinesio taping effect on quadriceps strength and lower limb function of healthy individuals: A blinded, controlled, randomized, clinical trial. *Phys. Ther. Sport* **2016**, *18*, 27–31. [CrossRef] [PubMed]
46. Al-Shareef, A.T.; Omar, M.T.; Ibrahim, A.H. Effect of kinesio taping on pain and functional disability in chronic nonspecific low back pain: A randomized clinical trial. *Spine* **2016**, *41*, E821–E828. [CrossRef] [PubMed]

International Journal of
Environmental Research and Public Health

MDPI

Article

Lung Diffusion in a 14-Day Swimming Altitude Training Camp at 1850 Meters

Iker García [1,2], Franchek Drobnic [3], Teresa Galera [1], Victoria Pons [2] and Ginés Viscor [1,*]

1 Secció de Fisiologia, Departament de Biologia Cel·lular, Fisiologia i Immunologia, Facultat de Biologia, Universitat de Barcelona, Av. Diagonal, 643, E-08028 Barcelona, Spain; ikergarciaalday@gmail.com (I.G.); teresa.galera@gmail.com (T.G.)

2 Centre d'Alt Rendiment (CAR) de Sant Cugat, Av. Alcalde Barnils s/n, E-08173 Sant Cugat del Vallés, 08174 Barcelona, Spain; vpons@car.edu

3 Medical Services Shenhua Greenland FC, Shanghai 201315, China; docdrobnic@gmail.com

* Correspondence: gviscor@ub.edu

Received: 26 March 2020; Accepted: 14 May 2020; Published: 17 May 2020

Abstract: Swimming exercise at sea level causes a transient decrease in lung diffusing capacity for carbon monoxide (DL_{CO}). The exposure to hypobaric hypoxia can affect lung gas exchange, and hypoxic pulmonary vasoconstriction may elicit pulmonary oedema. The purpose of this study is to evaluate whether there are changes in DL_{CO} during a 14-day altitude training camp (1850 m) in elite swimmers and the acute effects of a combined training session of swimming in moderate hypoxia and 44-min cycling in acute normobaric severe hypoxia (3000 m). Participants were eight international level swimmers (5 females and 3 males; 17–24 years old; 173.5 ± 5.5 cm; 64.4 ± 5.3 kg) with a training volume of 80 km per week. The single-breath method was used to measure the changes in DL_{CO} and functional gas exchange parameters. No changes in DL_{CO} after a 14-day altitude training camp at 1850 m were detected but a decrease in alveolar volume (VA; 7.13 ± 1.61 vs. 6.50 ± 1.59 L; $p = 0.005$; d = 0.396) and an increase in the transfer coefficient of the lung for carbon monoxide (K_{CO}; 6.23 ± 1.03 vs. 6.83 ± 1.31 $mL \cdot min^{-1} \cdot mmHg^{-1} \cdot L^{-1}$; $p = 0.038$; d = 0.509) after the altitude camp were observed. During the acute hypoxia combined session, there were no changes in DL_{CO} after swimming training at 1850 m, but there was a decrease in DL_{CO} after cycling at a simulated altitude of 3000 m (40.6 ± 10.8 vs. 36.8 ± 11.2 $mL \cdot min^{-1} \cdot mmHg^{-1}$; $p = 0.044$; d = 0.341). A training camp at moderate altitude did not alter pulmonary diffusing capacity in elite swimmers, although a cycling session at a higher simulated altitude caused a certain degree of impairment of the alveolar–capillary gas exchange.

Keywords: pulmonary diffusing capacity; DL_{CO}; altitude training; swimming; SIPO

1. Introduction

Swimming increases mechanical stress on the pulmonary system since it combines water immersion, exercise and breath-holding periods, leading to subtle changes in the permeability of the lungs [1]. Altitude exposure can be an added physiological challenge on the pulmonary system, raising the susceptibility to pulmonary oedema in combination with exercise, water immersion and hypoxia (Figure 1) [2].

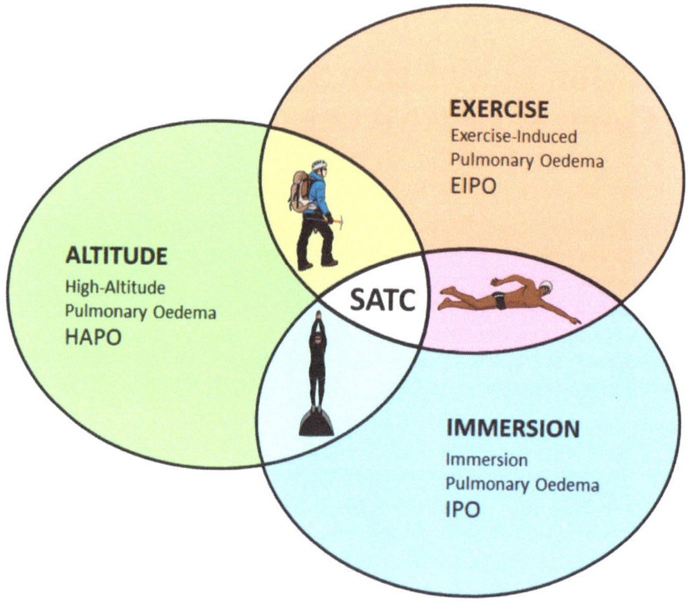

Figure 1. Schematic representation of external stimuli for the development of environmental-induced pulmonary oedema in healthy individuals. At high altitude, mountaineers are exposed to the effects of hypoxic pulmonary vasoconstriction, and increased pulmonary blood flow during exercise, thus developing the risk for high-altitude pulmonary oedema. Breath-holding divers suffer the simultaneous effects of hypoxia, central blood-shift, and chest compression. Swimmers experience hemodynamic changes in pulmonary circulation during exercise, due to regular breath-holding pattern and chest compression. SATC (swimming altitude training camp) combines all three forms of environmental stress that can elicit sub-clinical pulmonary oedema. Based on Marabotti et al. [2].

Endurance training at sea level triggers significant physiological adjustments among cardiovascular, musculoskeletal and haematological systems, but the structural and functional properties of the lung and airways do not change in response to training in land-based sports. However, aquatic sports such as swimming [3–5], artistic swimming [6], and apnoeic diving [7] elicit improvements of the lung capacity and diffusion. During exercise, swimmers are exposed to a reduced frequency breathing against the hydrostatic forces produced by the water, which requires larger inspiration, and it can mimic intermittent hypoxic training where hypercapnia and hypoxia occur [8].

The diffusion capacity for carbon monoxide (DL_{CO}) describes the conductance of gas from the alveolar air to the capillaries and provides a measure of gas transfer in the lungs [9]. Training camps at moderate altitudes are typically utilized among coaches to improve performance at sea level [10]. Different modalities of altitude training have been proposed [11] although Living High–Training High (LHTH) protocol is still the most feasible modality among swimmers due to the logistic limitation to locate an adequate swimming pool at a low altitude closer to the altitude training facility. A possible increase in lung diffusing capacity after altitude exposure would be a favourable adaptation in swimmers by allowing them to maintain gas exchange efficiency at a lower energy cost of breathing [12]. While a superior lung diffusing capacity has been reported in native highlanders [12], at the best of our knowledge, it remains unknown whether a short-term altitude training camp can achieve similar enhancements in pulmonary gas exchange in elite swimmers. Modifications of lung diffusing capacity in lowlanders sojourning at altitude still remain unclear with an overall pattern of minimal changes or a slight transient initial increase or decrease [13,14].

On the other hand, strenuous exercise at sea level may cause transient mild interstitial oedema [15,16], influenced by an increased pulmonary capillary pressure [17], which eventually causes leakage of fluid into the lung interstitium [18]. Accordingly, lung diffusing capacity measured after strenuous exercise at sea level has been reported to be decreased [19–21] which, normally, may not be an inconvenience in the highly-developed lungs from elite swimmers (unpublished) but it still remains unknown whether the exposure to swimming altitude training camps (SATCs) may impair the alveolar–capillary gas exchange. Pulmonary oedema has been related to outdoor swimming and also to high altitude exposure with different specific denominations: *high-altitude pulmonary oedema (HAPO)* and *swimming-induced pulmonary oedema (SIPO)*, although the occurrence rate of lung interstitial oedema under both conditions remains unclear [18,22,23]. The combination of hypoxic pulmonary vasoconstriction, basal hyperventilation at altitude and intense swimming may stress the respiratory system, limiting its functional capacity [24]. Subjects with higher FVC and VA showed more resistance to HAPO than counterparts suggesting that the compensatory rise in ventilation and pulmonary circulation could play a crucial role under environmental stress [25].

The question faced in this study is whether recurrent minor lung injuries could lead to long-term pulmonary deterioration. This could be of great practical importance, given the large number of competitive swimmers who are exposed themselves to repetitive environmental stress during altitude training camps [26]. Altitude training camps are extensively utilized by elite swimming coaches, but the possible modifications of the alveolar–capillary exchange are still unknown. Thus, the aim of this study is to evaluate the possible changes in lung diffusion capacity after 14 days of an altitude training camp in elite swimmers and the acute effects of a combined training session of swimming at 1850 m of real altitude (hypobaric hypoxia) and cycling at 3000 m simulated altitude (normobaric hypoxia). We hypothesize that a 14-day altitude training camp will increase lung diffusion capacity in swimmers, while the possible positive or detrimental effect of an acute combined training session is unknown.

2. Materials and Methods

2.1. Subjects

The participants were eight international level swimmers (5 females and 3 males) aged 17 to 24 years old. The average FINA (Fédération Internationale de Natation) points in their best event were 827 FINA points at the time of the study. The athlete's swim specialties were 6 middle-distance (200 or 400 m) and 2 long-distance (800 and 1500 m) swimmers. None of them suffered from asthma.

2.2. Experimental Design

The Altitude Training Camp was placed in the Centre National d'Entraînement en Altitude de Font-Romeu (France). The training schedule was 10 swimming sessions and 6 dry-land sessions per week throughout 30 h of training per week. The altitude training protocol utilized was the LHTH modality that is routinely used by the Royal Spanish Swimming Federation, where they lived at 1850 m during the whole altitude training camp. The weekly training volume was 80 kilometres, and the volume of swimming per session was 7000 to 9000 m. To evaluate the changes in lung diffusion induced by the altitude training camp, DL_{CO} was measured at rest 72 h after arrival to avoid the acute changes in diffusing capacity associated with hyperventilation produced as an immediate response to altitude exposure; then, a second DL_{CO} measurement was taken at rest the last day of the camp. The participants realized two measures before the beginning of the study to be familiar with the procedure. For the study of acute changes in lung diffusing capacity, the system was placed in a corner 10 m away from the pool where the swimmers did the training session to perform the measures before and after swimming training. Measurements were performed less than 5 min before the start of the warm-up and less than 5 min after the end of the training session.

The combined training Session was performed on the 10th day of the Altitude Training Camp. The protocol consisted of a first swimming training that covered 7500 m of moderate-intensity at a moderate altitude (1850 m). This was followed by a cycling exercise performed in a normobaric hypoxic room (3000 m) lasting 44 min. The system was moved out of the normobaric hypoxic chamber to evaluate the lung diffusion capacity at the end of the cycling session. Cycling exercise intensity alternated 8 min of moderate-intensity with 3 min of low-intensity until completing 4 series. All the participants were familiar with this protocol; they performed similar cycling sessions in the normobaric chamber in previous altitude training camps, and they performed 6 similar cycling sessions during the 14-day altitude training camp.

2.3. DL_{CO} Measurements

The procedure which was used for obtaining the diffusing lung capacity parameters was the single-breath method by means of a computerized spirometer (Easy One Pro, ndd Medical Technologies, Zurich, Switzerland) attached to a gas mixture cylinder. This method involves measuring the uptake of CO from the lung over a short breath-holding period. The recommendations made in a recent joint statement by the American Thoracic Society (ATS) and the European Respiratory Society (ERS) were followed [27]. The results obtained in DL_{CO} were adjusted for the change in PAo2 due to barometric pressure (DL_{CO} adj) and haemoglobin (Hb) concentration that was determined from a small blood sample obtained by venepuncture to adjust DL_{CO} to individual parameters before the beginning of the study and at the end of the study. The participants were placed in a seated position, with a mouthpiece and nose-clip in place throughout the test procedure. The test started with tidal breathing for 2–4 breaths until the subject felt comfortable with the mouthpiece. Then the DL_{CO} manoeuvre began with an unforced exhalation to residual volume (RV). At RV, the subject's mouthpiece was connected to a source of test gas, and the subject inhaled rapidly to maximal inspiration. After that, the participant was asked to hold their breath for 10 s and then exhale completely without interruption in less than 4 s and to continue with a tidal breath to finish the test. All measures considered were "grade A", as identified by the system [27], and DL_{CO} was corrected to the individual. A maximum of 3 trials was performed. At least 4 min was allowed between trials to ensure adequate washout of the gases. The test gas mixture used to evaluate the pulmonary function and diffusion capacity was 0.3% of CO, 11% of a tracer inert gas (He) used to measure alveolar volume (VA), and the initial alveolar CO, and a mixture of 20.9% of O_2 balanced with N_2. In addition, the transfer coefficient of the lung for carbon monoxide (K_{CO}), total lung capacity (TLC), vital capacity inspired (VC_{IN}), and residual volume (RV) were calculated.

2.4. Ethical Considerations

All procedures were in accordance with the ethical standards of the Clinical Research Ethics Committee at the *Direcció General de l'Esport* of the Catalonian Sports Council (05-2020-CEICEGC). The study followed the principles of the Declaration of Helsinki for human experimentation. Informed consent was obtained to perform any type of test and evaluation procedures from the participants or their parents as it is mandatory for the athletes pertaining to the national swimming team and training along the entire season at the National Olympic Training Center of Sant Cugat del Valles.

2.5. Statistical Analysis

The results are reported as mean values ± standard deviation (SD). Differences in pulmonary parameters between pre- and post-altitude training camp were assessed using a paired sample *t*-test. Differences in pulmonary parameters during the acute combined session (pre- to mid- to post-training) were analyzed using one-way repeated-measures analysis of variance (ANOVA). Effect size (Cohen's d) was calculated to estimate the magnitude of the difference between group means, with d = 0.2, 0.5, and 0.8 reflecting small, medium, and large effect sizes, respectively [28]. The level of significance was set at $p < 0.05$ for all statistical comparisons. The software package used for the statistical analysis was SPSS ver26 (IBM SPSS Statistics, Armonk, NY, USA).

3. Results

3.1. Anthropometrical Parameters

Table 1 shows the average values and SD of physical and anthropometrical data of our sample of elite swimmers. The participants show similar anthropometrical values compared to those found in elite open water swimmers [29] and young amateur swimmers [30]. Spirometric values were higher than predicted for their age and height in forced vital capacity (FVC) and forced expiratory volume in 1-s (FEV1), both females (FVC: 108 ± 10% and FEV1: 107 ± 7%; Table 1) and males (FVC: 114 ± 18% and FEV1: 108 ± 16%; Table 1).

Table 1. Anthropometrical and physical capacity parameters of the studied sample of elite swimmers.

Anthropometric and Spirometric Parameters (Units)	Elite Swimmers (n = 8)	
	Female (n = 5)	Male (n = 3)
Age (y)	18.2 ± 3.3	18.0 ± 1.7
Height (cm)	170.6 ± 4.7	178.3 ± 2.1
Body weight (Kg)	62.0 ± 3.9	69.0 ± 2.0
BMI	21.3 ± 0.5	21.7 ± 0.7
6 skinfolds	83.3 ± 13.5	49.3 ± 8.5
VO_2max ($mL \cdot Kg^{-1} \cdot min^{-1}$)	55.8 ± 2.1	59.2 ± 8.4
V_Emax ($L\ min^{-1}$)	110.4 ± 11.3	130.6 ± 13.6
FVC (L)	4.4 ± 0.4	5.8 ± 1.0
FVC (%-predicted)	108 ± 10	114 ± 18
FEV1 (L)	3.8 ± 0.4	4.6 ± 0.8
FEV1 (%-predicted)	107 ± 7	108 ± 16
FEV1/FVC	85.2 ± 2.5	79.5 ± 1.2
PEF ($L \cdot s^{-1}$)	7.3 ± 0.9	8.2 ± 0.9
MEF25-75 ($L \cdot s^{-1}$)	4.0 ± 0.7	4.3 ± 0.7

3.2. Changes in Lung Capacity and Function After 14-Day Altitude Training Camp at 1850 m

Table 2 shows the changes recorded in the different parameters of pulmonary function among the 14-day altitude training camp as mean ± SD. There were no changes in DL_{CO} adj after 14 days of altitude training camp in our sample of elite swimmers. However there were significant decreases in VA (7.13 ± 1.61 vs. 6.50 ± 1.59 L, *p*-value = 0.005; d = 0.396; Table 2) and TLC (7.28 ± 1.61 vs. 6.65 ± 1.59 L, *p*-value = 0.005; d = 0.396; Table 2) and a significant improvement in K_{CO} (6.23 ± 1.03 vs. 6.83 ± 1.31 $mL \cdot min^{-1} \cdot mmHg^{-1} \cdot L^{-1}$, *p*-value = 0.038; d = 0.509; Table 2).

Table 2. Lung capacity and pulmonary gas diffusion parameters before (day 3) and after (day 14) altitude training camp at 1850 m in elite swimmers.

Pulmonary Parameters (Units)	Elite Swimmers (n = 8)		
	Pre	Post	*p*-Value
DL_{CO} (mL·min^{-1}·mmHg^{-1})	44.8 ± 12.4	45.0 ± 14.3	0.974
DL_{CO} (%-predicted)	160 ± 33	159 ± 34	
DL_{CO} adj (mL·min^{-1}·mmHg^{-1})	40.4 ± 11.2	40.4 ± 12.8	0.966
DL_{CO} adj (%-predicted)	144 ± 30	143 ± 30	
K_{CO} (mL·min^{-1}·mmHg^{-1}·L^{-1})	6.23 ± 1.03	6.83 ± 1.31	**0.038**
K_{CO} (%-predicted)	126 ± 25	138 ± 29	
VA (L)	7.13 ± 1.61	6.50 ± 1.59	**0.005**
VA (%-predicted)	127 ± 18	116 ± 18	
TLC (L)	7.28 ± 1.61	6.65 ± 1.59	**0.005**
TLC (%-predicted)	127 ± 18	116 ± 18	
VC_{IN} (L)	4.76 ± 1.12	4.35 ± 1.52	0.130
RV (L)	2.51 ± 0.74	2.30 ± 0.57	0.381

Marginal significance (close to 0.05) in bold and italic characters.

3.3. *Changes in Lung Capacity and Function After a Combined Session of Swimming at 1850 m and Cycling at 3000 m*

When measuring DL_{CO} within a combined session of swimming at moderate altitude (1850 m) and cycling at high-altitude (3000 m) there were significant differences in DL_{CO} from post-swimming compared to post-cycling (40.6 ± 10.8 vs. 36.8 ± 11.5 mL·min^{-1}·mmHg^{-1}, *p*-value = 0.044; d = 0.341; Table 3) and K_{CO} was also slightly, but no significantly decreased after cycling (6.34 ± 1.00 vs. 6.27 ± 1.16 vs. 6.17 ± 1.13 mL·min^{-1}·mmHg^{-1}·L^{-1}, *p*-value = 0.053; d = 0.087; Table 3). Also, there was a decrease in RV from basal to post-cycling (2.37 ± 0.63 vs. 2.16 ± 0.65 vs. 1.78 ± 0.59 L, *p*-value = 0.001; d = 0.966; Table 3).

Table 3. Lung capacity and pulmonary gas diffusion parameters before and after a combined session (day 10) of swimming at 1850 m in hypobaric hypoxia and cycling at 3000 m in normobaric hypoxia.

Pulmonary Parameters (Units)	Elite Swimmers (n = 8)					
	Pre	Mid	Pre vs. Mid *p*-Value	Post	Pre vs. Post *p*-Value	Mid vs. Post *p*-Value
DL_{CO} (mL·min^{-1}·mmHg^{-1})	45.8 ± 14.5	45.2 ± 12.0	1.000	41.1 ± 12.8	0.156	**0.044**
DL_{CO} (%-predicted)	166 ± 30	165 ± 26		150 ± 32		
DL_{CO} adj (mL·min^{-1}·mmHg^{-1})	41.1 ± 13.0	40.6 ± 10.8	1.000	36.8 ± 11.5	0.153	**0.044**
DL_{CO} adj (%-predicted)	149 ± 27	148 ± 24		134 ± 29		
K_{CO} (mL·min^{-1}·mmHg^{-1}·L^{-1})	6.34 ± 1.00	6.27 ± 1.16	1.000	6.17 ± 1.13	1.000	***0.053***
K_{CO} (%-predicted)	132 ± 14	134 ± 28		126 ± 23		
VA (L)	6.53 ± 1.35	6.37 ± 1.24	1.000	5.66 ± 0.52	0.330	1.000
VA (%-predicted)	125 ± 18	123 ± 14		118 ± 18		
TLC (L)	6.68 ± 1.35	6.52 ± 1.24	1.000	5.81 ± 0.52	0.330	1.000
TLC (%-predicted)	124 ± 18	123 ± 14		118 ± 17		
VC_{IN} (L)	4.69 ± 1.15	4.73 ± 1.12	1.000	4.22 ± 0.31	0.823	1.000
RV (L)	2.37 ± 0.63	2.16 ± 0.65	1.000	1.78 ± 0.59	**0.001**	0.266

Marginal significance (close to 0.05) in bold and italic characters.

4. Discussion

This study shows that elite swimmers with previous experience in altitude training and extremely high basal values in DL_{CO} do not suffer any change in lung diffusing capacity after 14 days of altitude training camp. During acclimatization to altitude, organs that experience high O_2 demands, such as skeletal and cardiac muscle, are downregulated as a way of minimising hypoxic tissue injury and maximising the efficiency of O_2 utilization [31,32]. At the same time, organs involved in O_2 uptake, such as blood and the lungs, the alveolar–capillary gas exchange increases their capacities [33].

However, because these responses are limited, aerobic performance is impaired by a progressive reduction in maximum O_2 uptake (VO_2max) as altitude increases.

Our results show that DL_{CO} remains unaffected, although there is a decrease in VA and TLC, and an increase in K_{CO}, probably produced as a compensatory adaptive mechanism to keep DL_{CO} levels stable against a reduced alveolar expansion or alveolar damage [34]. The decrease in VA may be a consequence of a decrease in right ventricular function and cardiac output after altitude acclimatization, which produces longer pulmonary capillary erythrocyte transit time, resulting in less alveolar/end capillary diffusion unbalance [35,36]. Lungs may also have an anti-oedematous response with marked alveolar vasoconstriction triggering a decrease in pulmonary blood capillary volume (V_C) and an increase in membrane diffusive capacity (D_M) [37] when facing hypobaric hypoxia exposure, and a slight increase in hemoglobin concentration at the end of the altitude stay could also contribute to the increase in K_{CO} after the altitude training camp.

A 14-day exposure to moderate altitude training camp may not provide ventilatory stimuli enough to modify pulmonary function, by inducing lung growth or altering alveolar–capillary gas exchange associated with SATC. Most of the studies evaluating changes in diffusing capacity has been performed on active mountaineers at high altitude, a condition that differs considerably from the situation faced by elite trained subjects exercising at moderate altitude. Different studies have been conducted to assess the effect of hypobaric hypoxia in lung diffusion properties, yielding conflicting results. Lung diffusing capacity for carbon monoxide (DL_{CO}) has been reported to either increase or decrease after short- or long-term exposures to altitude. Faoro et al. [13] found that DL_{CO}, K_{CO} and VA increased after acute exposure to moderate altitude (2250 m) of only 1 h. DL_{CO} was also significantly increased after 9 days at 5150 m [38] and after three weeks at 5400 m [39]. Martinot et al. [40] showed an increase in DL_{CO} from sea level to days 2–3 at 4300 m, but there was a decrease to the sea level values in VA and K_{CO} from days 2–3 to 7–8. In contrast, DL_{CO} did not change after acclimatization in 5050 m, although VA was decreased after 2 weeks of exposure [41]. Diffusing capacity also remained unchanged during a rapid ascent (1–3 days) in control subjects [42] and after a moderate stance (7–10 days) [43] at 4559 m. Senn et al. [14] also showed a slight decrease after a rapid ascent (1–2 d) to 4559 m, and subjects suffering HAPO revealed a decrease in DL_{CO} of more than 10% before HAPO occurred. Inter-individual response, exposure time and different altitudes may explain the unclear results in DL_{CO} modifications.

In this study, we found that pulmonary function was not negatively affected by ~15 km/day of swimming training at moderate altitude after 14 days. Swimmers trained 80 km in the pool, around 30 h per week, during the whole altitude training camp, a remarkable program at altitude in opposition to mountaineer's expeditions. Tiller et al. [44] have also shown that pulmonary function responds well to chronic endurance exercise performed, running 10 marathons on 10 consecutive days at sea level. All the participants recruited in our study had previous experience in altitude training camps, and they also have much higher DL_{CO} basal values than predicted by their age and height, probably with very limited margin for improvement and an extraordinary capacity to face the environmental stress.

Exercise at hypoxia failed to elicit acute functional improvements in the pulmonary system in adults, suggesting that functional plasticity of the ventilatory muscles is limited in adulthood [45]. During somatic maturation, a relatively short period (5 months) of altitude exposure enhanced lung diffusing capacity for O_2 transport and metabolic efficiency in growing dogs [33], which was maintained after return to sea level (1–2 yr) suggesting that the functional improvement during maturation may be permanent [46]. It appears that altitude exposure accentuates active lung growth during maturation but may be insufficient to reinitiate lung growth in adulthood [47]. Therefore, altitude training in young swimmers could be an interesting strategy to develop lung functional development, but in highly developed lungs, elite adult swimmers may have no physiological effect.

Despite repeated coughs and feelings of dyspnoea, our subjects did not present a limited diffusion capacity after swimming training at 1850 m of altitude. Swimming training at sea level has been associated with a decrease in DL_{CO} (under review for publication). Therefore, the acute decrease in DL_{CO} after training was expected to be aggravated after altitude exposure as an added stressor. Surprisingly, in this study, there was not a reduction in DL_{CO} after swimming training at 1850 m. Most of the swimmers presented a certain breathing discomfort induced by swimming training and/or chlorine after the last training of the altitude training camp. A breathless athlete is challenging due to a non-specific nature of symptoms [48], such as cough and wheeze and poor predictive clinical signs, and we must be cautious before relating SIPO to the athlete's self-report of cough and breathlessness development. SIPO occurs when fluid accumulates in the lungs in the absence of water aspiration during swimming, causing acute shortness of breath and a cough productive of blood-tinged sputum [18].

Although DL_{CO} was not decreased after swimming training, there was an acute decrease in DL_{CO} (−10%) after cycling (3000 m), suggesting that 1850 m may be a safe altitude to practice endurance training but higher altitudes such as 3000 m may entail a risk for elite athletes training. The cause of the decrease of DL_{CO} after cycling is unknown, but a mild interstitial fluid accumulation may be the most suitable candidate [49]. Pulmonary capillary stress failure develops with intense exercise in healthy humans, and pulmonary vasoconstriction induced by alveolar hypoxia further augments the mechanical stress on capillary walls, leading to greater disruption of pulmonary blood–gas barrier integrity [50]. After cycling, there was also a severe decrease in RV after the combined training session (−33%), which is a compelling finding associated with a post-exercise response in altitude. Some studies have linked reductions in RV with the reversibility of obstructive lung disease [51] and the responsiveness after bronchodilator administration [52], but, to the best of our knowledge, this is the first time that a severe decrease in RV is described after exercise at high-altitude.

The most common medical problems occur at high altitudes above 2500 m [53], where a significant decrease in O_2 transport to the tissues occurs [54]. Although lower lung volumes are one determinant of the augmented pulmonary arterial pressures at altitude and the consequent susceptibility to HAPO [55], it has been reported that exercise at altitude may produce interstitial pulmonary oedema in cyclists [50] due to a substantial increase in pulmonary capillary hydrostatic pressure [56], increasing alveolar fluid flooding [57,58]. In fact, interstitial oedema has been presented whenever microvascular filtration is increased because it is the mechanism that protects against the development of severe oedema [22]. Therefore, interstitial lung oedema could be considered as the interface between tissue repair and the manifestation of a severe disease after exercise or altitude exposure [22]. Finally, a common pathophysiologic pathway seems to be shared by SIPO and HAPO, allowing translation of preventive and therapeutic strategies for HAPO such as progressive acclimatization, avoidance of excessive exertion, and use of drugs that increase the availability of nitric oxide into the unexplored field of SIPO prevention and treatment [2].

Strengths and Limitations

While DL_{CO} is consistent with an increase in extravascular lung water [42,59,60], a combination of indirect and direct techniques, such as sensitive lung function tests like DL_{CO}, and imaging techniques such as chest imaging or pulmonary echography, would be the most suitable approach to definitively demonstrate the presence of a mild perturbation in extravascular water balance [22]. The main value of this study resides in the integration of lung function measures and the collaboration with coaches for volume and intensity assignment in a susceptible environment, such as the altitude training stage.

Previous lung diffusing capacity for carbon monoxide (DL_{CO}) at sea level was not obtained, and as Martinot et al. [40] showed, there could be changes in DL_{CO} from sea level to day 3 after altitude arrival. However, the value of the data here presented relies on the analysis of conditions; milder symptoms may occur in order to reflect the true impact of SIPO in swimming [18].

This study was performed on a small sample of elite swimmers studied in their own environment under their own routines, which is very difficult to obtain. Measures of alveolar–capillary membrane conductance (D_M) or pulmonary capillary blood volume (V_C) were not obtained, which would have provided a deeper explanation of the changes in lung diffusion capacity. However, the changes in DL_{CO}

and K_{CO} are still relevant and coherent with those in VA as to be considered as a correct evaluation of lung diffusion capacity in elite swimmers.

5. Conclusions

A 14-days training camp at moderate altitude does not change lung diffusion capacity in elite swimmers, although there was a decrease in VA and an increase in K_{CO}, keeping DL_{CO} unaltered. An acute swimming session does not change lung diffusing capacity, but a posterior cycling session at normobaric-simulated 3000 m reduced DL_{CO} and RV in elite swimmers.

The high level of fitness and experience at altitude may have influenced these results. Although effect sizes oscillated in the range of small to medium effect, the number of participants in our study is rather limited. Further investigations should consider a larger sample size, with different levels of fitness and experience in altitude training, to confirm these results.

Author Contributions: Conceptualization, I.G. and G.V.; methodology, F.D. and G.V.; formal analysis, F.D. and G.V.; resources, I.G. and V.P.; data curation, I.G. and T.G.; writing—original draft preparation, I.G. and T.G.; writing—review and editing, F.D. and G.V.; supervision, G.V.; project administration, V.P. All authors have read and agreed to the published version of the manuscript.

Funding: This research received no external funding.

Acknowledgments: The authors would like to thank all participants for their time and commitment in undertaking this study and the coaches from the Catalonian Swimming Federation, Luis Rodriguez, and from the Sabadell Swimming Club, Alex Lopez, for their collaboration during the study. We would also like to thank Álvaro Sánchez–Nieva (Sanro Electromedicina) for the kind supply of the equipment to conduct this research. We are grateful to John Dannehl for his help in the editing of the manuscript.

Conflicts of Interest: The authors declare no conflict of interest.

References

1. Drobnic, F.; García-Alday, I.; Banquells, M.; Bellver, M. Interstitial Pulmonary Edema and Acetazolamide in High-Performance Sport: A Case Report. *Arch. Bronconeumol.* **2018**, *54*, 584–585. [CrossRef] [PubMed]
2. Marabotti, C.; Cialoni, D.; Pingitore, A. Environment-induced pulmonary oedema in healthy individuals. *Lancet Respir. Med.* **2017**, *5*, 374–376. [CrossRef]
3. Mickleborough, T.D.; Stager, J.M.; Chatham, K.; Lindley, M.R.; Ionescu, A.A. Pulmonary adaptations to swim and inspiratory muscle training. *Eur. J. Appl. Physiol.* **2008**, *103*, 635–646. [CrossRef] [PubMed]
4. Burtch, A.R.; Ogle, B.T.; Sims, P.A.; Harms, C.A.; Symons, T.B.; Folz, R.J.; Zavorsky, G.S. Controlled frequency breathing reduces inspiratory muscle fatigue. *J. Strength Cond. Res.* **2017**, *31*, 1273–1281. [CrossRef] [PubMed]
5. Rosser-Stanford, B.; Backx, K.; Lord, R.; Williams, E.M. Static and dynamic lung volumes in swimmers and their ventilatory response to maximal exercise. *Lung* **2019**, *197*, 15–19. [CrossRef] [PubMed]
6. Bjurstrom, R.L.; Schoene, R.B. Control of ventilation in elite synchronized swimmers. *J. Appl. Physiol.* **1987**, *63*, 1019–1024. [CrossRef] [PubMed]
7. Schagatay, E.; Richardson, M.X.; Lodin-Sundström, A. Size matters: Spleen and lung volumes predict performance in human apneic divers. *Front. Physiol.* **2012**, *3*, 173. [CrossRef]
8. Stavrou, V.; Toubekis, A.G.; Karetsi, E. Changes in respiratory parameters and fin-swimming performance following a 16-week training period with intermittent breath holding. *J. Hum. Kinet.* **2015**, *49*, 89–98. [CrossRef]
9. Hegewald, M.J. Diffusing capacity. *Clin. Rev. Allergy Immunol.* **2009**, *37*, 159–166. [CrossRef]
10. Lundby, C.; Robach, P. Does 'altitude training' increase exercise performance in elite athletes? *Exp. Physiol.* **2016**, *101*, 783–788. [CrossRef]
11. Rodríguez, F.A.; Iglesias, X.; Feriche, B.; Calderón-Soto, C.; Chaverri, D.; Wachsmuth, N.B.; Schmidt, W.; Levine, B.D. Altitude Training in Elite Swimmers for Sea Level Performance (Altitude Project). *Med. Sci. Sports Exerc.* **2015**, *47*, 1965–1978. [CrossRef] [PubMed]
12. Dempsey, J.A.; Reddan, W.G.; Birnbaum, M.L.; Forster, H.V.; Thoden, J.S.; Grover, R.F.; Rankin, J. Effects of acute through life-long hypoxic exposure on exercise pulmonary gas exchange. *Respir. Physiol.* **1971**, *13*, 62–89. [CrossRef]

13. Faoro, V.; Deboeck, G.; Vicenzi, M.; Gaston, A.F.; Simaga, B.; Doucende, G.; Hapkova, I.; Roca, E.; Subirats, E.; Durand, F.; et al. Pulmonary Vascular Function and Aerobic Exercise Capacity at Moderate Altitude. *Med. Sci. Sports Exerc.* **2017**, *49*, 2131–2138. [CrossRef] [PubMed]
14. Senn, O.; Clarenbach, C.F.; Fischler, M.; Thalmann, R.; Brunner-La Rocca, H.; Egger, P.; Maggiorini, M.; Bloch, K.E. Do changes in lung function predict high-altitude pulmonary edema at an early stage? *Med. Sci. Sports Exerc.* **2006**, *38*, 1565–1570. [CrossRef] [PubMed]
15. Hohmann, E.; Glatt, V.; Tetsworth, K. Swimming induced pulmonary oedema in athletes—A systematic review and best evidence synthesis. *BMC Sports Sci. Med. Rehabil.* **2018**, *3*, 18. [CrossRef]
16. Zavorsky, G.S.; Milne, E.N.C.; Lavorini, F.; Rienzi, J.P.; Lavin, K.M.; Straub, A.M.; Pistolesi, M. Interstitial lung edema triggered by marathon running. *Respir. Physiol. Neurobiol.* **2014**, *190*, 137–141. [CrossRef]
17. Hopkins, S.R. Point: Counterpoint: Pulmonary edema does/does not occur in human athletes performing heavy sea-level exercise. *J. Appl. Physiol.* **2010**, *109*, 1270–1275. [CrossRef]
18. Spencer, S.; Dickinson, J.; Forbes, L. Occurrence, Risk Factors, Prognosis and Prevention of Swimming-Induced Pulmonary Oedema: A Systematic Review. *Sport. Med. Open* **2018**, *4*, 43. [CrossRef]
19. Caillaud, C.; Serre-Cousine, O.; Anselme, F.; Capdevilla, X.; Prefaut, C. Computerized tomography and pulmonary diffusing capacity in highly trained athletes after performing a triathlon. *J. Appl. Physiol.* **1995**, *79*, 1226–1232. [CrossRef]
20. Manier, G.; Moinard, J.; Stoicheff, H. Pulmonary diffusing capacity after maximal exercise. *Am. Physiol. Soc.* **1993**, *75*, 2580–2585. [CrossRef]
21. Zavorsky, G.S.; Lands, L.C. Lung diffusion capacity for nitric oxide and carbon monoxide is impaired similarly following short-term graded exercise. *Nitric Oxide-Biol. Chem.* **2005**, *12*, 31–38. [CrossRef] [PubMed]
22. Cogo, A.; Miserocchi, G. Pro: Most climbers develop subclinical pulmonary interstitial Edema. *High Alt. Med. Biol.* **2011**, *12*, 121–124. [CrossRef] [PubMed]
23. Swenson, E.R. CON: Most climbers do not develop subclinical interstitial pulmonary Edema. *High Alt. Med. Biol.* **2011**, *12*, 125–128. [CrossRef] [PubMed]
24. McKenzie, D.C. Respiratory physiology: Adaptations to high-level exercise. *Br. J. Sports Med.* **2012**, *46*, 381–384. [CrossRef]
25. Gupta, R.K.; Soree, P.; Desiraju, K.; Agrawal, A.; Singh, S.B. Subclinical pulmonary dysfunction contributes to high altitude pulmonary edema susceptibility in healthy non-mountaineers. *Sci. Rep.* **2017**, *7*, 1–7. [CrossRef]
26. Mijacika, T.; Dujic, Z. Sports-related lung injury during breath-hold diving. *Eur. Respir. Rev.* **2016**, *25*, 506–512. [CrossRef]
27. Graham, B.L.; Brusasco, V.; Burgos, F.; Cooper, B.G.; Jensen, R.; Kendrick, A.; Macintyre, N.R.; Thompson, B.R.; Wanger, J. 2017 ERS/ATS standards for single-breath carbon monoxide uptake in the lung. *Eur. Respir. J.* **2017**, *49*, 1600016. [CrossRef]
28. Cohen, J. *Statistical Power Analysis for the Behavioral Sciences*; Academic Press: New York, NY, USA, 1977.
29. Shaw, G.; Mujika, I. Anthropometric profiles of elite open water swimmers. *Int. J. Sports Physiol. Perform.* **2018**, *13*, 115–118. [CrossRef]
30. Martinez, S.; Pasquarelli, B.; Romaguera, D.; Arasa, C.; Tauler, P.; Aguiló, A. Anthropometric characteristics and nutritional profile of young amateur swimmers. *J. Strength Cond. Res.* **2011**, *25*, 1126–1133. [CrossRef]
31. Hoppeler, H.; Kleinert, E.; Schlegel, C.; Claassen, H.; Howald, H.; Kayar, S.R.; Cerretelli, P., II. Morphological adaptations of human skeletal muscle to chronic hypoxia. *Int. J. Sports Med.* **1990**, *11*, 3–9. [CrossRef]
32. Bogaard, H.J.; Hopkins, S.R.; Yamaya, Y.; Niizeki, K.; Ziegler, M.G.; Wagner, P.D. Role of the autonomic nervous system in the reduced maximal cardiac output at altitude. *J. Appl. Physiol.* **2002**, *93*, 271–279. [CrossRef] [PubMed]
33. Hsia, C.C.W.; Johnson, R.L.; McDonough, P.; Dane, D.M.; Hurst, M.D.; Fehmel, J.L.; Wagner, H.E.; Wagner, P.D. Residence at 3800-m altitude for 5 mo in growing dogs enhances lung diffusing capacity for oxygen that persists at least 2.5 years. *J. Appl. Physiol.* **2007**, *102*, 1448–1455. [CrossRef] [PubMed]
34. Hughes, J.M.B.; Pride, N.B. Examination of the carbon monoxide diffusing capacity (DL CO) in relation to its KCO and VA components. *Am. J. Respir. Crit. Care Med.* **2012**, *186*, 132–139. [CrossRef] [PubMed]
35. Bebout, D.E.; Story, D.; Roca, J.; Hogan, M.C.; Poole, D.C.; Gonzalez-Camarena, R.; Ueno, O.; Haab, P.; Wagner, P.D. Effects of altitude acclimatization on pulmonary gas exchange during exercise. *J. Appl. Physiol.* **1989**, *67*, 2286–2295. [CrossRef] [PubMed]

36. Stembridge, M.; Ainslie, P.N.; Shave, R. Mechanisms underlying reductions in stroke volume at rest and during exercise at high altitude. *Eur. J. Sport Sci.* **2016**, *16*, 577–584. [CrossRef] [PubMed]
37. Beretta, E.; Lanfranconi, F.; Grasso, G.S.; Bartesaghi, M.; Alemayehu, H.K.; Miserocchi, G. Reappraisal of DL_{CO} adjustment to interpret the adaptive response of the air-blood barrier to hypoxia. *Respir. Physiol. Neurobiol.* **2017**, *238*, 59–65. [CrossRef] [PubMed]
38. Taylor, B.J.; Stewart, G.M.; Marck, J.W.; Summerfield, D.T.; Issa, A.N.; Johnson, B.D. Interstitial lung fluid balance in healthy lowlanders exposed to high-altitude. *Respir. Physiol. Neurobiol.* **2017**, *243*, 77–85. [CrossRef]
39. Agostoni, P.; Swenson, E.R.; Bussotti, M.; Revera, M.; Meriggi, P.; Faini, A.; Lombardi, C.; Bilo, G.; Giuliano, A.; Bonacina, D.; et al. High-altitude exposure of three weeks duration increases lung diffusing capacity in humans. *J. Appl. Physiol.* **2011**, *110*, 1564–1571. [CrossRef]
40. Martinot, J.-B.; Mulè, M.; De Bisschop, C.; Overbeek, M.J.; Le-Dong, N.N.; Naeije, R.; Guénard, H. Lung membrane conductance and capillary volume derived from the NO and CO transfer in high-altitude newcomers. *J. Appl. Physiol.* **2013**, *115*, 157–166. [CrossRef]
41. de Bisschop, C.; Martinot, J.B.; Leurquin-Sterk, G.; Faoro, V.; Guénard, H.; Naeije, R. Improvement in lung diffusion by endothelin A receptor blockade at high altitude. *J. Appl. Physiol.* **2012**, *112*, 20–25. [CrossRef]
42. Clarenbach, C.F.; Senn, O.; Christ, A.L.; Fischler, M.; Maggiorini, M.; Bloch, K.E. Lung function and breathing pattern in subjects developing high altitude pulmonary edema. *PLoS ONE* **2012**, *7*, 3–8. [CrossRef] [PubMed]
43. Kreuzer, F.; van Lookeren Campagne, P. Resting pulmonary diffusion capacity for CO and O_2 at high altitude. *J. Appl. Physiol.* **1965**, *20*, 519–524. [CrossRef] [PubMed]
44. Tiller, N.B.; Turner, L.A.; Taylor, B.J. Pulmonary and respiratory muscle function in response to 10 marathons in 10 days. *Eur. J. Appl. Physiol.* **2019**, *119*, 509–518. [CrossRef] [PubMed]
45. Thomas, R.G.; LaStayo, P.C.; Hoppeler, H.; Favier, R.; Ferretti, G.; Kayser, B.; Desplanches, D.; Spielvogel, H.; Lindstedt, S.L. Exercise training in chronic hypoxia has no effect on ventilatory muscle function in humans. *Respir. Physiol.* **1998**, *112*, 195–202. [CrossRef]
46. McDonough, P.; Dane, D.M.; Hsia, C.C.W.; Yilmaz, C.; Johnson, R.L., Jr. Long-term enhancement of pulmonary gas exchange after high-altitude residence during maturation. *J. Appl. Physiol* **2006**, *100*, 474–480. [CrossRef]
47. Guleria, J.S.; Pande, J.N.; Sethi, P.K.; Roy, S.B. Pulmonary diffusing capacity at high altitude. *J. Appl. Physiol.* **1971**, *31*, 536–543. [CrossRef]
48. Hull, J.H.; Wilson, M.G. The breathless swimmer: Could this be swimming-induced pulmonary edema? *Sport. Med. Open* **2018**, *4*, 8–10. [CrossRef]
49. Wagner, P. The lungs during exercise. *Physiology* **1987**, *2*, 6–10. [CrossRef]
50. Anholm, J.D.; Milne, E.N.C.; Stark, P.; Bourne, J.C., Friedman, P. Radiographic evidence of interstitial pulmonary edema after exercise at altitude. *J. Appl. Physiol.* **1999**, *86*, 503–509. [CrossRef]
51. McCartney, C.T.; Weis, M.N.; Ruppel, G.L.; Nayak, R.P. Residual volume and total lung capacity to assess reversibility in obstructive lung disease. *Respir. Care* **2016**, *61*, 1505–1512. [CrossRef]
52. Newton, M.F.; O'donnell, D.E.; Forkert, L. Response of lung volumes to inhaled salbutamol in a large population of patients with severe hyperinflation. *Chest* **2002**, *121*, 1042–1050. [CrossRef] [PubMed]
53. West, J.B. High-altitude medicine. *Lancet Respir. Med.* **2015**, *3*, 12–13. [CrossRef]
54. Hanel, B.; Teunissen, I.; Rabøl, A.; Warberg, J.; Secher, N.H. Restricted postexercise pulmonary diffusion capacity and central blood volume depletion. *J. Appl. Physiol.* **1997**, *83*, 11–17. [CrossRef] [PubMed]
55. Steinacker, J.M.; Tobias, P.; Menold, E.; Reißnecker, S.; Hohenhaus, E.; Liu, Y.; Lehmann, M.; Bärtsch, P.; Swenson, E.R. Lung diffusing capacity and exercise in subjects with previous high altitude pulmonary oedema. *Eur. Respir. J.* **1998**, *11*, 643–650.
56. Naeije, R.; Huez, S.; Lamotte, M.; Retailleau, K.; Neupane, S.; Abramowicz, D.; Faoro, V. Pulmonary artery pressure limits exercise capacity at high altitude. *Eur. Respir. J.* **2010**, *36*, 1049–1055. [CrossRef]
57. Sartori, C.; Rimoldi, S.F.; Scherrer, U. Lung fluid movements in hypoxia. *Prog. Cardiovasc. Dis.* **2010**, *52*, 493–499. [CrossRef]
58. Mutlu, G.M.; Koch, W.J.; Factor, P. Alveolar epithelial β2-adrenergic receptors: Their role in regulation of alveolar active sodium transport. *Am. J. Respir. Crit. Care Med.* **2004**, *170*, 1270–1275. [CrossRef]

59. Agostoni, P.; Cattadori, G.; Bianchi, M.; Wasserman, K. Exercise-Induced Pulmonary Edema in Heart Failure. *Circulation* **2003**, *108*, 2666–2671. [CrossRef]
60. Snyder, E.M.; Beck, K.C.; Hulsebus, M.L.; Breen, J.F.; Hoffman, E.A.; Johnson, B.D. Short-term hypoxic exposure at rest and during exercise reduces lung water in healthy humans. *J. Appl. Physiol.* **2006**, *101*, 1623–1632. [CrossRef]

International Journal of
Environmental Research and Public Health

MDPI

Article

Changes in Salivary Levels of Creatine Kinase, Lactate Dehydrogenase, and Aspartate Aminotransferase after Playing Rugby Sevens: The Influence of Gender

Álvaro González Fernández [1], Jose Enrique de la Rubia Ortí [2], Lorena Franco-Martinez [3], Jose Joaquín Ceron [3], Gonzalo Mariscal [1,*] and Carlos Barrios [1]

1 Institute for Research on Musculoskeletal Disorders, Catholic University of Valencia San Vicente Mártir, 46001 Valencia, Spain; alvaro.glez@mail.ucv.es (Á.G.F.); carlos.barrios@ucv.es (C.B.)
2 Department of Nursing, Catholic University of Valencia San Vicente Mártir, 46001 Valencia, Spain; joseenrique.delarubi@ucv.es
3 Interdisciplinary Laboratory of Clinical Analysis, Campus of Excellence Mare Nostrum, University of Murcia, 30100 Murcia, Spain; lorena.franco2@um.es (L.F.-M.); jjceron@um.es (J.J.C.)
* Correspondence: gonzalo.mariscal@mail.ucv.es

Received: 11 October 2020; Accepted: 2 November 2020; Published: 5 November 2020

Abstract: Rugby sevens is characterised by continuous exertion and great physical contact per unit of time, leading to muscle damage. It is important to identify markers that can quantify muscle damage in order to improve recovery strategies. The objective of this study was to evaluate the release dynamics of muscle damage markers creatine kinase (CK), lactate dehydrogenase (LDH), and aspartate aminotransferase (AST) in saliva samples when playing rugby sevens, analysing the influence of gender, during the rugby sevens university championship of Spain. The total sample included 27 athletes, divided into two teams of 14 men and 13 women between 18 and 31 years of age. CK, LDH, and AST were quantified from salivary samples collected from each athlete before and after three rugby sevens matches. The modified Borg scale of perceived exertion was also used after each match. When the results were analysed globally, there were no differences in CK and LDH before and after any match, but AST did show differences after two days of completing all matches. In terms of gender, the three enzymes showed different responses in men and women. Regarding the Borg scale, there were only significant differences between men and women after completing all mataches, with a greater perceived exertion in women. Based on our results, it can be stated that that serial matches of rugby sevens can cause changes of different magnitude in AST, CK and LDH activities in saliva, with AST showing the most significant variations and these changes are more pronounced in men than in women.

Keywords: rugby sevens; muscle damage; gender; creatine kinase; lactate dehydrogenase; aspartate aminotransferase

1. Introduction

Rugby is currently one of the most played and followed contact sports in the world [1]. There are two main kinds of rugby: rugby union and rugby sevens. In particular, rugby union is a team sport with great physical demand, including high intensity activities, such as sprinting, rucks, scrums, and tackles. It also includes low intensity activities, such as walking and jogging [2]. Rugby sevens is a traditional sport, but more attention has been paid to this form of rugby since it was included in the Olympics. In this modality, there are seven players on each team (three forwards and four backs), and the game lasts 15 min in total (two halves of seven minutes and a one-minute rest at the half-time break). This version, regarding Rugby League, increases both aerobic and anaerobic activity even more [3] with high speed fatigue [4], especially more than observed in rugby union. However, despite players possibly suffering less contact cruelty in narrow spaces than in rugby union, the fact that many rugby sevens competitions involve several matches played on consecutive days leads to greater impact in terms of neuromuscular damage and recovery [5]. Efficient muscle damage markers need to be identified in order to propose suitable recovery strategies due to this great contact. In addition, regarding these recovery strategies, rugby sevens has more and more followers, with exponential growth in the number of competitions and athletes who take part in both male and female elite competitions [6]. As a result, possible differences in muscle damage depending on gender would also be interesting. Therefore, recovery strategies can be adapted and, in this sense, athletes' performance would be improved.

Aetiology of muscle damage caused by physical exercise is mainly based on three mechanisms: mechanical fibre interruption, alterations of calcium homoeostasis, and inflammatory processes [7]. Within the inflammatory processes, measuring certain biomarkers in serum and plasma has been used to identify muscle damage. Among these biomarkers, the enzymes creatine kinase (CK), lactate dehydrogenase (LDH), or aspartate aminotransferase (AST) stand out as tools to determine skeletal muscle injury and tissue damage in the muscles [8]. These enzymes are found in the cytoplasmic matrix of muscle cells; therefore, their presence in serum or plasma are an indicator for cell lesions [9]. CK is considered to be one of the most important markers for muscle damage [10]. High levels of LDH specifically indicate muscle fatigue, while high levels of AST in the blood can be due to a wide range of clinical alterations; therefore, it is regarded as a more non-specific biomarker [11]. Quantification of these three molecules (CK, LDH, and AST) as markers of the response to exercise has not only been performed on blood samples but also from salivary samples [12]. In this sense, quantification in saliva has advantages over blood samples, highlighting that sample collection is a simple, safe, inexpensive, and non-invasive technique, thus reducing anxiety and discomfort in comparison to extracting blood [13]. From an analytical point of view, saliva contains less proteins than serum, so there is less risk of non-specific interference [14].

Regarding muscle damage response to physiological stress according to gender, we know that women are more resistant to neuromuscular fatigue during isolated isometric muscle contractions and of a similar intensity in comparison to men [15]. Nonetheless, if these contractions were caused with dynamic tasks, the answer is less clear, as they depend on the specific task and, therefore, on variables, such as shortening velocity and muscle group. In addition, rugby sevens players can be affected more uniformly by this contact cruelty and fatigue than in rugby union. It is for this reason that further studies are necessary to research the response in muscle damage according to the activity. In particular, this article delves into this point. The approach and originality of the study is to describe the kinetics of muscle damage by quantifying some related biomarkers after high intensity physical activity over two days, as represented with rugby sevens. Thus, the aim of this study is to establish the release dynamics of the muscle damage markers of the enzymes CK, LDH, and AST in saliva samples when playing rugby sevens, additionally to establishing the possible differences according to gender, which could establish different recovery strategies.

2. Material and Methods

2.1. Study Design

This is a cohort, observational, longitudinal, quantitative, and prospective pilot study with follow-up.

2.2. Subjects

The samples have been obtained from all the university rugby sevens players at the Catholic University of Valencia who voluntarily agreed to take part in this study. The study was carried out during the final stages of the rugby sevens university championship of Spain, both for women's and men's teams. All participants signed an informed consent form after being informed on the nature of the study. The total sample included 27 individuals between 18 and 31 years of age. Two cohorts were created: a male cohort including 14 athletes that were on the men's rugby sevens university team, and the female cohort including 13 athletes that were on the women's rugby sevens university team. All participants in the study followed the exact same guidelines for recovery and diet throughout the competition (without differentiation between men and women). These guidelines were designed and controlled by nutritionists and sports recovery specialists, both specialised in top-level sports competitions.

2.3. Procedure

The competition took place in Valencia in May 2019, with an environmental temperature of 24 °C. Two different championships were held, a women's and a men's. Six samples of saliva were collected from each participant during the tournament. As seen in Figure 1, the first sample was collected before match 1 on day 1 of the competition (9 a.m.) and the second aftermatch 1 (10 a.m.). The third and fourth samples were taken before and after match 2 (4:20 p.m. and 5:20 p.m., respectively). Finally, the fifth and sixth samples were obtained the following day, before and after each team's match 3 (11:00 a.m. and 12:00 p.m., respectively). The samples of saliva were collected 5 min before and 5 min after each match. Samples were collected from all participants in the study who needed to rinse their mouths with distilled water in order to avoid altering the samples with food left in the mouth that could contain a high content of acid or sugar. At least 2 mL of unstimulated saliva was collected in 10 mL sterile plastic tubes that were then stored in a container with ice. The procedure had an approximate total duration of 5 min. The samples were then centrifuged in the laboratory at 1500 g for 15 min, and the supernatant was frozen and stored in micro sample tubes at −20 °C until the samples were ready to be analysed.

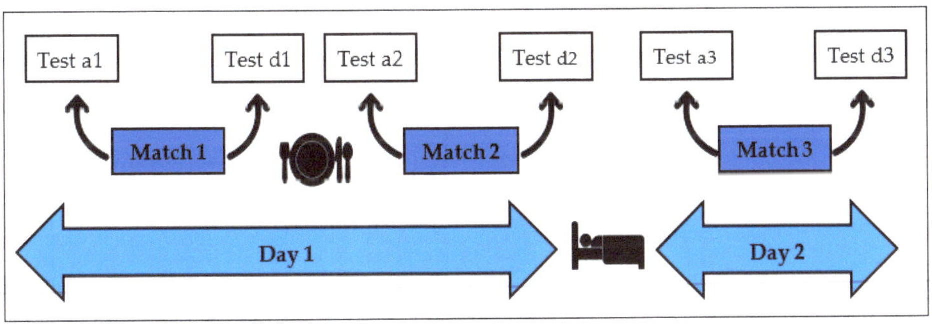

Figure 1. Timeline followed throughout both competitions (men and women) when collecting saliva samples.

In order to quantify the intensity of the exercise, perceived intensity was measured 10 min after exertion of each match using the modified 0–10 Borg scale, where 0 represents no exertion and 10 very, very hard exertion [16]. The players were familiar with this method before data were collected.

The players' position was not taken into account in this study due to the fact that physiological and performance characteristics in rugby sevens are relatively homogeneous in the different positions of the game [3,17], which is possibly associated with movement patterns in rugby sevens being less position-dependent than in rugby union [18].

Nonetheless, the 27 players took part in all the matches for at least 7 min and for a maximum of 9 min each.

2.4. Analysis of Salivary Samples

Immediately after collection, the samples were centrifuged (500× g for 10 min at 4 °C) and stored in a freezer at −80 °C until needed for analysing. Once the samples were thawed, they were thoroughly vortexed before analysis. CK was quantified by means of a commercial kit (Beckman Coulter, Brea, CA, USA), as well as LDH with a commercial kit (Biosystems, Barcelona, Spain) and AST with a commercial kit (Beckman Coulter, Brea, CA, USA). All tests were adapted in order to be used to collect saliva samples and were carried out in an automated biochemical analyser (Olympus A400, Beckman Coulter, Brea, CA, USA) at 37 °C.

2.5. Statistical Analysis

The statistical analysis was carried out with the SPSS 25 package for Windows (SPSS Inc., IBM Company, Armonk, NY, USA), with a level of significance of $p < 0.05$. After establishing the non-normality of the sample with the Kolmogorov-Smirnov test, the nonparametric Mann–Whitney U test was used and applied to two independent samples, while the Wilcoxon signed-rank test was used for related samples.

2.6. Ethical Concerns

The study was developed in accordance with the Declaration of Helsinki [19] with the prior approval of the protocol by the Ethical Committee of the Catholic University of Valencia (UCV/2019-2020/017). Participants were provided with a written informed consent form after being informed on the procedures and the nature of the study.

3. Results

The sociodemographic characteristics of the population sample of the study are demonstrated in Table 1, where no significant differences between men and women in terms of age were observed, yet, in terms of weight, a differentiation can be seen (Z = −3.88; $p < 0.05$), height (Z = −3.88; $p < 0.05$), and body mass index (BMI) (Z = −2.18; $p = 0.029$).

Table 1. Anthropometric and age data of the study population.

	Men'S Team ($n = 14$)	Women'S Team ($n = 13$)	Mann–Whitney U Test	
	Mean ± SD	Mean ± SD	Z	p
Age (years)	22.21 ± 3.07	21.85 ± 2.27	−0.25	0.807
Weight (kg)	81.04 ± 8.51	64.93 ± 13.17	−3.49	0.000 ***
Height (cm)	175.56 ± 7.32	162.38 ± 4.72	−3.88	0.000 ***
BMI (Kg/m^2)	26.27 ± 1.94	24.51 ± 3.81	−2.18	0.029 *

BMI: body mass index; * significant differences $p < 0.05$; *** significant differences $p < 0.001$.

When saliva enzymes were analysed in the whole sample of 27 athletes, CK and LDH did not show significant differences in activity before and after any of the 3 matches (Tables 2 and 3). However, there was a significant increase in AST after match 3 on the second day (Table 4).

Regarding gender, when comparing values between the men's and women's teams before and after each match, we could observe that CK showed significantly higher values in men before match 2 and after the match 3 (Table 2). AST, although showed significant increases after match 3 form men and women, it has significantly higher values in the men's team that in women after playing the three matches. (Table 4). LDH did not show significant differences between men and women in any of the three matches (Table 3).

Table 2. Statistical analysis of creatine kinase (CK) samples in saliva.

CK (ng/mL)	Total Sample Mean ± SD (Median)	Men Mean ± SD (Median)	Women Mean ± SD (Median)	Mann–Whitney U Test Z (p)
1A	68.815 ± 51.853 (73.5)	84.977 ± 62.088 (85.5)	52.654 ± 34.360 (45.3)	−1.436 (0.151)
1D	88.512 ± 82.388 (47.0)	108.136 ± 106.300 (68.4)	65.617 ± 31.787 (34.9)	−1.157 (0.247)
Wilcoxon signed-rank test Z (p)	−1.457 (0.145)	−0.524 (0.600)	−1.778 (0.075)	
2A	61.005 ± 51.114 (42.9)	92.489 ± 63.105 (86.1)	35.246 ± 12.493 (30.1)	−2.545 (0.011 *)
2D	74.515 ± 59.811 (58.1)	106.656 ± 76.478 (75.4)	48.218 ± 20.675 (53.9)	−1.557 (0.119)
Wilcoxon signed-rank test Z (p)	−1.923 (0.055)	−0.889 (0.374)	−1.867 (0.062)	
3A	59.744 ± 55.243 (58.9)	77.115 ± 69.830 (63.0)	40.925 ± 24.411 (36.2)	−1.034 (0.301)
3D	78.280 ± 69.106 (47.0)	109.069 ± 83.919 (73.3)	44.925 ± 20.071 (40.2)	−2.448 (0.014 *)
Wilcoxon signed-rank test Z (p)	−1.789 (0.074)	−1.852 (0.064)	−0.706 (0.480)	

A: before the match; D: after the match; * significant difference $p < 0.05$.

Table 3. Statistical analysis of lactate dehydrogenase (LDH) samples in saliva.

LDH (U/l)	Total Sample Mean ± SD (Median)	Men Mean ± SD (Median)	Women Mean ± SD (Median)	Mann–Whitney U Test Z (p)
1A	320.358 ± 299.804 (185.2)	341.000 ± 309.482 (209.3)	299.715 ± 300.919 (146.2)	−0.590 (0.555)
1D	360.635 ± 436.736 (192.2)	398.564 ± 538.385 (158.2)	316.383 ± 294.907 (106.2)	−0.669 (0.504)
Wilcoxon signed-rank test Z (p)	−0.175 (0.861)	−0.035 (0.972)	−0.078 (0.937)	
2A	306.565 ± 328.447 (201.2)	423.389 ± 423.862 (451.8)	210.982 ± 197.249 (132.7)	−0.570 (0.569)
2D	261.165 ± 252.243 (290.3)	377.089 ± 236.488 (328.5)	199.046 ± 161.811 (163.8)	−0.722 (0.470)
Wilcoxon signed-rank test Z (p)	−1.400 (0.161)	−1.481 (0.139)	−0.622 (0.534)	
3A	171.076 ± 250.427 (188.4)	134.792 ± 240.492 (70.7)	210.383 ± 265.507 (84.3)	−0.870 (0.384)
3D	279.904 ± 372.832 (220.1)	797.008 ± 488.854 (223.3)	153.042 ± 93.875 (122.5)	−0.598 (0.550)
Wilcoxon signed-rank test Z (p)	−1.816 (0.069)	−2.691 (0.007 ⁺)	−0.392 (0.695)	

A: before the match; D: after the match; ⁺ significant differences $p < 0.05$.

Table 4. Statistical analysis of aspartate aminotransferase (AST) samples in saliva.

AST (U/l)	Total Sample Mean ± SD (Median)	Men Mean ± SD (Median)	Women Mean ± SD (Median)	Mann–Whitney U Test Z (p)
1A	45.992 ± 57.848 (30.6)	67.700 ± 74.819 (36.8)	24.285 ± 18.781 (25.8)	−2.333 (0.020)
1D	57.727 ± 80.259 (19.1)	81.686 ± 101.581 (37.3)	29.775 ± 19.424 (15.2)	−1.260 (0.208 *)
Wilcoxon signed-rank test Z (p)	−0.646 (0.518)	−0.210 (0.834)	−0.941 (0.347)	
2A	42.530 ± 58.500 (18.3)	73.389 ± 78.034 (45.4)	17.282 ± 8.521 (14.6)	−1.824 (0.068)
2D	57.325 ± 92.423 (26.8)	99.300 ± 128.574 (45.6)	22.982 ± 11.026 (20.5)	−2.013 (0.044 *)
Wilcoxon signed-rank test Z (p)	−1.493 (0.135)	−0.889 (0.374)	−1.600 (0.110)	
3A	27.896 ± 37.218 (16.0)	41.262 ± 47.301 (43.1)	13.417 ± 11.900 (15.4)	−1.251 (0.211)
3D	47.496 ± 53.572 (22.1)	71.785 ± 65.588 (39.4)	21.183 ± 10.791 (18.4)	−2.284 (0.022 *)
Wilcoxon signed-rank test Z (p)	−2.879 (0.004 ⁺⁺)	−2.201 (0.028 ⁺)	−1.962 (0.048 ⁺)	

A: before the match; D: after the match; ⁺ significant differences $p < 0.05$, ⁺⁺ $p < 0.005$; * significant differences $p < 0.05$.

As far as the Borg scale, the mean values throughout the competition for men and women varied between 5.42 ± 1.34 and 7.25 ± 1.48, illustrating a perceived exertion between hard and very hard, respectively. Concerning differences between the men and women, there were only significant differences ($p < 0.008$) in match 3 with a higher perceived exertion in women (Figure 2).

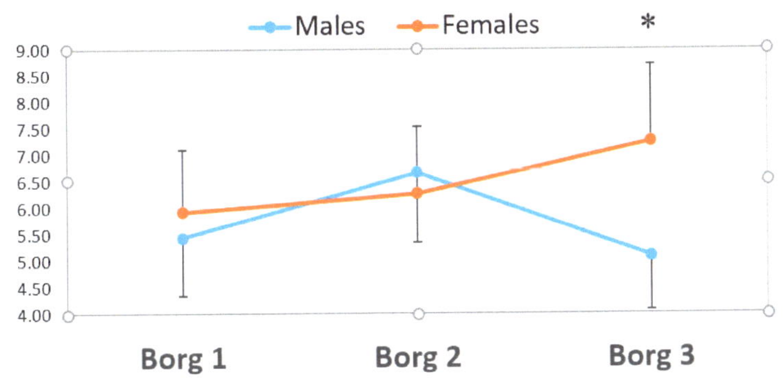

Figure 2. Comparison between men and men of perceived exertion as established by the modified Borg scale after the 3 matches. Borg: modified Borg scale of perceived exertion; * significant differences $p < 0.05$ with the Mann–Whitney U Test.

4. Discussion

Rugby sevens is characterised by quick and powerful muscle contractions, as well as continuous collisions between players, that can lead to muscle damage. In this sense, measuring activity of CK, LDH, and AST in serum can be used as a muscle injury marker [9], as they have been observed to increase in the blood after physical activities that cause intense muscle fatigue, such as running a mountain marathon [20] or resistance exercises [21]. These enzymes can also be quantified in saliva [22]. Therefore, CK, LDH, and AST were quantified in our study in saliva samples obtained before and after the rugby sevens matches. Despite the lack of studies of this nature that identify normal values of enzymes in saliva related to possible muscle damage, the values obtained in our study for AST and CK were higher than those described by Barranco T. et al., 2018, in healthy people and who had not performed any kind of previous exercise [23].

When analysing the possible changes in these enzymes total study population, no significant differences were observed for CK and LDH concentration levels before and after any of the 3 matches, despite the results of the Borg scale indicating a perceived exertion between hard and very hard, respectively. These results do not coincide with those obtained in another study, where there were significant changes in saliva after playing an indoor football match, registering an equally high perceived exertion (average of 7 on the Borg Scale) [24]. The fact that these results do not coincide could be due to the time when the samples were collected, as samples were taken immediately after physical activity in our study. However, in the study conducted by Barranco et al. [12], the samples were collected 30 min and 12 h after exertion. In this sense, we must outline that there has been evidence of a delay in the movement of some enzymes from blood to saliva, including CK [25]. In addition to this, it is precisely CK that takes time to increase in the blood after physical activity, as other authors observed a rise in plasma after 72 h after a football match [26]. In particular, when CK was measured after playing rugby, it was only increased in the blood after 30 min after the match [27], remaining high and even showing higher peaks after 24 h after finishing the sport [27,28]. Something similar was also registered for LDH, whose levels were seen to increase in the blood after 8, 24, and 48 h after exercise, coinciding with the feeling of muscle ache [29]. Yet, in saliva, the only published data indicate an increase 4 weeks after the aerobic exercise was carried out [30]. Nonetheless, we did observe a significant increase in AST after match 3 on the second day in our study. Curiously, this enzyme was seen to rise in the blood samples obtained immediately after a high intensity boxing match [31], which seems to confirm our results.

Nonetheless, this study has also assessed the possible differences in the response of the 3 enzymes according to gender. Authors, such as Franco Martínez L. et al. [32] and Souglis A. et al. [33,34], show in their studies that there is a different salivary proteome in men and women after exercising. They propose the idea to conduct further studies to learn what physiological changes are represented in the saliva of both men and women. In this sense, we observed that CK, AST, and LDH behaviour is different throughout the rugby sevens competition, showing generally higher enzyme levels in men, both before and after the matches.In particular, if the differences between pre- and post-match values between both men and women are analysed, CK shows higher levels in men before match 2 and after match 3. Something similar happens with AST, as match 1 displays these significant differences are always higher after the match. LDH is the only case where there are no differences in any match. This would indicate a different behavior of the enzymes analysed in our study according to gender.

Despite not being able to compare these results with previous ones, due to the lack of research analysing differences between men and women in terms of enzyme salivary secretion after physical activity, they were in line with a recent study where the values obtained in serum samples were compared. Specifically, after the Ecomotion Pro edition, significant increases in CK, AST, and LDH in serum were detected only in men, showing differences between men and women in the secretion of these enzymes [35]. These results show that behaviour in the face of stress is different in men and women. In addition the study conducted by O'Leary T.J. et al. [36] differences in the response to physiological stress afterload carriage was dectected regarding gender. It was specifically observed that, despite the fact that women had a higher heart rate and greater perceived exertion after activity, loss in strength of maximal isometric contraction was higher in men, therefore higher physiological stress during load carriage for women did not mean more severe muscle fatigue, showing more resistance towards said fatigue [36] and confirming what had been described in another prior study [15].

With regard to the Borg scale, perceived exertion implies a subjective assessment of strength, tension, discomfort and/or fatigue while exercising. Therefore, perception depends on physiological mediators grouped into central mediators (related to cardiorespiratory processes) and peripheral mediators (related to processes inherent to skeletal muscle, with blood acidosis, etc.) [37]. Concerning central mediators, important correlations between perceived exertion and heart rate have been established (between $r = 0.80$ and $r = 0.90$) [38]. However, this correlation is not as obvious in peripheral mediators, such as biomarker quantification. Thus, a close relation between concentration of blood lactate and the valuation of perceived exertion are established [39]. Nonetheless, other authors have found differences up to 3–4 points on the perceived exertion scale for the same value of concentration of blood lactate (4 mmol/L), in a maximal, progressive treadmill test [40]. This discrepancy between biomarkers and perceived exertion would be in line with our results, where female players show a higher perceived exertion than men, even though the levels of muscle damage markers are generally higher in men. On the other hand, delving into discrepancies in perceived exertion between men and women regardless of muscle damage, it does seem that it is higher in women, in accordance with studies published in other situations involving intense physical activity [41]. These results seem to be in accordance with those obtained in our study, where women show a significantly higher perceived effort than men in match 3.

The results of our study showed a high intersubject variability. In this sense, other authors have described that the values of muscle enzymes show this great variability between individuals and depend on the individual to a high degree, observing high variability between athletes who are even on the same team. This fact demonstrates the need for individualised follow-ups [42,43]. In terms of rugby, this variability has been previously verified in other enzymes, such as myoglobin. Lindsay A. et al. suggest that each subject should be analysed individually and not as a group, as rugby is a sport where muscle damage is highly variable, depending on the progression of the match [44]. Moreover, although this study used two complete teams, it would be necessary to increase the sample for future research as it is limited, analysing also the possible influence of match time on athletes. In addition since muscle damage leads to increase pain, this variable could be assessed through tests, such as vertical jumps, maximum isometric force, and subjective muscle pain measurements. Nonetheless, it would be interesting to do a longer follow up of the enzymes of our study after match in order to evaluate long-term changes in these analytes.

In terms of the interest that our study may have, the differences in the response to physiological stress may be related to the onset of injuries after exercise. In skeletal muscle, there have been described gender differences in muscle injuries with a decrease in the frequency of injuries in female rodents [45], with CK having lower increases in serum after injury in women than men [46] that would be in agreement with our findings. The enzymes CK, LDH (to a lesser degree as it seems less sensitive), and especially AST could be used as possible diagnostic tools to predict this risk of injury, which could help to improve young athletes' performance.

5. Conclusions

CK, AST, and LDH in saliva showed changes of different magnitude after serial matches of rugby seven, with AST showing the most significant variations. Differences in terms of gender were observed, with men showing increases of higher magnitude, mainly in AST after the matches. Due to the large variations in enzyme values between athletes, it would be recommended to monitor the changes so they can be carried out individually in order to determine the status and muscle damage more objectively.

Author Contributions: Conceptualization, C.B. and Á.G.F.; Data curation, L.F.-M., J.J.C.; Formal analysis, J.E.d.l.R.O. and G.M.; Funding acquisition, C.B. and Á.G.F.; Investigation, G.M., L.F.-M., J.J.C., and J.E.d.l.R.O; Methodology, L.F.-M., J.J.C.; Project administration, G.M.; Resources, C.B., Á.G.F.; Software, C.B.; Validation, G.M.; Writing—original draft, J.E.d.l.R.O.; Writing—review & editing, J.E.d.l.R.O., Á.G.F., and G.M. All authors have read and agreed to the published version of the manuscript.

Funding: This research was funded by the Catholic University Foundation San Vicente Mártir.

Acknowledgments: The authors would like to thank the participants for taking part in the study.

Conflicts of Interest: The authors declare no conflict of interest.

References

1. World Rugby. What is Rugby? Available online: https://www.world.rugby/welcome-to-rugby/what-is-rugby (accessed on 17 March 2020).
2. Roberts, S.P.; Trewartha, G.; Higgitt, R.J.; El-Abd, J.; Stokes, K.A. The physical demands of elite English rugby union. *J. Sports Sci.* **2008**, *26*, 825–833. [CrossRef] [PubMed]
3. Higham, D.G.; Pyne, D.B.; Anson, J.M.; Eddy, A. Movement patterns in rugby sevens: Effects of tournament level, fatigue and substitute players. *J. Sci. Med. Sport* **2012**, *15*, 277–282. [CrossRef] [PubMed]
4. Higham, D.G.; Pyne, D.B.; Anson, J.M.; Eddy, A. Physiological, anthropometric, and performance characteristics of rugby sevens players. *Int. J. Sports Physiol. Perform.* **2013**, *8*, 19–27. [CrossRef] [PubMed]
5. West, D.J.; Cook, C.J.; Stokes, K.A.; Atkinson, P.; Drawer, S.; Bracken, R.M.; Kilduff, L.P. Profiling the time-course changes in neuromuscular function and muscle damage over two consecutive tournament stages in elite rugby sevens players. *J. Sci. Med. Sport* **2014**, *17*, 688–692. [CrossRef]
6. World Rugby. The History of Rugby Sevens. Available online: https://www.world.rugby/sevens/history-of-sevens (accessed on 17 March 2020).
7. Clarkson, P.M.; Sayers, S.P. Etiology of exercise-induced muscle damage. *Can. J. Appl. Physiol.* **1999**, *24*, 234–248. [CrossRef]
8. Nie, J.; Tong, T.K.; George, K.; Fu, F.H.; Lin, H.; Shi, Q. Resting and post-exercise serum biomarkers of cardiac and skeletal muscle damage in adolescent runners. *Scand. J. Med. Sci. Sports* **2011**, *21*, 625–629. [CrossRef]
9. Brancaccio, P.; Maffulli, N.; Buonauro, R.; Limongelli, F.M. Serum Enzyme Monitoring in Sports Medicine. *Clin. Sports Med.* **2008**, *27*, 1–18. [CrossRef]
10. Brancaccio, P.; Maffulli, N.; Limongelli, F.M. Creatine kinase monitoring in sport medicine. *Br. Med. Bull.* **2007**, *81–82*, 209–230. [CrossRef]
11. Nathwani, R.A.; Pais, S.; Reynolds, T.B.; Kaplowitz, N. Serum alanine aminotransferase in skeletal muscle diseases. *Hepatology* **2005**, *41*, 380–382. [CrossRef]
12. Barranco, T.; Tvarijonaviciute, A.; Tecles, F.; Carrillo, J.M.; Sánchez-Resalt, C.; Jimenez-Reyes, P.; Rubio, M.; García-Balletbó, M.; Cerón, J.J.; Cugat, R. Changes in creatine kinase, lactate dehydrogenase and aspartate aminotransferase in saliva samples after an intense exercise: A pilot study. *J. Sports Med. Phys. Fit.* **2018**, *58*, 910–916. [CrossRef]
13. Lee, Y.H.; Wong, D.T. Saliva: An emerging biofluid for early detection of diseases. *Am. J. Dent.* **2009**, *22*, 241–248.
14. Mirzaii-Dizgah, I.; Jafari-Sabet, M. Unstimulated whole saliva creatine phosphokinase in acute myocardial infarction. *Oral Dis.* **2011**, *17*, 597–600. [CrossRef] [PubMed]
15. Hunter, S.K. Sex Differences in Human Fatigability: Mechanisms and Insight to Physiological Responses. *Acta Physiol.* **2014**, *210*, 768–789. [CrossRef]
16. Borg, G.; Ljunggren, G.; Ceci, R. The increase of perceived exertion, aches and pain in the legs, heart rate and blood lactate during exercise on a bicycle ergometer. *Eur. J. Appl. Physiol. Occup. Physiol.* **1985**, *54*, 343–349. [CrossRef]
17. Carreras, D.; Kraak, W.; Planas, A.; Martín, I.; Vaz, L. Analysis of International Rugby Sevens matches during tournaments. *Int. J. Perform. Anal. Sport* **2013**, *13*, 833–847. [CrossRef]
18. Fuller, C.; Taylor, A.; Molloy, M. Epidemiological study of injuries in internationalrugby sevens. *Clin. J. Sport Med.* **2010**, *20*, 179–184. [CrossRef]

19. World Medical Association. World Medical Association declaration of Helsinki: Ethical principles for medical research involving human subjects. *JAMA* **2013**, *310*, 2191–2194. [CrossRef]
20. Belli, T.; Macedo, D.V.; De Araújo, G.G.; dos Reis, I.G.M.; Scariot, P.P.M.; Lazarim, F.L.; Nunes, L.A.S.; Brenzikofer, R.; Gobatto, C.A. Mountain ultramarathon induces early increases of muscle damage, inflammation, and risk for acute renal injury. *Front. Physiol.* **2018**, *9*, 1–10. [CrossRef]
21. Isik, O.; Dogan, I. Effects of bilateral or unilateral lower body resistance exercises on markers of skeletal muscle damage. *Biomed. J.* **2018**, *41*, 364–368. [CrossRef] [PubMed]
22. Ovchinnikov, A.N.; Deryugina, A.V. Saliva as highly informative substrate for non-invasive analysis of lipoperoxide processes and muscle damage in highly skilled athletes. *Klin. Lab. Diagn.* **2019**, *64*, 405–408. [CrossRef] [PubMed]
23. Barranco, T.; Cerón, J.J.; López-Jornet, P.; Pastor, J.; Carrillo, J.M.; Rubio, M.; Tornel, P.L.; Cugat, R.; Tecles, F.; Tvarijonaviciute, A. Impact of Saliva Collection and Processing Methods on Aspartate Aminotransferase, Creatin Kinase and Lactate Dehydrogenase Activities. *Anal. Sci.* **2018**, *34*, 619–622. [CrossRef] [PubMed]
24. Moreira, A.; Arsati, F.; Lima-Arsati, Y.B.D.O.; de Freitas, C.G.; de Araújo, V.C. Salivary Immunoglobulin A Responses in Professional Top-Level Futsal Players. *J. Strength Cond. Res.* **2011**, *25*, 1932–1936. [CrossRef] [PubMed]
25. Foo, J.Y.Y.; Wan, Y.; Kostner, K.; Arivalagan, A.; Atherton, J.; Cooper-White, J.; Dimeski, G.; Punyadeera, C. NT-ProBNP Levels in Saliva and Its Clinical Relevance to Heart Failure. *PLoS ONE* **2012**, *7*, e48452. [CrossRef]
26. Ascensão, A.; Rebelo, A.; Oliveira, E.; Marques, F.; Pereira, L.; Magalhães, J. Biochemical impact of a soccer match—analysis of oxidative stress and muscle damage markers throughout recovery. *Clin. Biochem.* **2008**, *41*, 841–851. [CrossRef] [PubMed]
27. McLellan, C.P.; Lovell, D.I.; Gass, G. Creatine Kinase and Endocrine Responses of Elite Players Pre, During, and Post Rugby League Match Play. *J. Strength Cond. Res.* **2010**, *24*, 2908–2919. [CrossRef]
28. Taylor, T.; West, D.J.; Howatson, G.; Jones, C.; Bracken, R.M.; Love, T.D.; Cook, C.J.; Swift, E.; Baker, J.S.; Kilduff, L.P. The impact of neuromuscular electrical stimulation on recovery after intensive, muscle damaging, maximal speed training in professional team sports players. *J. Sci. Med. Sport* **2015**, *18*, 328–332. [CrossRef]
29. Tiidus, P.M.; Ianuzzo, C.D. Effects of intensity and duration of muscular exercise on delayed soreness and serum enzyme activities. *Med. Sci. Sports Exerc.* **1983**, *15*, 461–465. [CrossRef]
30. Alghadir, A.H.; Gabr, S.A.; Aly, F.A. The effects of four weeks aerobic training on saliva cortisol and testosterone in young healthy persons. *J. Phys. Ther. Sci.* **2015**, *27*, 2029–2033. [CrossRef]
31. Kılıc, Y.; Cetin, H.N.; Sumlu, E.; Pektas, M.B.; Koca, H.B.; Akar, F. Effects of boxing matches on metabolic, hormonal, and inflammatory parameters in male elite boxers. *Medicina* **2019**, *55*, 288. [CrossRef]
32. Franco Martínez, L.; González-Hernández, J.M.; Horvatić, A.; Guillemin, N.; Cerón, J.J.; Martínez-Subiela, S.; Sentandreu, M.Á.; Brkljačić, M.; Mrljak, V.; Tvarijonaviciute, A.; et al. Differences on salivary proteome at rest and in response to an acute exercise in men and women: A pilot study. *J. Proteom.* **2020**, *214*, 103629. [CrossRef]
33. Souglis, A.; Bogdanis, G.C.; Giannopoulou, I.; Papadopoulos, C.; Apostolidis, N. Comparison of Inflammatory Responses and Muscle Damage Indices Following a Soccer, Basketball, Volleyball and Handball Game at an Elite Competitive Level. *Res. Sports Med.* **2015**, *23*, 59–72. [CrossRef]
34. Souglis, A.; Bogdanis, G.C.; Chryssanthopoulos, C.; Apostolidis, N.; Geladas, N.D. Time Course of Oxidative Stress, Inflammation, and Muscle Damage Markers for 5 Days After a Soccer Match. *J. Strength Cond. Res.* **2018**, *32*, 2045–2054. [CrossRef]
35. Silva, R.P.M.; Vilaça, A.; Guerra, F.D.; Mundim, A.V.; de Agostini, G.G.; de Abreu, L.C.; Zhiguo, Z.; Sorpreso, I.C.; Valenti, V.E.; Penha-Silva, N. Sex Differences in Physiological Stress Induced by a Long-Lasting Adventure Race: A Prospective Observational Analytical Study. *Sportverletz Sportschaden* **2019**, *34*, 84–95. [CrossRef]
36. O'Leary, T.J.; Saunders, S.C.; McGuire, S.J.; Izard, R.M. Sex differences in neuromuscular fatigability in response to load carriage in the field in British Army recruits. *J. Sci. Med. Sport* **2018**, *21*, 591–595. [CrossRef]
37. Robertson, R.J.; Goss, F.L.; Metz, K.F. Perception of physical exertion during dynamic exercise: A tribute to Professor Gunnar, A. V. Borg. *Percept. Mot. Ski.* **1998**, *86*, 183–191. [CrossRef]
38. Arruza Gabilondo, J.; Alzate Sáez de Heredia, R.; Valencia Garate, J. Esfuerzo percibido y frecuencia cardiaca: El control de la intensidad de los esfuerzos en el entrenamiento de judo. *Rev. Psicol. Deporte* **1996**, *5*, 29–40.

39. Seip, R.L.; Snead, D.; Pierce, E.F.; Stein, P.; Weltman, A. Perceptual responses and blood lactate concentration: Effect of training state. *Med. Sci. Sports Exerc.* **1991**, *23*, 80–87. [CrossRef]
40. Held, T.; Marti, B. Substantial influence of level of endurance capacity on the association of perceived exertion with blood lactate accumulation. *Int. J. Sports Med.* **1999**, *20*, 34–39. [CrossRef] [PubMed]
41. Pincivero, D.M.; Coelho, A.J.; Campy, R.M. Gender Differences in Perceived Exertion during Fatiguing Knee Extensions. *Med. Sci. Sports Exerc.* **2004**, *36*, 109–117. [CrossRef] [PubMed]
42. Proia, P.; Bianco, A.; Schiera, G.; Saladino, P.; Pomara, F.; Petrucci, M.; Traina, M.; Palma, A. The effects of a 3-week training on basal biomarkers in professional soccer players during the preseason preparation period. *J. Sports Med. Phys. Fit.* **2012**, *52*, 102–126.
43. Thorpe, R.; Sunderland, C. Muscle damage, endocrine, and immune marker response to a soccer match. *J. Strength Cond. Res.* **2012**, *26*, 2783–2790. [CrossRef]
44. Lindsay, A.; Lewis, J.; Scarrott, C.; Draper, N.; Gieseg, S.P. Changes in acute biochemical markers of inflammatory and structural stress in rugby union. *J. Sports Sci.* **2015**, *33*, 882–891. [CrossRef]
45. Enns, D.L.; Tiidus, P.M. Estrogen influences satellite cell activation and proliferation following downhill running in rats. *J. Appl. Physiol.* **2008**, *104*, 347–353. [CrossRef] [PubMed]
46. Carter, A.; Dobridge, J.; Hackney, A.C. Influence of estrogen on markers of muscle tissue damage following eccentric exercise. *Fiziol. Cheloveka* **2001**, *27*, 133–137. [CrossRef]

Publisher's Note: MDPI stays neutral with regard to jurisdictional claims in published maps and institutional affiliations.

International Journal of
Environmental Research and Public Health

MDPI

Article

All-Time Best Norwegian Track and Field Athletes: To What Extent Did They Achieve Outstanding Results at The Ages of 15 and 18 Years?

Leif Inge Tjelta * and Ola Tjensvoll

Faculty of Arts and Education, University of Stavanger, 4036 Stavanger, Norway; olatjensvoll@hotmail.com
* Correspondence: leif.i.tjelta@uis.no; Tel.: +47-976-873-83

Received: 11 September 2020; Accepted: 28 September 2020; Published: 29 September 2020

Abstract: The aim of the study was to determine how many Norwegian athletes who, during all the times they had achieved the European Athletics Championship 2020—Entry Standards (EAC20ES), were also ranked among the 20 all-time-best athletes at the ages of 15 and 18 years. The number of athletes who achieved the EAC20ES during their career, and the percentage of those who were among top 20 in the age groups 15 and 18 years, were determined from the Norwegian all-time-best results lists. A total of 202 athletes achieved the EAC20ES in the studied time period. Of these, 14.4% and 42.1% were ranked among the top 20 all-time best in one or more events at the ages of 15 and 18 years, respectively. However, among those who had won an international gold medal, these percentages were much higher. Eight out of 12 champions (66.7%) were ranked among the top 20 all-time best in one or more event at 15 years of age, and 11 of 12 champions (91.6%) were ranked among the top 20 all-time best at 18 years of age. Athletes that went on to win international championships typically performed better as adolescents compared to other athletes who also reach an international level as seniors. However, due to the low number of international champions, the date should be interpreted with caution.

Keywords: elite athletes; athletics; youth performance; talent identification

1. Introduction

Exceptional sporting performance, often defined as winning a medal in an international competition, is dependent on motor and physical development over the lifespan [1]. Today, children often focus on training and competition in sports from an early age, in the hope that this will help them to reach an elite level as adults [2–4].

It is a debated topic whether long-term success in elite sports can be predicted from performance in youth competitions [5,6] and to what extent early specialization [7] or early diversification is key for success at senior level [8]. Early specialization has been defined as intensive training or competition in organized sport by prepubescent children (<12 years of age) for more than 8 months per year, with a focus on a single sport to the exclusion of other sports and free play [9].

The early specialization framework [7] postulates that training and development for 10,000 hours from early to middle childhood in the primary sport is necessary to achieve exceptional performance.

According to LaPrade, Agel, Baker, Brenner, Cordasco, Côté, Engebretsen, Feeley, Gould and Hainline [10], there is no evidence that young children will benefit from early sport specialization in the majority of sports. However, in some sports like golf, tennis and gymnastics, early specialization has been considered important for the development of certain skills [11]. Early specialization and intensive training during early adolescence can also result in an increased risk of injuries and a decrease in sport enjoyment [12,13].

The early diversification path recommends a greater involvement in a variety of sports before specializing [13,14]. Evidence has proved that the early diversification path where athletes had been engaged in deliberate play during childhood could lead to elite level of performance in sports [15–18].

Previous research has examined the relationship between youth and adult performance in different sports [19–22]. For example, Barreiros, Côté and Fonseca [21] found that only one in three athletes who competed at an international level at pre-junior level (≤16 years) in swimming, volleyball, judo or football, also competed internationally at senior level. Conversely, in a study of Norwegian road cyclists by Svendsen, Tønnesen, Tjelta and Ørn [19], race performance at age 18 was found to be the strongest predictor of success at senior level.

In the sport of track and field athletics, the International Association of Athletics Federations (IAAF) arranges the World Junior Championship every other year, for athletes under the age of 20. Hollings and Hume [23] retrospectively examined a cohort of 137 athletes who were Olympic or World Champions, and previous competitors in the World Junior Championship (WJC). Of these, 55% were former medalists and 80% were top eight finishers in WJC. However, a contrasting picture emerges from the same data analyzed prospectively, following 1054 medalists at World Junior Championships from 1986 to 2004. Of the 1054 junior medalists, only 34% became medalists or finalists in international competitions as seniors, whilst a further 12% competed at international level, but never made it to an international final. As many as 54% never participated in international competitions as senior athletes. In a study where the purpose was to examine the lifetime best performance of World Junior Championship finalists and Olympic Games finalists in athletic events, Foss, Sinex and Chapman [1] found that World Junior Championship finalists achieved their career-best performance at a younger age compared to Olympic Games finalists. They also had less performance improvement over the course of their career compared to Olympic Games finalists. Kearney and Hayes [24] conducted a retrospective study of top 20 ranked senior track and field athletes in the United Kingdom and found that performance during youth had only a weak relationship with performance at senior level.

Three Norwegian brothers who have all been European 1500 m champions, were found to have had very different athletic developments [20]. The oldest (HI) took part in football, cross-country skiing and distance running during his childhood, and is ranked among the top 10 all-time best in the 1500 m in Norway in the age groups 15, 16, 17 and 18 years. The 2016 European 1500 m champion (FI), played football from the age of 7 until the age of 16 and is not among the all-time top ten in any event in any age group from 13 to 18 years. The youngest brother (JI) however, has been the best runner in Norway in all age groups from the age of 13 years. FI's and, to some extent, HI's development is in accordance with the findings of Anderson and Mayo [25] who reported that many elite athletes specialize late, following diversification in other sports during their youth. JI on the other hand, focused on distance running from an early age [20]. This is in accordance with the findings of a review article by Coutinho, Mesquita and Fonseca [26], who claim there is considerable evidence in the literature that both early specialization and diversified experience in other sports can lead to elite development. A study of ten elite track and field athletes from Australia, who had all finished top ten at the Olympic Games and/or World Championships, indicates that the main factors accounting for success at senior level are high self-belief, high motivation with personal goals and achievement and athletics being a central part of their lives [27].

In athletics, performance can be quantitively measured in minutes and seconds or meters and centimeters, and to qualify for an international competition such as the European Championships 2020, an athlete has to achieve the European Athletics Championship 2020—Entry Standards (EAC20ES) [28] (Table 1). In Norway, the Norwegian Athletic Federation (Norges Friidrettsforbund—NFIF) registers all-time best results for seniors, juniors and boys and girls in all track and field events from the age of 13 years. The aim of this retrospective study was to determine how many of the all-time best Norwegian track and field athletes had performed at an international level (defined as having achieved the EAC20ES) and how many of these can also be found among the 20 all-time-best results for girls and boys at the ages of 15 and 18 years. In addition, we wished to examine to what extent Norwegian track and field gold medal winners in European Championships, World Championships and Olympic Games from 1980 to 2019 are represented in the top 20 all-time best lists for girls and boys at ages 15 and 18 years.

Table 1. European Athletics Championships 2020—Entry Standards (https://www.european-athletics.org).

Men	Discipline	Women
10.28	100 m	11.44
20.80	200 m	23.35
46.40	400 m	52.65
1:47.30	800 m	2:02.50
3:39.50	1500 m	4:11.00
13:44.00	5000 m	15:50.00
28:50.00	10,000 m	33:20.00
8:45.00	3000 m steeplechase	9:55.00
13.90	110 m hurdles/100 m hurdles	13:30
50.70	400 m hurdles	57.95
NES	Half-Marathon	NES
2.24	High Jump	1.90
5.60	Pole Vault	4.45
7.95	Long Jump	6.60
16.60	Triple jump	13.90
20.00	Shot Put	17.00
63.50	Discus	57.00
74.45	Hammer	69.00
80.50	Javelin	58.00
7850	Combined Events	5850

NES = No entry standard.

2. Materials and Methods

2.1. Data Sample

The present study was conducted in accordance with the declaration of Helsinki. Since data in the present study are based on publicaly available resources (https://www.friidrett.no/aktivitet/statistikk), no informed consent was obtained. The study was approved by the Norwegian social science data services.

The Norwegian Athletic Federation (Norges Friidrettsforbund—NFIF) register all-time best results for women and men, for juniors and for girls and boys in all track and field events from the age of 13. The number of athletes who achieved EAC20ES in sprint, middle distance, long distance, jumping, throwing and combined events, and their best results at 15 and 18 years of age are taken from these official lists, which were updated on the 31.12.2019.

To avoid an athlete who achieved the EAC20ES in more than one event being registered multiple times, athletes were divided into the following sub-groups: sprint and hurdles; middle and long distances; jumping; throwing; combined events. Athletes who, at the age of 15 and/or 18 years, were among the top 20 in more than one event are only registered once.

Norwegian gold medal winners in European Championships, World Championships and Olympic Games from 1980 to 2019 are also from The Norwegian Athletic Federation's (Norges Friidrettsforbund—NFIF) official statistics.

2.2. Different Equipment in the Throwing Events

Over the last 30 years, some changes have been made to the standards for throwing equipment in Norway in the age group of 15 years. In the hammer throw, the length of the hammer wire was 110 cm until the year 2000, after which it was increased to 119.5 cm. As such, the top 20 athletes in the age group of 15 years competing with both 110 cm and 119.5 cm hammer wire are registered. Athletes in the 15 years age group also competed with equipment of differing weights in the javelin, discus and shot-put events. The equipment weights most frequently registered for each event are included here. In shot put, this is 3.0 and 5.5 kg for girls and boys, respectively. In discus and javelin, equipment weights of 1 kg and 600 g, respectively, were used for both girls and boys. In the age group 18 years, the equipment is of the same weight and standard as that used at senior level.

2.3. Statistical Analyses

The number of men and woman who achieved the EAC20ES in the different subgroups, and the percentage of these who were ranked among the top 20 in the age groups 15 and 18 years, were calculated.

Descriptive statistics are presented as means and standard deviations (SD) for the age when Norwegian track and field gold medals winners in European Championships, World Championships, and Olympic Games won their first international title.

3. Results

Table 2 shows the total number of Norwegian athletes, and the number of male and female athletes, who have achieved the EAC20ES, and the number who have achieved the EAC20ES, in the following sub-groups: sprint and hurdle events (sprints), middle- and long-distances events (distances), jumping events (jumping), throwing events (throwing), and combined events. The number of these, and the percentage rank among the top 20 in the age groups 15 and 18 years, are also listed in Table 2.

Table 2. The number of Norwegian athletes who achieved the EAC20ES in sprints, distances, jumping, throwing and combined events, and the number and percentage (%) of these ranked among the top 20 in the age groups 15 and 18 years.

Group	Number of Norwegian Athletes Who Achieved EACS20ES			Number and Percentage (%) Ranked in the Top 20 Age 15			Number and Percentage (%) Ranked in the Top 20 Age 18		
	Total	Men	Women	Total	Boys	Girls	Total	Boys	Girls
sprints	31	15	16	4 (12.9%)	1 (6.7%)	3 (18.8%)	20 (64.5%)	9 (60.0%)	11 (68.8%)
distances	108	74	34	6 (5.6%)	4 (5.4%)	3 (8.8%)	24 (22.0%)	17 (22.9%)	7 (20.5%)
jumping	22	12	10	7 (31.8%)	4 (5.5%)	3 (30%)	16 (72.7%)	10 (83.4%)	6 (50%)
throwing	31	24	7	8 (25.8%)	5 (20.8%)	3 (42.9%)	21 (67.7%)	16 (66.7%)	5 (71.4%)
combined events	10	7	3	3 (30.0%)	2 (28.6%)	1 (33.34%)	4 (40.0%)	2 (28.6%)	2 (66.7%)
total	202	132	70	29 (14.4%)	16 (12.1%)	13 (18.6%)	85 (42.1%)	54 (40.9%)	31 (44.3%)

Norwegian athletes who became Olympic Champions (OC), World Champions (WC) and European Champions (EC) from 1980 to 2019 and their best ranking in any event at ages 15 and 18 years are listed in Table 3. In addition to the track and field events, marathon is also included. International champions in cross-country and road races are not included in Table 3. The ages at which the athletes won their first international title in track and field events or marathons are also included in Table 3.

Table 3. Norwegian athletes who have become OC, WC and/or EC from 1980 to 2019, their best ranking in any event at ages 15 and 18 years, and the age at which they won their first international title in track and field events or marathon. If their best ranking at ages 15 and 18 years is in another event than the one they have won an international title in, the event is noted in parentheses. M = male, F = female.

Athlete	Event	Year	OC	WC	EC	15 Years	18 Years	Age
GW (F)	marathon	1983		X			3 (1500 m)	30 **
IK (F)	10.000 m	1986, 1987		X	X	2 (1500 m)	*	30
EKH (F)	javelin	1993, 1997, 1994, 2000	X	XX	X	1	1	27
GM (M)	200 m	1994			X		16 (100 m)	25
SH (M)	High jump	1994			X	16	2	23
VR (M)	800 m	1996	X				5	24
HH (F)	high jump	1997		X		16	1	30
AT (M)	javelin	2004, 2008, 2006, 2010, 2009	XX	X	XX	4	1	24
HI (M)	1500 m	2012			X	9	2	21
FI (M)	1500 m	2016			X		14 (800 m)	23
JI (M)	1500 m, 5000 m	2018			X	1	1	18
KW (M)	400 m hurdles	2017, 2019, 2018		XX	X	2 (long jump)	1 (400 m)	21

* IK did not compete in athletics at the age of 18, but instead competed as an international cross-country skier at junior level. ** GW was also 5 times World Cross-Country Champion; the first time was in 1978 at the age of 25 years.

The average age at which the athletes listed in Table 3 won their first international title in track and field events or marathon was 24.7 ± 3.9 years.

4. Discussion

A total of 202 Norwegian track and field athletes have during all times achieved the EAC20ES (Table 1). Of these, 14.4% and 42.1% are ranked among the top 20 all-time best Norwegian athletes in one or more events at the ages of 15 and 18 years, respectively.

The data from the present study are in line with the findings of Kearney and Hayes [24] who conducted a retrospective study of the top 20 ranked senior track and field athletes in the United Kingdom. However, the percentage of top 20 ranked 15 and 18 year old boys and girls in the present study who later achieved the EAC20ES is even lower than the percentage of the top 20 ranked girls and boys at age 15 and 17 years who reached top 20 senior level in United kingdom [24]. In the study by Kearney and Hayes [24], 48% of boys and 58% of girls who were ranked top 20 at an age of 17 years were also among the top 20 ranked senior athletes. In the present study, more female athletes who achieved the EAC20ES are ranked in the top 20 at the age of 15 and 18 years than their male counterparts. This is in agreement with the findings in the study by Kearney and Hayes [24] and may be due to the fact that girls mature earlier than boys [29,30]. However, the absolute numbers of athletes having achieved the EAC20ES are in all groups, besides sprints, lower for women than for men.

The percentage of athletes ranked in the top 20 at age 15 who later went on to achieve EAC20ES is highest for jumping (31.8%), throwing (25.8%), and combined events (30%) and lowest for distance events (5.6%). For the sprint events, the percentage is 12.9%. At age 18, the percentage of top 20 athletes who later achieve EAC20ES for all events is much higher than at age 15. However, for the middle- and long-distance events, the percentage is still markedly lower than for the other events. This may be due to the fact that peak athletic performance in endurance events normally occurs at a later age than in explosive power/sprint events [31]. However, it has to be underlined that from the data in Table 1, no information can be drawn from the ranking in the lists to determine the amount of athletics training at ages 15 and 18 years, and to what extent the athletes at these ages also took part in other sports.

The percentage athletes who were ranked top 20 at the ages of 15 and 18 years is much higher for those who have won an international title: 66.7% (8 of 12 champions) in age group 15 years and 91.6% (11 of 12 champions) in age group 18 years. As such, it appears that results at a top national level at the age of 18 years may be a premise for becoming an international champion. This is in agreement with the findings of Svendsen et al. (2018), who found that the strongest predictor of senior success among Norwegian junior road cyclists was race performance at 18 years of age. However, it is in contrast to the findings of Foss, Sinex, and Chapman [1], who, after finding that World Junior Championship finalists in athletics reached their career-best performance at an earlier age and had less performance improvements during their careers than Olympic Games finalists, challenged the assertion that elite success at junior level is a prerequisite for success at senior level. It has to be underlined that, despite the fact that the Norwegian international champions listed in Table 3 showed excellent performance at the age of 18 years, only one of them (JI) won an international title at U20.

What more do we know about the 12 international athletic champions listed in Table 3? Is early specialization or early diversification the key for success as an elite senior athlete?

Among the two outstanding former world record holders and World Champions in distance running events GW and IK, we find similarities in training during their adolescence [32]. They both participated in an extensive range of sports. In addition to distance running, GW competed in sprints, jumps and throws, as well as playing handball during her early youth. IK participated in cross-country skiing and running. One difference between the two is that, up until senior level, GW did more anaerobic training than IK. The latter got her basic training through aerobics, cross-country skiing and trail running. GW achieved her best times in the 1500 m and the 3000 m. She was also best in the 800 m. IK was best over the longest distances. This might have been a consequence of differences in training during their youth and/or "genetic differences" [32]. We also know that the male distance runners included in Table 3 have taken part in a variety of sports during childhood and early adolescence. The 1996 Olympic Champion VR competed in both cross-country skiing and athletics up to the age of 16 years [33]. Of the three brothers, HI, FI, and JI, who are all European 1500 m champions, HI played football from the age of 10 to 14 years. From the age of 13 to 17 years he also competed in cross-country skiing during the winter season and in distance running during the summer season, and at the age of 17, became Norwegian junior cross-country skiing champion. FI played football from the age of ten, competed in cross-country skiing and did some track and field training. From the age of 17, he focused more and more on distance running. The youngest of the brothers, JI, started to train for athletics at the age of 7 years. He competed in sprints, hurdles, and jumps. He also competed in cross-country skiing at regional level until the age of 12. From that age he focused entirely on distance running [20].

The female and male javelin throwers in Table 3 have four and five international titles, respectively. They both showed an outstanding talent for javelin throwing from an early age and are number one and four in the all-time rankings at age 15, and both number one at age 18. However, EKH also played handball at a regional level during most of her career and after she retired as a javelin thrower.

The 400 m hurdler, twice World Champion and once European Champion, also achieved outstanding results in different track and field events from an early age. In the age group 15 years, he is ranked as the second-best long jumper in Norway of all time, and at the age of 17 years he became U18 World Champion in combined events (eight events).

Why do the international champions listed in Table 3 to a greater extent show outstanding results in their youth compared to the EAC20ES in Table 2? It is a frequent topic of discussion whether genes [34] or environment play the most important role in talent development [35]. Three of the 12 champions are brothers, which underlines the importance of favorable genes. But, in addition to genetic predisposition, these brothers are characterized by an active childhood, a gradual progression in training volume, strong family support, and mental toughness [20]. This is in agreement with Simonton [36] who argued that talent arises from dynamic processes and is a complex system beyond the environment vs. gender debate. Simonton [36] explains the development of talent from a mathematical model. In the model, different factors are weighted by importance, and include genetic dispositions, environmental (e.g., social and family support) and development constraints (e.g., structure of training and competition program). Simonton's model is in accordance with Mallett and Harrahan [27] who found that elite track and field athletes have, (1) high motivation with achievement and personal goals, (2) high self-belief, and (3) athletics being a central part of their lives.

5. Conclusions

In Norway, a total of 202 track and field athletes achieved the European Athletics Championship 2020—Entry Standards (EAC20ES) in one or more events during all times. Of these, 14.4% are ranked among the all-time top 20 athletes in Norway in one or more events in the age group 15 years, and 42.1% in the age group 18 years. However, there is no available information regarding the amount of athletics training at ages 15 and 18 years, or to what extent the athletes at these ages also took part in other sports.

During the last four decades, 12 Norwegian athletes have won one or more international titles in track and field events or marathons. Of these champions, the number who were ranked among the top 20 in the age groups 15 and 18 years is much higher: 66.7% and 91.6%, respectively. This could indicate that those who go on to become international champions perform at a higher level in adolescence than other athletes who also reach senior international level. However, due to the low number of international champions, the date should be interpreted with caution.

Author Contributions: Conceptualization, L.I.T.; methodology, L.I.T. and O.T.; formal analysis, L.I.T and O.T., data curation O.T. and L.I.T.; writing—original draft preparation; L.I.T.; writing—review and editing, L.I.T. and O.T.; supervision, L.I.T.; project administration, L.I.T. All authors have read and agreed to the published version of the manuscript.

Funding: This research received no external funding.

Conflicts of Interest: The author declares no potential conflicts of interest with respect to the research, authorship, and/or publication of this article.

References

1. Foss, J.L.; Sinex, J.A.; Chapman, R.F. Career performance progressions of junior and senior elite track and field athletes. *J. Sci. Sport Exerc.* **2019**, *1*, 168–175. [CrossRef]
2. Costa, M.J.; Marinho, D.; Bragada, J.A.; Silva, A.J.; Barbosa, T.M. Stability of elite freestyle performance from childhood to adulthood. *J. Sports Sci.* **2011**, *29*, 1183–1189. [CrossRef]
3. Ericsson, K.A.P. Deliberate practice and acquisition of expert performance: A general overview. *Acad. Emerg. Med.* **2008**, *15*, 988–994. [CrossRef] [PubMed]
4. Côté, J.; Baker, J.; Abernethy, B. Practice and play in the development of sport expertise. *Handb. Sport Psychol.* **2007**, *3*, 184–202.
5. Abbott, A.; Button, C.; Pepping, G.-J.; Collins, D.J. Unnatural selection: Talent identification and development in sport. *Nonlinear Dyn. Psychol. Life Sci.* **2005**, *9*, 61–88.
6. Davison, R.R. Talent identification and coaching in the Journal of Sports Sciences. *J. Sports Sci.* **2006**, *24*, 805. [CrossRef]
7. Ericsson, K.A.; Krampe, R.T.; Tesch-Römer, C. The role of deliberate practice in the acquisition of expert performance. *Psychol. Rev.* **1993**, *100*, 363. [CrossRef]
8. Huxley, D.J.; O'Connor, D.; Larkin, P. The pathway to the top: Key factors and influences in the development of Australian Olympic and World Championship Track and Field athletes. *Int. J. Sports Sci. Coach.* **2017**, *12*, 264–275. [CrossRef]
9. Popkin, C.A.; Bayomy, A.F.; Ahmad, C.S. Early sport specialization. *J. Am. Acad. Orthop. Surg.* **2019**, *27*, e995–e1000. [CrossRef]
10. Laprade, R.F.; Agel, J.; Baker, J.; Brenner, J.S.; Cordasco, F.A.; Côté, J.; Engebretsen, L.; Feeley, B.T.; Gould, D.; Hainline, B.; et al. AOSSM early sport specialization consensus statement. *Orthop. J. Sports Med.* **2016**, *4*. [CrossRef]
11. Feeley, B.T.; Agel, J.; Laprade, R.F. When is it too early for single sport specialization? *Am. J. Sports Med.* **2016**, *44*, 234–241. [CrossRef] [PubMed]
12. Wiersma, L.D. Risks and benefits of youth sport specialization: Perspectives and recommendations. *Pediatric Exerc. Sci.* **2000**, *12*, 13–22. [CrossRef]
13. Côté, J.; Lidor, R.; Hackfort, D. ISSP position stand: To sample or to specialize? Seven postulates about youth sport activities that lead to continued participation and elite performance. *Int. J. Sport Exerc. Psychol.* **2009**, *7*, 7–17.
14. Güllich, A.; Emrich, E. Considering long-term sustainability in the development of world class success. *Eur. J. Sport Sci.* **2014**, *14* (Suppl. 1), S383–S397.

15. Hayman, R.J.; Borkoles, E.; Taylor, J.A.; Hemmings, B.; Polman, R. From pre-elite to elite: The pathway travelled by adolescent golfers. *Int. J. Sports Sci. Coach.* **2014**, *9*, 959–974. [CrossRef]
16. Coutinho, P.; Mesquita, I.; Fonseca, A.M.; de Martin-Silva, L. Patterns of sport participation in Portuguese volleyball players according to expertise level and gender. *Int. J. Sports Sci. Coach.* **2014**, *9*, 579–592. [CrossRef]
17. Baker, J.; Côté, J.; Deakin, J. Expertise in ultra-endurance triathletes early sport involvement, training structure, and the theory of deliberate practice. *J. Appl. Sport Psychol.* **2005**, *17*, 64–78. [CrossRef]
18. Memmert, D.; Baker, J.; Bertsch, C. Play and practice in the development of sport-specific creativity in team ball sports. *High Abil. Stud.* **2010**, *21*, 3–18. [CrossRef]
19. Svendsen, I.S.; Tønnesen, E.; Tjelta, L.I.; Ørn, S. Training, performance, and physiological predictors of a successful elite senior career in junior competitive road cyclists. *Int. J. Sports Physiol. Perform.* **2018**, *13*, 1287–1292. [CrossRef]
20. Tjelta, L.I. Three Norwegian brothers all European 1500 m champions: What is the secret? *Int. J. Sports Sci. Coach.* **2019**, *14*, 694–700. [CrossRef]
21. Barreiros, A.; Côté, J.; Fonseca, A.M. From early to adult sport success: Analysing athletes' progression in national squads. *Eur. J. Sport Sci.* **2014**, *14* (Suppl. 1), S178–S182. [CrossRef] [PubMed]
22. Durandt, J.; Parker, Z.; Masimla, H.; Lambert, M. Rugby-playing history at the national U13 level and subsequent participation at the national U16 and U18 rugby tournaments. *South Afr. J. Sports Med.* **2011**, *23*. [CrossRef]
23. Hollings, S.; Hume, P. Is success at the World Junior Athletics Championships a prerequisite for success at World Senior Championships or Olympic Games?—Prospective and retrospective analyses. *New Stud. Athl.* **2010**, *25*, 65–77.
24. Kearney, P.E.; Hayes, P. Excelling at youth level in competitive track and field athletics is not a prerequisite for later success. *J. Sports Sci.* **2018**, *36*, 2502–2509. [CrossRef] [PubMed]
25. Anderson, D.I.; Mayo, A.M. A skill acquisition perspective on early specialization in sport. *Kinesiol. Rev.* **2015**, *4*, 230–247. [CrossRef]
26. Coutinho, P.; Mesquita, I.; Fonseca, A.M. Talent development in sport: A critical review of pathways to expert performance. *Int. J. Sports Sci. Coach.* **2016**, *11*, 279–293. [CrossRef]
27. Mallett, C.J.; Hanrahan, S.J. Elite athletes: Why does the 'fire' burn so brightly? *Psychol. Sport Exerc.* **2004**, *5*, 183–200. [CrossRef]
28. European Athletics. European Athletics Championship 2020-Entry Standards and Conditions. 2019. Available online: https://www.european-athletics.org/mm/Document/EventsMeetings/General/01/28/98/79/ECH2020-EntryStandardsandConditions_English.pdf (accessed on 28 September 2020).
29. Cumming, S.P.; Standage, M.; Gillison, F.B.; Malina, R.M. Sex differences in exercise behavior during adolescence: Is biological maturation a confounding factor? *J. Adolesc. Health* **2008**, *42*, 480–485. [CrossRef]
30. Tønnessen, E.; Svendsen, I.S.; Olsen, I.C.; Guttormsen, A.; Haugen, T. Performance development in adolescent track and field athletes according to age, sex and sport discipline. *PLoS ONE* **2015**, *10*, e0129014.
31. Allen, S.; Hopkins, W.G. Age of peak competitive performance of elite athletes: A systematic review. *Sports Med.* **2015**, *45*, 1431–1441. [CrossRef]
32. Tjelta, L.I.; Enoksen, E. Training volume and intensity. In *Running & Science—An Interdisiciplinary Perspective*; Bangsbo, J., Larsen, H.B., Eds.; Institute of Exercise and Sport Sciences, University of Copenhagen: Copenhagen, Denmark, 2001; pp. 149–177.
33. Leknes, T. The training prosess in 800 m from adolescent to intenational level. (in Norwegian: Treningsprosessen på 800 m fra ungdomsår til internasjonalt nivå). In *Endurance Training. Research and Best Practice (in Norwegian: Utholdenhetstrening. Forskning og beste praksis)*; Tjelta, L.I., Enoksen, E., Tønnesen, E., Eds.; Cappelen Damm Akademisk: Oslo, Norway, 2013; pp. 210–234.
34. Buxens, A.; Ruiz, J.R.; Arteta, D.; Artieda, M.; Santiago, C.; González-Freire, M.; Martínez, A.; Tejedor, D.; Lao, J.I.; Gómez-Gallego, F.; et al. Can we predict top-level sports performance in power vs endurance events? A genetic approach. *Scand. J. Med. Sci. Sports* **2011**, *21*, 570–579. [CrossRef] [PubMed]

35. Phillips, E.J.; Davids, K.; Renshaw, I.; Portus, M. Expert performance in sport and the dynamics of talent development. *Sports Med.* **2010**, *40*, 271–283. [CrossRef] [PubMed]
36. Simonton, D.K. Talent and its development: An emergenic and epigenetic model. *Psychol. Rev.* **1999**, *106*, 435–457. [CrossRef]

International Journal of *Environmental Research and Public Health*

MDPI

Article

The Acute Effect of Foam Rolling on Eccentrically-Induced Muscle Damage

Masatoshi Nakamura [1,2,*], Koki Yasaka [1], Ryosuke Kiyono [2], Remi Onuma [1], Kaoru Yahata [2], Shigeru Sato [2] and Andreas Konrad [3]

1 Department of Physical Therapy, Faculty of Rehabilitation, Niigata University of Health and Welfare, 1398 Shimami-cho, Kita-ku, Niigata City, Niigata 950-3198, Japan; hpa17114@nuhw.ac.jp (K.Y.); hpa17024@nuhw.ac.jp (R.O.)

2 Institute for Human Movement and Medical Sciences, Niigata University of Health and Welfare, 1398 Shimami-cho, Kita-ku, Niigata City, Niigata 950-3198, Japan; hpm19005@nuhw.ac.jp (R.K.); hpm20011@nuhw.ac.jp (K.Y.); hpm19006@nuhw.ac.jp (S.S.)

3 Institute of Sport Science, University of Graz, Mozartgasse 14, 8010 Graz, Austria; andreas.konrad@uni-graz.at

* Correspondence: masatoshi-nakamura@nuhw.ac.jp; Tel.: +81-25-257-4451

Abstract: Previous studies have shown significant improvement in muscle soreness and muscle function loss after 300-s foam rolling intervention two days after intense exercise. However, this duration is assumed to be too long, so investigating the effect of short-term duration foam rolling intervention on an eccentrically-damaged muscle is needed. This study aimed to eccentrically induce muscle damage in the leg extensors, and to detect the acute effect of 90-s foam rolling on muscle soreness and muscle function of the quadriceps muscle. We enrolled 17 healthy and nonathlete male volunteers. They performed a bout of eccentric exercise of the knee extensors with the dominant leg and received 90-s foam rolling intervention of the quadriceps two days after the eccentric exercise. The dependent variables were measured before the eccentric exercise (baseline), and before (preintervention) and after foam rolling intervention (postintervention), two days after the eccentric exercise. The results show that the preintervention muscle soreness and muscle strength values were significantly increased, compared with the baseline values, whereas the postintervention values were significantly decreased, compared with the preintervention values. Furthermore, 90-s of foam rolling intervention could improve muscle soreness and muscle function loss.

Keywords: muscle soreness; muscle strength; range of motion; knee extensor

Citation: Nakamura, M.; Yasaka, K.; Kiyono, R.; Onuma, R.; Yahata, K.; Sato, S.; Konrad, A. The Acute Effect of Foam Rolling on Eccentrically-Induced Muscle Damage. *Int. J. Environ. Res. Public Health* **2021**, *18*, 75. https://dx.doi.org/10.3390/ijerph18010075

Received: 22 November 2020
Accepted: 22 December 2020
Published: 24 December 2020

1. Introduction

Compared with resistance training emphasizing concentric contraction, it is well known that resistance training emphasizing eccentric contraction (ECC) allows for greater increases in muscle strength and muscle volume [1,2]. However, previous studies have shown the negative aspects, including delayed-onset muscle soreness (DOMS), muscle function loss (muscle strength or athletic performance), decrease in range of motion (ROM), and increase in muscle-tendon stiffness after performing ECC [3–7]. These muscle damage symptoms peaked in two days and remained for about one week [4,5]. Since DOMS and muscle function loss impair the individual's willingness to exercise, and inhibit the continuation of exercise for a certain period, it is necessary to establish effective intervention modalities to prevent or treat DOMS and muscle function loss after ECC [8].

In previous studies, the effective intervention modalities to prevent DOMS and muscle function loss were investigated, and a systematic review concluded that active recovery, massage, compression garments, immersion, contrast water therapy, and cryotherapy induced a small-to-large decrease in the magnitude of DOMS and muscle damage. However, there was no significant decrease in the effect of stretching on DOMS [8]. Furthermore, it is well known that a bout of ECC exercise confers protection against DOMS and muscle damage by ECC exercise following a subsequent bout of ECC exercise via the repeated-bout effect [9,10]. Conversely, to the best of our knowledge, the acute effect of some interventions on damaged muscle caused by ECC exercise has been investigated in a few studies. One study investigated the effect of static stretching on eccentrically-damaged muscle two days after ECC exercise and showed that there was an improvement in muscle soreness, ROM, and muscle-tendon stiffness after a static stretching intervention [7]. Additionally, the other studies showed that there was an improvement in muscle soreness and ROM after static stretching and hold–relax stretching interventions [11,12]. These results revealed that stretching intervention might not be effective in preventing DOMS, whereas a stretching intervention could be effective in improving muscle soreness and muscle function in eccentrically-damaged muscle.

Furthermore, many researchers have focused on the foam rolling effect using a foam roller, roller massage bars/sticks, or a ball. The foam rolling effects on muscle strength and athletic performance have not reached consensus [13–18]; however, previous studies have shown that a foam rolling intervention increased ROM and pain threshold [16,18,19]. Although Behm and Wilke pointed out that the evidence supporting the fact that the primary mechanisms underlying foam rolling are the release of myofascial restrictions is insufficient [20], foam rolling intervention could be useful in sports and rehabilitation settings, because of its increment effect on ROM and pain threshold. Regarding the recovery effects after foam rolling, previous studies have shown that foam rolling intervention aids in the recovery from muscle damage immediately after 24, 48, and 72 h after ECC exercise [21,22]. Moreover, Romero-Moraleda and colleagues investigated the effect of 300-s foam rolling on the damaged muscle two days after exercise, in which the symptoms of DOMS and muscle function loss peaked, and showed significant improvement in DOMS and function loss [23,24]. However, after specific ECC exercise studies, it was shown that the acute effect of foam rolling on DOMS is limited. Furthermore, Romero-Moraleda and colleagues used the 300-s foam rolling intervention duration, and showed that it is too long for clinical application in sports and rehabilitation settings. Hence, investigating the effect of a short-term duration of foam rolling intervention in the clinical settings is needed. One previous systematic review concluded that a reduction in pain/soreness could be achieved by >90-s foam rolling [25], and we believed that to change the DOMS and muscle function loss, >90-s foam rolling duration is required. This study aimed to eccentrically induce muscle damage of the leg extensors and to investigate the acute effect of 90-s foam rolling intervention on muscle soreness and loss of muscle function of the quadriceps muscle.

2. Materials and Methods

2.1. Participants

A total of 17 healthy and sedentary male volunteers (mean $\pm$ standard deviation (SD): age 21.1 $\pm$ 0.5 years; height, 170.9 $\pm$ 5.9 cm; weight, 61.1 $\pm$ 6.2 kg), who had not performed habitual exercise activities at least for the past six months before the measurements, were enrolled in this study. We excluded participants who had a history of neuromuscular disease or musculoskeletal injury on the lower extremity. All participants had not been involved in any regular resistance training or flexibility training. Previous studies have revealed that the repeated muscle contractions—especially ECC—could attenuate the muscle soreness and muscle function loss: the so-called "repeated-bout effect" [9,10]. Therefore, we included nontrained male participants in this study. All participants provided written informed consent. The study was approved by the Ethics Committee (#18220) and complies with the requirements of the Declaration of Helsinki.

2.2. Experimental Protocol

The participants performed a bout of eccentric exercise of the knee extensors with the dominant leg (preferred leg for kicking a ball), as described in the following (Figure 1), and received 90-s foam rolling intervention (30 s $\times$ three sets) of the quadriceps two days after the eccentric exercise [9–11]. The dependent variables included muscle soreness at contraction, palpation, and stretching, maximum voluntary isometric contraction (MVC-ISO) torque and maximum voluntary concentric contraction (MVC-CON) torque of knee extensors, and range of motion (ROM) of passive knee flexion. These variables were measured before the eccentric exercise (baseline), and before (preintervention) and after (postintervention) foam rolling intervention two days after the eccentric exercise. Immediately after the foam rolling intervention, we performed the postintervention measurements. All measurements were taken at the same time of the day for each participant between days. Furthermore, the participants practiced the foam rolling intervention on the opposite side (nondominant leg) before baseline and preintervention measurements. Additionally, the participants became familiarized with all measurements and ECC exercises before baseline measurement in the measurement leg (dominant leg).

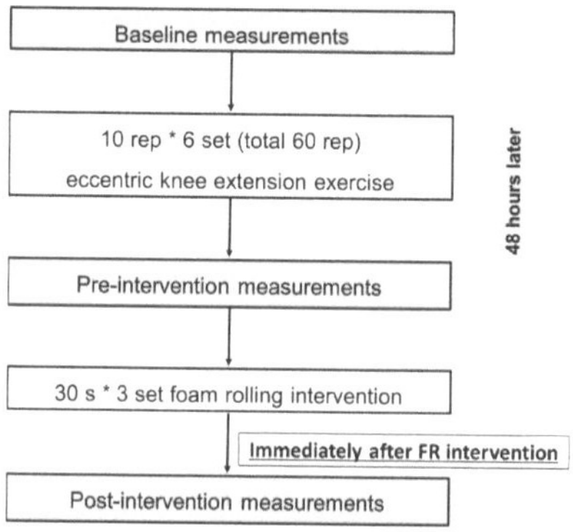

Figure 1. Experimental flowchart.

2.3. Eccentric Exercise

On an isokinetic dynamometer (Biodex System 3.0, Biodex Medical Systems Inc., Shirley, NY, USA), all participants performed six sets out of 10 maximal ECC of the unilateral knee extensors (dominant leg) [11,12]. Participants were seated in the dynamometer chair at an 80° hip flexion angle, with adjusted Velcro straps fixed over the trunk, pelvis, and thigh of the exercised limb. The exercised limb knee joint was aligned with the axis of rotation of the dynamometer. According to the previous studies [11,12], the participants were instructed to perform the maximal ECC from a slightly flexed position (20°) to a flexed position (110°) at an angular velocity of 60°/s. After each ECC, the lever arm passively returned the knee joint to the starting position at 10°/s, which gave a 9-s rest between contractions. Each set was repeated 10 times, and a 100-s rest was given between sets to complete the six sets. To generate maximum force, the participants received strong verbal encouragement during each ECC.

2.4. Foam Rolling Intervention

A foam roller (Gold's Gym 18 Foam Roller, Logan, UT, USA), with a total diameter of 12.7 cm consisting of a 5-mm thick hollow plastic core covered with a 12-mm layer of dense foam, was used to perform the foam rolling [26]. The subjects were instructed to perform three sets of 30-s foam rolling intervention with 30-s rest between each set. The participants were instructed to be in the plank position with the foam roller at the most proximal portion of the quadriceps of the dominant leg only (Figure 2). This study defined one cycle of foam rolling intervention as one distal rolling plus one subsequent proximal rolling movement, whereas the frequency was defined as 30 cycles per 1 min using a metronome (Smart Metronome; Tomohiro Ihara, Japan). In detail, 15 cycles for each set were completed. The foam rolling intervention was performed between the top of the patella and the anterior superior iliac spine under the direct supervision of investigators. Based on a previous study [27], the pressure was subjectively controlled with a target numerical rating scale rating of 7/10 (0 represents no discomfort and 10 represents maximal discomfort) during the intervention. Additionally, the participants were instructed to control the pressure with a target numerical rating scale rating of 7/10 before each set.

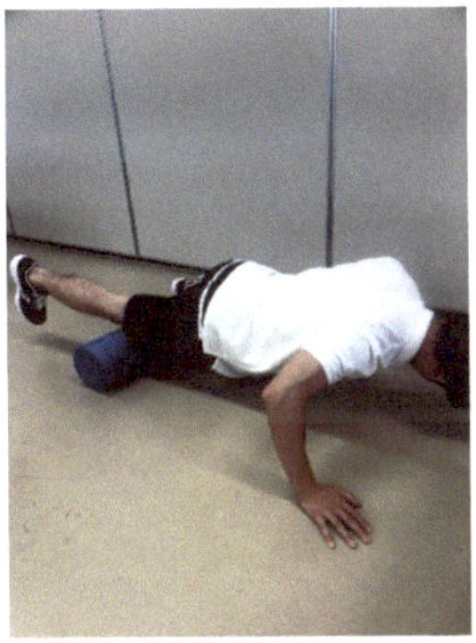

Figure 2. Foam rolling technique.

2.5. MVC-ISO and MVC-CON

MVC-ISO was measured at two different angles, such as 20° and 70° knee angles, with the same setup as the eccentric exercise using the dynamometer after gravity correction [28]. The participants were instructed to perform maximal contraction for 5 s at each angle two times with 60-s rest between trials, and the average value was adopted for further analysis.

MVC-CON was measured at the angular velocity of 60°/s for the ROM of 70° (20–90° knee angles) for five continuous maximal voluntary concentric contractions, for both directions [11,12]. The highest value among the five trials was adopted for further analysis. During all tests, verbal encouragement was provided consistently.

2.6. Knee Flexion ROM

Each participant was placed in a side-lying position on a massage bed, and the hip and knee of the nondominant leg were flexed at 90° to prevent the movement of the pelvis during ROM measurements. The investigator brought the dominant leg to full knee flexion with the hip joint in a neutral position. A goniometer was used to measure the knee flexion ROM twice, and the average value was used for further analysis [11,12].

2.7. Muscle Soreness

Using a visual analog scale that had a 100-mm continuous line with "not sore at all" on one side (0 mm) and "very, very sore" on the other side (100 mm), the magnitude of knee extensor muscle soreness was assessed by muscle contraction, stretching, and palpation [9,29]. Muscle soreness at contraction was assessed at both MVC-ISO and MVC-CON, and the average value was adopted for further analysis. For muscle soreness during palpation, participants laid supine on a massage bed, and the investigator palpated the proximal, middle, and distal points of the vastus medialis, vastus lateralis, and rectus femoris [28]. The average value of the knee extensor palpation points was used for further analysis. As for muscle soreness during stretching, muscle soreness during ROM measurement was measured twice, and the average value was used for further analysis.

2.8. Test–Retest Reliability of the Measurements

Using seven different healthy males other than those in this study (age, 21.3 ± 0.7 years; height, 173.2 ± 5.9 cm; weight, 62.8 ± 7.3 kg), the test–retest reliability of the measurement for MVIC-ISO, MVIC-CON, ROM, and muscle soreness at contraction, stretching, and palpation was determined by coefficient variation (CV) and intraclass correlation coefficient

(ICC), with 5-min rest interval between the two measures in damaged muscle after the same ECC exercise protocol. The CV of the measurements for MVIC-ISO, MVIC-CON, ROM, and muscle soreness at contraction, stretching, and palpation were 4.1% ± 4.1%, 9.2% ± 4.8%, 1.2% ± 0.8%, 10.1% ± 4.5%, 9.9% ± 4.5%, and 8.5% ± 4.2%, respectively, and the ICC for the measurements were 0.98, 0.80, 0.91, 0.96, 0.97, and 0.88, respectively.

2.9. Statistical Analysis

SPSS (version 24.0; SPSS Japan Inc., Tokyo, Japan) was used for statistical analysis. By analyzing the standardized residuals using a Shapiro–Wilk test, data were assessed for assumptions of normality. One-way repeated analysis of variance was used to assess significant differences in all variables. When a significant effect was found, the Bonferroni post hoc test was used to determine the differences between measurements taken at baseline, preintervention, and postintervention. Additionally, the effect size (d) was calculated as differences in the mean value divided by the pooled SD [30].

The relationship between changes from baseline to preintervention and from pre- to postintervention in muscle soreness during muscle contraction, stretching, and palpation was quantified using Pearson's product-moment correlation coefficient. Moreover, it was also used to quantify the relationship between relative changes (%) from baseline to preintervention and from pre- to postintervention in MVC-ISO, MVC-CON, and ROM. Data are presented as mean ± SD.

3. Results

Table 1 presents all variables in all groups. The one-way analysis of variance indicated the main effects for all variables. As a result of the post hoc test, muscle soreness at contraction, stretching, and palpation values was significantly increased at preintervention, compared with the baseline values ($p < 0.01$ and d = 1.19; $p = 0.012$ and d = 0.69, $p < 0.01$ and d = 1.57, respectively), whereas postintervention values were significantly decreased, compared with the preintervention values ($p < 0.01$ and d = 0.63; $p < 0.01$ and d = 1.02; $p < 0.01$ and d = 1.27, respectively).

Table 1. The changes in maximum voluntary isometric contraction (MVC-ISO) torque, maximum voluntary concentric contraction (MVC-CON) torque of knee extensors, and maximal voluntary range of motion (ROM) of passive knee flexion and muscle soreness at contraction, palpation, and stretching at baseline, before foam rolling intervention, and after foam rolling intervention.

	Baseline	Preintervention	Postintervention	F Value
MVC-ISO (Nm)	151.4 ± 22.8	96.8 ± 39.5 *	112.4 ± 30.0 *,†	22.6
MVC-CON (Nm)	147.1 ± 23.9	82.3 ± 30.7 *	100.3 ± 31.4 *,†	44.9
ROM (°)	145.6 ± 7.3	140.5 ± 6.3 *	149.2 ± 6.1 *,†	24.2
Muscle soreness				
At contraction (mm)	10.1 ± 8.6	25.3 ± 17.0 *	15.9 ± 12.9 †	10.2
At stretching (mm)	31.8 ± 23.1	47.6 ± 22.6 *	25.1 ± 21.5 †	13.5
At palpation (mm)	19.9 ± 14.4	44.1 ± 16.5 *	25.0 ± 13.6 †	26.5

* A significantly ($p < 0.05$) different from the baseline value; † A significantly ($p < 0.05$) different from the preintervention value.

Furthermore, the preintervention MVC-ISO and MVC-CON values were significantly decreased, compared with the baseline values ($p < 0.01$ and d = 1.75; $p < 0.01$ and d = 2.38, respectively), whereas the postintervention values were significantly increased, compared with the preintervention values ($p < 0.01$ and d = 0.45; $p < 0.01$ and d = 0.58, respectively). In addition, the postintervention MVC-ISO and MVC-CON values were significantly lower than the baseline values ($p < 0.01$ and d = 0.74; $p < 0.01$ and d = 0.85, respectively). Similarly, the preintervention ROM values were significantly decreased, compared with the baseline value ($p < 0.01$ and d = 0.75), whereas the postintervention ROM value was significantly increased, compared with the baseline and preintervention values ($p < 0.01$ and d = 0.27; $p < 0.05$ and d = 1.41, respectively).

Figures 3 and 4 show the associations between changes from baseline to preintervention and from pre- to postintervention. The results show that there were significant negative associations between changes (mm) in muscle soreness at muscle contraction, stretching, and palpation ($r = -0.722$ and $p < 0.01$; $r = -0.689$ and $p < 0.01$; $r = -0.647$ and $p < 0.01$, respectively) and relative changes (%) in MVC-ISO and ROM ($r = -0.641$ and $p < 0.01$; $r = -0.467$ and $p = 0.059$; $r = -0.488$ and $p = 0.047$, respectively).

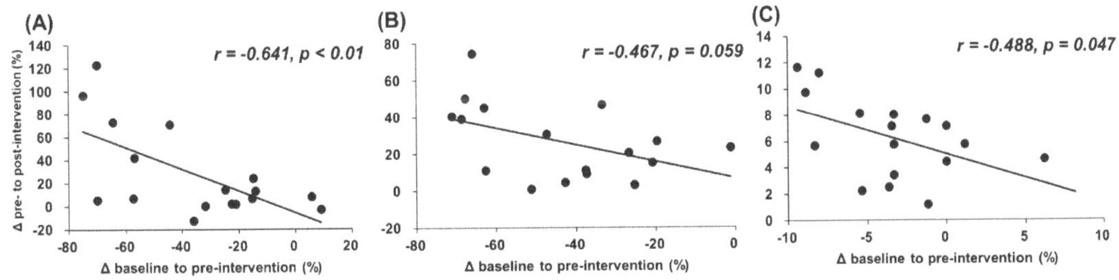

Figure 3. Relationships (Pearson r and p values) between changes from baseline to preintervention and from pre- to postintervention in muscle soreness at muscle contraction (**A**), stretching (**B**), and palpation (**C**).

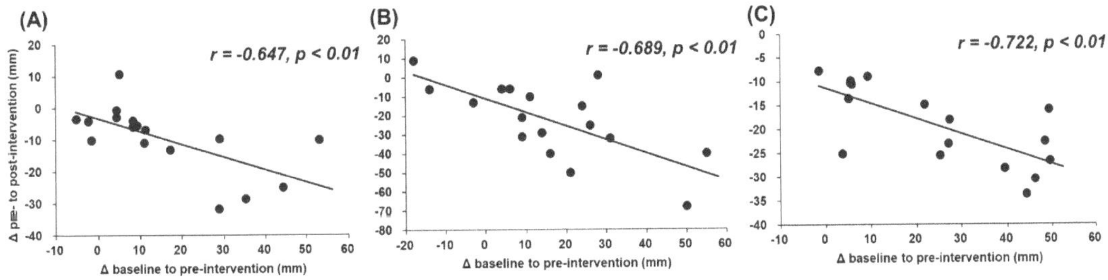

Figure 4. Relationships (Pearson r and p values) between relative changes (%) from baseline to preintervention and from pre- to postintervention in maximal voluntary isometric contraction (MVC-ISO) torque (**A**), maximum voluntary concentric contraction (MVC-CON) torque (**B**) of knee extensors, and range of motion (ROM) of passive knee flexion (**C**).

4. Discussion

This study investigated 90-s (30 s × three sets) foam rolling intervention on DOMS and muscle function loss 48 h after ECC exercise. The results revealed the following points: (1) The muscle strength loss was recovered after foam rolling intervention, whereas the postintervention values were still lower than the baseline values (MVC-ISO: −25.7%, MVC-CON: −31.9%). (2) After foam rolling intervention, DOMS was recovered, which was similar to the baseline value. (3) After foam rolling, the loss of flexibility was recovered, which was higher than the baseline value. (4) Lastly, the abovementioned foam rolling effect was significantly greater in the participants with higher DOMS and function loss. Romero-Moraleda and colleagues showed that 300-s foam rolling intervention improved DOMS and muscle function loss after intense exercises [23,24]. To the best of our knowledge, this is the first study to investigate the effect of 90-s foam rolling intervention on the damaged muscle that could be applied in the sports and rehabilitation settings.

Our results support and expand the previous works investigating the effect of 300-s foam rolling [23,24]. Interestingly, there is a dose–response relationship between foam rolling duration and foam rolling intervention effect. Moreover, Hughes and Ramer, in their systematic review (2019), showed that >90-s foam rolling intervention could relieve pain/soreness [25]. In this study, DOMS was similarly improved in muscles with eccentrically-induced muscle damage after 90-s foam rolling intervention. The proposed global pain modulatory by foam rolling intervention might be involved with the gate control theory of pain, diffuse noxious inhibitory control, or parasympathetic nervous system alteration [20]. Although the mechanism underlying pain modulatory by foam rolling intervention has been unclear, in this study, 90-s foam rolling intervention could cause pain modulatory and reduce the muscle soreness in eccentrically-damaged muscle.

The findings showed that both MVC-ISO and MVC-CON were improved by foam rolling intervention, which was consistent with the previous studies [23,24]. However, although no significant difference in muscle soreness was observed between baseline and postintervention, there were still significant decrements in MVC-ISO and MVC-CON at postintervention, rather than at baseline, which showed that there could not be a full recovery at baseline. The discrepancy between changes in muscle soreness and function loss after foam rolling intervention has been unclear. Previous studies have shown that >90-s foam rolling could achieve a short-term reduction in pain/soreness [25], but the effects of foam rolling intervention on muscle strength and athletic performance have been debated [13–18]. Therefore, although muscle soreness improvement during muscle contraction by the foam rolling intervention improved both MVC-ISO and MVC-CON, the improvement effects on both MVC-ISO and MVC-CON might not be lower than that in muscle soreness.

Interestingly, Matsuo and colleagues (2015) investigated the effect of 300-s static stretching on eccentrically-damaged muscle and revealed that static stretching intervention improved DOMS, whereas there were no significant changes in muscle strength [7]. Generally, muscle strength and athletic performance decrease immediately after static stretching. Therefore, the previous study stated that the possibility of decreased pain sensation counteracted the force loss of eccentrically-damaged muscle after a static stretching intervention [7]. Conversely, although the effects of foam rolling intervention on muscle strength and athletic performance have been debated [13–18], to the best of our knowledge, a study showing the decrement effect after foam rolling intervention has not been conducted yet. Therefore, foam rolling intervention for eccentrically-damaged muscle could improve muscle strength loss by improving DOMS. Altogether, the foam rolling intervention could be an effective recovery tool superior to static stretching as an intervention modality for eccentrically-damaged muscle in the sports and rehabilitation settings. In future studies, a comparison of the effects of foam rolling and static stretching on the eccentrically-damaged muscles is needed.

This study revealed that there was a significant negative correlation between the deterioration of DOMS and muscle function loss by ECC exercise and the improvement effect of foam rolling intervention (Figures 3 and 4). These results showed that the subjects with greater muscle soreness or decreased muscle function loss after the ECC exercise were shown to improve greatly after foam rolling intervention. As mentioned above, ECC exercise can be expected to have a great muscle strengthening/muscular hypertrophy effect; however, it has the problem of causing muscle soreness and prolonged muscle function loss. From these study results, since foam rolling intervention on eccentrically-damaged muscle could improve and attenuate the DOMS and muscle function loss, the foam roller can be used as a recovery tool for eccentrically-damaged muscle, controlling the muscle soreness and muscle function loss in sport and rehabilitation settings, especially for the subjects with greater muscle soreness or decreased muscle function loss after the ECC exercise.

There are some limitations to the present study. First, there was no control group (no foam rolling intervention group) in this study. However, the high reliabilities for all measurements were confirmed in the eccentrically-induced damaged muscles. Therefore, there was a possibility that the changes in muscle soreness and muscle function loss could be involved by 90-s foam rolling intervention. Second, since only the acute effect of 90-s foam rolling intervention was investigated in this study, the sustained effect and/or dose–response relationship for foam rolling intervention still is unclear. To clarify the sustained effect or dose–response relationship of foam rolling on eccentrically-damaged muscle, future studies are needed. Moreover, to investigate the effect of foam rolling on eccentrically-damaged muscle in the athletic population, further studies are needed, since the participants of this study were sedentary and nonathletes.

5. Conclusions

In conclusion, we investigated the effect of 90-s foam rolling intervention on eccentrically-damaged muscle. The study results indicate that muscle soreness and muscle function loss were improved, and the effect was greater in the subjects with greater muscle soreness and decreased muscle function by the ECC exercise. Therefore, foam rolling is an effective recovery tool for eccentrically-damaged muscles in sports and rehabilitation settings.

Author Contributions: Conceptualization: M.N., K.Y. (Koki Yasaka), R.K., and A.K.; formal analysis: M.N. and K.Y. (Koki Yasaka); investigation: M.N., K.Y. (Koki Yasaka), R.K., R.O., K.Y. (Kaoru Yahata), and S.S.; methodology: M.N., K.Y. (Koki Yasaka), R.K., R.O., K.Y. (Kaoru Yahata), and S.S.; supervision: M.N. and A.K.; writing—original draft: M.N., K.Y. (Koki Yasaka), R.K., and K.Y. (Koki Yasaka), writing—review and editing: M.N., K.Y. (Koki Yasaka), R.K., R.O., K.Y. (Kaoru Yahata), S.S., and A.K. All authors have read and agreed to the published version of the manuscript.

Funding: This study was supported by a grant (Project P 32078-B) from the Austrian Science Fund FWF.

Institutional Review Board Statement: The study was approved by the Ethics Committee (#18220) and complies with the requirements of the Declaration of Helsinki.

Informed Consent Statement: Informed consent was obtained from all participants involved in the study.

Data Availability Statement: All data generated or analyzed during this study are included in this published article.

Acknowledgments: The authors gratefully acknowledge all participants involved in this study.

Conflicts of Interest: The authors declare no conflict of interest.

References

1. Tseng, W.-C.; Nosaka, K.; Tseng, K.-W.; Chou, T.-Y.; Chen, T.C. Contralateral Effects by Unilateral Eccentric versus Concentric Resistance Training. *Med. Sci. Sports Exerc.* **2020**, *52*, 474–483. [CrossRef] [PubMed]
2. Katsura, Y.; Takeda, N.; Hara, T.; Takahashi, S.; Nosaka, K. Comparison between eccentric and concentric resistance exercise training without equipment for changes in muscle strength and functional fitness of older adults. *Graefe's Arch. Clin. Exp. Ophthalmol.* **2019**, *119*, 1581–1590. [CrossRef] [PubMed]
3. Clarkson, P.M.; Nosaka, K.; Braun, B. Muscle function after exercise-induced muscle damage and rapid adaptation. *Med. Sci. Sports Exerc.* **1992**, *24*, 512–520. [CrossRef] [PubMed]
4. Cleak, M.; Eston, R. Delayed onset muscle soreness: Mechanisms and management. *J. Sports Sci.* **1992**, *10*, 325–341. [CrossRef] [PubMed]
5. Armstrong, R.B. Mechanisms of exercise-induced delayed onset muscular soreness: A brief review. *Med. Sci. Sports Exerc.* **1984**, *16*, 529–538. [CrossRef] [PubMed]
6. Nosaka, K.; Clarkson, P.M.; McGuiggin, M.E.; Byrne, J.M. Time course of muscle adaptation after high force eccentric exercise. *Graefe's Arch. Clin. Exp. Ophthalmol.* **1991**, *63*, 70–76. [CrossRef]
7. Matsuo, S.; Suzuki, S.; Iwata, M.; Hatano, G.; Nosaka, K. Changes in force and stiffness after static stretching of eccentrically-damaged hamstrings. *Graefe's Arch. Clin. Exp. Ophthalmol.* **2015**, *115*, 981–991. [CrossRef]
8. Dupuy, O.; Douzi, W.; Theurot, D.; Bosquet, L.; Dugué, B. An Evidence-Based Approach for Choosing Post-exercise Recovery Techniques to Reduce Markers of Muscle Damage, Soreness, Fatigue, and Inflammation: A Systematic Review with Meta-Analysis. *Front. Physiol.* **2018**, *9*, 403. [CrossRef]
9. Chen, T.C.; Nosaka, K.; Sacco, P. Intensity of eccentric exercise, shift of optimum angle, and the magnitude of repeated-bout effect. *J. Appl. Physiol.* **2007**, *102*, 992–999. [CrossRef]
10. Chen, T.C.; Chen, H.-L.; Lin, M.-J.; Wu, C.-J.; Nosaka, K. Potent Protective Effect Conferred by Four Bouts of Low-Intensity Eccentric Exercise. *Med. Sci. Sports Exerc.* **2010**, *42*, 1004–1012. [CrossRef]

11. Yahata, K.; Sato, S.; Kiyono, R.; Inaba, K.; Sutoh, S.; Hiraizumi, K.; Nakamura, M. The acute effect of stretching on eccentrically-damaged muscle: Analysis of differences between Hold relax stretching and modified PNF stretching. *Jpn. J. Phys. Fit. Sports Med.* **2020**, *69*, 157–164. [CrossRef]
12. Suzuki, D.; Nakamura, M.; Ohya, S.; Aoki, T.; Edama, M. The acute effect of stretching on eccentrically-damaged muscle: Analysis of differences between hold-relax and static stretching. *Jpn. J. Phys. Fit. Sports Med.* **2019**, *68*, 117–123. [CrossRef]
13. Halperin, I.; Aboodarda, S.J.; Button, D.C.; Andersen, L.L.; Behm, D.G. Roller massager improves range of motion of plantar flexor muscles without subsequent decreases in force parameters. *Int. J. Sports Phys. Ther.* **2014**, *9*, 92–102. [PubMed]
14. Peacock, C.A.; Krein, D.D.; Silver, T.A.; Sanders, G.J.; Von Carlowitz, K.-P.A. An Acute Bout of Self-Myofascial Release in the Form of Foam Rolling Improves Performance Testing. *Int. J. Exerc. Sci.* **2014**, *7*, 202–211. [PubMed]
15. Macdonald, G.Z.; Penney, M.D.; Mullaley, M.E.; Cuconato, A.L.; Drake, C.D.; Behm, D.G.; Button, D.C. An Acute Bout of Self-Myofascial Release Increases Range of Motion Without a Subsequent Decrease in Muscle Activation or Force. *J. Strength Cond. Res.* **2013**, *27*, 812–821. [CrossRef]
16. Sullivan, K.M.; Silvey, D.B.; Button, D.C.; Behm, D.G. Roller-massager application to the hamstrings increases sit-and-reach range of motion within five to ten seconds without performance impairments. *Int. J. Sports Phys. Ther.* **2013**, *8*, 228–236.
17. Behara, B.; Jacobson, B.H. Acute Effects of Deep Tissue Foam Rolling and Dynamic Stretching on Muscular Strength, Power, and Flexibility in Division I Linemen. *J. Strength Cond. Res.* **2017**, *31*, 888–892. [CrossRef]
18. Wiewelhove, T.; Döweling, A.; Schneider, C.; Hottenrott, L.; Meyer, T.; Kellmann, M.; Pfeiffer, M.; Ferrauti, A. A Meta-Analysis of the Effects of Foam Rolling on Performance and Recovery. *Front. Physiol.* **2019**, *10*, 376. [CrossRef]
19. Phillips, J.; Diggin, D.; King, D.L.; Sforzo, G.A. Effect of Varying Self-myofascial Release Duration on Subsequent Athletic Performance. *J. Strength Cond. Res.* **2018**. [CrossRef]
20. Behm, D.G.; Wilke, J. Do Self-Myofascial Release Devices Release Myofascia? Rolling Mechanisms: A Narrative Review. *Sports Med.* **2019**, *49*, 1173–1181. [CrossRef]
21. Drinkwater, E.J.; Latella, C.; Wilsmore, C.; Bird, S.P.; Skein, M. Foam Rolling as a Recovery Tool Following Eccentric Exercise: Potential Mechanisms Underpinning Changes in Jump Performance. *Front. Physiol.* **2019**, *10*, 768. [CrossRef] [PubMed]
22. Naderi, A.; Rezvani, M.H.; Degens, H. Foam Rolling and Muscle and Joint Proprioception After Exercise-Induced Muscle Damage. *J. Athl. Train.* **2020**, *55*, 58–64. [CrossRef] [PubMed]
23. Romero-Moraleda, B.; González-García, J.; Cuéllar-Rayo, Á.; Balsalobre-Fernández, C.; Muñoz-García, D.; Morencos, E. Effects of Vibration and Non-Vibration Foam Rolling on Recovery after Exercise with Induced Muscle Damage. *J. Sports Sci. Med.* **2019**, *18*, 172–180. [PubMed]
24. Romero-Moraleda, B.; La Touche, R.; Lara, S.L.; Ferrer-Peña, R.; Paredes, V.; Peinado, A.B.; Muñoz-García, D. Neurodynamic mobilization and foam rolling improved delayed-onset muscle soreness in a healthy adult population: A randomized controlled clinical trial. *PeerJ* **2017**, *5*, 3908. [CrossRef] [PubMed]
25. Hughes, G.A.; Ramer, L.M. Duration of myofascial rolling for optimal recovery, range of motion, and performance: A systematic review of the literature. *Int. J. Sports Phys. Ther.* **2019**, *14*, 845–859. [CrossRef]
26. Richman, E.D.; Tyo, B.M.; Nicks, C.R. Combined Effects of Self-Myofascial Release and Dynamic Stretching on Range of Motion, Jump, Sprint, and Agility Performance. *J. Strength Cond. Res.* **2019**, *33*, 1795–1803. [CrossRef]
27. Krause, F.; Wilke, J.; Niederer, D.; Vogt, L.; Banzer, W. Acute effects of foam rolling on passive stiffness, stretch sensation and fascial sliding: A randomized controlled trial. *Hum. Mov. Sci.* **2019**, *67*, 102514. [CrossRef]
28. Mavropalias, G.; Koeda, T.; Barley, O.R.; Poon, W.C.K.; Fisher, A.J.; Blazevich, A.J.; Nosaka, K. Comparison between high- and low-intensity eccentric cycling of equal mechanical work for muscle damage and the repeated bout effect. *Graefe's Arch. Clin. Exp. Ophthalmol.* **2020**, *120*, 1015–1025. [CrossRef]
29. Chen, T.C.; Lin, K.-Y.; Chen, H.-L.; Lin, M.-J.; Nosaka, K. Comparison in eccentric exercise-induced muscle damage among four limb muscles. *Graefe's Arch. Clin. Exp. Ophthalmol.* **2010**, *111*, 211–223. [CrossRef]
30. Cohen, J. (Ed.) *Statistical Power Analysis for the Behavioral Sciences*, 2nd ed.; Routledge: Hillsdale, MI, USA, 1988.

International Journal of
Environmental Research and Public Health

MDPI

Article

A Novel mHealth Monitoring System during Cycling in Elite Athletes

Alexandros Iliadis [1], Milena Tomovic [1], Dimitrios Dervas [1], Markella Psymarnou [2], Kosmas Christoulas [3], Evangelia Joseph Kouidi [1] and Asterios Pantazis Deligiannis [1,*]

1 Sports Medicine Laboratory, Department of Physical Education and Sports Science, Aristotle University of Thessaloniki, 57001 Thessaloniki, Greece; alexcyclist@hotmail.com (A.I.); milenatomovic83@gmail.com (M.T.); dimdervas@gmail.com (D.D.); kouidi@phed.auth.gr (E.J.K.)
2 Vidavo S.A., Balkan Center, 57001 Thessaloniki, Greece; markella@vidavo.eu
3 Laboratory of Evaluation of Human Biological Performance, Department of Physical Education and Sports Science, Aristotle University of Thessaloniki, 57001 Thessaloniki, Greece; kchristo@phed.auth.gr
* Correspondence: adeligia@phed.auth.gr; Tel.: +30-6945151398

Abstract: Background: Cycling is a very demanding physical activity that may create various health disorders during an athlete's career. Recently, smart mobile and wearable technologies have been used to monitor physiological responses and possible disturbances during physical activity. Thus, the application of mHealth methods in sports poses a challenge today. This study used a novel mobile-Health method to monitor athletes' physiological responses and to detect health disorders early during cycling in elite athletes. Methods: Sixteen high-level cyclists participated in this study, which included a series of measurements in the laboratory; health and performance assessments; and then application in the field of mHealth monitoring in two training seasons, at the beginning of their training period and in the race season. A field monitoring test took place during 30 min of uphill cycling with the participant's heart rate at the ventilatory threshold. During monitoring periods, heart rate, oxygen saturation, respiratory rate, and electrocardiogram were monitored via the mHealth system. Moreover, the SpO_2 was estimated continuously, and the symptoms during effort were reported. Results: A significant correlation was found between the symptoms reported by the athletes in the two field tests and the findings recorded with the application of the mHealth monitoring method. However, from the pre-participation screening in the laboratory and from the spiroergometric tests, no abnormal findings were detected that were to blame for the appearance of the symptoms. Conclusions: The application of mHealth monitoring during competitive cycling is a very useful method for the early recording of cardiac and other health disorders of athletes, whose untimely evaluation could lead to unforeseen events.

Keywords: mHealth; tele-monitoring; cycling; health disorders

Citation: Iliadis, A.; Tomovic, M.; Dervas, D.; Psymarnou, M.; Christoulas, K.; Kouidi, E.J.; Deligiannis, A.P. A Novel mHealth Monitoring System during Cycling in Elite Athletes. *Int. J. Environ. Res. Public Health* **2021**, *18*, 4788. https://doi.org/10.3390/ijerph18094788

Academic Editor: Shaher A.I. Shalfawi

Received: 4 April 2021
Accepted: 26 April 2021
Published: 30 April 2021

1. Introduction

Acute health disorders, such as musculoskeletal injuries, cardiovascular events, etc., may occur during long-distance competitive cycling due to prolonged strenuous exercise and sometimes environmental conditions [1]. Health disorders are more common in young athletes and particularly at the beginning of the training season [2]. This highly demanding sport discipline often leads to dehydration that can be further followed by hypotension; decreased coordination; fatigue; and, in some cases, fainting episodes [3]. More severe events attributed to cycling include arrhythmias, hypoxia, hypoglycemia, hyperventilation, and inappropriate dyspnea [4–9].

During a sports competition in real time, e-health monitoring is beneficial for determining the athlete's response to the load of the exercise; assessing fatigue; and minimizing the risk of injury, cardiac problems, and other disorders [10,11]. Conventional measures of exercise load include power output, speed, time-motion analysis, global positioning system

(GPS) parameters, and accelerometer-derived parameters [11,12]. Moreover, monitoring some hemodynamic responses, the cardiac rhythm, respiratory and metabolic indices, body temperature, and other settings is essential for safe exercise [10,11]. Smart mobile devices and wearable technologies are becoming increasingly useful for monitoring athletes' physical activity and health disorders in sports. The World Health Organization has defined mHealth as the "use of mobile and wireless technologies to support the achievement of health objectives". Mobile health (mHealth)-related applications are popular in health and fitness, according to recent studies [13,14]. However, there is a lack of continuous and comprehensive measurement of physiological parameters during cycling by such methods in elite athletes [15]. The application of such methods in competitive cycling is a challenge because of the sport's characteristics.

The present study aimed to evaluate the application of a novel mobile telemetric procedure to monitor elite cyclists' physiological parameters during strenuous cycling to detect health disorders that may appear or evolve during exercise in two training periods.

2. Materials and Methods

Sixteen high-level male cyclists aged 18–33 years from cycling clubs in Northern Greece with the best ranking participated in the study. Cyclists are ranked by the Greek Cycling Federation according to their position in domestic competitions (national and local championships, cups, inter-club competitions, cycling rounds) and abroad (Olympic Games and world championships, international rounds, Mediterranean and Balkan championships) on track, road, and mountain terrain. The design of the study included a series of measurements in the laboratory and then the application of the mHealth monitoring method in the field in two training seasons: firstly, at the beginning of the training cycle (November), and secondly at the end of the preparation period (during competition season—May and June). All measurements were taken in the morning (between 09:00 and 11:00 a.m.), while athletes abstained from alcohol and coffee at least 24 h before the tests. All the athletes were healthy, as evidenced by their history and the pre-participation health screening that took place in the Sports Medicine Laboratory of the Aristotle University of Thessaloniki; were not taking any medications; and completed the informed consent form. The University Ethics Committee approved the study protocol following the Helsinki Declaration for human research.

2.1. Laboratory Measurements

Participants were asked to fill in a pre-participation medical history questionnaire (including demographic, training, personal, and family medical history data). Then, anthropometric measurements (weight and BMI by FORA TN'G, Moorpark, CA, USA) and physical examinations were performed. Moreover, glucose measurement (Easy2Check Card Guard) and resting 12-lead electrocardiograms (ECG-PMP SelfCheck ECG Card Guard, Rehovot, Israel) were carried out. Finally, a maximal cardiopulmonary exercise test (CPET) via a breath-by-breath gas analyzing system (Ultima Series Med Graphics, Saint Paul, MN, USA) was contacted on a Seca Cardiotest 100 cycle ergometer, (Vogel & Halke Gmbh & Co, Hamburg, Germany). They performed the following maximal ramp exercise protocol until exhaustion: preheating (5 min at 100 W and 3 min at 150 W); test (3 min at 200 W, 3 min at 250 W); and then an increase of 25 W every minute to exhaustion. The pedaling speeds used were 80 to 90 ramp per minute. The athletes' maximal oxygen consumption (VO_2 max), maximal heart rate (HR max), and ventilator threshold (VT) were obtained. The HR at the VT point (HRVT) was also detected. All the pre-participation data were transferred to the previously generated electronic file for each cyclist. The exercise test was repeated before the second monitoring procedure.

2.2. mHealth Monitoring Procedure

The e-health system architecture, provided by Vidavo SA, a Greek e-Health company, was composed of four parts (Figure 1): (1) four sensors, suitable for a secure biomedical wireless transmission, mounted in a specific wearable belt (Vidavo SA, Zephyr BioHarness, Annapolis, MD, USA), placed on each cyclist's chest under the papilla; (2) a receptor on-board to a Smartphone, where an embedded software allowed the pre-processing of acquired body sensor data. The Android Studio, which was the official IDE for Android development, and included everything someone needed to build Android apps, was used to build the software. In addition, some features were designed: the acquisition of data via Bluetooth, view of these data, control of the sensors, signaling the presence of noise; (3) a mobile Smartphone (Google Nexus S Android 4.0 operating system, Mountain View, CA, USA), which had GPS and Bluetooth connection managing the real-time data transmitting with the receptor and a GSM for real time data transmitting to the server; (4) a Linux based data server (laptop computer—Samsung Galaxy Book, Suwon, South Korea) oriented to store, process, and manage all data. Pilot studies of the mHealth system were performed before the study to check its reliability.

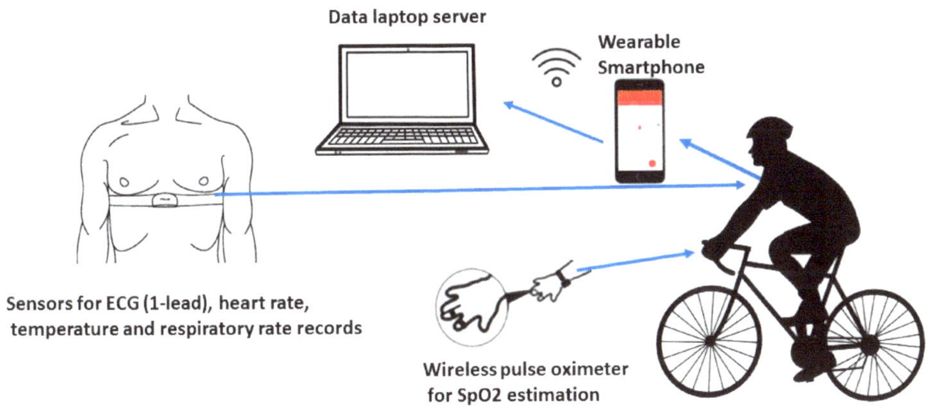

Figure 1. mHealth monitoring methodology.

Within a week after the pre-participation examination, the cyclists were tested in the field. The field training test included 30 min of strenuous uphill cycling at each athlete's HRVT after a warm up of 10 min of low-intensity straight path cycling. Perceived exertion, using Borg scale, speed, cadence, and heart-rate measurement via a monitoring system, was used to measure their effort during field training to maintain the desired level of cycling intensity. During cycling, each athlete's ECG (1-lead), heart rate, temperature, and respiratory rate were recorded via the sensors. Simultaneously, SpO2 was recorded by a wireless pulse oximeter (OxyPro, Card Guard, Neuhausen am Rheinfall, Switzerland) placed on each athlete's wrist and connected to the cover on the top of the finger. While recording, all available data were automatically transferred through the mobile phone, which was in the pocket of every cyclist, to the car escort's laptop and stored in the electronic file of each cyclist. Moreover, at rest and at the end of each monitoring test, blood pressure (Omron M7 Intelli IT Comfort, Hoofddorp, Netherlands), glucose (Easy2Check Card Guard, Rehovot, Israel), and hemoglobin levels (Hemosmart Apex Biotechnology Corporation, Hsinchu City, Taiwan) were measured and simultaneously transferred to the athlete's e-file. The same monitoring test was repeated at the end of the racing period. In case of a technical problem, such as the inability to communicate between the sensors and the mobile phone, the measurement was repeated the next day, as happened in one case.

A primary target of the study was to assess the data quality issues on our mHealth monitoring. Thus, the data collection rate, performance of body sensors, quantity of data to be pre-processed and transferred (i.e., respecting data quote), as well as the quality of communication were evaluated. During the field effort, the participants were asked to report any of the experienced exercise-related symptoms, such as fatigue, dyspnea, inappropriate tachycardia, and dizziness. The reported symptoms were also automatically noted in the electronic file of each athlete. For the accurate evaluation of the m-health system measurements' quality, the results of the two field monitoring tests and the athletes' symptoms were correlated with the data from the pre-participation screening and the corresponding spiroergometric estimations (VO_2max) in the laboratory.

Descriptive statistics were used to describe categorical variables. Continuous variables were expressed as mean ± SD. The Shapiro–Wilk test was used for testing the normality of all data. The differences between values registered during the two testing periods were evaluated using the paired sample *t*-test. Relationships between categorical variables were tested using the Chi- Square statistic. For statistical analysis, the SPSS statistical program (Social Package for Social Sciences, Chicago, IL, USA, version 20.0) was used. A $p < 0.05$ was accepted as statistically significant.

3. Results

All 16 cyclists participated in all phases of the study. However, six athletes in each field training test interrupted their effort, due to the appearance of abnormal findings in mHealth monitoring. These were added in the results. All the cyclists had at least 5 years of racing experience, and they were trained more than five times per week. The demographic characteristics and the training habits of the participants are listed in Table 1. The data from the two maximal cardiopulmonary exercise tests, as well as from the two field monitoring tests, are presented in Tables 2 and 3.

Table 1. Cyclists' demographic and training history data.

Age (years)	24.1 ± 4.5
Weight (Kg)	76.0 ± 6.9
Height (cm)	179.3 ± 5.2
BMI	23.3 ± 1.5
Years of training (years)	5.6 ± 1.9
Frequency of training (times/week)	5.3 ± 0.9
Heart rate at rest (b/min)	56.2 ± 5.5
Systolic blood pressure at rest (mm/Hg)	125.8 ± 8.4
Diastolic blood pressure at rest (mm/Hg)	73.8 ± 10.0

Table 2. Results of the two maximal cardiopulmonary exercise tests.

Physiological Parameters	Beginning of Training Period	Racing Season
Heart Rate at rest (b/min)	71.4 ± 6.5	68.6 ± 8.7
Systolic Blood Pressure at rest (mm/Hg)	126.8 ± 7.1	125.8 ± 6.5
Diastolic Blood Pressure at rest (mm/Hg)	76.6 ± 9.4	75.7 ± 7.8
Heart Rate max (b/min)	195.7 ± 9.6	195.4 ± 10.0
Systolic Blood Pressure max (mm/Hg)	195.4 ± 6.4	194 ± 3.9
Diastolic Blood Pressure max (mm/Hg)	72.6 ± 2.9	71.8 ± 2.3
Time to fatigue (min)	11.69 ± 1.8	13.72 ± 1.3 *
Max Power (Watts)	354.7 ± 46.7	403.1 ± 30.1 *
HR_{VT} (b/min)	176.6 ± 8.7	175.6 ± 9.6
VO_2max (mL/kg/min)	55.4 ± 5.3	63.4 ± 6.9 *

HR_{VT}: Heart rate at the ventilatory threshold; VO_2max: maximal oxygen consumption. * $p < 0.05$.

From the first continuous field monitoring of cyclists' physiological parameters, three cases of athletes' peripheral capillary oxygen saturation of 88.5% were detected who also reported dyspnea, two cases of hypotension were detected who reported dizziness, and one case of paroxysmal supraventricular tachycardia was detected who reported palpitations at the beginning of the training period. Moreover, in the training period, field monitoring detected two athletes with hypotension appearing dizzy, two athletes with SpO_2 90% who reported dyspnea, and two athletes with extrasystoles in ECG describing palpitations (Figure 2).

Table 3. Results of the two field monitoring tests.

Physiological Parameters	Start of the Training Period		Racing Season	
	Rest	Max	Rest	Max
Systolic Blood Pressure (mm/Hg)	131.2 ± 8.8	148.3 ± 13.6	130.8 ± 7.5	147.5 ± 8.3
Diastolic Blood Pressure (mm/Hg)	77.8 ± 9.4	76.3 ± 6.3	78 ± 8.5	77.8 ± 8.7
Heart Rate (b/min)	68.4 ± 6.4	165.6 ± 6.6	67.8 ± 6.2	163.6 ± 8.4
Hemoglobin (g/dL)	15.4 ± 1.5	14.5 ± 1.4 [a]	15.2 ± 1.3	14.7 ± 1.2 [b]
Hematocrit (%)	46.2 ± 4.5	43.4 ± 4.1 [a]	45.5 ± 3.8	44.2 ± 3.8 [b]
Glucose (mg/dL)	105.3 ± 8.4	100.7 ± 8.6 [a]	99.8 ± 6.4 [c]	94.8 ± 5.7 [b]
Oxygen saturation	99.1 ± 0.7	96.4 ± 0.6 [a]	98.7 ± 0.7 [c]	96.9 ± 0.8 [b]

[a] $p < 0.05$ between rest and max in the preparation period; [b] $p < 0.05$ between rest and max in the racing season; [c] $p < 0.05$ between rest in the preparation period and in the racing season.

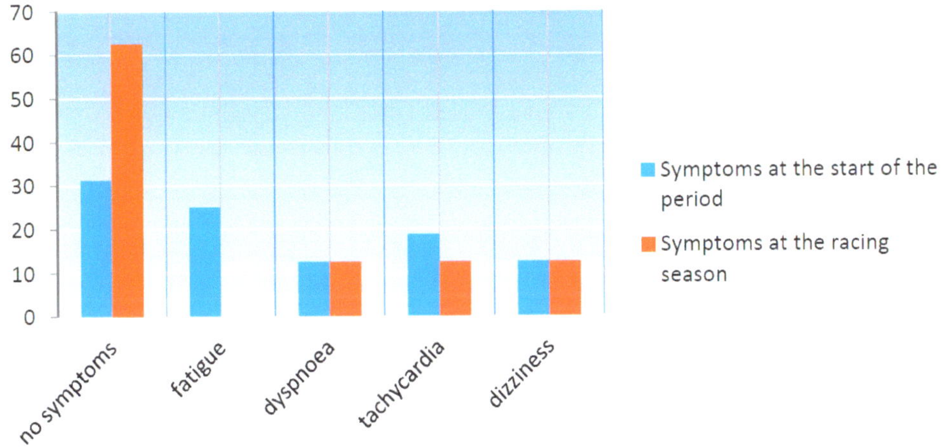

Figure 2. Percentage of athletes that reported health related symptoms during the two monitoring field tests.

One cyclist who developed hypotension was the same with a similar finding on the first measurement, an athlete who had a feeling of pallor had shown it during the initial evaluation, and an athlete with dyspnea had a decrease in O_2 saturation during the first procedure. There were no correlations between the above findings and the medical history, clinical screening, and laboratory evaluation of the athletes. Specifically, the athletes with the abnormal symptoms from e-health monitoring do not have different values in VO2 max in comparison with the rest. All the athletes reported positive feedback for applying the e-health monitoring system, which gave them a feeling of security. All the athletes reported that the system was easy to use, and did not cause them problems in their movement. All the vital signs recorded via the monitoring system were legible, without noises.

4. Discussion

The present study results show that the mHealth monitoring system could effectively and quickly detect health disorders during strenuous cycling training. This leads to a timely cessation of the athlete's effort to prevent possible dangerous incidents. At the beginning of the racing season, training adaptations allowed the better management of the training load and less frequent health-related problems. Observed physiological changes were not significant, due to the elite level of the included cyclist and their long-term involvement in sport.

e-Health monitoring, a modern approach in ambulatory health disorder detection and management of an athlete or a patient during exercise effort, has demonstrated the potential for considerable clinical utility in sports medicine [10]. Among other benefits, it provides ease of use; is relatively inexpensive; and is highly effective in supporting the diagnosis of various cardiac, metabolic, musculoskeletal, and other complications, especially those appearing during strenuous exercise [11]. A monitoring system based on an e-Health sensor board has been implemented before; it provides follow-up on athletes and measures vital physiological parameters [10–12]. In recent decades, many e-Health systems and applications have been developed in sports [10–12,16,17]. The devices in this class of monitoring can be divided into three categories: wearable-based, ambient-based (i.e., sensor-based approach), and camera-based (i.e., vision-based approach) [18]. Wearable detection approaches use sensors, such as accelerometers and gyroscopes, to detect and measure motion, location, and posture by measuring acceleration and orientation [19]. Ambient detection approaches use devices, such as pressure sensors, for movement detection [20]. They also rely on audio and vibration data analysis. The camera and vision detection approach, implemented in video tracking systems, relies on video data processing, such as activities in extreme conditions [21]. Wearable sensors have been embedded into watches, shirts, belts, etc. Such sensors provide real-time physiological information related to the health condition of the monitored subject. Various biosensors are used, such as electrocardiography sensors (ECG) used to monitor cardiac activity, electroencephalography sensors (EEG) used to monitor brain activity, electromyography sensors (EMG) used to monitor muscle activity, and electrooculography sensors (EOG) used to monitor eye movements [11,12]. Pulse oximeters are used to measure the oxygen level of the blood (i.e., oxygen saturation), while plethysmography sensors (EPG) are used to monitor the rate of blood flow [22]. Other biomedical parameters can also be evaluated using CO_2 gas sensors to evaluate gaseous carbon dioxide levels to monitor respiration. Bluetooth communications were integrated to link the system to commercial medical devices for measuring blood pressure, blood glucose levels, etc. [11]. Data can be generated based on three event types: constant, interval, or instant [23]. Constant events ensure that data are continuously transmitted. The wearable sensors and mobile devices gathered biological signals and were connected to a personal digital assistant. The assistant held and processed biological signals and communicated with a computer server for additional processing, such as database services.

A number of smart e-platforms have been proposed to monitor a lot of events in cycling [24–26]. The feedback provided by these platforms is however not sufficient in real-time efforts. Recently, the CONAMO project (CONtinuous Athlete MOnitoring), which combined the Wireless Personal-Area Network (WPAN) technology, widely used in cycling and the 6TiSCH network, has provided a dynamic, real-time, and reliable novel sensing system that can be used for covering cycling events, in amateur or professional cycling [25]. Gaidos and dos Sandos [26] designed and developed a system of mobile-Health monitoring and training for cyclists. The hardware application contained sensors for heart rate, oxygen percentage, speed, distance, time, and room temperature, during and after the training.

Our proposed mHealth monitoring system is very similar to many modern applications existing in smartphones. Using various sensors allowed exercising users to perform personal health checks based on their vital signs sent from sensors to the assistant. It can measure four parameters via biosensors (one lead ECG, heart rate, temperature, and respiratory rate) and the other four parameters (SPO_2, blood pressure, glucose, and hemoglobin levels) by e-health application devices. Besides, it uses security to send the information and it could be implemented in teams of cyclists due to its easy scalability and cost-effectiveness. For the sports industry, wearable technology will always have extensive research in the microcontroller, power management of integrated circuits, and how sensor signal conditioning occurs. When these three are defined, the compatibility of sensory elements can be known for a required application, such as our mHealth system. Compared with other mobile health systems, our system has some advantages; it has a user-friendly operation process and lightweight on-body monitoring sensors. The physiologic parameters are measured by a wearable belt-like sensor and recorded by an Android smartphone via a specific software program, offering a real-time response for the abnormal situation. Such approaches provide several quality criteria to qualify data, such as accuracy, completeness, timeliness, relevance, legibility, accessibility, and usefulness [27]. In the previous studies [24,25] the sensors provided real-time feedback about the cyclists' heart rate and heart rate training zones only, helping to coach and improving cycling experience and performance. The strength of our study was to investigate a wearable mHealth system to monitor a lot of physiological parameters of cyclists during intensive and strenuous training, in order to detect any health disorders early that may appear or progress during a race competition which demands an extreme body and mind effort. In comparison to a similar e-monitoring system for cyclists of Gaidos and Santos [26], there are some differences regarding the architecture of the mobile system as well as the ability to measure certain parameters. They monitored the saturation of oxygen; ambient temperature; and speed, distance, and altitude of the athlete. In addition, using the Karvonen formula, the maximum and minimum heart rate training range was calculated. Other researchers used a similar smart phone-based sensor interface technology to monitor some biological signals, specifically heart rate and body temperature during cycling, as well as riding and geographical information [28]. One of the results of the mHealth system developed in this project is the additional specialized examination of athletes that can lead to deeper insights, which are currently analyzed manually with wide margins of error. The results of biomedical information led to the conclusion that the developed system can be used to significantly increase speed and improve the quality and accuracy of monitoring during exercise. Finally, its management through the cloud facilitates its integration across platforms. Regarding data collection, the frequency of receiving data plays an essential role in overall system performance.

Continuous field monitoring during the two field tests revealed arrhythmias, hypotension, and hypoxemia, which were confirmed by the athletes' reported symptoms. Vigorous physical activity in susceptible individuals activates specific mechanisms that can lead to serious cardiac events [29,30] with cycling being the sporting activity with the highest number of adverse cardiac events according to a study by Vicent et al. [31]. Additionally, demanding endurance events followed by electrolyte imbalance and increased sympathetic activation in some cases can lead to transit myocardial ischemia and repolarization changes which are the ground base of severe arrhythmias [29]. Recent research by Breedt [1] and Killops et al. [4] concluded that medical complaints in cycling predominantly refer to sustained injuries which are followed by cardiovascular symptoms with the incidence of life-threatening medical encounters of 0.5 per 1000 athletes. Our study data showed that symptoms of increased fatigue and tachycardia appeared more commonly at the beginning of the training season indicating that the telemetric monitoring of elite cyclists should be considered from the start of the macrocycle. These performance-related and detraining-induced self-reported symptoms of fatigue and palpitations can be explained with literature data on injury and illnesses in armature cyclists [32,33]. Namely, these two studies showed that medical covering of recreational cycling events should consider heat, fatigue, and abdominal-related non-traumatic injuries. Dyspnea registered in our cyclists also at the beginning of the training season correlates with data from the study by McGrath et al., who found asthma and other respiratory-related symptoms to form 25% of all reported illnesses during mountain cycling events [34]. The results of the two CPETs also confirmed the high performance of our study's participants, since the accomplished VO_2max was above 55.4 mL/kg/min during the first assessment and 63.4 mL/kg/min during the second. These values are in agreement with the study by Buck and McNaughton [35], who found an average VO_2max of 57.5 mL/kg/min in high-level cycling athletes. Notably, the above abnormal findings during mHealth monitoring at the fields were not expected, since the pre-participation screening of the cyclists at baseline did not reveal any pathological condition. Most of the athletes that had symptoms in their first attempt on the field had reappearing symptoms during their second effort. The above highlights the system's usefulness in the early detection of disorders during the intense exercise of "healthy" athletes. However, we should emphasize that we were strict in our decision to interrupt the effort in some athletes with mild symptoms, because our primary concern in this experimental study was to assess the sensitivity of the mHealth system. Furthermore, our study data confirm the conclusion of a study on the medical coverage of cycling events that emphasizes the importance of communication systems between individual medical staff, race officials, and local emergency medical services [36].

The results of our study should be interpreted in light of some limitations. The main limitation is that only males and high-level cyclists participated in the study. Moreover, continuous monitoring was applied during an experimental strenuous cycling effort and not during a competitive cycling race, considering that the race-related stress may pose an additional health risk.

5. Conclusions

In conclusion, the use of the novel described mHealth monitoring system in sports such as cycling was a feasible and usable method. Such monitoring during competitive cycling is an advantageous method for the early recording of cardiac and other health disorders of athletes, whose untimely evaluation could lead to unforeseen events.

Author Contributions: Conceptualization, A.I., D.D., M.P., K.C., E.J.K. and A.P.D.; Formal analysis, A.I., M.T., D.D. and M.P.; Investigation, A.I.; Methodology, M.P., K.C. and E.J.K.; Supervision, E.J.K. and A.P.D.; Validation, K.C., E.J.K. and A.P.D.; Writing—original draft, A.I. and M.T.; Writing—review & editing, M.T., D.D. and E.J.K. All authors have read and agreed to the published version of the manuscript.

Funding: This research received no external funding.

Institutional Review Board Statement: The study was conducted according to the guidelines of the Declaration of Helsinki, and approved by the Institutional Ethics Committee of Aristotle University (Approval number EC-10/2020, Thessaloniki, 27 February 2020).

Informed Consent Statement: Informed consent was obtained from all subjects involved in the study.

Data Availability Statement: The data presented in this study are available on request from the corresponding author. The data are not publicly available due to privacy of included athletes.

Conflicts of Interest: The authors and the company declare no conflict of interest.

References

1. Breedt, M.; Janse van Rensburg, D.C.; Fletcher, L.; Grant, C.C.; Schwellnus, M.P. The Injury and Illness Profile of Male and Female Participants in a 94.7 Km Cycle Race: A Cross-Sectional Study. *Clin. J. Sport Med. Off. J. Can. Acad. Sport Med.* **2019**, *29*, 306–311. [CrossRef]
2. Helzer-Julin, M. Sun, Heat, and Cold Injuries in Cyclists. *Clin. Sports Med.* **1994**, *13*, 219–234. [CrossRef]
3. Powers, S.K.; Dodd, S.; Lawler, J.; Landry, G.; Kirtley, M.; McKnight, T.; Grinton, S. Incidence of Exercise Induced Hypoxemia in Elite Endurance Athletes at Sea Level. *Eur. J. Appl. Physiol.* **1988**, *58*, 298–302. [CrossRef] [PubMed]
4. Killops, J.; Schwellnus, M.; Janse van Rensburg, D.C.; Swanevelder, S.; Jordaan, E. Medical Encounters, Cardiac Arrests and Deaths during a 109 Km Community-Based Mass-Participation Cycling Event: A 3-Year Study in 102,251 Race Starters—SAFER IX. *Br. J. Sports Med.* **2020**, *54*, 605. [CrossRef] [PubMed]
5. Serrano Ostariz, E.; López Ramón, M.; Cremades Arroyos, D.; Izquierdo Álvarez, S.; Catalán Edo, P.; Baquer Sahún, C.; Legaz Arrese, A. Post-Exercise Left Ventricular Dysfunction Measured after a Long-Duration Cycling Event. *BMC Res. Notes* **2013**, *6*, 211. [CrossRef] [PubMed]
6. Woodward, A.; Tin Tin, S.; Doughty, R.N.; Ameratunga, S. Atrial Fibrillation and Cycling: Six Year Follow-up of the Taupo Bicycle Study. *BMC Public Health* **2015**, *15*, 23. [CrossRef] [PubMed]
7. Jordaens, L.; Missault, L.; Pelleman, G.; Duprez, D.; De Backer, G.; Clement, D.L. Comparison of Athletes with Life-Threatening Ventricular Arrhythmias with Two Groups of Healthy Athletes and a Group of Normal Control Subjects. *Am. J. Cardiol.* **1994**, *74*, 1124–1128. [CrossRef]
8. Endo, M.Y.; Shimada, K.; Miura, A.; Fukuba, Y. Peripheral and Central Vascular Conductance Influence on Post-Exercise Hy-potension. *J. Physiol. Anthropol.* **2012**, *31*, 32. [CrossRef] [PubMed]
9. Felig, P.; Cherif, A.; Minagawa, A.; Wahren, J. Hypoglycemia during Prolonged Exercise in Normal Men. *N. Engl. J. Med.* **1982**, *306*, 895–900. [CrossRef]
10. Deligiannis, P.; Deligiannis, A.-S.; Kouidi, E. Trends in E-Health Monitoring Implementation in Sports. *Sport Prav.* **2011**, *41*, 34–37. [CrossRef]

11. do Nascimento, L.M.S.; Bonfati, L.V.; Freitas, M.L.B.; Mendes Junior, J.J.A.; Siqueira, H.V.; Stevan, S.L. Sensors and Systems for Physical Rehabilitation and Health Monitoring—A Review. *Sensors* **2020**, *20*, 4063. [CrossRef] [PubMed]
12. Skarbalius, A.; Vidunaite, G.; Kniubaite, A.; Reklaitiene, D.; Simanavicius, A. Importance of Sport Performance Monitoring for Sports Organization. *Transform. Bus. Econ.* **2019**, *18*, 279–303.
13. Dallinga, J.; Janssen, M.; van der Werf, J.; Walravens, R.; Vos, S.; Deutekom, M. Analysis of the Features Important for the Effectiveness of Physical Activity-Related Apps for Recreational Sports: Expert Panel Approach. *JMIR MHealth UHealth* **2018**, *6*, e143. [CrossRef] [PubMed]
14. Gorski, M.A.; Mimoto, S.M.; Khare, V.; Bhatkar, V.; Combs, A. Real-Time Digital Biometric Monitoring during Elite Athletic Competition: System Feasibility with a Wearable Medical-Grade Sensor. *Digit. Biomark.* **2021**, *5*, 37–43. [CrossRef] [PubMed]
15. Kolsung, E.B.; Ettema, G.; Skovereng, K. Physiological Response to Cycling With Variable versus Constant Power Output. *Front. Physiol.* **2020**, *11*, 1098. [CrossRef]
16. Samaras, T.; Karavasiliadou, S.; Kouidi, E.; Sahalos, J.N.; Deligiannis, A. Transtelephonic Electrocardiographic Transmission in the Preparticipation Screening of Athletes. *Int. J. Telemed. Appl.* **2008**, *2008*, 217909. [CrossRef]
17. Kouidi, E.; Farmakiotis, A.; Kouidis, N.; Deligiannis, A. Transtelephonic Electrocardiographic Monitoring of an Outpatient Cardiac Rehabilitation Programme. *Clin. Rehabil.* **2006**, *20*, 1100–1104. [CrossRef]
18. Mubashir, M.; Shao, L.; Seed, L. A Survey on Fall Detection: Principles and Approaches. *Neurocomputing* **2013**, *100*, 144–152. [CrossRef]
19. Seshadri, D.R.; Li, R.T.; Voos, J.E.; Rowbottom, J.R.; Alfes, C.M.; Zorman, C.A.; Drummond, C.K. Wearable Sensors for Moni-toring the Internal and External Workload of the Athlete. *NPJ Digit. Med.* **2019**, *2*, 71. [CrossRef]
20. Uddin, M.Z.; Khaksar, W.; Torresen, J. Ambient Sensors for Elderly Care and Independent Living: A Survey. *Sensors* **2018**, *18*, 2027. [CrossRef]
21. Jung, S.; Cho, Y.; Kim, D.; Chang, M. Moving Object Detection from Moving Camera Image Sequences Using an Inertial Measurement Unit Sensor. *Appl. Sci.* **2020**, *10*, 268. [CrossRef]
22. Castaneda, D.; Esparza, A.; Ghamari, M.; Soltanpur, C.; Nazeran, H. A Review on Wearable Photoplethysmography Sensors and Their Potential Future Applications in Health Care. *Int. J. Biosens. Bioelectron.* **2018**, *4*, 195–202. [CrossRef]
23. Chen, Y.-C.; Peng, W.-C.; Lee, S.-Y. Mining Temporal Patterns in Time Interval-Based Data. *IEEE Trans. Knowl. Data Eng.* **2015**, *27*, 3318–3331. [CrossRef]
24. De Brouwer, M.; Ongenae, F.; Daneels, G.; Municio, E.; Famaey, J.; Latré, S.; De Turck, F. *Personalized Real-Time Monitoring of Amateur Cyclists on Low-End Devices*; ACM Press: New York, NY, USA, 2018; pp. 1833–1840.
25. Municio, E.; Daneels, G.; De Brouwer, M.; Ongenae, F.; De Turck, F.; Braem, B.; Famaey, J.; Latré, S. Continuous Athlete Mon-itoring in Challenging Cycling Environments Using IoT Technologies. *IEEE Internet Things J.* **2019**, *6*, 10875–10887. [CrossRef]
26. Gaidos Rosero, O.F.; Santos, I. Mobile System of Monitoring and Training Cyclists with Smartphone. In *VI Latin American Congress on Biomedical Engineering CLAIB 2014, Paraná, Argentina 29, 30–31 October 2014*; Springer: Cham, Switzerland, 2015; Volume 49, pp. 59–62. ISBN 978-3-319-13116-0.
27. Aroganam, G.; Manivannan, N.; Harrison, D. Review on Wearable Technology Sensors Used in Consumer Sport Applications. *Sensors* **2019**, *19*, 1983. [CrossRef]
28. Lee, Y.; Jeong, J. Design and Implementation of Monitoring System Architecture for Smart Bicycle Platform. *Procedia Comput. Sci.* **2018**, *134*, 464–469. [CrossRef]
29. Wundersitz, D.; Williamson, J.; Nadurata, V.; Nolan, K.; Lavie, C.; Kingsley, M. The Impact of a 21-Day Ultra-Endurance Ride on the Heart in Young, Adult and Older Adult Recreational Cyclists. *Int. J. Cardiol.* **2019**, *286*, 137–142. [CrossRef] [PubMed]
30. Thompson, P.D.; Franklin, B.A.; Balady, G.J.; Blair, S.N.; Corrado, D.; Estes, N.A.M.; Fulton, J.E.; Gordon, N.F.; Haskell, W.L.; Link, M.S.; et al. Exercise and Acute Cardiovascular Events Placing the Risks into Perspective: A Scientific Statement from the American Heart Association Council on Nutrition, Physical Activity, and Metabolism and the Council on Clinical Cardiology. *Circulation* **2007**, *115*, 2358–2368. [CrossRef] [PubMed]
31. Vicent, L.; Ariza-Solé, A.; González-Juanatey, J.R.; Uribarri, A.; Ortiz, J.; López de Sá, E.; Sans-Roselló, J.; Querol, C.T.; Codina, P.; Sousa-Casasnovas, I.; et al. Exercise-Related Severe Cardiac Events. *Scand. J. Med. Sci. Sports* **2018**, *28*, 1404–1411. [CrossRef] [PubMed]
32. Roi, G.S.; Tinti, R. Requests for Medical Assistance during an Amateur Road Cycling Race. *Accid. Anal. Prev.* **2014**, *73*, 170–173. [CrossRef]
33. Pommering, T.L.; Manos, D.C.; Singichetti, B.; Brown, C.R.; Yang, J. Injuries and Illnesses Occurring on a Recreational Bicycle Tour: The Great Ohio Bicycle Adventure. *Wilderness Environ. Med.* **2017**, *28*, 299–306. [CrossRef]
34. McGrath, T.M.; Yehl, M.A. Injury and Illness in Mountain Bicycle Stage Racing: Experience from the Trans-Sylvania Mountain Bike Epic Race. *Wilderness Environ. Med.* **2012**, *23*, 356–359. [CrossRef] [PubMed]
35. Buck, D.; McNaughton, L.R. Changing the Number of Submaximal Exercise Bouts Effects Calculation of MAOD. *Int. J. Sports Med.* **1999**, *20*, 28–33. [CrossRef] [PubMed]
36. Martinez, J.M. Medical Coverage of Cycling Events. *Curr. Sports Med. Rep.* **2006**, *5*, 125–130. [CrossRef] [PubMed]

International Journal of
Environmental Research and Public Health

MDPI

Article

Role of Type and Volume of Recreational Physical Activity on Heart Rate Variability in Men

Shaea Alkahtani [1,*], Andrew A. Flatt [2], Jawad Kanas [1], Abdulaziz Aldyel [1] and Syed Shahid Habib [3]

1 Department of Exercise Physiology, College of Sport Sciences and Physical Activity, King Saud University, Riyadh 11451, Saudi Arabia; Jawad-Kanas@outlook.sa (J.K.); aldayel@ksu.edu.sa (A.A.)
2 Department of Health Sciences and Kinesiology, Biodynamics and Human Performance Center, Georgia Southern University – Armstrong, Savannah, GA 31419, USA; aflatt@georgiasouthern.edu
3 Department of Physiology, College of Medicine & King Khalid University Hospital, King Saud University, Riyadh 11461, Saudi Arabia; sshahid@ksu.edu.sa
* Correspondence: shalkahtani@ksu.edu.sa

Received: 26 March 2020; Accepted: 14 April 2020; Published: 15 April 2020

Abstract: The aim of this study was to investigate the effect of recreational aerobic physical activity (PA) type and volume on heart rate variability (HRV) in Arab men. This was a retrospective, cross-sectional study, and included men (n = 75, age = 37.6 ± 7.1 years, body mass index (BMI) = 26.7 ± 3.1 kg/m^2) who were members of a walking group, cycling group, or were inactive controls. Monthly distances from the past three months were obtained from walking and cycling groups, and the volume of PA was classified into three subgroups (high, moderate, low). HRV was measured using a computerized electrocardiographic data acquisition device. R–R interval recordings were performed while participants rested in a motionless supine position. RR intervals were recorded for 15 minutes, and a five-minute segment with minimal ectopic beats and artifacts was selected for HRV analysis. Time-domain parameters included the mean R–R interval, standard deviation of the mean R–R interval (SDNN), and root-mean-squared difference of successive RR intervals (RMSSD). The frequency-domain parameters included high-frequency power (HF), low-frequency power (LF), and LF to HF ratio (LF/HF). Results showed that there were no significant differences between walking, cycling, and control groups for all HRV parameters. Time-domain analyses based on PA volume showed that age-adjusted SDNN for the high-active group was greater than the low-active group (P = 0.03), and RMSSD for the moderate-active group was greater than the control group (P = 0.009). For the frequency domain, LF for the high-active group was greater than the low-active and control groups (P = 0.006), and HF for the moderate-active group was greater than the low-active group (P = 0.04). These data indicate that walking >150 km per month, or cycling >100 km per month at a speed >20 km/h may be necessary to derive cardiac autonomic benefits from PA among Arab men.

Keywords: sedentary; walking; cycling; time and frequency domains; blood pressure

1. Introduction

Heart rate variability (HRV) is a valid marker that reflects cardiac modulation by sympathetic and parasympathetic components of the autonomic nervous system (ANS) [1]. The clinical applications of HRV are mainly associated with the prediction of sudden cardiac death and assessing the progression of cardiovascular and metabolic conditions [2]. Indeed, lower vagal-related HRV indices are associated with elevated markers of inflammation, blood lipids and triglycerides, blood pressure, and blood glucose [3]. Computerized electrocardiographic (ECG) recordings are typically used to monitor HRV. Cardiac cycle length (R–R interval) in relation to the immediately preceding R–R interval can be converted to a scatter plot. Using specialized software, artifacts and ectopic beats are filtered prior to computation of time- and frequency-domain parameters of HRV. These methods of evaluating HRV are generally accepted for reflecting cardiac parasympathetic nervous system activity (PNSA) [4]. Interactions between sympathetic and parasympathetic activity can be assessed by low-frequency power/high-frequency power ratio (LF/HF) [2]. Low-frequency power (LF) from 0.04 to 0.15 Hz is related to baroreceptor sensitivity mediated by vagal and sympathetic systems, whereas high-frequency power is influenced by respiratory sinus arrhythmia [5].

Physical activity (PA) guidelines for adults consider the volume of PA performed at low–moderate intensities, which improves many health parameters [6]. Whether such guidelines are applicable for improving HRV has been the topic of recent investigation. While high-intensity training has been shown to improve HRV, findings pertaining to the effects of low- and moderate-intensity PA are inconsistent. For example, the use of high-intensity interval exercise performed at maximal, near-maximal, or supramaximal aerobic power may have a greater effect on HRV [7]. Another study found that high-intensity interval training at 130% of maximal oxygen uptake (VO_{2max}) for three weeks increased HRV threshold [8]. On the other hand, training at moderate intensity levels for 24 sessions increased (VO_{2max}) by 11% among sedentary middle-age men, but did not increase vagal modulation as measured using HRV [9]. Similar outcomes were observed after an eight-week exercise intervention among old adults [10]. Factors such as age and duration of the intervention were hypothesized to explain these findings [1]. Thus, while athletes can safely train at ≥ maximal intensities, which improves HRV [11], there are many precautions for performing high-intensity exercise for the general public [6]. This highlights a need for examining the role of low–moderate-intensity PA on HRV, which remains inconclusive.

Aerobic training such as walking and cycling are the predominant modes of PA among active groups with voluntary membership in Saudi Arabia. However, key variables for improving HRV such as intensity and duration of these free-living activities are rarely well-supervised [12]. A six-month randomized active-controlled trial showed that structured PA can improve HRV to a greater extent than unstructured PA in adolescents [13]. Therefore, recreationally active groups may be less consistent than athletes in performing PA, which may limit the positive effects of training on HRV. Ethnicity is an additional factor that may influence HRV, with possible implications for metabolic and psychological outcomes [14,15]. With a lack of studies investigating HRV and PA among Saudis and Arabs [16], it is important to examine how HRV is affected by regular recreational PA among this underrepresented population.

Given the association between HRV and various health markers, further investigation into modifiable factors that can potentially improve HRV is warranted. Performing more PA is a potential lifestyle intervention that individuals can adopt to improve HRV, although how factors such as type and volume of PA effect cardiac autonomic function, particularly among individuals of Saudi-Arabian descent, requires further investigation. Therefore, the current study aimed to examine the effect of recreational aerobic PA type and volume on HRV in Arab men living in Saudi Arabia. We hypothesized that men who performed regular walking and cycling would exhibit higher levels of HRV compared to age- and body composition-matched inactive men. A secondary hypothesis was that higher volumes of PA would be associated with greater HRV, independent of PA type.

2. Materials and Methods

2.1. Study Design

This was a retrospective cross-sectional study. HRV parameters were dependent variables and the volume and type of PA were independent variables.

2.2. Participants

Study participants included men ($n = 75$, age = 37.6 ± 7.1 years, body mass index (BMI) = 26.7 ± 3.1 kg/m^2, fat percent = 24.1% ± 5.4%) without any chronic medications and with normal resting heart rate

(HRrest), and systolic (SBP) and diastolic (DBP) blood pressure (HRrest = 59.7 ± 6.0 b·min^{-1}, SBP = 115.3 ± 14.2 mmHg, DBP = 82.6 ± 13.2 mmHg). Participants were members of the general public and were categorized according to PA type which included a walking group (Riyadh Walkers), a cycling group (Saudi Cyclists), and an inactive control group. To meet inclusion criteria, it was required that volunteers must: have engaged in regular PA for the past 3 months (for walking and cycling groups); be non-smokers; be <60 years old; have a BMI <30 kg/m^2; and be free from injury or a newly diagnosed chronic illness within the past year. Figure 1 shows the flowchart of participants' inclusion/exclusion in the study. Participants voluntarily expressed their interest by contacting the principal researcher or research assistant. Study aims and instructions for participation were provided by the researchers to prospective individuals. All participants signed a consent form of voluntary participation. This study was approved by the institutional review board (IRB) of King Saud University (IRB No. E-18-3381) and conformed with the guidelines provided by the Declaration of Helsinki.

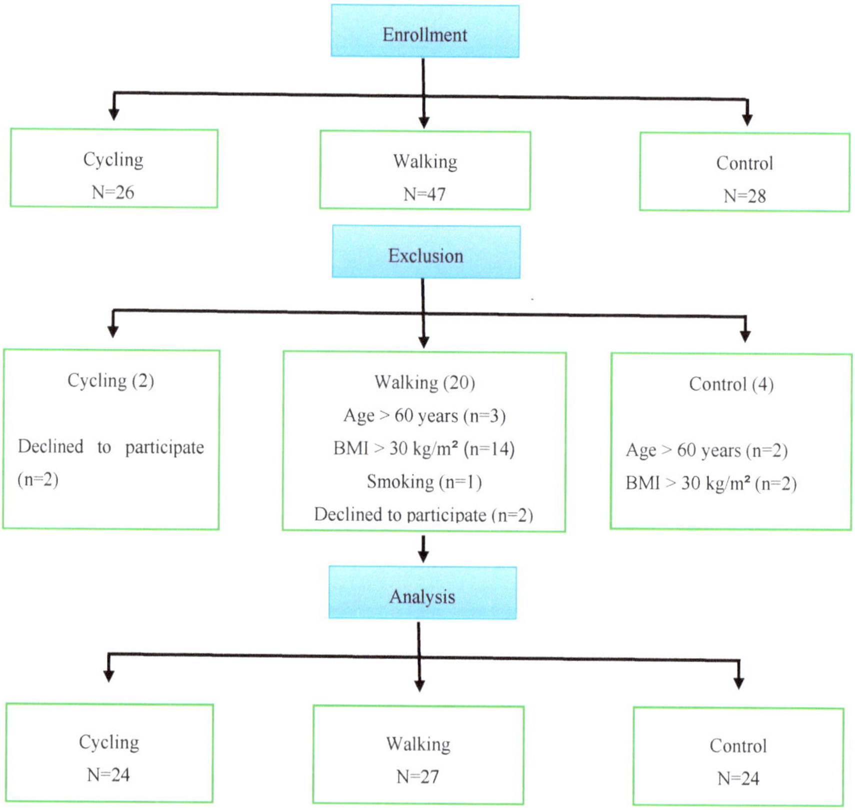

Figure 1. Flowchart of participants' recruitment and exclusion process.

2.3. Pre-Screening Procedures

Study measures were obtained in the Exercise Physiology Laboratories within the Department of Exercise Physiology at the College of Sport Sciences and Physical Activity at King Saud University. All participants were pre-screened for any cardiac abnormalities related to rhythm, ischemia, or heart size with a standard 12 lead ECG prior to HRV acquisition. All subjects that were included in the study had normal resting ECG. SBP and DBP were measured using an automatic brachial sphygmomanometer (Omron HEM-7121, Omron Healthcare manufacturing, Japan).

Participants were instructed to maintain their habitual lifestyle and declare if they experienced greater than usual stress during the testing period. They were also asked to limit excess caffeine consumption and refrain from exercising 24 h prior to testing. Data collection took place early in the morning, at least 4 h post-prandial, and before interacting in their daily life commitments. Study measures included body composition and HRV.

2.4. Study Variable Measures

Study variables included laboratory measures and field measures. Laboratory measures included body composition and HRV, whereas field measures included self-monitored distances of walking and cycling.

2.4.1. Body Composition

Height was measured to the nearest 0.1 cm using a stadiometer (Seca 213, Seca GmbH & Co., Hamburg, Germany), and body weight was measured to the nearest 0.1 kg using a digital scale (PD100 ProDoc, Detecto Scale, Cardinal, Webb City, MO, USA). Body mass index (BMI) was calculated by dividing body weight in kg by height in square meters. Body composition was measured using multi-frequency bioelectrical impedance analysis (BIA) (MC-980MA, Tanita Corporation, Tokyo, Japan) where participants stood barefoot on the scale while holding the handles for approximately 60 sec. Upon completion of the test, body fat percentage (BF%) was recorded for analysis.

2.4.2. Heart Rate Variability

HRV parameters were measured using a computerized ECG data acquisition device with 16 analog input channels (PL3516 PowerLab 16/35, ADInstruments Pty Ltd. New South Wales, Australia). R–R interval filtering of artifacts and ectopic beats and computation of time- and frequency-domain parameters was performed using customized software (LabChart v. 8.1.13 Windows, ADInstruments Pty Ltd. New South Wales, Australia). Time-domain parameters included the mean R–R interval, standard deviation of the mean R–R interval (SDNN), and root-mean-squared difference of successive RR intervals (RMSSD). The frequency-domain parameters included high-frequency power (HF) from 0.15 to 0.40 Hz, low-frequency power (LF) from 0.04 to 0.15 Hz, and LF to HF ratio (LF/HF).

R–R interval recordings were performed in a quiet room with dim lighting while participants rested in a motionless supine position. Use of electrical devices (e.g., smartphones) was prohibited during ECG recordings. Three electrodes were applied on the chest following the Einthoven triangle. Leads were connected from the device to the electrodes to record HRV. A trained instructor supervised the procedure and did not talk with the participants during the test. Participants were asked to breathe naturally and avoid swallowing during the recording. Following a 5-minute stabilization period, RR intervals were recorded for 15 minutes while the researcher monitored signal quality. From the 15-minute recording, a 5-minute segment with minimal ectopic beats and artifacts was selected for HRV analysis.

2.4.3. Volume of Physical Activity for Walking and Cycling Participants

PA volume was measured with smartphone tracking applications used by the walking (i.e., Nike Inc.) and cycling (i.e., Strava Inc.) groups. Walkers and cyclists were members of private communication forums within the applications where they announced their monthly distances to encourage less-active members to maintain and improve their PA levels. This strategy had been implemented among the groups for a year prior to the current study. The average distance from the past 3 months of 51 participants was automatically obtained from the application by walking and cycling group supervisors. Classification of PA volume was standardized independently for walking and cycling groups to account for the different modalities. The volume of PA for walking was divided into 3 levels as follows: low (50–<150 km/month), moderate (150–<300 km/month), and high (≥300 km/month). Whereas the volume of PA for cycling participants was divided into 3 levels as follows: low (50–<100 km/month, at average speed 17 ± 2 km/h), moderate (100–<300 km/month, at average speed 23 ± 2 km/h), and high (>400 km/month, at average speed 30 ± 4 km/h).

2.5. Statistical Analysis

Data were analyzed using SPSS (version 21, IBM). Continuous data were presented as mean ± standard deviation (SD) for normally distributed variables, and as median and (25th and 75th) percentiles for non-normal variables. All continuous variables were checked for normality using the Kolmogorov–Smirnov test. Logarithmic transformations were applied to non-normal variables. Univariate analysis of variance (ANOVA) was used to determine the effect of PA type (walking vs. cycling vs. control) and volume (high vs. moderate vs. low vs. control) on HRV parameters. If known confounders, such as age or BF%, differed between groups, analysis of covariance (ANCOVA) was performed using the significant confounder (e.g., age of BF%) as a covariate. The estimate of effect size was assessed for all parameters. *P*-values < 0.05 were considered statistically significant.

3. Results

Results based on activity type are presented in Table 1. There were no significant differences between groups for age or BF%. Although mean values for all time- and frequency-domain HRV parameters were higher for walking and cycling groups relative to the control group (or lower for LF/HF), there were no statistically significant differences between groups.

Table 1. Comparison between physical activity types (walking, cycling, non-active control) for time- and frequency-domain parameters.

Parameters	Walking	Cycling	Non-Active	Effect Size	*P*-Value
N	27	24	24		
Age	38.0 ± 8.4	39.3 ± 7.5	35.5 ± 4.4	0.047	0.180
Fat (%)	24.4 ± 6.1	22.4 ± 4.9	25.7 ± 4.6	0.061	0.105
Ln-RR interval (sec)	1.05(0.91–1.12)	1.06 (1.0–1.1)	0.99 (0.92–1.1)	0.035	0.292
Ln-SDNN (ms)	53.3(31.1–69.9)	52.6(35.7–73.8)	45.8(37.9–54.9)	0.017	0.563
Ln-RMSSD (ms)	47.5(26.9–71.2)	39.4 (31.9–60.4)	35.2 (22.1–46.5)	0.039	0.250
Ln-LF (ms^2)	918(246–2110)	764(230–1838)	594(414–1069)	0.009	0.765
Ln-HF (ms^2)	786(310–2444)	609(345–1352)	408(223–1937)	0.038	0.317
Ln-LF/HF ratio	0.88(0.45–1.2)	0.76 (0.53–1.3)	1.07 (0.70–2.01)	0.025	0.464

Note: Data presented as mean ± SD for normal variables or median (25th–75th) percentile for non-normal variables; *P*-values < 0.05 considered significant.

Results based on PA volume are presented in Table 2. There was no significant effect for BF%. However, age significantly differed between groups. Therefore, age-adjusted values were determined for HRV parameters. The time-domain analysis showed that after controlling for age, SDNN for the high-active group was significantly greater than the low-active group ($P < 0.05$). In addition, RMSSD for the moderate-active group was significantly greater than the control group ($P < 0.01$). For the frequency domain, LF for the high-active group was significantly greater than the low-active and control groups ($P < 0.01$). Additionally, HF for the moderate-active group was significantly greater than the low-active group ($P < 0.05$). There were no significant differences between the moderate- and high-active groups or between the low- and inactive control groups for all variables. No between-group differences were observed for the R–R interval or LF/HF ratio ($P > 0.05$).

Table 2. Comparison of physical activity (PA) volume between groups (low-, moderate-, high-, and non-active control) for time- and frequency-domain parameters.

Parameters	Volume of Physical Activity				Effect Size	*P*-Value	Adjusted for Age
	Low	Moderate	High	Control			
N	13	24	14	24			
Age	33.3 ± 9.3	40.0 ± 7.4^A	41.1 ± 5.0^A	35.5 ± 4.4	0.174	0.003	
Fat (%)	23.4 ± 7.0	23.9 ± 4.9	22.6 ± 5.6	25.7 ± 4.6	0.054	0.349	0.279
Ln-RR interval (sec)	1.0 (0.9–1.1)	1.08 (0.9–1.1)	1.06 (1.01–1.12)	0.99 (0.92–1.08)	0.096	0.074	0.201
Ln-SDNN (ms)	41.9 (30.9–63.3)	52.9 (32.2–69.9)	67.3 (44.1–77.9)^A	45.8 (37.9–54.9)	0.079	0.135	0.025
Ln-RMSSD (ms)	32.6(18.6–52.9)	47.7 (35.3–69.6)	44.0 (32.5–73.1)	35.2 (22.1–46.5)^B	0.066	0.198	0.009
Ln-LF (ms^2)	338.7(196.6–764)	790 (203–2110)	1759(922–4942)^A	594 (414–1069)^C	0.183	0.006	< 0.001
Ln-HF (ms^2)	481 (151.7–832)	676 (365–4347)^A	838 (391–3109)	406 (223–1189)	0.163	0.014	0.004
Ln-LF/HF ratio	0.73 (0.46–1.18)	0.75 (0.40–0.95)	1.19 (0.59–2.1)	1.07 (0.70–2.01)	0.103	0.092	0.096

Note: Data presented as mean ± SD for normal variables or median (25th–75th) percentile for non-normal variables; $P < 0.05$ was considered statistically significant. ^{A} represents a significant difference relative to the low-active group; ^{B} represents a significant difference relative to the moderately-active group; and ^{C} represents a significant difference relative to the high-active group.

4. Discussion

This study evaluated differences in HRV based on the type and volume of PA among Arab men. In disagreement with our first hypothesis, there were no significant differences between walking, cycling, and inactive control groups for all indices of HRV. In agreement with our second hypothesis, significant differences were observed between groups based on PA volume, independent of known confounders such as age and body fat. These findings suggest that the volume of PA could be an important determinant of HRV in recreationally active Saudi-Arabian men, regardless of PA type.

Unexpectedly, HRV parameters did not differ between active and inactive groups (Table 1). Conflicting findings have been reported within the available literature. For example, some studies have shown no differences in HRV between active and in active groups [17,18], while others found differences favoring active groups [19,20]. Some investigations have reported that even low PA can improve HRV to a greater extent than being sedentary. For example, a cross-sectional study of 84 adults suggested that aerobic exercise increased vagal HRV for all levels of PA [21]. Another investigation compared HRV between a sedentary group and two middle-aged groups with equivalent weekly PA energy expenditure, but different intensities. They found that HRV indices were greater in the two active groups compared to the sedentary group [20]. A recent study showed that even slight increments in PA are beneficial for cardiac autonomic regulation among young men, as RMSSD significantly increased according to PA categories from low, moderate, high, to highest. The multivariable linear regression analysis showed a significant positive relationship between self-reported PA and Ln-RMSSD, independent of BMI, waist circumference and BF% [22]. In short, we found no differences between active and inactive groups, which may be explained by the considerable heterogeneity in PA volume among active groups, which was subsequently found to account for differences in HRV (Table 2). In addition, despite being described as inactive controls, this group exhibited similar BF% values relative to both walking and cycling groups (Table 1). This may indicate comparable metabolic health profiles among groups, which may also help explain a lack of between-group differences in HRV [23].

As hypothesized, we observed significant between-group differences in HRV based on PA volume classifications (Table 2). This finding is in agreement with several previous studies. For example, a systematic review reported positive associations between moderate-to-vigorous PA and RMSSD [24]. In a study that measured HRV over five consecutive days in 37 men with a mean age of 33 years, participants were categorized as having low, medium, or high self-reported PA. Significantly higher HRV (Ln-RMSSD, R–R interval) was observed in the moderate- and high-PA groups compared with the low PA group [19]. Similarly, we found that recreationally moderate- and high-PA groups showed comparable levels of time- and frequency-domain HRV. Likewise, inactive and low-active groups showed comparable levels of time- and frequency-domain HRV, which were significantly lower than either moderate- or high- active groups.

Our findings indicate that walking up to 150 km per month, or cycling up to 100 km per month at a speed slower than 20 km/h, were insufficient for improving HRV in the current population. This finding suggests that a PA volume- or intensity-related threshold likely exists that must be met to improve HRV. In support of this postulation regarding intensity, a recent investigation demonstrated a dose–response relationship for the effects of very vigorous PA (>8 metabolic equivalents) on HRV in 1040 adult men and women [25]. Participants were stratified into quintiles according to min per week of very vigorous PA. Group 5 was greater than Groups 1–3, but did not differ from Group 4 in any HRV indices, suggesting similar effects at the top quantiles of very vigorous PA [25]. The volume of PA that improves physical fitness and health markers such as body composition and blood pressure has been described based on pedometer-derived daily step counts [26], or intensity and duration of PA per week (e.g., 75 to 150 minutes of high-intensity PA and 150 to 300 minutes of moderate-intensity PA) [27]. However, the volume of PA that improves HRV is less clearly defined. Thus, further research is needed to determine volume-based thresholds for PA that increases HRV, particularly for members of the population where higher intensity exercise may be contraindicated.

The main limitation of the current study was that we did not measure the intensity of walking. This factor has been addressed in many previous studies. For example, a five-year follow up from a large prospective study showed that walking distance and pace were positively associated with higher SDNN and ultra LF power [28]. It was also found that walking pace may contribute to less erratic sinus patterns and lower cardiovascular mortality, whereas general total leisure activity time did not show a similar association [28]. In another investigation, leisure-time PA, quantified as the hours of metabolic equivalent per week (MET.hr/week), and five-minute HRV were recorded for adults. There were significant linear trends of higher LF power with the highest quartile of vigorous activity, and lower HR with increasing quartile of moderate activity, suggesting that vigorous activity showed a possible mechanism by which PA reduces coronary heart disease risk [29].

In conclusion, the current study found that HRV among regular walking and cycling groups did not significantly differ from age- and body fat-matched inactive controls. However, when stratified by PA volume, greater HRV parameters were observed among moderate- and high-PA groups. From a practical perspective, the current findings indicate that walking >150 km per month, or cycling >100 km per month at a speed >20 km/h, may be necessary to derive cardiac autonomic benefits from PA. While further investigation is needed to identify more specific volume-related thresholds for improving HRV, these PA benchmarks may provide practical aiming points for healthy adult men seeking to improve cardiovascular health.

Ethical Approval: All procedures performed in studies involving human participants were in accordance with the ethical standards of the institutional and/or national research committee (King Saud University, IRB no. E-18-3381) and with the 1964 Helsinki declaration and its later amendments or comparable ethical standards.

Author Contributions: Conceptualization, S.A., A.F., J.K., A.A. and S.S.H.; methodology, S.A., A.A.F., and J.K.; formal analysis, S.A., A.A., and S.S.H.; investigation, S.A., and J.K.; resources, S.A. and A.A.; data curation, J.K. and A.A.; writing—original draft preparation, S.A., A.A.F., and A.A.; writing—review and editing, S.A., A.A.F., and S.S.H.; project administration, S.A.; funding acquisition, S.A. All authors have read and agreed to the published version of the manuscript.

Funding: The authors extend their appreciation to the International Scientific Partnership Program (ISPP) at King Saud University for funding this research work through ISPP - 141.

Acknowledgments: The authors are highly grateful to the Riyadh walkers and Saudi cyclists who contributed to the study by contacting their members. Thanks go to all participants and research assistants particularly Ahmed Al Gazwani, Ahmed Sunbea, Abdulrahman Al Shebl and Ali Al Dakkan.

Conflicts of Interest: The authors declare no conflict of interest.

References

1. Aubert, A.; Seps, B.; Beckers, F. Heart rate variability in athletes. *Sports Med.* **2003**, *33*, 889–919. [CrossRef] [PubMed]
2. Sondermeijer, H.P.; van Marle, A.G.; Kamen, P.; Krum, H. Acute effects of caffeine on heart rate variability. *Am. J. Cardiol.* **2002**, *90*, 906–907. [CrossRef]
3. Jarczok, M.N.; Koenig, J.; Wittling, A.; Fischer, J.E.; Thayer, J.F. First evaluation of an index of low vagally-mediated heart rate variability as a marker of health risks in human adults: Proof of concept. *J. Clin. Med.* **2019**, *8*, 1940. [CrossRef] [PubMed]
4. Force, T. Heart rate variability: Standards of measurement, physiological interpretation, and clinical use. task force of the European society of cardiology the north American society of pacing electrophysiology. *Circulation* **1996**, *93*, 1043–1065.
5. Yeragani, V.K.; Krishnan, S.; Engels, H.J.; Gretebeck, R. Effects of caffeine on linear and nonlinear measures of heart rate variability before and after exercise. *Depress. Anxiety* **2005**, *21*, 130–134. [CrossRef]
6. Garber, C.E.; Blissmer, B.; Deschenes, M.R.; Franklin, B.A.; Lamonte, M.J.; Lee, I.-M.; Nieman, D.C.; Swain, D.P. American college of sports medicine position stand. Quantity and quality of exercise for developing and maintaining cardiorespiratory, musculoskeletal, and neuromotor fitness in apparently healthy adults: Guidance for prescribing exercise. *Med. Sci. Sports Exerc.* **2011**, *43*, 1334–1359. [CrossRef]

7. Bonato, M.; Meloni, A.; Merati, G.; La Torre, A.; Agnello, L.; Vernillo, G. Effect of repeated-sprints on the reliability of short-term parasympathetic reactivation. *PLoS ONE* **2018**, *13*, e0192231. [CrossRef]
8. Fronchetti, L.; Nakamura, F.; De-Oliveira, F.; Lima-Silva, A.; De Lima, J. Effects of high-intensity interval training on heart rate variability during exercise. *J. Exerc. Physiol. Online* **2007**, *10*, 1–9.
9. Boutcher, S.H.; Stein, P. Association between heart rate variability and training response in sedentary middle-aged men. *Eur. J. Appl. Physiol. Occup. Physiol.* **1995**, *70*, 75–80. [CrossRef]
10. Perini, R.; Fisher, N.; Veicsteinas, A.; Pendergast, D. Aerobic training and cardiovascular responses at rest and during exercise in older men and women. *Med. Sci. Sports Exerc.* **2002**, *34*, 700–708.
11. Bonato, M.; Agnello, L.; Galasso, L.; Montaruli, A.; Roveda, E.; Merati, G.; La Torre, A.; Vitale, J.A. Acute modification of cardiac autonomic function of high-intensity interval training in collegiate male soccer players with different chronotype: A cross-over study. *J. Sports Sci. Med.* **2017**, *16*, 286. [PubMed]
12. Vitale, J.A.; Bonato, M.; La Torre, A.; Banfi, G. Heart rate variability in sport performance: Do time of day and chronotype play a role? *J. Clin. Med.* **2019**, *8*, 723. [CrossRef] [PubMed]
13. Sharma, V.K.; Subramanian, S.K.; Radhakrishnan, K.; Rajendran, R.; Ravindran, B.S.; Arunachalam, V. Comparison of structured and unstructured physical activity training on predicted VO2max and heart rate variability in adolescents–a randomized control trial. *J. Basic Clin. Physiol. Pharmacol.* **2017**, *28*, 225–238. [CrossRef] [PubMed]
14. Williams, E.D.; Steptoe, A.; Chambers, J.C.; Kooner, J.S. Ethnic and gender differences in the relationship between hostility and metabolic and autonomic risk factors for coronary heart disease. *Psychosom. Med.* **2011**, *73*, 53–58. [CrossRef]
15. Hill, L.K.; Hu, D.D.; Koenig, J.; Sollers III, J.J.; Kapuku, G.; Wang, X.; Snieder, H.; Thayer, J.F. Ethnic differences in resting heart rate variability: A systematic review and meta-analysis. *Psychosom. Med.* **2015**, *77*, 16. [CrossRef]
16. Al-Fehaid, A.F.; Alkahtani, S.A.; Al-Sunni, A.A.; Yar, T. Role of the work-to-rest ratio in high-intensity interval exercise on heart rate variability and blood pressure in sedentary obese men. *Saudi J. Health Sci.* **2018**, *7*, 83.
17. Loimaala, A.; Huikuri, H.; Oja, P.; Pasanen, M.; Vuori, I. Controlled 5-mo aerobic training improves heart rate but not heart rate variability or baroreflex sensitivity. *J. Appl. Physiol.* **2000**, *89*, 1825–1829. [CrossRef]
18. Migliaro, E.; Contreras, P.; Bech, S.; Etxagibel, A.; Castro, M.; Ricca, R.; Vicente, K. Relative influence of age, resting heart rate and sedentary life style in short-term analysis of heart rate variability. *Braz. J. Med Biol. Res.* **2001**, *34*, 493–500. [CrossRef]
19. Melanson, E.L. Resting heart rate variability in men varying in habitual physical activity. *Med. Sci. Sports Exerc.* **2000**, *32*, 1894–1901. [CrossRef]
20. Buchheit, M.; Simon, C.; Charloux, A.; Doutreleau, S.; Piquard, F.; Brandenberger, G. Heart rate variability and intensity of habitual physical activity in middle-aged persons. *Med. Sci. Sports Exerc.* **2005**, *37*, 1530–1534. [CrossRef]
21. Soares-Miranda, L.; Sandercock, G.; Valente, H.; Vale, S.; Santos, R.; Mota, J. Vigorous physical activity and vagal modulation in young adults. *Eur. J. Cardiovasc. Prev. Rehabil.* **2009**, *16*, 705–711. [CrossRef]
22. Tornberg, J.; Ikäheimo, T.M.; Kiviniemi, A.; Pyky, R.; Hautala, A.; Mäntysaari, M.; Jämsä, T.; Korpelainen, R. Physical activity is associated with cardiac autonomic function in adolescent men. *PLoS ONE* **2019**, *14*, e0222121. [CrossRef] [PubMed]
23. Yoo, H.J.; Hwang, S.Y.; Choi, K.M.; Baik, S.H.; Lee, E.M.; Kim, E.J.; Rha, S.-W.; Park, C.G.; Oh, D.J.; Seo, H.S. Clinical implication of body size phenotype on heart rate variability. *Metabolism* **2016**, *65*, 1589–1596. [CrossRef] [PubMed]
24. Oliveira, R.S.; Barker, A.R.; Wilkinson, K.M.; Abbott, R.A.; Williams, C.A. Is cardiac autonomic function associated with cardiorespiratory fitness and physical activity in children and adolescents? A systematic review of cross-sectional studies. *Int. J. Cardiol.* **2017**, *236*, 113–122. [CrossRef] [PubMed]
25. De Sousa, T.L.W.; Ostoli, T.L.V.d.P.; Sperandio, E.F.; Arantes, R.L.; Gagliardi, A.R.d.T.; Romiti, M.; da Silva, R.P.; Dourado, V.Z. Dose-response relationship between very vigorous physical activity and cardiovascular health assessed by heart rate variability in adults: Cross-sectional results from the EPIMOV study. *PLoS ONE* **2019**, *14*, e0210216. [CrossRef] [PubMed]
26. Bravata, D.M.; Smith-Spangler, C.; Sundaram, V.; Gienger, A.L.; Lin, N.; Lewis, R.; Stave, C.D.; Olkin, I.; Sirard, J.R. Using pedometers to increase physical activity and improve health: A systematic review. *JAMA* **2007**, *298*, 2296–2304. [CrossRef] [PubMed]

27. Piercy, K.L.; Troiano, R.P.; Ballard, R.M.; Carlson, S.A.; Fulton, J.E.; Galuska, D.A.; George, S.M.; Olson, R.D. The physical activity guidelines for Americans. *JAMA* **2018**, *320*, 2020–2028. [CrossRef]
28. Soares-Miranda, L.; Sattelmair, J.; Chaves, P.; Duncan, G.E.; Siscovick, D.S.; Stein, P.K.; Mozaffarian, D. Physical activity and heart rate variability in older adults: The Cardiovascular Health Study. *Circulation* **2014**, *129*, 2100–2110. [CrossRef]
29. Rennie, K.L.; Hemingway, H.; Kumari, M.; Brunner, E.; Malik, M.; Marmot, M. Effects of moderate and vigorous physical activity on heart rate variability in a British study of civil servants. *Am. J. Epidemiol.* **2003**, *158*, 135–143. [CrossRef]

International Journal of
Environmental Research and Public Health

MDPI

Article

Systematic Observation of the Verbal Behavior of Families of Youth Athletes in Grassroots and Team Sports

Elisa I. Sánchez-Romero [1,*], Francisco J. Ponseti Verdaguer [2], Pere A. Borràs [2] and Alejandro García-Mas [3]

1 Department of Social, Legal and Business Sciences, Catholic University of Murcia (UCAM), 30107 Murcia, Spain
2 Department of Pedagogy, University of the Balearic Islands, 07122 Palma, Spain; xponseti@uib.es (F.J.P.V.); pa-borras@uib.es (P.A.B.)
3 Department of Psychology, University of the Balearic Islands, 07122 Palma, Spain; alex.garcia@uib.es
* Correspondence: eisanchez@ucam.edu; Tel.: +34-968278181

Received: 9 January 2020; Accepted: 15 February 2020; Published: 17 February 2020

Abstract: Some of the more protective and favorable factors for the development and health in children and teenagers are family and sport, so family involvement in the children's sports activities is vital in their sports process. The purpose of this study was to analyze the verbal behavior (positive, negative, and neutral comments) of family spectators of school-age athletes regarding sociodemographic and sporting variables. The sample consisted of 190 family spectators of 215 male and female (M_{age} = 11.66; SD = 1.60) football, basketball, and volleyball players. The Parents' Observation Instrument at Sport Events (POISE) was used for the observation and LINCE was used to codify the verbal comments made. After registering 38,829 comments, the results showed statistically significant differences in relation to the comments made and the gender of athletes, geographical area, kind of sport, and the sporting category. The findings highlight that in a competitive environment, the comments made by spectators related to athletes do not seem to be initiators of potentially violent situations but rather are dependent on the atmosphere in question. Further research is required in this area to foster positive conduct relating to grassroots sports.

Keywords: physical activity; grassroots sports; clubs sports; school sport; families; spectators; verbal behavior; competitive environment

1. Introduction

In recent years, family participation in grassroots sport has increased significantly [1,2], so that the verbal behavior of parents is the main method of family participation in children's sporting events [3]. In this sense, one of the consequences is the increase of inappropriate comments by family members and spectators [4]. Thus, Walters et al. [5] recorded over ten thousand verbal comments made by coaches in grassroots sports, of which 35.4% were positive, 21.6% negative, and 43% neutral. The media has also recorded an increase in aggressive behavior and/or violence in sport [6,7]. In this regard, several studies have observed parents that incite aggressiveness in the playing field [8], authoritarian parents who severely sanctioned children in the case of not winning [9], and even parents who exercise violent behavior in the sports field [10,11].

The comments made and the behavior and attitudes shown have an influence on the wellbeing and future performance of athletes [12]. Although it has not been possible to establish a cause-and-effect relationship between inappropriate comments and violent behavior in sport, there is no doubt that such inappropriate comments generate an aggressive atmosphere that, on occasions, can lead to violent behavior. Parental and spectator pressure in games and matches may cause athletes to doubt their moral decisions on behavior, in line with the ethical foundations of the sport [13]. Parents are the most relevant socioeducational agents in sport, so the most successful athletes received more support from their parents [14,15]. Positive parental behavior toward the sporting activity of their children has been found to be associated with the attainment of the values of the sport transmitted by parents [16], evidencing that the family participation in the sports practiced by their children is vital in the sporting process of young athletes [17]. Thus, Witt and Dangi [18] suggest undertaking an intervention with parents to help them to be better s9pectators and, therefore, not to negatively affect performance or athlete attitudes. With the aim of optimizing the integral and sport development of young athletes, these kinds of programs are highly beneficial in sport, given that families are key elements in terms of their influence on athletes, both in a personal and sporting sense [19].

Hence, the aim of this study was to analyze the verbal behavior (categorized into three kinds of comments: positive, negative, and neutral) of family spectators of school-age (9–15 years old) sports teams as well as to study potential sociodemographic and sport-related differences (sex of player, geographical area, sports club, sport modality, and age group). According to previous studies [20–23], the preliminary hypothesis is: (1) the number of negative comments made in matches played in rural areas will be greater than the number recorded in urban areas; (2) in the verbal behavior of family spectators at basketball games, there will be a higher number of comments (positive, negative, and neutral) compared with the other sports analyzed; and, (3) the number of negative comments made by family spectators will rise as the sporting category increases.

2. Materials and Methods

2.1. Design

This study corresponds to a predictive correlational design. The possible influence of certain demographic and sporting variables in the verbal behavior of the athletes' relatives who were watching the matches or games of the grassroots sports teams was measured. The study design allows collecting data and describes connections between two or more variables at a specific point in time [24]. Furthermore, these research designs offer efficiency in the collection of extensive data on a particular subject, while obtaining highly realistic content, which is inherently appealing in solving practical problems. As such, this kind of research design is rarely criticized for being artificial [25]. Therefore, non participant systematic observation was used as a data collection technique [20]. The observation technique is widely used and accepted in studying changeable social problems in a context of spontaneousness or naturalness of the behavior observed [20,26–29].

2.2. Participants

One hundred and ninety spectators (64 male, 33.7%; 126 female, 66.3%) of 215 athletes of both sexes (164 male, 74.3%; 51 female, 23.7%), aged between 9 and 15 years (M = 11.66 years old; SD = 1.60), participated in this study. All athletes belonged to 11 sports clubs (68.2% in urban areas; 31.8% rural areas), three grassroots sports: football (50.7%), basketball (14%), volleyball (35.3%), established in different categories: Under-11s (34.4%), Under-13s (49.8%), and Under-16s (15.8%).

Ethical Considerations

Authorization to conduct the research was granted by the Regional Government of the Balearic Islands (Spain) in its project, Posam Valors a l'esporty. Furthermore, the Department of Physical Education and Sport of the University of the Balearic Islands (UIB) contacted the different corresponding federations to obtain their authorization and that of their clubs.

This study analyzes the verbal behavior of human beings and, as such, it must meet the ethical principles of respect for human dignity, confidentiality, and non-discrimination. A favorable report by the ethics committee of the University of the Balearic Islands (UIB-93CER18) has been obtained regarding the conducting of this study. Therefore, this study was undertaken in accordance with the 1975 Declaration of Helsinki, revised in 2000.

2.3. Instruments

To measure the verbal behavior of the participants, two instruments were used: one for the observation and another to code the behavior observed. Furthermore, sociodemographic and sporting data were asked by researchers (geographical area, sex, sports club, the kind of sport, and sporting category).

To observe the comments made, the Parents' Observational Instrument at Sport Events (POISE) [30] was used. Designed to register the verbal behavior of spectators at sports events, it comprises four areas of observation: (1) Nature of the comment (positive, neutral, negative) (Table 1); (2) Target of the comment (players, teams, coaches, officials, other parents, children, spectators, individuals); (3) Event unfolding (ball in play-goal-penalty); and (4) Match or game result (win, loss). It includes a categorization of possible kinds of behavior for each area observed (this study focused on area of observation 1: Nature of the verbal comment made (positive, neutral, negative) and area 4: The match or game result, although it was extended to sporting performance measured in the final classification (low, medium, high). This instrument has an inter-observer and intra-observer reliability rate of 92% and 97%, respectively [31].

To code the comments of family spectators, LINCE [32] was used. LINCE is a coding software that provides computerized procedures in observation methods, facilitating the registering of match actions or spectator comments during the visualization of different match recordings on the same screen. LINCE also helps to simultaneously code match actions and comments to verify the quality of observer data and to export the results obtained to other computer programs for additional analysis [33].

Furthermore, all the match recordings were made using a Toshiba Camileo X-200 video camera (Toshiba Europe GmbH, Madrid, Spain).

Table 1. Categories of the kind of comments made by family spectators [30].

Positive	Neutral	Negative
- Reinforcing: comments aimed at reinforcing and supporting the behavior of athletes (e.g., "well done"). - Hustle: done with the aim of encouraging athletes so that they improve performance (e.g., "go on, go on, go on").	- Instructing: telling players what to do (e.g., "play up the field/court"). - Direct question (e.g., "Do you want to come off?"). - Indirect question: aimed at a player, but not relating to the event (e.g., "Who will be at training next week?"). - Rhetorical question: one that does not require a response (e.g., "Where was the movement today?"). - Social: any comment not related to the event (e.g., "Let's get a coffee later"). - Other: any other comment that does not fit into another category.	- Correction: comments changing specific behavior. The comment is usually directly related to the subject (e.g., "John, arms up"). - A telling off: a comment indicating that the performance was not good enough. Comments displeasure with the circumstance (e.g., "Don't sit there, get up"). - Witticism: a comment that often involves sarcasm or ridicule (e.g., "Your dad could hit it better than that"). - Contradicting: comments that could vary and that players could find confusing ("hit the ball toward the center. You should have hit it to the right-hand side!").

2.4. Procedure

To analyze the verbal comments of family spectators in the stands at matches, 22 observations were carried out through the POISE, which made one recording per match. It took twenty-two hours and twenty minutes (1332 min) to complete the observation from the stands at the matches of different sports: football (U11s, 60 min; U13s, 72 min); basketball (48 min); and volleyball (average of 60 min per match).

One of the researchers captured all the entries with a video camera. The researcher only registered audio recordings of the comments made by family spectators at matches and games. Furthermore, if any family member watching the match or game had an issue with the presence of the video camera, the researcher reminded them of the main aim of the study. In terms of the recordings, the researcher was careful to be positioned between the fans of both clubs, depending on the team to be recorded. The researcher always arrived 15 min before the start of each match to detect the location of the family spectators of both teams.

2.5. Statistical Analysis

All the statistical analyses were conducted using the SPSS program (IBM, SPSS v.22.0, Armonk, NY, USA). After the verbal behavior of family spectators was registered, it was coded and tabulated to represent the nature of the comments made (positive, neutral, negative). To establish the prevalence of the variable under the study, descriptive statistics (average and standard deviation) and the percentage of comments made by family spectators at grassroots sports team matches and games were calculated. Furthermore, Pearson's Chi-squared (χ^2) distribution was used to compare the division of categorical variables into three sports. The Poisson regression model was used to estimate the comments according to the variables to compare: geographic area, sex of the player, sports club, kind of sport practiced, sporting category, and sport performance (using the Wald Chi-Squared Test or the Wald χ^2 test). For all statistical tests, the level adopted for significance was a two-tailed $p < 0.05$. The effects of the variables of the geographical area, sex of the player, sports club, kind of sport practiced, sporting category, and sports performance in the ratio of comments made by family spectators were also analyzed through the Poisson regression model.

3. Results

3.1. Prevalence of the Comments Made by Family Spectators

The total of all the comments made per sport is set out in Table 2. A total of 38829 were registered in 22 matches or games observed (11 football, 4 basketball, 7 volleyball) at a rate of 29.15 (95% confidence interval (CI): 22.45–37.82) comments per minute (ratio). The highest number of registered comments made by family spectators at matches or games corresponded to football (n = 18,024), which also had a higher play-observation time (720 min), followed by volleyball (n = 12527; 420 min) and, lastly, basketball games, with the lowest rate (n = 8278; 192 min). However, the highest number of comments per minute was registered in basketball matches (43.10; 95% CI: 10.92–75.58), followed by volleyball games (29.83; 95% CI: 16.04–43.67), and lastly by football matches (25.03; 95% CI: 14.28–36.81). That said, no statistically significant differences were observed between the number of comments made per minute (ratio) in the three sports observed (Wald $\chi^2_{(2)}$ test (n = 22) = 2.42, $p > 0.05$).

Table 2. Games and matches, comments, minutes, and ratio of comments observed per minute.

Sport	Matches/Games	Comments	Minutes	Ratio * (95% CI)
Football	11	18024	720	25.03 (14.28–36.81)
Basketball	4	8278	192	43.10 (10.92–75.58)
Volleyball	7	12527	420	29.83 (16.04–43.67)
Total	22	38829	1332	29.15 (22.45–37.82)

* Comments per minute.

In terms of the nature (positive, neutral, negative) of all the comments made, the highest rate corresponded to neutral comments (n = 21081; 54.29%), followed by positive comments (n = 13053; 33.62%) and, lastly, negative comments (n = 4695; 12.09%). After establishing the comments made according to their nature and classifying them by sport, volleyball registered the highest percentage of neutral comments (n = 7153; 57.10%) and a lower rate of negative comments (n = 1346; 10.74%) compared with the other sports observed. The sport that registered the highest percentage of positive comments was football (n = 6427; 35.66%), while basketball registered the highest number of negative comments (n = 1194; 14.43%) (Table 3). In this respect, statistically significant differences were detected between the comments made by family spectators (positive, neutral, negative), according to the sport of the matches or games observed (Pearson's $\chi^2_{(4)}$ test (n = 38829) = 44.00, $p < 0.001$; Cramer's V = 1.00, $p < 0.001$).

Table 3. Average, standard deviation, number, and percentage of comments (according to their nature and established by sport).

	Comments						
	Positive		Neutral		Negative		Total
Sport	*M* ± *SD*	*n* (%)	*M* ± *SD*	*n* (%)	*M* ± *SD*	*n* (%)	*n* (%)
Football	9.09 ± 4.23	6427 (35.66%)	3.18 ± 4.07	9442 (52.39%)	13.18 ± 10.90	2155 (11.96%)	18024
Basketball	13.75 ± 6.13	2598 (31.39%)	6.25 ± 6.19	4486 (54.20%)	23.25 ± 9.18	1194 (14.43%)	8278
Volleyball	9.57 ± 5.06	4028 (32.15%)	3.14 ± 2.61	7153 (57.10%)	17.14 ± 9.19	1346 (10.74%)	12527
Total	10.09 ± 4.94	13053 (33.62%)	3.73 ± 4.10	21081 (54.29%)	16.27 ± 10.36	4695 (12.09%)	38829

3.2. *Effects of the Variables in the Positive Comments Made by Family Spectators*

After conducting the Poisson regression analysis (n = 22), statistically significant differences were detected in the relationship between the variable of positive comments made by family spectators and that of the kind of sport practiced (Wald $\chi^2_{(2)}$ test = 6.50, $p < 0.05$).

With regard to the kind of sport practiced (football, basketball, or volleyball), using football as the point of reference, the incidence rate [Exp (β)] of positive comments was 1.51 (95% CI: 1.09–2.10) for basketball. That entails that when basketball games were played, the rate of positive comments made by family spectators increased 51% on average compared with football matches.

However, no statistical differences were detected in relation to the variable of positive comments made by family spectators and the geographical area variable (Wald $\chi^2_{(1)}$ test = 0.04, $p > 0.05$), the variable of the sex of players (Wald $\chi^2_{(1)}$ test = 2.47, $p > 0.05$), the sporting category variable (Wald $\chi^2_{(2)}$ test = 6.35, $p > 0.05$), and the sports club variable (Wald $\chi^2_{(10)}$ test = 24.27, $p > 0.05$).

3.3. *Effects of the Variables in the Neutral Comments Made by Family Spectators*

The Poisson regression analysis (n = 22) produced statistically significant differences in the relationship between the variable of neutral comments made by family spectators and: (1) the variable of sex of the players (Wald $\chi^2_{(1)}$ test = 8.05, $p < 0.05$); (2) the sporting category variable (Wald $\chi^2_{(2)}$ test = 7.80, $p < 0.05$); and (3) the sport practiced variable (Wald $\chi^2_{(2)}$ test = 8.04, $p < 0.05$).

With regard to the sex of players, using the male sex as a reference, the incidence rate [Exp (β)] of neutral comments was 1.89 (95% CI: 1.22–2.93) in female matches and games. That means that when female teams played, the rate of neutral comments made by family spectators increased 89% on average compared with football matches played by male teams.

In terms of sporting category (U11s, U13s, and U16s), using the U11s as a reference category, the incidence rate [Exp (β)] of neutral comments was 0.18 (95% CI: 0.04–0.77) for the U16s. That means that in U16 matches or games, the rate of neutral comments made by family spectators fell 82% on average compared with those of the U11s.

With regard to the kind of sport practiced (football, basketball, or volleyball), using football as the reference category, the incidence rate [Exp (β)] of positive comments was 1.96 (95% CI: 1.18–3.28) for basketball. That means that when basketball games were played, the rate of neutral comments made by family spectators increased 96% on average compared with football matches.

No statistically significant differences were detected in the relationship between the neutral comments of family spectators and the geographical area variable (Wald $\chi^2_{(1)}$ test = 0.05, $p > 0.05$) and the sports club variable (Wald $\chi^2_{(10)}$ test = 23.34, $p > 0.05$).

3.4. Effects of the Variables in the Negative Comments Made by Family Spectators

After undertaking the Poisson regression analysis ($n = 22$), statistically significant differences were detected in the relationship between the variable of negative comments made by family spectators and: (1) the geographical area variable (Wald $\chi^2_{(1)}$ test = 15.62, $p < 0.001$); (2) the sporting category variable (Wald $\chi^2_{(2)}$ test = 15.75, $p < 0.001$); and (3) the sport practiced variable (Wald $\chi^2_{(2)}$ test = 18.38, $p < 0.001$).

In terms of the geographical area (urban and rural areas), using the urban areas the reference category, the incidence rate [Exp (β)] of negative comments was 1.53 (95% CI: 1.24–1.89) in games or matches played in urban area. That means that when the games or matches were played in rural areas, the rate of negative comments made by family spectators increased 53% on average compared with the games or matches in urban areas.

In terms of the sporting category (U11s, U13s, and U16s), using the U11s as a reference, the incidence rate [Exp (β)] of negative comments was 1.28 (95% CI: 1.02–1.66) for the U13s. In this regard, when U13 games or matches were played, the rate of negative comments made by family spectators increased 28% on average compared with U11 games or matches.

With regard to the kind of sport practiced (football, basketball, or volleyball), using football as the reference category, the incidence rate [Exp (β)] of negative comments was 1.76 (95% CI: 1.40–2.29) for basketball. As such, when basketball games were played, the rate of negative comments made by family spectators increased by 76% on average compared with football matches.

However, no statistically significant differences were detected in relation to the variable of negative comments of family spectators, the variable of sex of the players (Wald $\chi^2_{(1)}$ test = 2.51, $p > 0.05$), and the sports club variable (Wald $\chi^2_{(10)}$ test = 75.81, $p > 0.05$).

4. Discussion

The aim of this study was to analyze the verbal behavior (categorized into three kinds of comments: positive, negative, and neutral) of family spectators of school-age (9–15 years old) sports teams as well as to study potential sociodemographic and sport-related differences (sex of player, geographical area, sports club, sport modality, and age group).

The results obtained allow us to ensure that hypothesis 1 has been confirmed. In effect, there are statistically significant differences in the negative comments made, according to the geographical area variable, with a 53% increase in games and matches in rural areas. In this sense, it coincides with previous authors [20], who have concluded that the sociocultural context is an important variable between the behavior of spectators at sporting events and how sporting success is interpreted. The reason is due to the urban areas are characterized by having a higher population density and human diversity. Conversely, in rural areas availability, people manage to create and develop a sense of belonging to the territory. Moreover, results have shown that, according to previous studies [20], some clear connections between the comments made by family spectators and the sport atmosphere.

Furthermore, the second hypothesis has been confirmed, because in basketball the most of comments were negative, in contrast with previous studies about other psychosocial factors [21,22]. Moreover, a higher percentage of comments was observed (51% positive; 96% neutral; and 76% negative) compared with the other sports, showing statistically significant differences. Basketball is a sport in which there is constant physical contact between players, as well as blocks, and covering with and without the ball, which leads to numerous heated moments. Furthermore, spectators are very close to the court, which, together, could generate more emotion in the stands, producing a higher number of comments as a result. It is evident, however, that clarification is required on this shift through further studies, as it is still to be "observed" by the general media. Negative comments from parents cause more pressure, insecurity, anxiety, and feelings of guilt, leading to a reduced sporting performance [20], while also may generate negative psychosocial effects in their kids [10].

The third hypothesis was also confirmed, given that statistically significant differences were identified in the negative comments made according to the sporting category (28% more were registered in the U13s than in the U11s category). In contrast with our findings, in recent studies [23,34], no association between the age of athletes and the verbal aggression of spectators was found, related to some theories about [35].

Finally, our results have shown that the comments with the greatest prevalence during games and matches were the neutral ones, followed by positive and, lastly, negative comments, which coincides with Reference [5]. In terms of the kind of sport, the highest percentage of positive comments was in football, while basketball had the highest number of negative comments, contrary to general belief. This "shift" has already been observed in antisocial situations, such as in the willingness to accept gamesmanship and cheating [22]. In terms of the number of comments made per minute (ratio), the highest number was in the basketball games, followed by volleyball games and, lastly, in the football matches. This distribution is fairly similar, excluding the theoretical distances, to the average observations made with the CBAS (Cognitive-Behavioral Approach Skills) regarding coaches and the kind of instructions they give to their players [21].

Limitations and Future Developments

The verbal behavior of family members in the stands is an important form of communication, as it represents their main method of participation in their children's sporting events [3]. These same authors suggest that the description of these kinds of behavior in games and matches could be an aspect of improving knowledge of parent–child relations, as well as the rules and expectations experienced by parents in organized youth sports.

It is important, therefore, to conduct research focused on analyzing not only comments but also the behavior of family members, spectators, and sport-related agents at school-age sports games and matches. The use of non-participant systematic observation in the research provides an approach to social problems in a natural context of observed behavior [20]. To do that, studies based on observation and description of this kind of aspect, as considered in this research, would serve as a starting point from which to discover the current situation regarding the atmosphere that surrounds athletes on the field of play. This kind of studies could also lead to the implementation and development of observation and registration protocols, as well as to their validation, in multiple areas of sport and physical activity, such as fair play in youth football [36], the influence of contextual variables in the efficiency of handball goalkeepers [37], and sports leadership behavior in youth football coaches [22,38].

Furthermore, as suggested by Walters et al. [5], the rate of negative comments observed in all sports is cause for concern, particularly considering the young ages of the child athletes. Even though, in this study, the percentage of negative comments (12.09%) was below those of neutral and positive comments, fostering positive behavior (verbal and non-verbal) in everything that surrounds the physical activity and sport of children is important.

Similarly, analyzing comments according to the sex of family members is an interesting line to consider for future research. However, due to the number of comments registered in this study (n = 38,829), coding this variable was too difficult or challenging. As such, there is the possibility of conducting future observations based on verbal comments (and other variables and aims geared toward their children's sport) of a smaller number of parents, previously selected, and carried out with other data collection techniques, such as semi-structured interviews, like those conducted in Reference [3]. The findings show that when female teams played, the rate of neutral comments made by family spectators significantly increased by 89% on average compared with matches played by male teams. The question of gender, therefore, is a variable to study, due not only to the comments received by female athletes but also to the comments made by male and female in the stands. However, the two future studies that we believe most promising that can be developed in the short term are: 1) take into account the changes in the score of the matches (raw performance) to check if there is a correlation between the result and the typology of the comments of the parents/spectators at any given time [3]; and 2), since it has been proven that the collective efficacy can predict the performance of a team -in semi-professional football players, it would be very interesting to study whether individual and collective effectiveness is modified according to the nature of the comments made from the sideline, considering that it can be understood as one of the basic sources of self-efficacy (verbal persuasion).

5. Conclusions

The main conclusion that can be taken from this study, conducted with a rather complex method of observation in real competition situations, is that the comments made by family spectators do not appear to be "initiators" of potentially violent on-pitch or court situations, but rather they depend on the atmosphere created, which can include group pressure, cognitive dissonance, and involvement. Therefore, from an applied perspective, psychoeducational endeavors, until now exclusively aimed at coaches and parents, should be geared toward the sporting culture and structures of clubs. Club sports participation may be an important component in the promotion of physical fitness and healthy at younger ages [39]. The way in which spectators create their reference framework for interpreting sporting success is mediated by sociocultural context, regarding which the media has an important role to play [25].

Author Contributions: Conceptualization, E.I.S.-R., F.J.P.V., and A.G.-M.; methodology, E.I.S.-R. and F.J.P.V.; software, F.J.P.V. and P.A.B.; formal analysis, E.I.S.-R.; investigation, E.I.S.-R., F.J.P.V., P.A.B., and A.G.-M.; resources, P.A.B. and A.G.-M.; data curation, E.I.S.-R.; writing—original draft preparation, E.I.S.-R. and F.J.P.V.; project administration, P.A.B. and A.G.-M.; funding acquisition, F.J.P.V., P.A.B., and A.G.-M. All authors have read and agreed to the published version of the manuscript.

Funding: This research was funded by the program Erasmus Sport of the project PsyTool—Sport Psychology as a Strategic Tool for Prevention and training on Grassroots Sports (grant numbers: 567199-EPP-1-2015-2-ES-SPO-SCP) and the program Posam Valors a l'Esport (Values in Sport; Conselleria de Transparència, Cultura i Esports. Govern de les Illes Balears).

Conflicts of Interest: The authors declare no conflict of interest.

References

1. Qurban, H.; Wang, J.; Siddique, H.; Morris, T.; Qiao, Z. The mediating role of parental support: The relation between sports participation, self-esteem, and motivation for sports among Chinese students. *Curr. Psychol.* **2019**, *38*, 308–319. [CrossRef]
2. Strandbu, A.; Stefansen, K.; Smette, I.; Sandvik, M.R. Young people's experiences of parental involvement in youth sport. *Sport Educ. Soc.* **2019**, *24*, 66–77.
3. Dorsch, T.E.; Smith, A.L.; Wilson, S.R.; McDonough, M.H. Parent Goals and Verbal Sideline Behavior in Organized Youth Sport. *Sport Exerc. Perform. Psychol.* **2015**, *4*, 19–35. [CrossRef]
4. Alzina, A. Una aproximación histórica a la violencia en el deporte. A historical approach to violence in sport. *Rev. Hum. Cult.* **2019**, *1*, 199–211.
5. Walters, S.R.; Schluter, P.J.; Oldham, A.R.; Thomson, R.W.; Payne, D. The sideline behaviour of coaches at children's team sports games. *Psychol. Sport Exerc.* **2012**, *13*, 208–215. [CrossRef]
6. Menéndez-Ferreira, R.; Ruiz, R.; Maldonado, A.; Camacho, D. Análisis y Propuesta de Una Herramienta Basada en Gamificación Para la Educación en Valores Dentro del Deporte. Analysis and Proposal of a Tool Based on Gamification for Education in Values within Sport. Available online: https://sci2s.ugr.es/caepia18/proceedings/docs/CAEPIA2018_paper_245.pdf (accessed on 17 February 2020).
7. Young, K. *Sport, Violence and Society*, 2nd ed.; Routledge: London, UK, 2019.
8. Calvo, G.; García, D. Manual para padres: Deporte y valores. Cómo sacar al deporte el máximo partido en la educación de tus hijos. In *Handbook for Parents: Sport and Values. How to Get the Most Out of Your Children's Education*; Fundación MutuaMadrileña: Madrid, Spain, 2017.
9. McMahon, J.A.; Penney, D. Sporting parents on the pool deck: Living out a sporting culture? *Qual. Res. Sport Exerc. Health* **2014**, *7*, 153–169. [CrossRef]
10. González-García, H.; Pelegrín, A.; Carballo, J. Protective Parents, Democratic Parents and Support to Physical Activity and Sport. *Cult. Cien. Deporte* **2019**, *14*, 51–59. [CrossRef]
11. Bean, C.N.; Tosoni, S.; Baker, J.; Fraser-Thomas, J. Negative parental behaviour in Canadian youth hockey: Expert insiders' perceptions and recommendations. *PHEnex J.* **2016**, *7*, 1–20.

12. O'Rourke, D.J.; Smith, R.E.; Smoll, F.L.; Cumming, S.P. Relations of Parent-and Coach-Initiated Motivational Climates to Young Athletes' Self-Esteem, Performance Anxiety, and Autonomous Motivation: Who Is More Influential? *J. Appl. Sport Psychol.* **2014**, *26*, 395–408. [CrossRef]
13. Spruit, A.; Kavussanu, M.; Smit, T.; IJntema, M. The relationship between moral climate of sports and the moral behavior of young athletes: A multilevel meta-analysis. *J. Youth Adolesc.* **2019**, *48*, 228–242. [CrossRef]
14. Simón, J.A. Percepciones de los Deportistas Sobre los Factores Que Contribuyen a la Excelencia en el Deporte Perceptions of Athletes about the Factors that Contribute to Excellence in Sport. Unpublished Thesis, University of Castilla-la Mancha, Toledo, Spain, 2009.
15. Visscher, C.; Elferink-Gemser, M.T.; Lemmink, K.A.P.M. Role of parental support in sports success of talented young Dutch athletes. In *Youth Sports. Participation, Trainability and Readiness*; Coelho, M.J., Silva, A.J., Figueiredo Elferink-Gemser, M.T., Malina, R.M., Eds.; Coimbra University Press: Coimbra, Portugal, 2009.
16. Danioni, F.; Barnib, D.; Rosnatia, R. Transmitting Sport Values: The Importance of Parental Involvement in Children's Sport Activity. *Eur. J. Psychol.* **2017**, *13*, 75–92. [CrossRef] [PubMed]
17. Romani, A.Q. Parental behaviour and children's sports participation: Evidence from a Danish longitudinal school study. *Sport Educ. Soc.* **2019**, 1–17. [CrossRef]
18. Witt, P.A.; Dangi, T.B. Helping Parents be Better Youth Sport Coaches and Spectators. *J. Park Recreat Admi* **2018**, *36*, 200C208. [CrossRef]
19. Rodríguez, M.; Cruz, F.; Torregrosa, M. Programa de intervención con entrenadores y padres de familia: Efectos en las conductas del entrenador y el clima motivacional del equipo Intervention program with coaches and parents: Effects of the coach's behavior and the team's motivational climate. *Rev. Psicol. Deporte* **2017**, *26*, 181–187.
20. Carriedo, A.; Cecchini, J.A.; González, C. Soccer in the mass media: Examining the role of metaperceptions of goal orientation on spectators' moral functioning. *J. Hum. Sport Exerc.* **2019**, *14*, 571–583. [CrossRef]
21. Cruz, J.; Mora, À.; Sousa, C.D.P.; Alcaraz, S. Effects of an individualized program on coaches' observed and perceived behavior. *Rev. Psicol. Deporte* **2016**, *25*, 137–144.
22. Ponseti, F.J.; Cantallops, J.; Borrás, P.A.; García, A. Does cheating and gamesmanship to be reconsidered regarding fair-play in grassroots sports? *Rev. Psicol. Deporte* **2017**, *26*, 28–32.
23. Wann, D.L.; Sherman, M.R. The Verbal Aggression of Spectators at Youth Baseball Games: Investigating the Impact of Competition Level, Team Identification, and Fan Dysfunction. *J. Amat. Sport* **2019**, *5*, 96–112. [CrossRef]
24. Hernández-Sampieri, R.; Fernández-Collado, C.; Baptista, P. *Metodología de la Investigación Investigation Methodology*, 4th ed.; McGraw-Hill: New York, NY, USA, 2006.
25. Polit, D.F.; Hungler, B.P. *Investigación Científica en Ciencias de la Salud Scientific Research in Health Sciences*, 6th ed.; McGraw-Hill: New York, NY, USA, 2000.
26. Gamonales, J.M.; León, K.; Muñoz, J.; González-Espinosa, S.; Ibáñez, S.J. Validation of the IOLF5C Instrument for the Efficacy of Shooting on Goal in Football for the Blind. *Rev. Int. Med. Cienc. Act. Fis. Deporte* **2018**, *18*, 361–381. [CrossRef]
27. Lefebvre, J.S.; Turnnidge, J.; Côté, J. A Systematic Observation of Coach Leadership Behaviours in Youth Sport. *J. Appl. Sport Psychol.* **2019**. [CrossRef]
28. Fahlén, J.; Stenling, C. Conceptualizing institutional change in sport management contexts: The unintended consequences of sport organizations' everyday organizational life. *Eur. Sport Manag. Q.* **2019**, *19*, 265–285. [CrossRef]
29. Jones, G.J.; Carlton, T.; Hyun, M.; Kanters, M.; Bocarro, J. Assessing the contribution of informal sport to leisure-time physical activity: A new perspective on social innovation. *Manag. Sport Leis.* **2019**. [CrossRef]
30. Kidman, L.; McKenzie, A. Parents' verbal comments at sporting events. In *Investing in Children, Primary Prevention Strategies: Proceedings of the Children's Issues Centre inaugural Child and Family Policy Conference*; Taylor, N.J., Smith, A.B., Eds.; Children's Issues Centre: Dunedin, New Zealand, 1996.
31. Siedentop, D. *Developing Teaching Skills in Physical Education*, 3rd ed.; Mayfield: Palo Alto, CA, USA, 1991.
32. Gabín, B.; Camerino, O.; Anguera, M.T.; Castañer, M. Lince: Multiplatform sport analysis software. *Procedia. Soc. Behav. Sci.* **2012**, *46*, 4692–4694. [CrossRef]
33. Hernández, A.; Castellano, J.; Camerino, O.; Jonsson, G.; Blanco, A.; Lopes, A.; Anguera, M.T. Programas informáticos de registro, control de calidad del dato, y análisis de datos Observational software, data quality control and data analysis. *Rev. Psicol. Deporte* **2014**, *23*, 111–121.

34. Courtney, J.J.; Wann, D.L. The relationship between sport fan dysfunction and bullying behaviors. *N. Am. J. Psychol.* **2010**, *12*, 191–198.
35. Dimmock, J.A.; Grove, J.R. Relationship of fan identification to determinants of aggression. *J. Appl. Sport Psychol.* **2005**, *17*, 37–47. [CrossRef]
36. Sáenz, A.; Gimeno, F.; Gutiérrez, H.; Lacambra, D. Evaluation of the Sportsmanship-Aggression Continuum in Youth Football. *J. Appl. Sport Psychol.* **2019**, *28*, 33–40.
37. Modolo, F.; Menezes, R.P. Características técnico-táticas dos goleiros de handebol da categoria sub-16: Opinião de treinadores brasileiros U-16 Handball goalkeepers' technical and tactical characteristics: Brazilian coaches' opinions. *CPD* **2019**, *19*, 206–221. [CrossRef]
38. Turnnidge, J.; Côté, J. Observing Coaches' Leadership Behaviours: The Development of the Coach Leadership Assessment System (CLAS). *Meas. Phys. Edu. Exerc. Sci.* **2019**. [CrossRef]
39. Drenowatz, C.; Greier, K.; Ruedl, G.; Kopp, M. Association between Club Sports Participation and Physical Fitness across 6- to 14-Year-Old Austrian Youth. *Int. J. Environ. Res. Public Health* **2019**, *16*, 3392. [CrossRef]

International Journal of
Environmental Research and Public Health

MDPI

Article

Effects of a Physical Education Intervention on Academic Performance: A Cluster Randomised Controlled Trial

Rodrigo Antunes Lima [1,2,*], Fernanda Cunha Soares [2], Jorge Bezerra [2] and Mauro Virgílio Gomes de Barros [2]

1 Institute of Sport Science, University of Graz, Mozartgasse 14, 8010 Graz, Austria
2 Research Group on Lifestyles and Health, University of Pernambuco, Arnóbio Marquês Street, 310, Recife 50100-130, PE, Brazil; fercsoares@gmail.com (F.C.S.); jorge.bezerra@upe.br (J.B.); mauro.barros@upe.br (M.V.G.d.B.)
* Correspondence: rodrigoantlima@gmail.com

Received: 18 May 2020; Accepted: 12 June 2020; Published: 16 June 2020

Abstract: Background: We investigated the effects of three different interventions on academic performance in students enrolled in the first year of high school. Methods: This was a cluster randomised controlled trial conducted with 1200 students enrolled in the first year of high school. Schools were randomly assigned to: 1. Doubling physical education (PE) classes (3:20 h of PE/week); 2. workshop with the PE teachers; 3. workshop with the PE teachers and doubling the PE classes; and 4. control group (1:40 h of PE/week). We assured that the schools within the groups were equal regarding: The structural condition of the sports court; number of PE teachers; number of school classes; and the average number of students per classroom. Results: Overall, the intervention was not effective in improving the students' academic performance. However, the subgroup analysis showed that the workshop intervention group increased the academic performance of students who had failed an academic year (from 16 years of age), compared to their peers in the doubling the PE classes (1.3 points on average) and the control groups (1.4 points on average). Conclusions: Enhancing the pedagogical skills of the teachers is a promising approach in improving the academic performance of students who failed an academic year.

Keywords: adolescent; physical activity; intervention study

1. Introduction

Although schools are identified as an ideal setting for stimulating children and adolescents' development and health [1], there are a limited number of randomised controlled trials evaluating the impact of school-based physical activity interventions on the students' academic performance [2]. Since observational cohort studies and small controlled laboratory studies showed some promising positive associations between higher physical activity, motor competence and fitness, and better academic performance [2–9], it is plausible that school-based interventions via the physical education lessons impact the students' academic performance. However, large school-based intervention studies reported conflicting results [10–15].

Most school-based interventions focused on improving the academic performance of the students by increasing the amount and/or enhancing the quality of the physical education (PE) classes [10–15], whereas other investigations implemented multicomponent interventions [16–19]. Independent of the intervention approach, results were inconsistent. Null, positive, and negative effects on academic performance were reported [2–4,13]. It was not clear which approach was more appropriate at influencing the students' academic performance. In addition, some studies only observed effects on academic performance in a subgroup of students [15,17,19]. For example, Resaland et al. (2016) reported higher academic performance after a physical activity intervention only in students with the poorest academic performance at baseline [17]. Interestingly, the 2019 Nobel Prize of economics valued the contributions of three scientists who conducted a series of studies targeting poverty [20,21]. Among several means of diminishing poverty, focusing on the students in the worst situation was one of the most effective approaches in improving the students' academic performance [20–23]. Therefore, besides evaluating the effects of school-based interventions on the students' academic performance, it was necessary to evaluate whether students with problems at school (i.e., older students who have failed an academic year) were benefiting from the interventions. Thus, we investigated the effects of three different interventions on the academic performance of students enrolled in the first year of high school. In addition, we also evaluated the effects of the interventions on the academic performance of students based on their age at the beginning of the academic year, as an indicator that the student has missed an academic year.

2. Materials and Methods

This was a cluster randomised controlled trial, part of the SACODE Project, which was an intervention in physical education classes to reduce sedentary behaviour and improve cognitive function. A total of eleven high schools were in the vale do Capibaribe region in the Pernambuco state in Brazil, and all were eligible for participating in the study. The protocol was approved by the Human Research Ethics Committee of the University of Pernambuco (protocol no. 55741016.0.0000.5207) and registered in the Brazilian Clinical trial registry: RBR-88tgky.

2.1. Randomisation

A researcher randomly assigned schools ensuring that groups would be equal in regards to: (1) The structural condition of the sports court (covered or uncovered); (2) number of PE teachers; (3) number of school classes; and (4) the average number of students per classroom. This categorisation resulted in three homogenous groupings of schools based on the aforementioned criteria, which is illustrated in Figure 1. After grouping the schools, we randomly assigned schools within each grouping to the following groups: Control group, doubling PE classes; workshop with the PE teachers; and workshop with PE teachers + doubling PE classes (Figure 1).

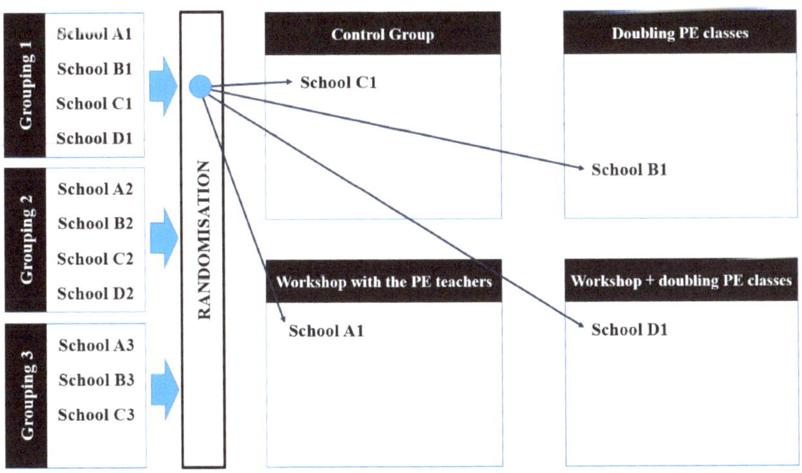

Figure 1. Randomisation of the schools.

2.2. Participants

All the 1474 students enrolled in the first year of high school were invited to participate. At the baseline, 1296 students (572 boys and 724 girls) who have returned the informed consent signed by their parents/guardians were included in the SACODE Project. However, after baseline measures, one school that should have doubled the amount of PE classes did not agree to implement the intervention and was excluded from this study. Therefore, 96 students who were enrolled in this school were excluded. Figure 2 presents a flowchart containing information on the number of adolescents with complete data in each step of the study.

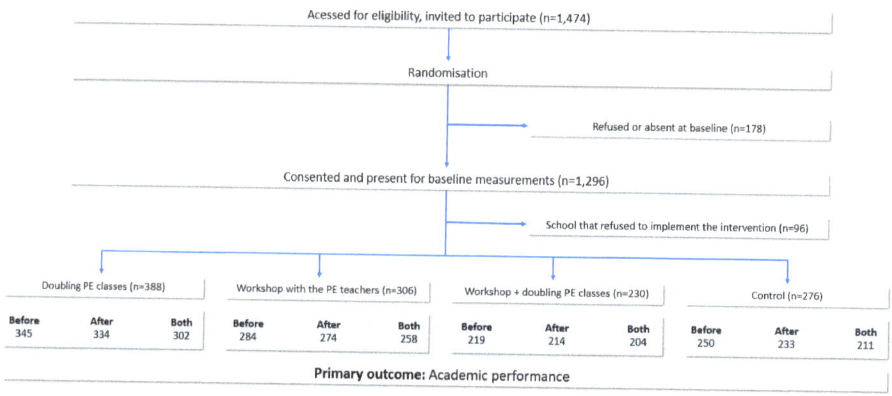

Figure 2. Flow of individual participants through the study with primary outcome measures.

2.3. Intervention

The intervention was implemented between April and October. However, the students were on holidays in July, resulting in six months of intervention. Schools that doubled the PE classes augmented from two classes to four classes per week, increasing from 1:40 h of PE classes to 3:20 h of PE classes per week for four months. The workshop with the PE teachers consisted of five lectures, lasting 4 h on average. Each workshop was structured to present pedagogical and health-related topics to the PE teachers. After the five workshops, an additional session took place to receive feedback on the teachers' experiences regarding the implementation and development of the contents in the PE classes. Table 1 describes the subjects introduced in each of the five workshops. In summary, the research team decided on the most relevant pedagogical and health-related topics for the workshops with the PE teachers. The third intervention group (workshop + doubling PE classes) implemented the same protocol described in the two abovementioned intervention groups. Schools in the control group maintained their habitual routine regarding their PE classes, which consisted of 1:40 PE h per week. Figure 3 presents a detailed description of the timeline of the intervention and measurements.

Table 1. Date and content of the workshop sessions for the workshop with the PE teachers and the workshop + doubling PE classes intervention groups.

Date of the Sessions	Topics	
	Pedagogical	**Health-Related**
2 June 2017	Current scenario and future prospects of the physical education in Brazil	Physical activity and physical fitness in the physical education classes
30 June 2017	Challenges in the physical education classes in high school	Sedentary behaviours
28 July 2017	Designing objectives and selecting topics (educational contents)	The teenage brain

Table 1. *Cont.*

Date of the Sessions	Topics	
	Pedagogical	Health-Related
2 June 2017	Current scenario and future prospects of the physical education in Brazil	Physical activity and physical fitness in the physical education classes
30 June 2017	Challenges in the physical education classes in high school	Sedentary behaviours
28 July 2017	Designing objectives and selecting topics (educational contents)	The teenage brain
1 September 2017	The importance of methodological strategies and process evaluation	Mental health and psychosocial stress indicators
22 September 2017	The importance of the motivational atmosphere and the perceived competence for the development and learning processes	Health eating and sleep quality
27 October 2017	Session for receiving feedback on the teachers' experiences regarding the implementation and development of the contents in the PE classes	

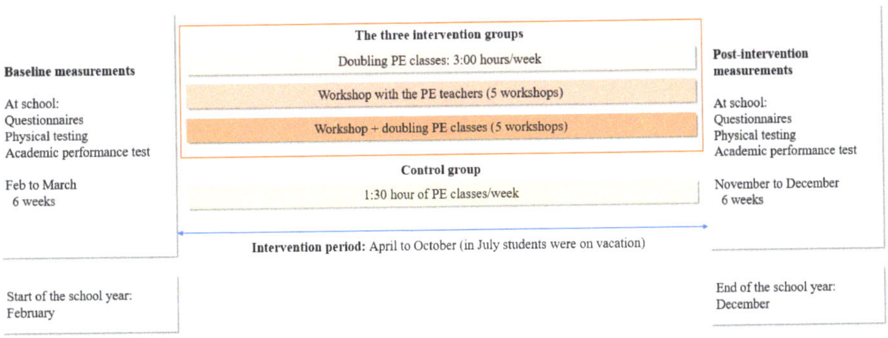

Figure 3. Content and timetable of intervention and measurements.

2.4. Measures

Only the variables included in the present study will be detailed in this manuscript. Baseline data were collected during March and April in 2017 (summer and autumn). The postintervention measures occurred between October and December in 2017 (spring and summer). All the measures were performed by a trained group of researchers that consisted of Master's and PhD students and PhDs from the University of Pernambuco.

2.5. Primary Outcome

Academic performance was assessed by two different tests in mathematics consisting of 10 questions each. The score of each question depended on their level of difficulty. The academic performance score was the standardised sum of the 10 questions, ranging from 0 to 10 points. The questions for the academic performance tests were withdrawn from the database of questions from the Ministry of Education. This database contains questions used in the national surveys evaluating the educational system in Brazil [24].

2.6. Covariates

We used a questionnaire to obtain information on sex (male, female), age, and maternal education level (≤8 years of education, >8 years of education). Maternal educational is a proxy measure of the students' socioeconomic status and it was used as an adjustment in the main analysis.

2.7. Statistical Analyses

All statistical analyses were conducted in STATA 15 for windows (StataCorp LP, College Station, TX, USA). The Fisher chi-square test assessed differences in the proportion of boys and girls and maternal educational level (<8 years of education and 8+ years of education) between intervention groups. One-way ANOVA evaluated differences in the variances of age by the intervention group. The Bonferroni post hoc analysis was used to indicate differences between groups.

The linear mixed model evaluated the effects of the intervention groups on the academic performance after the intervention period. The analysis was adjusted for academic performance at the baseline, sex, age, maternal educational level (≤8 years of education, >8 years of education), the structural condition of the sports court (with and without roof coverage), and the cluster structure of the data (individuals nested within classrooms). Subgroup analyses evaluated the effect of the intervention on the participants' academic performance at postintervention by the age group (in years) using the linear mixed model. The subgroup analysis was adjusted for academic performance at the baseline, sex, maternal educational level (≤8 years of education, >8 years of education), the structural condition of the sports court (with and without roof coverage), and the cluster structure of the data (individuals nested within classrooms). We accepted a 5% error in all analyses.

3. Results

From the 1200 students included in the study, 56.42% were females. Most of the students were between 14 and 16 years of age (89.6%), whereas 3.6% were 13 years of age, and 6.8% were older than 16 years of age at baseline. Students from the workshop with the PE teachers group were younger than their peers in the other groups at baseline (Table 2).

Table 2. Descriptive characteristics of 1200 students in the first year of high school at baseline according to the intervention group. Values are numbers and (percentages) unless stated otherwise.

Title	Doubling PE Classes	Workshop with the PE Teachers	Workshop + Doubling PE Classes	Control	Total	p
Age, in years Mean (SD)	15.08 (1.19)	14.66 (0.97)	15.07 (0.76)	15.15 (1.02)	14.99 (1.04)	<0.001 *
Female	201 (51.80)	177 (57.84)	133 (57.83)	166 (60.14)	677 (56.42)	0.149 §
<8 years of maternal education	139 (41.49)	93 (34.07)	84 (39.62)	108 (43.55)	424 (39.70)	0.130 §

Legend: * One-way ANOVA test; § Fisher chi-square test.

The academic performance at baseline was similar across groups. The intervention was not effective in increasing the academic performance of the participants (Table 3). However, subgroup analyses showed that one intervention arm increased the academic performance of the students who had failed an academic year (students older than 15 years at baseline). More specifically, we did not observe group differences in the academic performance of the students younger than 16 years of age. From 16 years of age, students from the workshop intervention group presented higher academic performance in comparison to their peers in the doubling PE classes (1.3 points on average) and the control groups (1.4 points on average). The academic performance was always similar between the workshop and the workshop + doubling PE classes intervention groups (Figure 4). See Table 4 for a detailed description of the predictive academic performance for each age and intervention group.

Table 3. Academic performance score in relation to the intervention group at baseline and postintervention and the adjusted difference of the academic performance at postintervention.

Intervention Group	Academic Performance at Baseline, Mean (SD)	Academic Performance at Postintervention, Mean (SD)	Adjusted Difference in Academic Performance at Postintervention in Relation to the Control Group*			ICC
			Coefficient	(95% CI)	*p*	
Control (*n* = 188)	3.50 (1.81)	3.64 (2.26)				
Doubling PE classes (*n* = 242)	3.65 (1.87)	3.82 (2.16)	−0.355	(−1.121 to 0.410)	0.363	0.092
Workshop with the PE teachers (*n* = 198)	3.89 (2.08)	4.45 (2.70)	0.361	(−0.387 to 1.110)	0.345	
Workshop + doubling PE classes (*n* = 152)	3.62 (1.93)	3.80 (2.01)	0.292	(−0.496 to 1.079)	0.468	

Legend: * Adjusted difference in scores of the academic performance at postintervention between the intervention groups and the control group; adjusted for academic performance at the baseline, sex, age, maternal educational level (≤8 years of education, >8 years of education), the structural condition of the sports court (with and without roof coverage), and the cluster structure of the data (students nested within classrooms).

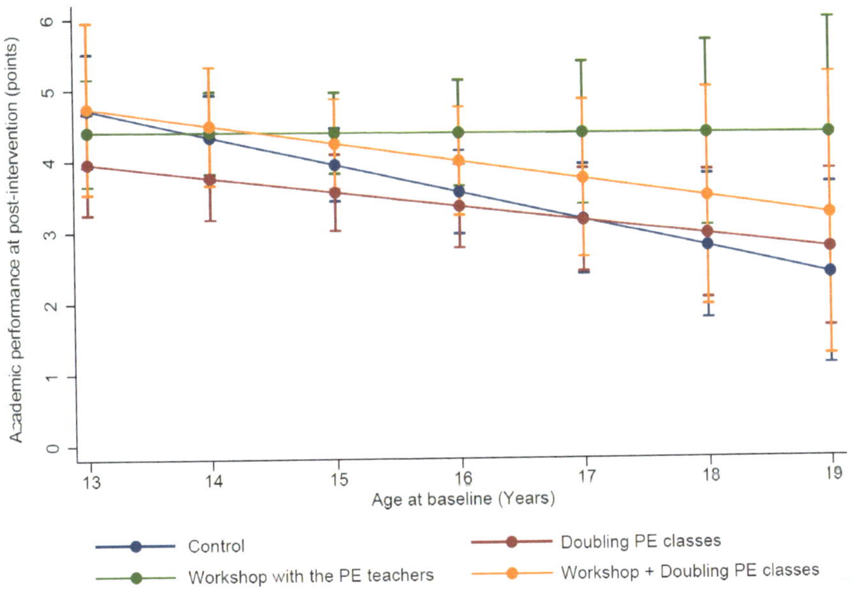

Figure 4. Predicted academic performance at postintervention of students from the first year of high school according to the intervention group and age. Legend: Adjusted for academic performance at the baseline, sex, maternal educational level (≤8 years of education, >8 years of education), the structural condition of the sports court (with and without roof coverage), and the cluster structure of the data (students nested within classrooms).

Table 4. Predicted academic performance of the first year high school students at postintervention (points), standard deviations (SD), and 95% confidence intervals (CI) for each age and intervention groups.

Age	Intervention Group	Predicted Academic Performance	(95% CI)	Difference in Relation to the Control
13	Control	4.72	(3.92 to 5.51)	
	Doubling PE classes	3.96	(3.25 to 4.67)	−0.76
	Workshop with the PE teachers	4.40	(3.65 to 5.16)	−0.31
	Workshop + doubling PE classes	4.74	(3.53 to 5.95)	0.02

Table 4. *Cont.*

Age	Intervention Group	Predicted Academic Performance	(95% CI)	Difference in Relation to the Control
14	Control	4.33	(3.73 to 4.92)	
	Doubling PE classes	3.75	(3.17 to 4.33)	−0.57
	Workshop with the PE teachers	4.39	(3.82 to 4.97)	0.07
	Workshop + doubling PE classes	4.48	(3.65 to 5.32)	0.16
15	Control	3.93	(3.42 to 4.45)	
	Doubling PE classes	3.55	(3.01 to 4.08)	−0.39
	Workshop with the PE teachers	4.38	(3.81 to 4.96)	0.45
	Workshop + doubling PE classes	4.23	(3.60 to 4.86)	0.30
16	Control	3.54	(2.96 to 4.13)	
	Doubling PE classes	3.34	(2.76 to 3.93)	−0.20
	Workshop with the PE teachers *	4.37	(3.63 to 5.12)	0.83
	Workshop + doubling PE classes	3.98	(3.22 to 4.73)	0.43
17	Control	3.15	(2.38 to 3.92)	
	Doubling PE classes	3.14	(2.42 to 3.86)	−0.01
	Workshop with the PE teachers *	4.36	(3.36 to 5.36)	1.21
	Workshop + doubling PE classes	3.72	(2.62 to 4.82)	0.57
18	Control	2.76	(1.75 to 3.77)	
	Doubling PE classes	2.93	(2.04 to 3.83)	0.17
	Workshop with the PE teachers *	4.35	(3.05 to 5.65)	1.59
	Workshop + doubling PE classes	3.47	(1.94 to 4.99)	0.70
19	Control	2.37	(1.10 to 3.65)	
	Doubling PE classes	2.73	(1.63 to 3.83)	0.36
	Workshop with the PE teachers *	4.34	(2.73 to 5.95)	1.97
	Workshop + doubling PE classes	3.21	(1.23 to 5.19)	0.84

Legend: * Higher academic performance in comparison to the doubling PE classes and control groups.

4. Discussion

Overall, none of the intervention arms, in comparison to the control group, increased the academic performance of the students. However, providing a workshop for the PE teachers positively affected the academic performance of the students who had failed an academic year in comparison to their peers in the control group. Moreover, we observed that a workshop updating pedagogical and health-related topics for PE teachers seemed a better approach in improving the academic performance than doubling the amount of PE classes for students who failed an academic year. At the end of the academic year, students who had failed an academic year (older than 15 years of age) presented lower academic performance compared to the younger peers, except for students exposed to the workshop with the PE teachers group, in which the academic performance was similar for older and younger students.

Resaland et al. (2016) [17] did not observe an effect of a multicomponent intervention on academic performance. However, authors reported that students with the poorest academic performance at baseline benefited from the effects of the intervention, which consisted of three different actions aiming at increasing the students' physical activity level during school and at home. In addition, another study that implemented a quasi-experimental multicomponent intervention reported higher math scores in low income elementary school children [19]. It is possible that students who needed the most help are the ones benefiting from the interventions.

Our results reinforce this theory. Students over 15 years of age in the beginning of the first year of high school were students who failed an academic year. Although, the academic performance at baseline did not differ between older and younger students, we observed that in the end of the curricular year older students had lower academic performance in comparison to the youngest peers, except for students exposed to the workshop with the PE teachers group (Figure 4). The grade retention is harmful for the social, emotional, and self esteem of the students [25]. Students who fail an academic year have a low self image and popularity with their peers. Repeaters often do not get social support and become more reserved and unfriendly with their class fellows [26]. In addition to updating the teachers in regards to several pedagogical skills, one of the workshop sessions dealt with the teachers on how to promote a greater integration of these students in the physical education classes. It is possible that students in the workshop intervention group felt more integrated and this may have helped their academic performance.

Importantly, failing an academic year has short- and long-term consequenes. There is a higher chance of dropping school and developing behavioural problems [23,27] for those students. Moreover, academic failure is associated with higher rates of infertility, mortality, and unemployment (see the 2018 World Development Report for review [23]). In addition, students with lower grades have lower earnings even nine years after finishing high school [28]. Therefore, the impact of upgrating the PE teacher skills on academic performance for students who failed an academic year should be further evaluated because of the potential attenuating effects on well-known consequences of academic failure.

Overall, our intervention did not affect the academic performance of the students independent of their age. Bugge et al. (2018) observed no improvements in academic performance in Danish students in an intervention that provided training sessions for the PE teachers in addition to exposing students to 4.5 h of PE lessons a week, whereas students in the control schools were exposed to 1.5 h of PE lessons a week [13]. Bugge et al. (2018) [13] suggested that the lack of improvements in physical activity and aerobic fitness was one of the main reasons for the nonsignificant effect on academic performance in their investigation.

In line with this theory, previous observational and controlled laboratory interventional studies observed a relationship between physical activity, aerobic fitness, and academic performance [2,4,7,8,29]. More specifically, Coe et al. (2006) only observed higher academic performance in children who met the recommendation for vigorous physical activity in comparison to children who did not perform any vigorous physical activity [15]. It is possible that effects on academic performance are dependent on improvements in physical activity and aerobic fitness levels.

Most multicomponent interventions suffered in improving students' academic performance [13,16–19], although studies that trained teachers to incorporate physical activity in their lessons (i.e., mathematics or language) showed encouraging effects on academic performance [30,31]. School-based interventions that both increased the time in the PE classes and enhanced PE classes by either training PE teachers or by specialised professionals showed conflicting results [10,12–14,16]. Our results suggested that single intervention strategies seemed more effective in improving the students' academic performance.

Strengths and Limitations

Some of the highlighted strengths in our study include the randomised design, the large sample size, and the national standardised tests as a measure of the students' academic performance. However, some limitations should be considered in the interpretation of our results. First, the study evaluated a short intervention period. Ideally, a longer intervention could have enhanced the interventions effects and other differences could have been observed between the intervention groups. Second, we did not assess the follow-up intervention effects in the current study. Third, we did not assess the content of the physical education lessons during the intervention period. Finally, adding other academic subjects as measures of academic performance would have been ideal.

5. Conclusions

Overall, the intervention was not effective in improving the students' academic performance. However, the workshop with the PE teachers improved the academic performance of students who had failed an academic year. It seems that providing a workshop for the PE teachers is an effective approach in avoiding the lower academic performance of the older students at the end of the curricular year. Based on our results and the existing literature, we believe that enhancing the pedagogical skills of the teachers is a promising path for improving the students' academic performance, especially the ones who need it the most.

Author Contributions: Conceptualization, R.A.L., F.C.S., J.B., M.V.G.d.B.; data curation, R.A.L. and F.C.S.; formal analysis, R.A.L.; funding acquisition, F.C.S., J.B., and M.V.G.d.B.; investigation, R.A.L. and F.C.S.; project administration, F.C.S., J.B., and M.V.G.d.B.; resources, M.V.G.d.B.; supervision, M.V.G.d.B.; writing—original draft,

R.A.L.; writing—review and editing, R.A.L., F.C.S., J.B., and M.V.G.d.B. All authors have read and agreed to the published version of the manuscript.

Funding: This study was financed in part by the Coordenação de Aperfeiçoamento de Pessoal de Nível Superior—Brasil (CAPES: 1900/2017). It was also supported by the Conselho Nacional de Desenvolvimento Científico e Tecnológico—Brasil (CNPQ: APQ 428203/2016-7), and Fundação de Amparo à Ciência e Tecnologia do Estado de Pernambuco (FACEPE: BCT 0233-4.09/17 and BFP 0029-4.09/16). The funders had no role in any aspect of the study beyond funding.

Acknowledgments: We would like to thank the municipalities, school staff, participants, and their families involved in this project. Open Access Funding by the University of Graz.

Conflicts of Interest: The authors report no conflict of interest.

Data Availability Statement: The dataset related to this manuscript can be made available under a reasonable request.

Abbreviations

PE refers to physical education.

References

1. Hills, A.P.; Dengel, D.R.; Lubans, D.R. Supporting Public Health Priorities: Recommendations for Physical Education and Physical Activity Promotion in Schools. *Prog. Cardiovasc. Dis.* **2015**, *57*, 368–374. [CrossRef]
2. Donnelly, J.E.; Hillman, C.H.; Castelli, D.; Etnier, J.L.; Lee, S.; Tomporowski, P.; Lambourne, K.; Szabo-Reed, A.N. Physical Activity, Fitness, Cognitive Function, and Academic Achievement in Children: A systematic review. *Med. Sci. Sport. Exerc.* **2016**, *48*, 1197–1222. [CrossRef] [PubMed]
3. Singh, A.; Uijtdewilligen, L.; Twisk, J.W.R.; Van Mechelen, W.; Chinapaw, M.J.M. Physical Activity and Performance at School. *Arch. Pediatr. Adolesc. Med.* **2012**, *166*, 49. [CrossRef] [PubMed]
4. Fedewa, A.L.; Ahn, S. The Effects of Physical Activity and Physical Fitness on Children's Achievement and Cognitive Outcomes: A Meta-Analysis. *Res. Q. Exerc. Sport* **2011**, *82*, 521–535. [CrossRef] [PubMed]
5. Chaddock, L.; Erickson, K.I.; Prakash, R.S.; Kim, J.S.; Voss, M.W.; Vanpatter, M.; Pontifex, M.B.; Raine, L.B.; Konkel, A.; Hillman, C.H.; et al. A Neuroimaging Investigation of the Association between Aerobic Fitness, Hippocampal Volume, and Memory Performance in Preadolescent Children. *Brain Res.* **2010**, *1358*, 172–183. [CrossRef] [PubMed]
6. Sibley, B.A.; Etnier, J. The Relationship between Physical Activity and Cognition in Children: A Meta-Analysis. *Pediatr. Exerc. Sci.* **2003**, *15*, 243–256. [CrossRef]
7. Lima, R.A.; Larsen, L.R.; Bugge, A.; Andersen, L.B. Physical Fitness Is Longitudinally Associated With Academic Performance During Childhood and Adolescence, and Waist Circumference Mediated the Relationship. *Pediatr. Exerc. Sci.* **2018**, *30*, 317–325. [CrossRef] [PubMed]
8. Lima, R.A.; Pfeiffer, K.A.; Møller, N.C.; Andersen, L.B.; Bugge, A. Physical Activity and Sedentary Time Are Positively Associated With Academic Performance: A 3-Year Longitudinal Study. *J. Phys. Act. Health* **2019**, *16*, 177–183. [CrossRef] [PubMed]
9. Lima, R.A.; Stodden, D.F.; Pfeiffer, K.A.; Larsen, L.R.; Barros, M.V.G.; Bugge, A.; Andersen, L.B. Dynamic balance, but not precision throw, is positively associated with academic performance in children. *Int. J. Environ. Res. Public Health* **2020**, *17*, 2790. [CrossRef]
10. Kall, L.B.; Nilssin, M.; Linden, T. The Impact of a Physical Activity Intervention Program on Academic Achievement in a Swedish Elementary School Setting. *J. Sch. Health* **2014**, *84*, 473–480. [CrossRef]
11. Ericsson, I.; Karlsson, M.K. Motor skills and school performance in children with daily physical education in school - a 9-year intervention study. *Scand. J. Med. Sci. Sports* **2014**, *24*, 273–278. [CrossRef] [PubMed]
12. Sallis, J.F.; Lewis, M.; McKenzie, T.L.; Kolody, B.; Marshall, S.; Rosengard, P. Effects of health-related physical education on academic achievement: Project spark. *Res. Q. Exerc. Sport* **1999**, *70*, 127–134. [CrossRef] [PubMed]
13. Bugge, A.; Möller, S.; Tarp, J.; Hillman, C.H.; Lima, R.A.; Gejl, A.K.; Klakk, H.; Wedderkopp, N. Influence of a 2- to 6-year physical education intervention on scholastic performance: The CHAMPS study-DK. *Scand. J. Med. Sci. Sports* **2018**, *28*, 228–236. [CrossRef] [PubMed]

14. Telford, R.D.; Cunningham, R.B.; Fitzgerald, R.; Olive, L.S.; Prosser, L.; Jiang, X.; Telford, R.M. Physical Education, Obesity, and Academic Achievement: A 2-Year Longitudinal Investigation of Australian Elementary School Children. *Am. J. Public Health* **2012**, *102*, 368–374. [CrossRef]
15. Coe, D.; Pivarnik, J.; Womack, C.; Reeves, M.; Malina, R. Effect of Physical Education and Activity Levels on Academic Achievement in Children. *Med. Sci. Sport. Exerc.* **2006**, *38*, 1515–1519. [CrossRef]
16. Ahamed, Y.; Macdonald, H.M.; Reed, K.; Naylor, P.-J.; Liu-Ambrose, T.; McKay, H. School-Based Physical Activity Does Not Compromise Children's Academic Performance. *Med. Sci. Sport. Exerc.* **2007**, *39*, 371–376. [CrossRef]
17. Resaland, G.K.; Aadland, E.; Moe, V.F.; Aadland, K.N.; Skrede, T.; Stavnsbo, M.; Suominen, L.; Steene-Johannessen, J.; Glosvik, Ø.; Andersen, J.R.; et al. Effects of physical activity on schoolchildren's academic performance: The Active Smarter Kids (ASK) cluster-randomized controlled trial. *Prev. Med.* **2016**, *91*, 322–328. [CrossRef]
18. Tarp, J.; Domazet, S.L.; Froberg, K.; Hillman, C.H.; Andersen, L.B.; Bugge, A. Effectiveness of a School-Based Physical Activity Intervention on Cognitive Performance in Danish Adolescents: LCoMotion-Learning, Cognition and Motion—A Cluster Randomized Controlled Trial. *PLoS ONE* **2016**, *11*, e0158087. [CrossRef]
19. Hollar, D.; Messiah, S.E.; Lopez-Mitnik, G.; Hollar, T.L.; Almon, M.; Agatston, A.S. Effect of a two-year obesity prevention intervention on percentile changes in body mass index and academic performance in low-income elementary school children. *Am. J. Public Health* **2010**, *100*, 646–653. [CrossRef]
20. Johnson, S. Pollard Niklas Trio Wins Economics Nobel for Science-Based Poverty Fight—Reuters. Available online: https://www.reuters.com/article/us-nobel-prize-economics/trio-wins-economics-nobel-for-science-based-poverty-fight-idUSKBN1WT17L (accessed on 15 October 2019).
21. Harrison, D.; Hannon, P. Nobel Prize in Economics Awarded for Work on Poverty—WSJ. Available online: https://www.wsj.com/articles/nobel-prize-in-economics-awarded-11571046679 (accessed on 15 October 2019).
22. Kremer, M. Randomized Evaluations of Educational Programs in Developing Countries: Some Lessons. *Am. Econ. Rev.* **2003**, *93*, 102–106. [CrossRef]
23. World Bank Group. *World Development Report: Learning to Realize Education's Promise*; World Bank Group: Washington, DC, USA, 2018.
24. Ministry of Education of Brazil Matrizes e Escalas—Instituto Nacional de Estudos e Pesquisas Educacionais Anisio Teixeira (INEP). Available online: http://portal.inep.gov.br/educacao-basica/saeb/matrizes-e-escalas (accessed on 3 June 2019).
25. Stearns, E.; Moller, S.; Blau, J.; Potochnick, S. Staying Back and Dropping out: The Relationship between Grade Retention and School. *Sociol. Educ.* **2007**, *80*, 210–240. [CrossRef]
26. Chohan, B.I.; Qadir, S.A. Self Esteem of the Repeaters: A Mixed Method Study of Elementary Grade Students. *Pak. J. Psychol. Res.* **2013**, *28*, 277–296.
27. Crosnoe, R. High School Curriculum Track and Adolescent Association with Delinquent Friends. *J. Adolesc. Res.* **2002**, *17*, 143–167. [CrossRef]
28. Miller, S.R. Shortcut: High School Grades As a Signal of Human Capital. *Educ. Eval. Policy Anal.* **1998**, *20*, 299–311. [CrossRef]
29. Booth, J.N.; Leary, S.D.; Joinson, C.; Ness, A.R.; Tomporowski, P.D.; Boyle, J.M.; Reilly, J.J. Associations between Objectively Measured Physical Activity and Academic Attainment in Adolescents from a UK Cohort. *Br. J. Sports Med.* **2014**, *48*, 265–270. [CrossRef]
30. Mullender-Wijnsma, M.J.; Hartman, E.; De Greeff, J.W.; Bosker, R.J.; Doolaard, S.; Visscher, C. Improving Academic Performance of School-Age Children by Physical Activity in the Classroom: 1-Year Program Evaluation. *J. Sch. Health* **2015**, *85*, 365–371. [CrossRef]
31. Donnelly, J.E.; Greene, J.L.; Gibson, C.A.; Smith, B.K.; Washburn, R.A.; Sullivan, D.K.; DuBose, K.; Mayo, M.S.; Schmelzle, K.H.; Ryan, J.J.; et al. Physical Activity Across the Curriculum (PAAC): A Randomized Controlled Trial to Promote Physical Activity and Diminish Overweight and Obesity in Elementary School Children. *Prev. Med.* **2009**, *49*, 336–341. [CrossRef]

International Journal of
Environmental Research and Public Health

MDPI

Article

Long-Term Influence of the Practice of Physical Activity on the Self-Perceived Quality of Life of Women with Breast Cancer: A Randomized Controlled Trial

Jose L. García-Soidán [1], Ignacio Pérez-Ribao [1], Raquel Leirós-Rodríguez [2,*] and Anxela Soto-Rodríguez [3]

1 Faculty of Education and Sport Sciences, University of Vigo, Campus a Xunqueira, s/n. 36005 Pontevedra, Spain; jlsoidan@uvigo.es (J.L.G.-S.); grupomovetesl@gmail.com (I.P.-R.)

2 Faculty of Physical Therapy, University of Vigo, Campus a Xunqueira, s/n. 36005 Pontevedra, Spain

3 Health Service from Galicia (SERGAS), Galician Health Services—Ourense Hospital, 32005 Ourense, Spain; anxelasoro@hotmail.com

* Correspondence: rleiros@uvigo.es; Tel.: +34-986-801-750

Received: 28 May 2020; Accepted: 9 July 2020; Published: 10 July 2020

Abstract: *Background:* There is still no consensus on the most suitable interventions for exercise practice in breast cancer survivors. Therefore, the aim of this study was to evaluate the effect of a two-year physical activity intervention (strength, aqua fitness and aerobic exercise programs) on the self-perceived quality of life and physical functionality of female breast cancer survivors. *Methods:* A randomized, controlled, experimental trial with a sample of 316 women (63 ± 7 years), who had been diagnosed with breast cancer. The evaluations were performed using the Rikli & Jones Senior Fitness Test, and the Short Form 12 Health Survey (SF-12). *Results:* The participants in the strength program showed statistically significant improvements in all the items of the SF-12. The aqua fitness program obtained significant improvements in Physical Functioning and Limitations, Pain and Emotional Limitations, General Health, Vitality, Social Functioning and the physical and mental components of the SF-12. The participants in the aerobic program showed a progressive deterioration of Vitality and Mental Health. *Conclusion:* When assigning breast cancer survivors to an exercise program, the preferential or predominant activity should include strength exercises. On the other hand, as the second choice, those patients with particularly low levels of Vitality or Physical Limitations will show greater improvement with an aqua fitness program.

Keywords: breast neoplasms; survival; exercise; quality of life; aged; women

1. Introduction

Breast cancer is among the main causes of morbidity and mortality all over the world, with approximately 14 million new cases and more than 8 million deaths each year [1]. In the female population, the most prevalent forms of cancer are breast, colorectal, lung, cervical and stomach cancer [2]. The relative survival 5 years after diagnosis is above 80% in developed countries, which, in turn, are also the ones that implement systematized mammography-screening programs [3].

Although the aim of reaching 100% survival in women with breast cancer is still being pursued [4], improving the quality of life and restoring the optimal functionality levels of the patients are also objects of study nowadays [5,6].

The benefits of practicing physical activity (PA) on the general population at the physical and emotional level have been extensively studied [7,8], and cancer patients can also benefit from all those positive health effects [6]. At the physical level, PA practice in cancer survivors facilitates the recovery of the previous functional capacity, strength and flexibility levels, the healthy parameters of body composition, as well as the reduction of neutropenia, anemia, thrombocytopenia, pain and fatigue (the latter five are frequent side effects of aggressive cancer treatments) [9,10]. Based on these benefits and recommendations, there is value to the efforts being made to connect breast cancer survivors to high-quality strength training programs [11]. Traditionally, more research has been done on the effects of aerobic exercise on patients with malignant disease. That said, more attention is currently being paid to the effects of other training modalities (such as strength training or aqua fitness) on the physical work capacity of cancer patients or survivors. In any case, PA programs should be evaluated and implemented for their positive effects on muscle atrophy induced by the treatments and sedentary habits of breast cancer survivors [12]. Aerobic training protocols involve short periods of exercise at a vigorous intensity, followed by brief, low intensity recovery breaks, which permit the relief from symptoms such as dyspnea and leg fatigue. Aerobic programs have been tolerated in a wide range of patient groups, including individuals with chronic obstructive pulmonary disease, metabolic syndrome, heart failure and obesity. Furthermore, the aerobic interval exercise programs are safe, and caused low levels of cardiac stress [13]. However, some particularities must be taken into account when designing interventions aimed at cancer patients, such as avoiding movements that cause pain, sudden or big changes in blood pressure and heart rate, and the reaching of high levels of dyspnea [5].

In addition to the benefits for the physical clinical parameters, it is important to highlight that, since the diagnosis of cancer represents a situation of considerable emotional stress, the benefits of PA practice at the psychological level (such as the reduction of depression levels and the improvement of strength, self-esteem and emotional control) are of special interest in cancer patients [14,15].

However, there is still no consensus on the most suitable interventions and specific training parameters for PA practice in breast cancer survivors. Therefore, the aim of this study was to evaluate the effect of a two-year PA practice program on the self-perceived quality of life and physical functionality of female breast cancer survivors, and to determine the existence of differences between three different interventions (strength, aqua fitness and aerobic exercise programs).

2. Materials and Methods

2.1. Experimental Design and Sample

This was a randomized, controlled, experimental trial with a 3 × 3 design. The sample consisted of 316 women (mean age: 63 ± 7 years) from the region of Ourense (Spain), who had been diagnosed with breast cancer, surgically treated, and subjected to chemotherapy, which they had completed in the previous six months. The selection criteria excluded those patients who had heart or coronary diseases that contraindicated the practice of exercise, hypertension, severe anemia, risk of fracture, disabling osteoarticular pathology, diabetes or other disabling diseases.

These were distributed in four groups of activity as shown in the flow diagram of Figure 1. For this research, a program for the promotion of PA and health was designed for women with cancer promoted through informative posters placed in different social centers and public boards (throughout the six months prior to the intervention), distributed by all the districts of the city. Participation was voluntary throughout the program, and distribution in all three physical activity groups and the control group was performed randomly among the participants. There was an initial medical evaluation confirming that all participants were able to participate in the intervention program.

The evaluators that recorded data in the different evaluation sessions did not know to which intervention group the participants belonged. Furthermore, during the statistical analysis, the authors who calculated the results also did not know how the intervention groups were categorized.

Patients who met the inclusion criteria were randomly assigned to one of four groups. Blank folders were numbered from 1 to 316, and were given concealed codes for the assigned group, determined by a random-number generator. When a patient was eligible and gave consent to participate, the treating monitor drew the next folder from the file, which determined the group of assignment.

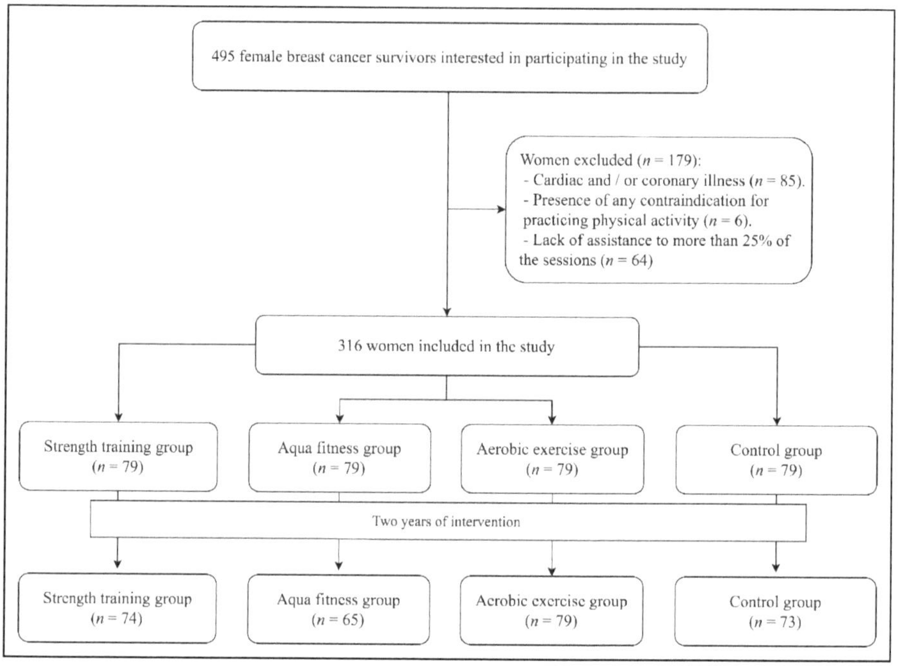

Figure 1. CONSORT flow diagram.

All of them signed informed consent in accordance with the Declaration of Helsinki (rev. 2013) and the Data Protection Act 15/1999. This research received ethical approval from the Commission of Ethics of the Faculty of Sciences of Education and Sport of the University of Vigo (Pontevedra, Spain) (code: 3-0504-16).

2.2. Procedure

The evaluations were performed using the Rikli & Jones Senior Fitness Test [16,17], which evaluated functional fitness, and the Short Form 12 Health Survey (SF-12) Questionnaire [18–20] that measured quality of life in relation to health. The strength and flexibility of the upper and lower extremities were extracted from the Rikli & Jones Senior Fitness Test as study variables (strength is quantified according to the number of repetitions and flexibility is quantified in centimeters, through four simple tests) [16,17]. On the other hand, the following variables were extracted from the SF-12 Questionnaire: the pain, the vitality, the physical and social functions, the general and mental health; the physical and emotional limitations; and two global scores on the physical and mental components of health (all the variables provided by this questionnaire are quantified in score points) [18–20].

During the investigation, three data points were taken: (a) Pre-test, prior to the start of the program, a doctor checked the health status of the participants and the possible limitations or contraindications to their performance of any of the program's activities. Then the anthropometric measures of height, weight and body mass index (BMI) were taken. Finally, the Rikli & Jones Senior Fitness Test (SFT) and the SF-12 Questionnaire were applied to the participants; (b) Intermediate test, at 12 months of onset (the same measurements were taken as at the beginning, except for the medical interview); (c) Post-test, at 24 months from the beginning, with identical parameters to those employed in the intermediate test. All evaluations were performed by qualified professionals with training in these procedures, who did not know which intervention group each of the participants belonged to. The participants who abandoned the study or missed over 25% of the sessions were removed from the final database.

2.3. Programs of PA

All participants were divided into four groups: one as control (who should not make any changes in their lifestyle, incorporating any new physical activity) and three activity groups of 79 people each. For the realization of the classes, the groups were divided into subgroups of 17–18 women. All programs consisted of two weekly sessions with two weeks of rest at Christmas, one week of rest at Easter and one month of rest in summer (August). Each year, 45 weeks of training were held and, in total, the women had to attend a minimum of 135 of the 180 sessions held within the intervention period. The different programs were given by monitors, who were graduates in PA and Sports Sciences, and were previously trained for the study.

(a) Strength group: Participants in this activity had a mean age of 63 ± 7 years. The activity sessions lasted 55–60 min. The work with gym machines had a progression adapted to the tests performed by the participants. During the first six weeks, the sessions consisted of an initial warm-up time of 10 min, performing general mobility exercises and stretching, followed by horizontal training with gym machines of 30–40 min, where the functioning of each muscle machine was progressively taught, which together formed a circuit of 8 exercises that worked the large muscle groups of the upper and lower limbs. Two sets of 12 repetitions with loads of 50–60% of the maximum resistance test (MR) were performed, and the 10 min at the end were dedicated to the stretching of the muscle groups worked during the session. From the seventh week loads increased, and maximum strength tests (MR) were performed to find out the individual work percentages. The strength program was initiated in the seventh week, at 60% of MR, then the repetitions were increased to 20 at weeks 7 and 8, and finally during the last four weeks the participants completed circuits of 3 series between 60% and 80% of the MR, with 10 repetitions per set and 2-minute breaks between each set.

(b) Aqua fitness Group: Participants in this activity had a mean age of 62 ± 6 years. The pool used had a depth of 1.4 m at the central area, and 1.75 m at the end. The classes lasted 55 min and the timing of this activity was as follows: An initial period of 2 weeks of low intensity. This initial period served to evaluate the average level of each group. They then went on to an improvement stage, where the repetitions, and then the intensity, were progressively increased between weeks 3 and 12. The basic structure of the sessions consisted of 5 initial minutes of joint mobility and warm-up outside the pool, followed by aerobic and choreographed exercises (25 min), strength-resistance work (10 min) in which the body regions varied according to the purpose of the session (e.g., chest, shoulder and dorsal region, arm and forearm region, lower limbs and muscles of the abdomen region), games (10 min), and finally stretches (5 min).

(c) Aerobic exercise group: This was formed of participants with a mean age of 64 ± 7 years. These lasted for 55 min, with a minimum warm-up time of 10 min (with choreographed basic aerobic steps focusing on mobility and short displacements), and 5 min of stretches at the end. All sessions also included a central component of 40 min in which mainly choreographed aerobic exercises (performed with a symmetric methodology) and, eventually, some strengthening exercises without loads, were performed (2 sets of 12 repetitions for each large muscle groups of the upper and lower limbs).

2.4. Data Analysis

The statistical package SPSS (version 22, SPSS Inc., Chicago, IL, USA) was used for the treatment of the data. The variables showed a normal distribution according to the Kolgomorov–Smirnov test ($p > 0.05$), and there was homogeneity of variances, determined by applying the Levene test. A factorial, repeated measures ANOVA compared the evolution of each activity group throughout the program, and to compare the effect of the different exercise programs we used the ANOVA statistic with the Bonferroni correction. The level of significance was set at $p < 0.05$.

3. Results

3.1. Strength Program

The participants in the strength program showed statistically significant improvements in all the items of the SF-12 (Table 1), except in Vitality, in which they obtained a significant worsening at the end of the intervention ($p < 0.05$). The results of Social Functioning, Physical and Emotional Limitations and Pain showed a progressive improvement ($p < 0.001$), which was more pronounced after the second year of the intervention (Figure 2). Physical Functioning obtained better results at the end of the study, although the benefits in this aspect were greater after the first year of the intervention ($p < 0.05$). Lastly, Global and Mental Health, and the physical and mental components of the SF-12, showed worse results after the first year of the intervention; however, there were significant improvements in these parameters at the end of the intervention, with respect to the initial state of the participants ($p < 0.05$).

In the SFT, the participants obtained significantly better results relating to the strength of the lower limbs after the intervention ($p < 0.001$) (Table 1), although this parameter showed worse results after the first year of the intervention (Figure 3). The flexibility of all the extremities increased significantly ($p < 0.001$). On the other hand, no improvement was found in the strength of the upper limbs in any of the two re-evaluations. Body weight and BMI were significantly lower after the intervention ($p < 0.01$).

3.2. Aqua Fitness Program

The participants in the aqua fitness program obtained progressive improvements in Physical Functioning and Limitations, Pain and Emotional Limitations ($p < 0.01$) (Table 1). In General Health, Vitality, Social Functioning and the physical and mental components of the SF-12, the participants completed the intervention with significantly better results ($p < 0.01$), although they obtained worse results in all of them after the first year of the intervention (Figure 2). Lastly, there were no significant changes in Mental Health. Regarding the SFT, the participants of the aqua fitness group obtained a significant improvement in flexibility ($p < 0.001$), although their upper limb strength decreased significantly ($p < 0.001$). On the other hand, lower limb strength, body weight and BMI showed no changes after the intervention (Figure 3).

3.3. Aerobic Exercise Program

The participants in the aerobic exercise program showed progressive improvements in Emotional Limitations ($p < 0.001$). On the other hand, they obtained a progressive deterioration of Vitality and Mental Health ($p < 0.01$). Physical Functioning, after the intervention, showed significantly better results ($p < 0.05$) (Table 1), although such improvement was greater after the first year of the intervention (Figure 2). Physical Limitations and Pain improved after the first year of the intervention, and showed an even greater improvement after the second year ($p < 0.05$). Lastly, General Health, Social Functioning and the physical and mental components of the SF-12 obtained significantly better results after the intervention ($p < 0.01$), although they showed worse results after the first year.

Regarding the results of the SFT, the participants of the aerobic exercise program obtained a significant improvement in the strength and flexibility of their lower limbs ($p < 0.05$); however, they showed a decrease in the strength and flexibility of their upper limbs ($p < 0.001$). The body weight and BMI of these participants increased after the intervention, although not significantly (Figure 3).

Table 1. Descriptive analysis of the sample by groups (mean ± standard deviation).

	Strength Group		Aqua Fitness Group		Aerobic Group		Control Group	
	Pre-Test	**Post-Test**	**Pre-Test**	**Post-Test**	**Pre-Test**	**Post-Test**	**Pre-Test**	**Post-Test**
Survival (n)	79	74	79	65	79	72	79	73
Age (years)	63 ± 7	65 ± 7	62 ± 6.8	64 ± 6.8	64 ± 7.1	66 ± 7.1	63 ± 4.6	65 ± 4.6
Weight (kg)	69 ± 11	67.7 ± 10.2 $^{\#**+}$	70.5 ± 11	71.2 ± 10.9 $^{\%\%**\$\$\$}$	65.7 ± 9.8	66 ± 10.5 $^{\&\&+\$\$\$}$	69.5 ± 10.6	69.7 ± 10.6 $^{\#\%\%\&\&}$
BMI (kg/m^2)	29.4 ± 8.5	28.8 ± 9 $^{\#**+}$	29.8 ± 9.6	30.2 ± 9.5 $^{\%\%**\$\$\$}$	27.7 ± 8.3	27.9 ± 9.1 $^{\&\&+\$\$\$}$	28.5 ± 9.4	28.6 ± 9.3 $^{\#\%\%\&\&}$
SF-12 health survey								
PF	50.8 ± 9.2	53.1 ± 6.6	49.8 ± 8.1	53 ± 7.2	51.5 ± 7.7	52.7 ± 6.7	53.2 ± 9.1	53.6 ± 7
PL	38.7 ± 1.3	34.4 ± 19.7 $^{\#++}$	38.7 ± 1.4	34 ± 21.9 $^{\%\%\%\$\$\$}$	38.7 ± 1.4	43.7 ± 23.7 $^{++\$\$\$}$	38.9 ± 22.9	44 ± 21 $^{\#\%\%\%}$
Pain	36 ± 13.7	34.1 ± 8.4 $^{\#\#**++}$	39.4 ± 13.7	37.1 ± 1.4 **	34.6 ± 11.5	37.1 ± 1.4 $^{++}$	27.2 ± 1.3	37.3 ± 1.6 $^{\#\#}$
GH	41.8 ± 9.3	44.4 ± 13.7 $^{\#\#**+}$	38.1 ± 8.3	39.8 ± 13.7 $^{\%\%\%**\$\$}$	40.3 ± 9.9	43 ± 11.5 $^{\&\&+\$\$}$	42.3 ± 9.3	25.6 ± 15.2 $^{\#\#\%\%\%\&\&}$
Vitality	41.4 ± 5.8	39.2 ± 9.3 **	43.2 ± 12.1	46.5 ± 8.3 $^{\%\%**\$\$}$	41.6 ± 14.2	38.7 ± 9.9 $^{\&\$\$}$	38.3 ± 12.9	40.7 ± 9.8 $^{\%\%\&}$
EL	54.4 ± 6.4	39.8 ± 5.8 $^{\#\#*}$	53 ± 4.1	41.6 ± 12.1 $^{\%\%*\$}$	54.4 ± 10.9	40 ± 14.2 $^{\&\&\$}$	54.5 ± 6.4	36.7 ± 13.1 $^{\#\#\%\%\&\&}$
SF	20.2 ± 3.9	52.8 ± 6.4 $^{\#\#\#*}$	20.7 ± 4.3	51.4 ± 4.1 $^{\%\%\%*\$}$	21.4 ± 4.5	52.8 ± 10.9 $^{\&\&\$}$	20.9 ± 3.9	50.9 ± 7 $^{\#\#\#\%\%\%\&\&}$
MH	49.1 ± 7.8	58.6 ± 3.9 $^{\#\#\#***+++}$	49.4 ± 7	49.1 ± 4.3 $^{\%\%\%***\$\$\$}$	48.9 ± 8.5	45.8 ± 4.5 $^{\&\&+++\$\$\$}$	48.5 ± 7.8	49.3 ± 3.6 $^{\#\#\#\%\%\%\&\&}$
SF12-P	45.6 ± 4.2	47.5 ± 7.8 $^{\#}$	45.1 ± 4.1	47.8 ± 7 $^{\%\%}$	44.8 ± 3.8	47.3 ± 8.5 $^{\&}$	43.8 ± 4.5	46.9 ± 7.4 $^{\#\%\%\&}$
SF12-M	38.4 ± 1.4	44 ± 4.5 $^{\#+}$	38.9 ± 4.2	43.5 ± 4.1 $^{\%}$	39 ± 4.5	43.2 ± 3.8 $^{+}$	38.1 ± 5.4	42.2 ± 4.5 $^{\#}$
Senior Fitness Test								
LLS	16.2 ± 0.6	18.3 ± 1	17.7 ± 4.5	18.2 ± 1.4	17.1 ± 4.9	18.8 ± 1.7 $^{\&}$	17.6 ± 5.8	17.2 ± 1.3 $^{\&}$
ULS	20.2 ± 7.6	19.2 ± 0.6 $^{\#\#**+++}$	20.9 ± 5.5	16.7 ± 4.5 **	20.2 ± 5.5	16.1 ± 4.9 $^{+++}$	19.6 ± 9.6	16.6 ± 4.9 $^{\#\#}$
LLF	−0.7 ± 5.2	19.2 ± 7.6 $^{\#}$	0.2 ± 8.5	19.9 ± 5.5 $^{\%\%}$	0.7 ± 8.8	19.2 ± 5.5	−0.1 ± 9	18.6 ± 5.8 $^{\#\%\%}$
ULF	−5.5 ± 7.4	0 ± 9.4 $^{\#\#+++}$	−5.7 ± 12	0.5 ± 10.2 $^{\%\%\$\$}$	−5.5 ± 13.3	−6.8 ± 8.8 $^{\&\&+++\$\$}$	−10.1 ± 4.9	−2 ± 9.8 $^{\#\#\%\%\&\&}$

BMI: body mass index; PF: physical function; PL: physical limitations; GH: general health; EL: emotional limitations; SF: social function; MH: mental health; SF12-P: SF12 physical component; SF12-M: SF12 mental component; LLS: lower limbs strength; ULS: upper limbs strength; LLF: lower limbs flexibility; ULF: upper limbs flexibility. Comparison between strength vs. control groups: $^{\#}$ $p < 0.05$; $^{\#\#}$ $p < 0.01$; $^{\#\#\#}$ $p < 0.001$. Comparison between aqua fitness vs control groups: $^{\%}$ $p < 0.05$; $^{\%\%}$ $p < 0.01$; $^{\%\%\%}$ $p < 0.001$. Comparison between aerobic vs control groups: $^{\&}$ $p < 0.05$; $^{\&\&}$ $p < 0.01$; $^{\&\&\&}$ $p < 0.001$. Comparison between strength vs. aqua fitness groups: * $p < 0.05$; ** $p < 0.01$; *** $p < 0.001$. Comparison between strength vs. aerobic groups: $^{+}$ $p < 0.05$; $^{++}$ $p < 0.01$; $^{+++}$ $p < 0.001$. Comparison between aqua fitness vs. aerobic groups: $^{\$}$ $p < 0.05$; $^{\$\$}$ $p < 0.01$; $^{\$\$\$}$ $p < 0.001$.

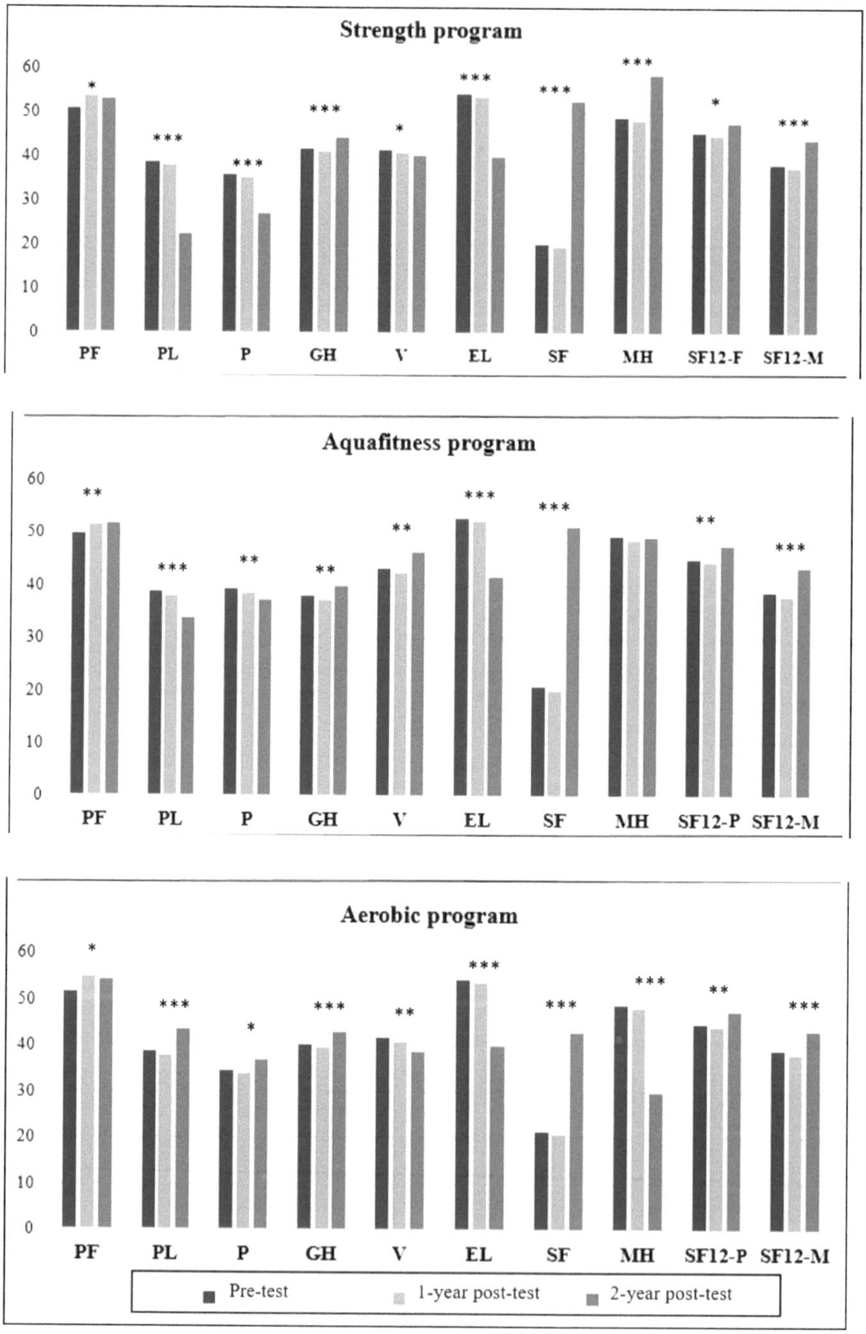

Figure 2. SF-12 survey results by intervention group. (PF: physical function; PL: physical limitations; P: pain; GH: general health; V: vitality; EL: emotional limitations; SF: social function; MH: mental health; SF12-P:SF12 physical component; SF12-M: SF12 mental component). Comparison between initial test vs. final test: * $p < 0.05$; ** $p < 0.01$; *** $p < 0.0001$.

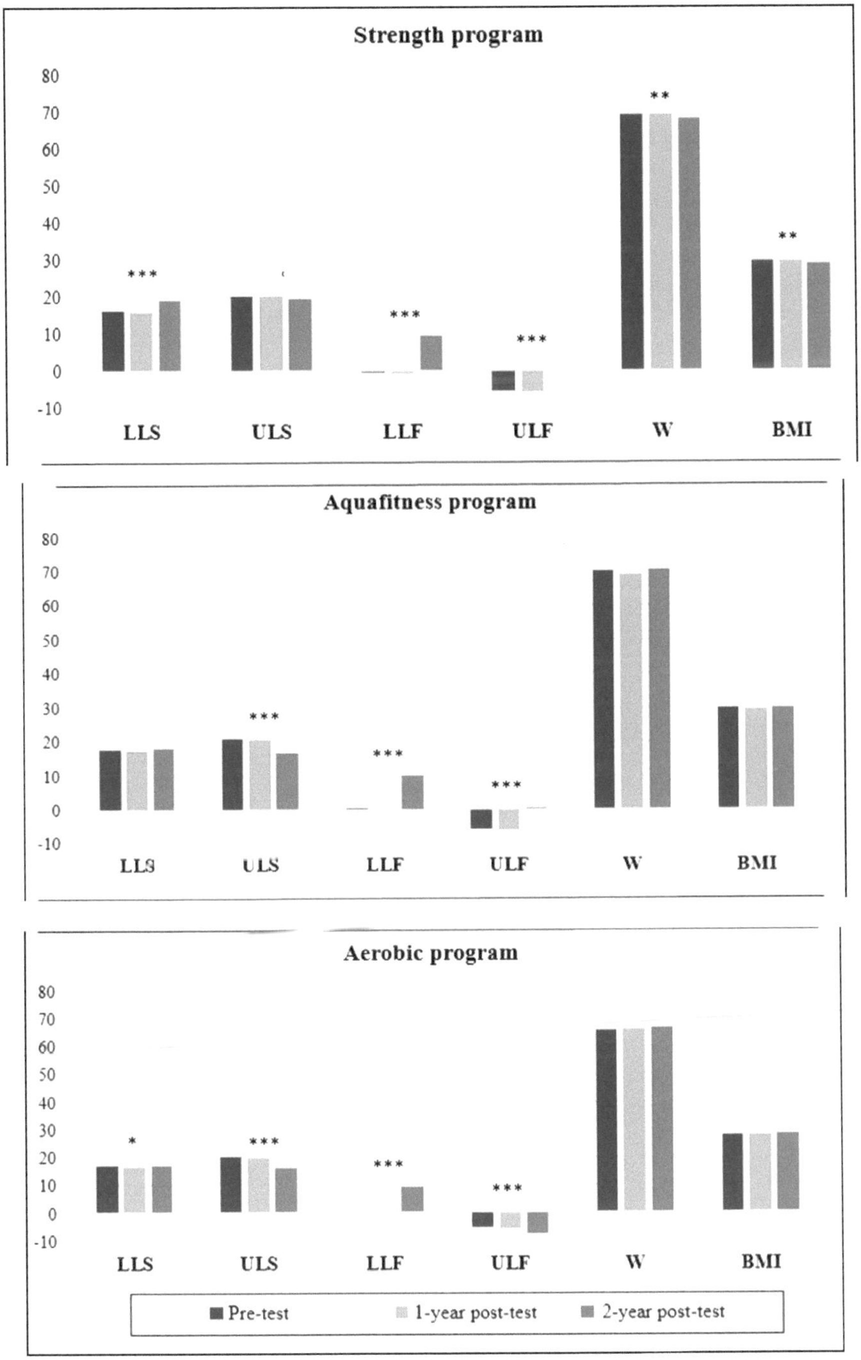

Figure 3. Senior Fitness Test, weight and body mass index results by intervention group. (LLS: lower limbs strength; ULS: upper limbs strength; LLF: lower limbs flexibility; ULF: upper limbs flexibility; W: weight; BMI: body mass index). Comparison between initial test vs. final test: * $p < 0.05$; ** $p < 0.01$; *** $p < 0.0001$.

3.4. Comparative Results between Groups

The results of the strength program group were positive in all the analyzed variables, except Vitality, which showed worse results at the end of the intervention with respect to the baseline levels. Moreover, the results of the strength group were significantly higher than those of the other two programs in body weight, BMI, Emotional Limitations, Social Functioning, Mental Health and the mental components of the SF-12. It was also the intervention that achieved the best results in the SFT battery, except for the flexibility of the lower limbs, which obtained its best improvement in the aqua fitness program.

Among the three different interventions, the aqua fitness group showed the best results in Physical Functioning, Physical Limitations, Vitality, Pain and the physical component of the SF-12. On the other hand, upper limb strength was the only variable with worse results at the end of this intervention.

Lastly, the aerobic exercise group obtained the best results in General Health. In contrast, it was the only group with worse results in body weight, BMI, Physical Limitations, Pain, Vitality, Mental Health, and upper limb flexibility and strength; in fact, the results of the last two variables after the two years of intervention were worse than those of the control group.

4. Discussion

The aim of this study was to evaluate the effect of a two-year PA practice program on the self-perceived quality of life and physical functioning of female breast cancer survivors, and to determine the existence of differences between different exercise-based interventions. After the analysis of the obtained data, we can conclude that the female breast cancer survivors benefit from PA practice. In addition, the design of such intervention programs has a considerable impact on the reachable benefits.

In general, the strength program provided the best, and the most, benefits, especially in the parameters of physical health, such as body weight, BMI, general health, pain, lower limb strength and the flexibility of all extremities. These findings are congruent, since strength programs are the ones that provide the greatest benefits to those who practice them, through the development of the functional capacity (respiratory and movement capacity), the prevention of sarcopenia and the reduction of weakness, pain and other side effects derived from medical cancer treatments [21,22]. Regarding the emotional scope, the strength program induced the greatest benefits in emotional limitations and mental health, which is in line with the results of previous studies in older populations [23] and women without cancer [24], with the exception that the vitality of the participants also improved. However, it is important to take into account that, in cancer survivors, emotional aspects such as self-perceived vitality can be strongly affected by the psycho-somatic impact of the disease [25,26].

In any case, if the initial valuation of the self-perceived health state of a breast cancer survivor obtains bad results in Vitality, the results of this study indicate that the most adequate intervention is that of aqua fitness. However, in the objective valuation of the physical health state through the SFT, the aqua fitness program only obtained positive results in the flexibility of the limbs, and limb strength did not improve in any case. This may be due to the fact that aquatic exercises are especially recommended to improve fatigue levels [27] (a variable of great interest in cancer survivors [28,29]) and abilities like coordination and balance [30]. This explains the positive results obtained in this study for Physical Functioning and Limitations via the aqua fitness program: by improving fatigue and coordination, the self-perceived impact on the development of the activities of daily living may be greater than the impact identified as a consequence of the specific improvement of upper limb strength (as was the case in the strength program group).

Lastly, the intervention based on aerobic exercise obtained the worst results. This program induced a worsening in the physical limitations, vitality, mental health, pain and upper limb strength and flexibility, reaching lower values than the control group in some of these parameters. It is important to highlighting that aerobic exercise programs can improve two physical capacities: aerobic capacity and limb movement range [31,32]. Since such improvements can also be obtained with the other two PA programs, it can be confirmed that aerobic exercise programs should not be considered as the first choice when incorporating PA practice after the active treatment of breast cancer, unless the patient has a special preference for this type of physical activity.

Therefore, when assigning breast cancer survivors to a PA program, the preferential or predominant activity should include strength exercises. Moreover, if their initial results are worse as regards pain, general and mental health of the SF-12 or limb strength and flexibility, they are likely to further benefit from strength training. On the other hand, as the second choice, those patients with particularly low levels of vitality or physical limitations will show greater improvements under a PA program that includes aquatic activities, such as aqua fitness. Lastly, if these two options are not suitable for the patient, an aerobic exercise program can be considered, whose benefits on general health, emotional limitations and social functioning are greater than those obtained by the aqua fitness program. It is worth highlighting that the three interventions proved to be safe; no adverse effects were reported by the participants in any of the exercise sessions throughout the two-year period of the programs (such as lymphedema, which did not appear in any of the participants). However, it is important to mention that the mortality of the participants was significantly higher in the aqua fitness group, although this is a multi-factor phenomenon that is beyond the scope of the present investigation.

Regarding the limitations of this study, more sensitive and specific objective measurements should have been included (such as cardiovascular and laboratory tests). However, this is the first study to carry out PA interventions comparatively, using a randomized and controlled methodology for a period of time long enough to obtain reliable results that can also be extrapolated to those of other populations of female breast cancer survivors.

Considering future research lines, similar studies could be conducted in other populations to improve the evidence of the findings presented in this work, including, if possible, medical laboratory tests, to compare the self-perceived changes of the participants.

5. Conclusions

PA practice in female breast cancer survivors has multiple and considerable health benefits. Strength training programs obtained the best, and the most, benefits in the quality of life related to self-perceived health and general physical state. Other valid strategies for the increase of PA practice for these patients include aqua fitness programs and, as the last option, aerobic exercise programs, unless the patient has especially important afflictions pertaining to physical limitations and social functioning, in which case the practice of aerobic exercise should be the first choice.

Author Contributions: I.P.-R., J.L.G.-S., R.L.-R. and A.S.-R. conceptualized and designed the study, drafted the initial manuscript, designed the data collection instruments, collected data, carried out the initial analyses, and critically reviewed the manuscript for important intellectual content. All authors approved the final manuscript as submitted and agree to be accountable for all aspects of the work. All authors have read and agreed to the published version of the manuscript.

Funding: This research received no external funding.

Conflicts of Interest: The authors declare no conflict of interest.

References

1. McGuire, S. *World Cancer Report 2014*; World Health Organization, International Agency for Research on Cancer; WHO Press: Geneva, Switzerland, 2015.
2. Carlson, C.L. Effectiveness of the World Health Organization cancer pain relief guidelines: An integrative review. *J. Pain Res.* **2016**, *9*, 515–534. [CrossRef]
3. Allemani, C.; Matsuda, T.; Di Carlo, V.; Harewood, R.; Matz, M.; Nikšić, M.; Bonaventure, A.; Valkov, M.; Johnson, C.; Estève, J.; et al. Global surveillance of trends in cancer survival 2000–14 (CONCORD-3): Analysis of individual records for 37,513,025 patients diagnosed with one of 18 cancers from 322 population-based registries in 71 countries. *Lancet* **2018**, *391*, 1023–1075. [CrossRef]

4. Rugo, H.S.; Finn, R.S.; Gelmon, K.; Joy, A.A.; Harbeck, N.; Castrellon, A.; Mukai, H.; Walshe, J.M.; Mori, A.; Gauthier, E.; et al. Progression-free survival outcome is independent of objective response in patients with estrogen receptor-positive, human epidermal growth factor receptor 2-negative advanced breast cancer treated with palbociclib plus letrozole compared with letrozole: Analysis from PALOMA-2. *Clin. Breast Cancer* **2019**, *20*, e173–e180. [CrossRef] [PubMed]
5. Irwin, M.M.L.; American College of Sports Medicine. *ACSM's Guide to Exercise and Cancer Survivorship*; Human Kinetics: Champaing, IL, USA, 2012.
6. Wattanapisit, A. Physical activity for adult cancer survivors: A literature review. *Walailak J. Sci. Technol.* **2017**, *14*, 1–10. [CrossRef]
7. World Health Organization. *Global Recommendations on Physical Activity for Health*; World Health Organization: Geneva, Switzerland, 2010.
8. World Health Organization. *Global Action Plan on Physical Activity 2018–2030: More Active People for a Healthier World*; World Health Organization: Geneva, Switzerland, 2019.
9. Betof, A.S.; Dewhirst, M.W.; Jones, L.W. Effects and potential mechanisms of exercise training on cancer progression: A translational perspective. *Brain Behav. Immun.* **2013**, *30*, S75–S87. [CrossRef] [PubMed]
10. Cave, J.; Paschalis, A.; Huang, C.; West, M.; Copson, E.; Jack, S.; Grocott, M.P.W. A systematic review of the safety and efficacy of aerobic exercise during cytotoxic chemotherapy treatment. *Support. Care Cancer* **2018**, *26*, 3337–3351. [CrossRef]
11. Schmitz, K.H. Incorporating strength training into cancer care: Translating PAL into the strength after Breast Cancer Program. *Obesity* **2017**, *25*, S32–S33. [CrossRef]
12. De Luca, V.; Minganti, C.; Borrione, P.; Grazioli, E.; Cerulli, C.; Guerra, E.; Bonifacino, A.; Parisi, A. Effects of concurrent aerobic and strength training on breast cancer survivors: A pilot study. *Public Health* **2016**, *136*, 126–132. [CrossRef]
13. Dolan, L.B.; Campbell, K.; Gelmon, K.; Neil-Sztramko, S.; Holmes, D.; McKenzie, D.C. Interval versus continuous aerobic exercise training in breast cancer survivors: A pilot RCT. *Support. Care Cancer* **2016**, *24*, 119–127. [CrossRef]
14. Ax, A.; Johansson, B.; Carlsson, M.; Nordin, K.; Börjeson, S. Exercise: A positive feature on functioning in daily life during cancer treatment–Experiences from the Phys-Can Study. *Eur. J. Oncol. Nurs.* **2020**, *44*, 101713. [CrossRef]
15. Mustian, K.; Alfano, C.; Heckle, C.; Kleckner, A.S.; Kleckner, I.R.; Leach, C.R.; Mohr, D.; Palesh, O.G.; Peppone, L.J.; Piper, B.F.; et al. Clinical benefits of exercise and psychological interventions in patients with cancer-related fatigue. *JAMA Oncol.* **2017**, *3*, 961–968. [CrossRef] [PubMed]
16. Rikli, R.E.; Jones, C.J. Development and validation of a functional fitness test for community-residing older adults. *J. Aging Phys. Act.* **1999**, *7*, 129–161. [CrossRef]
17. Rikli, R.E.; Jones, C.J. *Senior Fitness Test Manual*; Human Kinetics: Champaing, IL, USA, 2013.
18. Jenkinson, C.; Layte, R.; Jenkinson, D.; Lawrence, K.; Petersen, S.; Paice, C.; Stradling, J. A shorter form health survey: Can the SF-12 replicate results from the SF-36 in longitudinal studies? *J. Public Health* **1997**, *19*, 179–186. [CrossRef] [PubMed]
19. Gandek, B.; Ware, J.E.; Aaronson, N.K.; Apolone, G.; Bjorner, J.B.; Brazier, J.E.; Bullinger, M.; Kaasa, S.; Leplege, A.; Prieto, L.; et al. Cross-validation of item selection and scoring for the SF-12 Health Survey in nine countries: Results from the IQOLA Project. *J. Clin. Epidemiol.* **1998**, *51*, 1171–1178. [CrossRef]
20. Vilagut, G.; Valderas, J.M.; Ferrer, M.; Garin, O.; López-García, E.; Alonso, J. Interpretation of SF-36 and SF-12 questionnaires in Spain: Physical and mental components. *Med. Clin.* **2008**, *130*, 726–735. [CrossRef]
21. Winters-Stone, K.M.; Lyons, K.S.; Dobek, J.; Dieckmann, N.F.; Bennett, J.A.; Nail, L.; Beer, T.M. Benefits of partnered strength training for prostate cancer survivors and spouses: Results from a randomized controlled trial of the Exercising Together project. *J. Cancer Surviv.* **2016**, *10*, 633–644. [CrossRef]
22. Pronk, N.P.; Bender, E.G.; Katz, A.S. Health, function, and performance benefits of workplace strength training programs. *ACSM's Health Fit. J.* **2016**, *20*, 69–71. [CrossRef]
23. Seguin, R.; Nelson, M.E. The benefits of strength training for older adults. *Am. J. Prev. Med.* **2003**, *25*, 141–149. [CrossRef]
24. Leirós-Rodríguez, R.; Romo-Pérez, V.; Pérez-Ribao, I.; García-Soidán, J.L. A comparison of three physical activity programs for health and fitness tested with older women: Benefits of aerobic activity, aqua fitness, and strength training. *J. Women Aging* **2019**, *31*, 419–431. [CrossRef]

25. Nikendei, C.; Terhoeven, V.; Ehrenthal, J.C.; Maatouk, I.; Wild, B.; Herzog, W.; Friederich, H.C. Depression profile in cancer patients and patients without a chronic somatic disease. *Psychooncology* **2018**, *27*, 83–90. [CrossRef]
26. Zhukova, G.; Shikhlyarova, A.; Shirnina, E.; Zinkovich, M.; Maschenko, N.; Zlatnik, E.; Pyltsin, S.; Anistratov, P.; Bragina, M.I.; Zhadobina, A.; et al. Characteristics of the psychosomatic state of patients with lung cancer. *Ann. Oncol.* **2018**, *29*, viii561. [CrossRef]
27. Boguszewski, D.; Adamczyk, J.G.; Ochal, A. The role of pilates and aquafitness exercises in sustaining the health and fitness of elderly women. *Sport Sci. Rev.* **2012**, *21*, 127–138. [CrossRef]
28. Salmon, M.; Blanchin, M.; Rotonda, C.; Guillemin, F.; Sébille, V. Identifying patterns of adaptation in breast cancer patients with cancer-related fatigue using response shift analyses at subgroup level. *Cancer Med.* **2017**, *6*, 2562–2575. [CrossRef] [PubMed]
29. Pyszora, A.; Budzyński, J.; Wójcik, A.; Prokop, A.; Krajnik, M. Physiotherapy programme reduces fatigue in patients with advanced cancer receiving palliative care: Randomized controlled trial. *Support. Care Cancer* **2017**, *25*, 2899–2908. [CrossRef]
30. Vécseyné, M.; Kopkáné, J.; József, B.; Olvasztóné, Z.; Barthalos, I. Effects of pilates and aqua fitness training on older adults' physical functioning and quality of life. *Biomed. Hum. Kinet.* **2013**, *4*, 22–27. [CrossRef]
31. Kitzman, D.W.; Brubaker, P.; Morgan, T.; Haykowsky, M.; Hundley, G.; Kraus, W.E.; Eggebeen, J.; Nicklas, B.J. Effect of caloric restriction or aerobic exercise training on peak oxygen consumption and quality of life in obese older patients with heart failure with preserved ejection fraction: A randomized clinical trial. *JAMA* **2016**, *315*, 36–46. [CrossRef]
32. Zheng, G.; Xia, R.; Zhou, W.; Tao, J.; Chen, L. Aerobic exercise ameliorates cognitive function in older adults with mild cognitive impairment: A systematic review and meta-analysis of randomised controlled trials. *Br. J. Sports Med.* **2016**, *50*, 1443–1450. [CrossRef]

International Journal of
Environmental Research and Public Health

MDPI

Study Protocol

Impact of Aquatic-Based Physical Exercise Programs on Risk Markers of Cardiometabolic Diseases in Older People: A Study Protocol for Randomized-Controlled Trials

José Pedro Ferreira [1,*], Ana Teixeira [1], João Serrano [2], Carlos Farinha [1], Hélder Santos [3], Fernanda M. Silva [1], Márcio Cascante-Rusenhack [1,4] and Paulo Luís [5]

1 FCDEF-UC, CIDAF, University of Coimbra, 3040-248 Coimbra, Portugal; ateixeira@fcdef.uc.pt (A.T.); cmnfarinha@gmail.com (C.F.); geral.fernandasilva@gmail.com (F.M.S.); marciocascante@gmail.com (M.C.-R.)
2 Sport, Health & Exercise Research Unit (SHERU), Polytechnic Institute of Castelo Branco, 6000-266 Castelo Branco, Portugal; j.serrano@ipcb.pt
3 Coimbra College of Health Technology—IPC, 3046-854 Coimbra, Portugal; heldersantos98@gmail.com
4 School of Physical Education and Sports, University of Costa Rica (UCR), San José 11501-2060, Costa Rica
5 Municipality of Sertã, 6100-738 Sertã, Portugal; pauloluis@cm-serta.pt
* Correspondence: jpferreira@fcdef.uc.pt; Tel.: +351-926-294-135

Received: 22 October 2020; Accepted: 18 November 2020; Published: 23 November 2020

Abstract: Cardiometabolic diseases are one of the primary causes of mortality and morbidity worldwide and sedentary lifestyles are contributing factors to these pathologies. Physical exercise has been recognized as an important tool in the prevention and treatment of these diseases. However, there are still some doubts about the efficacy of certain type of physical exercise programs for older participants. The main goal of this study is to assess the impact of different aquatic-based physical exercise programs on risk markers of cardiometabolic diseases in older people. The study group will consist of non-institutionalized individuals, within the age group of 65 or older. The sample will be randomly divided into four groups, three experimental groups (EG) and one control group (CG). Participants from the EGs will be exposed to three physical aquatic-based exercise programs for a period of 28 weeks (continuous aerobic, interval aerobic and combined). The evaluated parameters include anthropometry, physical functions, mental health, cognitive function, carotid arteries intima-media thickness, heart rate variability and biochemical markers. The results will allow an interpretation of the impact of different aquatic-based physical exercise programs on cardiometabolic diseases markers and can also be used as a tool for professionals to prescribe adequate and more efficient physical exercise programs.

Keywords: exercise; aquatic-based; hydro gymnastics; elderly; cardiometabolic diseases

1. Introduction

Ageing is considered a progressive and inevitable phenomenon, where the reduction in various physical and metabolic functions occurs [1]. As they age, humans become increasingly sensitive to certain pathologies such as cardiometabolic diseases. These diseases are considered to be the main cause of mortality and morbidity worldwide and have attracted great interest in various fields of scientific investigation. The World Health Organization (WHO) reports that cardiometabolic diseases are responsible for 63% of 57 million annual deaths, with a significant correlation of 6 to 10% of these deaths due to physical inactivity [2].

Nowadays, more than 60% of the elderly population live a sedentary lifestyle [3]. This contributes to physical and mental frailty. Physical frailty is characterized by a reduction in physical activity levels, unintended weight loss, fatigue, reduction in handgrip strength, and a decrease in walking speed [4]. The same authors characterize cognitive frailty as the decline in all functional mental abilities that regulate the lifestyle of an individual. These mental activities range from simple to complex. Both types of frailty are associated to the process of physical and mental decline, with a deterioration in physical and mental capabilities that may lead to a serious decrease in health conditions, loss of autonomy, institutionalization and mortality [5]. To counteract sedentary lifestyles, WHO has developed strategies for a more active and healthy society. These strategies include the creation of guidelines that state the frequency, duration, intensity, type and amount of physical activity that are recommended for different age groups. Such guidelines target the prevention of non-transmissible chronic diseases [6]. Simultaneously, there has been an increase in research using a set of variables that are related to these types of pathologies, such as body composition [7], functional fitness [8], and variables related to the cardiovascular [9], cognitive [4] and immune systems [10].

Physical exercise is considered an effective tool during the process of ageing, as it helps to stabilize the loss of physical and metabolic capacities, mitigates the overall progress of ageing and enables more autonomy. Various studies indicate that regular physical exercise plays an important role in the prevention and treatment of cardiometabolic and cognitive diseases [10–14].

Different studies have been conducted recently to verify the efficacy of various physical exercise programs (aerobic, muscular strength and combined) on variables related to these pathologies. Such studies have analyzed the impact of exercise on cognition, cardiovascular, metabolic, immunological, functional and mental levels [15–18]. However, most of these studies have focused on land-based exercise and have not involved specific aquatic exercise programs, which are popular and successful among older participants.

The present investigation and its specific experimental design using different types of aquatic-based exercise programs aims to assess the impact of different aquatic-based physical exercise programs on risk markers of cardiometabolic diseases in older people.

2. Materials and Methods

2.1. Design

This investigation will be based on a randomized intervention, using three different aquatic-based exercise programs conducted in parallel for 28 weeks. The three programs include a continuous aerobic program, an interval aerobic program and a combined (aerobic and muscular strength) program. Variables related to cardiometabolic diseases will be evaluated, i.e., cardiovascular, mental health, and cognitive variables and biochemical markers.

All exercise programs will be conducted at the Piscina Muncipal da Sertã, two times a week (non-consecutive days), with 45-min sessions. All variables related to cardiometabolic diseases will be evaluated at two specific assessment moments: M1, before implementation of the physical exercise programs (baseline) and M2, after the conclusion of the 28 weeks aquatic-based physical exercise programs (post-intervention).

Each evaluation will be divided into three phases: Phase 1—Anthropometry evaluation, physical functions, cognitive and mental health levels; Phase 2—Evaluation of carotid arteries' intima-media thickness and heart rate variability; and Phase 3—Evaluation of biochemical markers.

The blood collection for biochemical analysis will be conducted by a specialized and certified lab. The measurement of the carotid arteries intima-media thickness will be conducted by a specialist in the area of cardiology. All the remaining data will be collected and organized by the research team members.

2.2. Participants

The participants were recruited in the central area of Portugal, more specifically in the region of Sertã. The sample was recruited by the non-probabilistic method for convenience. One hundred and fifty individuals from the community were personally invited, but only 102 agreed to participate in the study (mean age of 72.32 ± 5.2 and BMI 29.47 ± 4.85). Participants will be selected according to the following inclusion criteria: individual of both genders; age equal to or above 65 years of age; non-institutionalized individuals; they give permission to be part of the study and if the participant presents with a clinical condition or comorbidity, it must be stable and enable participation in aquatic-based exercises classes as approved by local medical staff. The exclusion criteria are: individuals less than 65 years of age; individuals with medical diagnosed pathologies that jeopardize their health while preforming aquatic based exercises, participants that attend less than 50% of all the sessions and participants who cannot complete all of the proposed tests.

The participants will be distributed randomly into different exercise groups based on their registration for one of the schedules offered for the hydro-gymnastics sessions. There will be three distinct schedules (9.00, 9.50 and 10.40), with the constraint being that the participants must attend the same schedule for the whole year. The 9.00 session includes the continuous aerobic program, the 9.50 session includes the interval aerobic program, and the 10.40 session includes the combined exercise program. This information will not be provided to participants before they register for the sessions so it will not be possible to establish any association between the schedule and the different exercises programs. Such information will be communicated later in the study. The control group will be randomly recruited from the community and will include those individuals that have not been involved in any kind of physical exercise during the last year.

Before each assessment moment, participants will be taken to a testing room, where the assessment tests will be performed. The room will be large and isolated, and the temperature will be controlled, and each assessment stages should be organized to provide maximum comfort and privacy to the participants during the tests. The research team will give the participants information about the tests they will perform for data collection, explain the purpose of each test, and explain the order and duration of the tests. Participants will be able to question researchers about any doubts that they may have regarding the tests and any possible consequences. During the assessment, participants may pause the evaluation and continue on another day if they feel very fatigued or if they are not able to complete all the tests at that time. In this situation, a new date will be scheduled to continue the tests.

2.3. Protocols

The percentage of adherence to the physical exercise programs, for each program, will be calculated considering the total attended sessions: (S × 100)/T, where "S" indicates the number of sessions that have been attended by the participant during the study and "T" indicates the total number (56) of physical exercise sessions. The participants' attendance will be recorded in a database. If a participant has two consecutive absences, they will be contacted and given motivational reinforcement to incentivize them to resume their physical exercise sessions.

During the study period, all adverse effects or health problems attributed to the physical exercise sessions or evaluation tests will be reported. Parameters such as muscle pain, excessive fatigue and general pain will also be reported and inserted in a database. Exercise technicians and researchers will be responsible for data collection as well as for gathering and communicating all relevant data.

Three physical exercise programs will be conducted for a time period of 28 weeks, two times per week (non-consecutive days) and have the following common characteristics: all sessions will have a duration of 45 min, taking into account previous studies [10] that suggest sessions of this duration seem to be sufficient to provide changes in several parameters in the elderly population; they will be aquatic-based (the water level will be between 0.80 and 1.20 m with a temperature of approximately 32 °C); and they will be conducted to the rhythm of music (bpm) that can be adjusted to achieve the target HR. Sessions are divided into three parts: the initial part, main part and final part, with common exercises in the initial and final part of the three programs. The initial part or warm-up has a duration of 10 min and the purpose is to assist participants to adapt to the water environment, more specifically, for participants' to acclimatize and prepare for muscular and metabolic stimulation. Simple aquatic-based exercises will be conducted, e.g., displacement and isolated movements. The exercises increase in complexity and intensity during this initial phase. The final part has a duration of 5 min. This part will be divided into two phases: return to calm (relaxation) where relaxing exercises are conducted with the purpose of returning the participants' heart rate (HR) value to a resting level. The second phase is composed of stretching routines that stretch the most exercised muscle groups stimulated in the main part of the session and reduce the level of lactic acid and the occurrence of post-exercise pain. The main part is different in the three physical exercise programs and their characteristics are described in Table 1. All physical exercise programs will be planned and implemented according to the recommendations of the American College of Sports Medicine [19] and conducted by specialized physical exercise technicians (with a degree in sports science) with specialization in hydro-gymnastics (instructor course—level 1).

Table 1. Characteristics of the three physical exercise programs applied for 28 weeks (continuous aerobic, interval aerobic and combined).

Program	Description	Intensity (Week 1–13)	Intensity (Week 14–28)	Exercises
Continuous Aerobic	30 min exercise aerobic (moderate intensity)	60–65% maximum HR	65–70% maximum HR	Basic hydro-gymnastics exercise, with some variations: running, bounce, kicking, pendulum jumping, skiing, twister and horse.
Interval Aerobic	10 min exercise aerobic (moderate intensity)	60–65% maximum HR	65–70% maximum HR	Basic hydro-gymnastics exercise, with some variations: running, bounce, kicking, pendulum jumping, skiing, twister and horse.
	5 min exercise aerobic (high intensity)	70–75% maximum HR	75–80% maximum HR	
	10 min exercise aerobic (moderate intensity)	60–65% maximum HR	65–70% maximum HR	
	5 min exercise aerobic (high intensity)	70–75% maximum HR	75–80% maximum HR	
Combined	15 min exercise aerobic (moderate intensity)	60–65% maximum HR	65–70% maximum HR	Basic hydro-gymnastics exercise, with some variations: running, bounce, kicking, pendulum jumping, skiing, twister and horse.
	15 min muscular strengthening exercises	2 steps 12 repetitions	3 steps 16 repetitions	Exercises with auxiliary equipment (dumbbells, pool noodles, etc.): elbow extension/flexion; shoulder extension/flexion; shoulder abduction/adduction; hip abduction/adduction; hip flexion/extension; knee flexion/extension; dorsal and plantar flexion of the ankle.

HR monitors (Polar V800) will be used on the participants during all sessions of the different physical exercise program. The intensity of each exercise program will be monitored using the data provided by the Polar V800 and adjusted accordingly. As a precaution and safety measure, the intensity will be indirectly calculated using the following equation [20]:

$$Target\ HR = ((Maximum\ HR - Resting\ HR)\ \%\ intensity) + Resting\ HR \quad (1)$$

Maximum HR is calculated with the following equation for senior populations [21]:

$$Maximum\ HR = 207 - (0.7 \times age) \quad (2)$$

The control group consists of non-institutionalized individual participants who have not partaken in any physical exercise during the preceding year. These participants will be encouraged to conduct their daily activities as usual, except for the data collection (M1 and M2) organized by the researchers.

2.4. Instruments

2.4.1. Individual Characterization

In the first assessment moment (M1), all participants will fill in a clinical survey to help with the clinical characterization of each participant. This document includes the following information: civil status, regular medication, infections, allergies, diseases, annual doctor consultations, average hours of daily sleep, supplement use, latest blood panel, information on dietary habits, smoking habits and drug use.

2.4.2. Environmental Characteristics

The physical exercise programs are aquatic-based, and will take place in water at temperatures that follow regional health guidelines (30–32 degrees Celsius) in the swimming pool complex of Piscina Municipal da Sertã (indoor pool), Portugal. During the study, daily monitoring of parameters such as the pool water temperature, free chlorine, combined chlorine, pH, relative humidity and pier external temperature will be conducted and the results will be inserted in a database by two facility staff members. An external certified company will conduct a bi-weekly analysis of the following parameters: pH, conductivity, free chlorine, total chlorine, temperature and, bacteriological tests (total germs, total coliforms, Escherichia coli, fecal enterococci, total staphylococci, coagulase-producing staphylococci, and pseudomonas aeruginosa).

2.4.3. Anthropometry

Anthropometric measurements will be conducted by a certified investigator by FCDEF-UC. The following parameters will be evaluated: (i) stature, using a portable stadiometer, Seca Bodymeter® (model 208, Hamburg, Germany) with a precision of 0.1 cm; (ii) weight, body mass index (BMI), visceral fat, percentage of fat and muscle mass using a portable scale from Seca® (model 770, Hamburg, Germany) with 0.1 kg accuracy; and (iii) waist circumference, arms and legs using a retractable fiberglass tape (model Hoechst mass-Rollfix®, Sulzbach, Germany) with an accuracy of 0.1 cm.

2.4.4. Physical Function

Physical function will be assessed using the Senior Fitness Test, developed and reviewed by Rikli and Jones [22] and validated for the Portuguese population [23]. It is composed of the following test items:

- Chair stand, assesses lower body strength and consists of the maximum number of full stands that can be concluded in 30 s. Necessary equipment: chair and stopwatch.
- Arm curl, assesses upper body strength and consists of the maximum number of bicep curls that can be completed in 30 s while holding a hand weight. Necessary equipment: 2.27 kg hand weight for women and 3.63 kg for men, chair and stopwatch.
- 2-min step, assesses aerobic endurance and consists of maximum number of full steps completed in 2 min, a full step is recorded when each knee reaches the point midway between the patella (kneecap) and iliac crest (top hip bone). Necessary equipment: stopwatch, sticky-tape and ruler.
- Chair sit and reach, assesses lower body flexibility and is conducted from a sitting position where one of the participant's legs is extended while the other is flexed and where hands are reaching towards the toes. This test is assessed in cm and is positive (+) if the extended fingers pass the tip of the toes or negative (−) if the extended fingers do not pass the tip of the toes. Necessary equipment: chair and ruler.
- Back scratch, assesses upper body flexibility and is conducted with one hand reaching over the shoulder in the direction of the floor and the other hand up the middle of the back in the direction of the head. This test is assessed in cm and is positive (+) if both hands overlap and is negative (−) if overlapping does not occur. Necessary equipment: ruler.

- Timed up and go, assesses agility and dynamic balance and is conducted from a starting sitting position where the participant stands up and walks, as fast as possible, to and from a distance 2.44 m (marked by a cone). Necessary equipment: chair, cone and stopwatch.
- Hand grip, assesses hand grip strength and consists of asking the participant to grip a dynamometer with maximum achievable force, the output value of the device is then registered. Necessary equipment: Lafayette hydraulic manual dynamometer (model J00105).

2.4.5. Cognitive Function

Cognitive function will be assessed with the Portuguese version of the Mini Mental State Examination (MMSE) [24]. The MMSE, evaluates the following cognitive areas: orientation, short term memory, attention and calculation capacities, long term memory and language capabilities. The final score has a maximum of 30 points, and scores below 24 can be used as an aid in the assessment of dementia. The test will be used as an instrument to create a cognitive profile with the following criterium [25]: severe cognitive impairment (scores between 1 and 9 points); moderate cognitive impairment (scores between 10 and 18 points); mild impairment (score between 19 and 24 points), normal cognitive profile (scores between 25 and 30 points).

2.4.6. Mental Health

Mental health will be assessed using the following scales and questionnaires validated for the Portuguese population: the Rosenberg Self-Esteem Scale (RSES) [26]; Physical Self-Perception Profile for Clinical Populations (CPSPP) [27]; World Health Organization Well-Being Index (WHO-5) [28]; Satisfaction With Life Scale (SWLS) [29]; EuroQol (EQ-5D) [30]; Geriatric Depression Scale (GDS) [31] and; Perceived Stress Scale (PSS) [32].

- RSES, assesses global self-esteem and is composed of 10 items that are answered using a 4-point Likert scale, the answers vary from "I totally agree" to "I totally disagree". In items 1, 2, 4, 6 and 7 the score is reversed. Global self-esteem is represented by the summation of all individual scores, providing a final score ranging from 10 to 40 points, where higher scores indicate higher self-esteem.
- CPSPP, is an instrument designed to provide a self-assessment summary of the physical characteristics of elderly groups in clinical and rehabilitation settings. A scale is defined by six subscales of three items that evaluate the following subdomains: functionality, physical health, sports competence, physical attractiveness, physical strength and physical self-worth. Answers to the items are displayed in an alternative structured format that is designed to eliminate social desirability bias. The score can vary between 3 to 12, with higher scores representing better performance.
- WHO-5, is an instrument that assesses psychological well-being. It is a self-administrated short questionnaire composed of 5 items with positive words, these words are related to a positive mood (good mood, relaxation), vitality (being active and waking up fresh and rested) and general interests. Each item is classified on a 5-point Likert scale, ranging from 0 (not present) to 5 (constantly present). The scores are summed, with the final score ranging from 0 to 25 points. The final score is then converted to a scale of 0 to 100 (by multiplying by 4), where higher scores represent a higher level of well-being and better quality of life. A final score equal to or below 50 points represents poor well-being but does not necessarily mean depression. A final score equal to or below 28 possibly indicates clinical depression.
- SWLS, assesses global cognitive parameters of life satisfaction. It is composed of 5 items with a 7-point Likert scale. The answers indicate the level of agreement the participant feels with each item. The final score ranges from 1 to 35 points, where higher final scores indicate higher satisfaction with life.
- EQ-5D, is an instrument that assesses general health status. It consists of two parts: the EQ-5D health descriptive system and the EQ visual analogue scale. The descriptive system consists of

five dimensions (mobility, personal care, usual activities, pain/discomfort and anxiety/depression). The participant is asked to indicate their health status by selecting the most appropriate options in the five dimensions. The visual analogue is self-assessed and is conducted in a scale from the lowest rate (0) "the worst health you can imagine" to the highest rate (100) "the best health you can imagine".

- GDS, assesses life satisfaction, interruptions in activities, annoyances, isolation, energy, joy and memory problems. It consists of fifteen easy to understand questions and has a binary answer system (0 or 1 point) for answers of "no" and "yes", respectively. A participant who obtains a final score between 0 and 5 points is considered healthy; scores between 6 and 10 points indicate signs of mild to moderate depression; scores between 11 and 15 points indicate signs of severe depression.
- PSS, is an instrument to measure perceptions of stress. It is composed of 14 items, where 7 items are considered as positive aspects while the rest are considered as negative aspects. The questions are about feelings and thoughts during the last month. A point reversal is conducted on items 4, 5, 6, 7, 9, 10 and 13. The final score may vary between 14 and 70 points and a higher score indicates higher stress levels.

2.4.7. Assessment of Carotid Arteries Intima-Media Thickness

The carotid arteries intima-media thickness assessment takes place with the participant lying down in a dorsal position. Then, the following parameters are evaluated using a sphygmomanometer from Riester (Model RI-championN®, Jungingen, Germany): heart rate (HR), systolic blood pressure (SP) and diastolic blood pressure (DP). The intima-media thickness of the right and left carotid arteries are measured with a Doppler two-dimensional ultrasound and are assessed with the AIRC study protocol [33]. The following values are then recorded through a portable ultrasound from General Electric® (VIDe, Vancouver, Canada) with probe linear 11 L: Intima-media thickness (IMT); systolic diameter (SD), diastolic diameter (DD), peak systolic velocity (PSV) and end-diastolic velocity (EDV).

2.4.8. Heart Rate Variability (HRV) Measurement

HRV will be assessed according to the procedures of Abad et al. [34] using Polar V800 heart rate monitors. Participants will place the sensor, which is synchronized with the V800 clock, on their chest beneath their pectoral muscles. Then, the participants will be asked to lie down in a dorsal position, in silence, with open eyes and with a calm respiration. The test will have a duration of 10 min in a calm, silent and low-light environment. After the conclusion of the test, HRV measurement data are downloaded from the Polar Flow Web Service.

2.4.9. Biochemical Markers

Blood samples will be drawn via venipuncture from fasting participants. For each participant a total of 18.5 mL of blood will be drawn. Of the 18.5 mL, 3.5 mL will be used by the clinic to assess lipid panel values (HDL, LDL, glucose, triglycerides). The remaining 15 mL, processed by the college laboratory, will be divided into three tubes: two serum separator tubes and one ethylenediaminetetraacetic acid (EDTA) tube. Once the test tubes arrive at the university laboratory a complete blood count (CBC) will be conducted using an automatic hematology analyzer Coulter Act Diff, Beckman Coulter, USA. Next, the test tubes are centrifuged for10 min at 3500× *g* rotations per minute and stored in cryogenic test tubes. Levels of HbA1C, IL-1, IL-1ra, IL-6, IL-10, TNF-alpha, Adiponectin, Leptin, MIP-1alpha, MCP-1, SOD, MMP-9, are subsequently analyzed with ELISA Invitrogen® CA kits (Bender MedSystems GmbH, Vienna, Austria).

2.5. Ethical Aspects

The researcher will be responsible for the data integrity and validity during the entire study. All data collected will be confidential and used exclusively for scientific purposes. Anonymization procedures will be conducted under the Data Protection Regulation of 25 May 2018. Data anonymization will be implemented by attributing a code to each participant. Each participant will receive a unique identification code that will correspond to their process; this code will be visually accessible with the use of "code cards". These "code cards" will be used by the participants during data collection. Once the data collection is finalized the participants will be asked to destroy their "code cards", thus finalizing the anonymization process.

Data will be stored in an Excel Microsoft Office 2016 database. Access to this database will be protected with a password and will be restricted to the main researcher responsible for the data collection. Data backups will be carried out regularly by the main researcher.

Participation in this study is purely voluntary, with no reprisals for non-participation. All subjects will be asked for their informed consent before they start participating in the study. The study will be conducted in accordance with the Declaration of Helsinki, and the protocol was approved by the Ethics Committee for Health of the Faculty of Sport Sciences and Physical Education of the University of Coimbra (reference: CE/FCDEF-UC/00462019).

The results from this study will be disseminated through publication in various scientific journals. The participants, if desired, will receive a copy of the main results and publications.

2.6. Statistical Analysis

The size and statistical power of the sample will be calculated using the G*Power software application [35]. The following parameters will be considered: F test (ANOVA); effect size: 0.25; α-level: 0.05; statistical power: 0.95; number of groups: 4; number of measures: 2 (pré and post intervention); a 30% margin for possible losses and refusals. Therefore, the initial size of the total sample was estimated at 76 participants.

The collected data will be subjected to descriptive statistical analysis where values such as maximum, minimum, mean and standard deviation will be calculated for each variable in each assessment moment. Afterwards, data normality will be tested by considering the response to three conditions: z-values from Skewness and Kurtosis tests; *p*-value from Shapiro-Wilk test; and visual inspection of generated histograms. Parametric data will be analyzed using the Student's *t*-test for independent samples to compare the groups and two paired samples to compare the different moments (M1 and M2). Nonparametric data will be analyzed using the Mann–Whitney U test to compare the groups and the Wilcoxon test to compare the different moments (M1 and M2). Statistical analysis will be performed using the Statistical Package for the Social Sciences (SPSS) statistical software, version 25.0. The level of significance used will be $p \leq 0.05$.

3. Expected Results/Discussion

The main aim of this study is to assess the impact of different aquatic exercise programs (a continuous aerobic program, aerobic interval program and combined program) on risk markers of cardiometabolic diseases in older people. The study is guided by scientific-based evidence on the practice of physical exercise in the elderly population [11,36].

The practice of regular physical exercise is considered as the optimum tool in the prevention and treatment of various types of cardiometabolic diseases. Thus, it is important that research on this topic continues; by doing so, new intervention methods can be identified and their efficacy validated. The offer of aquatic physical exercise programs is highly successful among the elderly because they transform physical exercise into something more pleasant and suitable for this particular population. However, the high costs of maintaining aquatic environments and the additional difficulties associated with assessment methodologies and specific equipment needed to monitor exercise in aquatic environments, means this topic not yet been sufficiently explored in the literature.

After completion of the data collection and analysis, the participants in the experimental groups are expected to show positive developments with regard to the anthropometric level, physical function, the intima-media thickness of the carotid arteries, heart rate variability, cognitive function, mental health and a number of biochemical markers. It is also expected that statistically significant differences will be found between the exercise groups for some of the variables. In the control group, no changes are expected in the analyzed variables. It is believed that the expected results can be attributed to the physical and physiological effects of the aquatic environment associated with the different proposed exercise protocols. The results will be published after the study is completed.

Author Contributions: Design and coordination, J.P.F., A.T. and J.S.; methods, J.P.F., A.T. and C.F.; resources, C.F., F.M.S., M.C.-R., H.S. and P.L.; first draft preparation, C.F.; reviewing and editing, J.P.F.; A.T. and J.S. All the authors have made a substantial contribution in their respective areas of expertise, critically revised the work, approved the final version, and agreed to be accountable for all aspects of the work. All authors have read and agreed to the published version of the manuscript.

Funding: This research received no external funding.

Acknowledgments: The authors wish to show appreciation for all the support and cooperation provided by the Research Unit for Sport and Physical Activity (CIDAF), Faculty of Sport Sciences and Physical Education (FCDEFUC), Municipality of Sertã, Clinic Affidea-Sertã and Higher School of Health Technologies of Coimbra.

Conflicts of Interest: The authors declare no conflict of interest.

References

1. Filho, M.; Zanella, A.; Aidar, F.; Silva, A.; Salgueiro, R.; Matos, D. Atividade física e envelhecimento humano: A busca pelo envelhecimento saudável. *Rev. Bras. Ciências Envelhec. Hum.* **2010**, *7*, 97–106. [CrossRef]
2. Roque, F.; Hernanz, R.; Salaices, M.; Briones, A. Exercise training and cardiometabolic diseases: Focus on the vascular system. *Curr. Hypertens. Rep.* **2013**, *15*, 204–214. [CrossRef] [PubMed]
3. Collard, R.; Boter, H.; Schoevers, R.; Voshaar, R. Prevalence of frailty in community-dwelling older persons: A systematic review. *J. Am. Geriatr. Soc.* **2012**, *60*, 1487–1492. [CrossRef]
4. Furtado, G.; Caldo, A.; Rieping, T.; Filaire, E.; Hogervorst, E.; Teixeira, A.; Ferreira, J. Physical frailty and cognitive status over-60 age populations: A systematic review with meta-analysis. *Arch. Gerontol. Geriatr.* **2018**, *78*, 240–248. [CrossRef]
5. Jang, I.; Kim, H.; Lee, E.; Jung, H.; Park, H.; Cheon, S.; Lee, Y.; Park, Y. Impact of a Wearable Device-Based Walking Programs in Rural Older Adults on Physical Activity and Health Outcomes: Cohort Study. *JMIR mHealth uHealth* **2018**, *6*, e11335. [CrossRef] [PubMed]
6. WHO. *Global Action Plan on Physical Activity 2018–2030: More Active People for a Healthier World*; Wold Health Organization: Geneva, Suiça, 2018; ISBN 9789241514187.
7. Arazi, H.; Asadi, R.; Taati, B. Exercise training in thermo-mineral spring water has beneficial effects on hemodynamic and health-related factors in young-older hypertensive women: A randomized control trial. *J. Women Aging* **2018**, 1–13. [CrossRef]
8. Sykes, K.; Roberts, A. The Chester step test-a simple yet effective tool for the prediction of aerobic capacity. *Physiotherapy* **2004**, *90*, 183–188. [CrossRef]
9. Pereira, T.; Pereira, T.; Santos, H.; Correia, C.; Cardoso, J. Arterial pulse pressure waveform monitoring by novel optical probe. *Int. J. Cardiol.* **2015**, *179*, 95–96. [CrossRef]
10. Teixeira, A.; Ferreira, J.; Hogervorst, E.; Braga, M.; Bandelow, S.; Rama, L.; Figueiredo, A.; Campos, M.; Furtado, G.; Chupel, M.; et al. Study Protocol on Hormonal Mediation of Exercise on Cognition, Stress and Immunity (PRO-HMECSI): Effects of Different Exercise Programmes in Institutionalized Elders. *Front. Public Health* **2016**, *4*, 1–13. [CrossRef]
11. Chupel, M.; Direito, F.; Furtado, G.; Minuzzi, L.; Pedrosa, F.; Colado, J.; Ferreira, J.; Filaire, E.; Teixeira, A. Strength training decreases inflammation and increases cognition and physical fitness in older women with cognitive impairment. *Front. Physiol.* **2017**, *8*, 1–13. [CrossRef]

12. Furtado, G.; Chupel, M.; Carvalho, H.; Souza, N.; Ferreira, J.; Teixeira, A. Effects of a chair-yoga exercises on stress hormone levels, daily life activities, falls and physical fitness in institutionalized older adults. *Complement. Ther. Clin. Pract.* **2016**, *24*, 123–129. [CrossRef] [PubMed]
13. Novaes, G.; Novaes, J.; Garrido, N.; Reis, V. Chronic Effects of Strength Training Vs. Hydro Aerobics on Functional and Cardiorespiratory Ability in Postmenopausal Women. *J. Hum. Kinet.* **2014**, *43*, 57–66. [CrossRef]
14. Reis, V.M. Effects of Exercise on Biomarkers in Health and Disease: Some New Insights with Special Focus on Extreme Exercise and Healthy Ageing. *Int. J. Environ. Res. Public Health* **2020**, *17*, 1986. [CrossRef]
15. Timmons, J.; Minnock, D.; Hone, M.; Cogan, K.; Murphy, J.; Egan, B. Comparison of Time-Matched Aerobic, Resistance, or Concurrent Exercise Training in Older Adults. *Scand. J. Med. Sci. Sport* **2018**, *28*. [CrossRef]
16. Morat, M.; Faude, O.; Hanssen, H.; Ludyga, S.; Zacher, J.; Eibl, A.; Albracht, K.; Donath, L. Agility training to integratively promote neuromuscular, cognitive, cardiovascular and psychosocial function in healthy older adults: A study protocol of a one-year randomized-controlled trial. *Int. J. Environ. Res. Public Health* **2020**, *17*, 1853. [CrossRef]
17. Melro, F.; Mesquita, P.; Carvalho, H.; Filaire, E.; Teixeira, A.; Ferreira, J. Metabolic health indicators and perceived quality of life in active versus inactive older adults: The Funchal community based intervention study. *Asian J. Gerontol. Geriatr.* **2016**, *11*, 1–8.
18. Furtado, G.; Carvalho, H.; Loureiro, M.; Patrício, M.; Uba-Chupel, M.; Colado, J.; Hogervorst, E.; Ferreira, J.; Teixeira, A. Chair-based exercise programs in institutionalized older women: Salivary steroid hormones, disabilities and frailty changes. *Exp. Gerontol.* **2020**, *130*, 110790. [CrossRef]
19. ACSM. *Diretrizes do ACSM Para Os Testes de Esforço e Sua Prescrição, 10ath ed.*; Guanabara Koogan LTDA: Philadelphia, PA, USA, 2016.
20. Karvonen, M.; Kentala, E.; Mustala, O. The effects of training on heart rate; a longitudinal study. *Ann. Med. Exp. Biol. Fenn.* **1957**, *35*, 307–315.
21. Franklin, B.; Whaley, M.; Howley, E.; Balady, G. ACSM's Guidelines for Exercise Testing and Prescription. 2000. Available online: http://books.google.com/books?id=_g5sAAAAMAAJ (accessed on 22 February 2020).
22. Rikli, R.; Jones, J. Development and validation of a functional fitness test for a community-residing adults. *J. Aging Phys. Act.* **1999**, *7*, 129–161. [CrossRef]
23. Baptista, F.; Sardinha, L. *Avaliação da Aptidão Física e do Equilíbrio de Pessoas Idosas: Baterias de Fullerton*; Faculdade de Motricidade Humana: Cruz Quebrada, Portugal, 2005.
24. Morgado, J.; Rocha, C.; Maruta, C.; Guerreiro, M.; Martins, I. Novos valores Normativos do mini-mental state examination. *Sinapse* **2009**, *9*, 10–16.
25. Mungas, D. In-office mental status testing: A practical guide. *Geriatrics* **1991**, *46*, 54–58,63,66. [PubMed]
26. Neto, F. Correlates of social blushing. *Pers. Individ. Dif.* **1996**, *20*, 365–373. [CrossRef]
27. Ferreira, J.; Cruz, M.; Salgueiro, T.; Fox, K. Propriedades psicométricas do perfil físico de autopercepção: Versão clínica curta em populações geriátricas. *EUJAPA* **2017**, *10*, 3–13.
28. Canavarro, M.; Serra, A.; Simões, M.; Rijo, D.; Pereira, M.; Gameiro, S.; Quartilho, M.; Quintais, L.; Carona, C.; Paredes, T. Development and psychometric properties of the world health organization quality of life assessment instrument (WHOQOL-100) in Portugal. *Int. J. Behav. Med.* **2009**, *16*, 116–124. [CrossRef]
29. Neto, F.; Oliveira, J. Satisfação Com a Vida Conforme a Religião e a Cultura. *Psicol. Educ. Cult.* **2004**, *6*, 349–361.
30. Ferreira, P.; Ferreira, L.; Pereira, L. Contributos para a validação da versão Portuguesa do EQ-5D. *Acta Med. Port.* **2013**, *26*, 664–675.
31. Apóstolo, J.; Loureiro, L.; Reis, I.; Silva, I.; Cardoso, D.; Sfetcu, R. Contribuição para a adaptação da Geriatric Depression Scale-15 para a língua portuguesa. *Rev. Enferm. Ref.* **2014**, 65–73. [CrossRef]
32. Trujillo, H.; Cabrera, J. Psychometric properties of the Spanish version of the Perceived Stress Scale (PSS). *Psicol. Conductual* **2007**, *15*, 457–477.
33. Stein, J.; Korcarz, C.; Hurst, R.; Lonn, E.; Kendall, C.; Mohler, E.; Najjar, S.; Rembold, C.; Post, W. Use of Carotid Ultrasound to Identify Subclinical Vascular Disease and Evaluate Cardiovascular Disease Risk: A Consensus Statement from the American Society of Echocardiography Carotid Intima-Media Thickness Task Force Endorsed by the Society for Vascular. *J. Am. Soc. Echocardiogr.* **2008**, *21*, 93–111. [CrossRef]
34. Abad, C.; Kobal, R.; Kitamura, K.; Gil, S.; Pereira, L.; Loturco, I.; Nakamura, F. Heart rate variability in elite sprinters: Effects of gender and body position. *Clin. Physiol. Funct. Imaging* **2017**, *37*, 442–447. [CrossRef]

35. Franz, F.; Erdfelder, E.; Buchner, A. G*Power 3: A flexible statistical power analysis program for the social, behavioral, and biomedical sciences. *J. Mater. Environ. Sci.* **2007**, *7*, 3759–3766. [CrossRef]
36. Furtado, G.; Chupel, M.; Minuzzi, L.; Patrício, M.; Loureiro, M.; Bandelow, S.; Hogervorst, E.; Ferreira, J.; Teixeira, A. Exploring the potential of salivary and blood immune biomarkers to elucidate physical frailty in institutionalized older women. *Exp. Gerontol.* **2020**, *129*. [CrossRef]

International Journal of
Environmental Research and Public Health

MDPI

Article

Acute Effects of Brief Mindfulness Intervention Coupled with Carbohydrate Ingestion to Re-Energize Soccer Players: A Randomized Crossover Trial

Yuxin Zhu [1], Fenghua Sun [1,*], Chunxiao Li [2] and Daniel Hung Kay Chow [1]

1 Department of Health and Physical Education, The Education University of Hong Kong, Hong Kong, China; im.usinzu@gmail.com (Y.Z.); danielchow@eduhk.hk (D.H.K.C.)
2 School of Physical Education & Sports Science, South China Normal University, Guangzhou 510631, China; cxlilee@gmail.com
* Correspondence: fhsun@eduhk.hk; Tel.: +852-2948-7854

Received: 18 November 2020; Accepted: 1 December 2020; Published: 4 December 2020

Abstract: *Background:* This field experiment investigated the acute effects of brief mindfulness-based intervention (MBI) coupled with carbohydrate (CHO) intake on players' recovery from half-time break in a simulated soccer competition. *Methods:* In a single-blinded randomized crossover experiment, 14 male players received 3 treatments (Control: non-carbohydrate solution + travelling introduction audio; CHO: CHO–electrolyte solution + travelling introduction audio; and CHO_M: CHO–electrolyte solution + MBI) during simulated half-time breaks. Vertical jump, sprint performance, mindfulness level, rate of perceived exertion, muscle pain, mental fatigue, blood glucose, and lactate were measured immediately before, during, and after the exercise. *Results:* (1) MBI significantly increased participants' mindfulness level (Control vs. CHO_M, $p < 0.01$; CHO vs. CHO_M, $p < 0.01$) and decreased mental fatigue for CHO_M condition (pre vs. post, $p < 0.01$); (2) participants in the CHO_M condition performed better in the repeated sprint tests than in the Control and CHO condition (Control vs. CHO_M, $p = 0.02$; CHO vs. CHO_M, $p = 0.02$). *Conclusion:* Findings of this study provide preliminary evidence of the positive effect of MBI coupled with CHO ingestion on athletes' recovery from fatigue in the early stage of the second half of a game.

Keywords: recovery; team sport; fatigue

1. Introduction

The game of soccer involves high-intensity intermittent exercise that can cause physiological and mental fatigue [1]. Physiological fatigue is generally defined as maximal voluntary muscle force reduction caused by exercise, while mental fatigue refers to a psychobiological status involving feelings of tiredness and lack of energy [1]. Laboratory-based research has demonstrated that both types of fatigue could adversely affect athletic performance. For example, muscle damage, resulting in physiological fatigue, impairs an athlete's performance by increasing muscle pain and decreasing muscle force [2]. Meanwhile, research has shown that mental fatigue causes altered attentional focus and reduces the speed and preciseness of responses [3]. Thus, fast recovery from fatigue is crucial to an athlete's performance. In soccer, the half-time break has been regarded as a good opportunity to recover from fatigue [4]. Therefore, it is necessary to investigate whether any strategies could facilitate soccer players' recovery from physiological and mental fatigue during that critical period.

Fluid intake in the form of common sports drinks is one of the most popular recovery strategies, as it prevents excessive dehydration and provides various nutrients for recovery. Nutrients with fluids, such as carbohydrate (CHO), have been found to be important for both anaerobic and aerobic energy systems [5]. Research suggests that CHO ingestion during a soccer match maintains the blood glucose concentration and spares muscle glycogen, which may improve performance in soccer [6].

Although numerous studies have investigated the effects of fluid intake on recovery from physiological fatigue, little attention has been paid to understand the recovery of mental fatigue. Recently, the potential benefits of mindfulness have been researched widely by scholars in a diverse number of fields, including psychology, education, healthcare, and sports (e.g., athletes' sleep [7,8] and burnout [9]). Mindfulness is defined as the awareness that emerges from paying attention to objects on purpose and without judging the unfolding of experience moment by moment [10]. The mindfulness-based intervention (MBI) programs that typically last for 8–12 weeks have been shown to reduce stress, anxiety, burnout, and pain [11]. In addition, brief MBI (i.e., 5–20 min/session) programs have been found to reduce chronic pain or increase pain tolerance [12,13], benefit cardiovascular and respiratory modulation [14], and help physiological relaxation responses [15].

To date, MBI has not been studied as a recovery tool in the context of sports competition. Considering the effectiveness of MBI in improving psychological outcomes [12–17], it is highly possible that MBI may provide beneficial effects in fatigue recovery after a 45 min soccer match. The present study therefore investigated the effect of brief MBI as an adjunct to CHO fluid intake to reenergize soccer players during half-time breaks. We hypothesized that the combination strategy would yield the best effect on recovery when compared with the other two conditions, i.e., CHO fluid intake with control audio and non-CHO fluid intake with control audio, respectively.

2. Materials and Methods

2.1. Participants

In total, 18 male soccer players were recruited, of which 14 completed the whole experiment (age: 24.3 ± 3.7 year, height: 1.74 ± 0.05 cm, weight: 68.3 ± 5.1 kg, VO_{2max}: 47.0 ± 4.4 mL/kg/min; average training years: 2.5 years; drop-out rate: 22%). Participants reported no history of MBI practice. The present research was approved by the University Human Research Ethics Committee (Ref. no. 2018-2019-0221). All the participants gave their written consent prior to joining the experiment.

2.2. Experimental Protocol

A 3-treatment, single-blinded, randomized, crossover design was used [17]. All the participants completed 1 pretrial and 3 main trials in 1 month. To prevent a carry-over effect and the effect of individual differences in recovery, washout periods of at least 72 h were arranged [2]. On the trial day, participants were refrained from ingesting any food or drink with caffeine, alcohol, or nicotine. In addition, they had restrictions on performing heavy exercises on the day before the main trial. For the main trials, participants were allocated to different small groups based on their maximal oxygen consumption (VO_{2max}), i.e., participants with similar VO_{2max} were assigned to the same group. Each participant was randomized to a sequence of three treatments (i.e., Control; CHO; CHO_M) by using Excel (Microsoft, Redmond, WA, USA).

2.2.1. Pretrial

To estimate VO_{2max} in the pretrial, the participants were instructed to finish a 20 m beep test (starting at 8.0 km/h and increasing by 0.5 km/h for each one-minute stage) after a warm-up session [18]. The warm-up protocol involved running for five laps around the field (i.e., 600 m) with low to moderate intensity, both static and dynamic stretching, 20 m of running at 55% VO_{2max}, 20 m of running at 95% VO_{2max}, and vertical jump (as high as possible) for three times. Participants could change warm-up intensity and time based on their personal habits, as long as it was finished within ten minutes. After that, participants had their body height and weight measured, and a detailed demographic information form completed. Furthermore, participants read the hard copy of the experimental protocol of the main trial to familiarize themselves with the study procedures.

2.2.2. Main Trial

The main trials were conducted during the daytime (i.e., 9:00 a.m.–5:30 p.m.). The average temperature was 28.9 ± 5.2 °C and average air humidity was 75.7% ± 5.8%. Two hours before entering the test field, participants were instructed to drink 500 mL of plain water to be normally hydrated [19]. Bladders were to be completely emptied before the main trials

The Loughborough Intermittent Shuttle Test [20] was selected, given that it is a reliable action mode to simulate athletic performance in soccer matches. The protocol consists of six 15-min blocks of exercise separated by 3-min rest periods. The exercises of each block include 10–12 cycles of different activities (i.e., a 20-min walk, 20-min maximal sprint, 4-s standing rest, 20-min run at approximately 55% VO_{2max} pace, and 20-min run at approximately 95% VO_{2max} pace). In the main trials, participants were instructed to finish the first 3 blocks of protocol to simulate the exercise intensity of the first half of a soccer match, and to finish the Stroop test on screen during the interval of each block to simulate the cognitive consumption of playing a soccer match. [21].

Participants' blood samples in the pretest were collected after they arrived at the test field. Then they were instructed to complete a 10-min warm-up following a standard protocol as described in pretrial. Subsequently, the warm-up vertical jump, 20-m sprint, rating of perceived exertion (RPE), muscle pain, and mental fatigue were measured. During the break between two blocks, participants were asked to report their RPE level (i.e., second and third tests) and complete one Stroop test to induce mental fatigue.

After finishing the first 3 blocks of exercise protocol, all participants had a half-time break that simulated the half-time break of a real soccer match. At the start of half-time, participants were asked to report their RPE (i.e., fourth test), provide a blood sample (i.e., mid-test), and drink a beverage. There were 2 different beverages (i.e., with and without CHO) contained in unmarked paper cups. Then they were required to listen to a 6-min audio labelled with numbers followed by the report of mindfulness level, muscle pain and mental fatigue. To avoid injury and maintain sport performance, they were instructed to do a standardized warm-up for 3 min (i.e., 200 m running, dynamic stretches, a 90% VO_{2max} sprint for 50 m and 2 vertical jumps) before the posttest for vertical jump and sprint performance. The processes of post tests were the same as those of the pretest except that the sprint performance test was repeated 6 times with a 30-s interval. Finally, participants' RPE (posttest) and blood samples (i.e., posttest) were collected. The protocol is illustrated in Figure 1.

2.3. *Treatment*

In the half-time break, three different treatments (i.e., CHO, CHO_M, and Control, as defined below) were applied.

Treatment CHO involved a CHO-electrolyte solution (Aquarius®, Coca-Cola Co., Hong Kong, China), contained with 4.2 g CHO, 30 mg sodium, 7 mg potassium, 0.7 mg calcium, 1.1 mg magnesium, and 18 kca energy, 3 mL/kg of which was to be consumed by the participants in each trial [22]. In addition, the researchers instructed them to listen to a 6-min travelling introduction, an audio recording of a Chinese tourist attraction, without mindfulness content, as an active control.

Treatment CHO_M involved the same CHO-electrolyte solution as well as a 6-min MBI comprising mindful breathing and body scanning.

The Control treatment involved the same electrolyte solution but without CHO and energy (Aquarius Zero®, Coca-Cola Co., Hong Kong, China), with the same volume, time, and steps, as stated in CHO treatment.

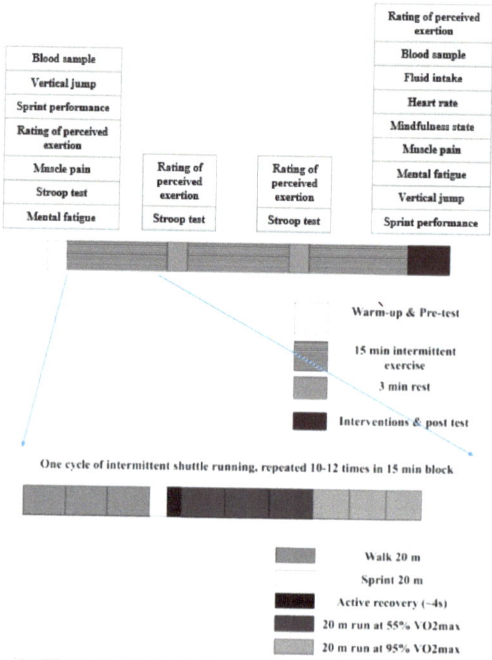

Figure 1. Adopted from the Loughborough Intermittent Shuttle Test.

2.4. Measurements

2.4.1. Heart Rate

The researchers recorded the heart rate (HR) during the half-time using an HR monitor (Polar H10, Polar Electro Oy, Kempele, Finland) and an iPad (2018 version, Apple Inc., Cupertino, CA, USA).

2.4.2. Blood Samples

Blood glucose was measured using a portable glucose analyzer (Accu-Chek Performa Nano, Roche, Germany). Blood lactate was assessed using a handheld portable lactate analyzer (Lactate Plus, Nova Biomedical, Waltham, MA, USA).

2.4.3. Vertical Jump

Vertical jump performance (i.e., jump height, flight time, velocity, force, and power) was assessed through the application "My Jump II" on the iPad (2018 version, Apple Inc., Cupertino, CA, USA). Jump height is determined by the app using the equation $h = t^2 \times 1.22625$, described by Bosco et al., where h stands for the jump height and t for flight time [23]. All collections were made with the same iPad and by the same researcher with no professional experience in video analysis. The researcher was always recording from the same position and with the same distance from the participants (i.e., 1.5 m). The validity and reliability of the application has previously been proven [24].

2.4.4. Sprint Performance

The 20-m sprint performance was measured using the Kinematic Measurement System ((KMS) Innervation, Perth, Australia), a visible red-light system modulated by a single beam with 2 sets of gates and polarizing filters. The time between the points when the participants passed through the first and second gates was recorded as the sprint performance.

2.4.5. Mindfulness State

Similar to other studies [17], the researchers asked the participants to answer 2 statements ("I felt in touch with my body" and "I focused on my breathing") as a manipulation check of mindfulness induction immediately after completing the treatments. A 7-point Likert scale, ranging from 0 (very slightly or not at all) to 6 (extremely), was used for responses. A higher mindfulness score by averaging the two responses indicated a higher mindfulness level.

2.4.6. Muscle Pain

Levels of muscle pain were evaluated by a pain intensity scale ranging from 0 (no pain at all) to 10 (extremely unbearable), as used in previous research [25].

2.4.7. Perceived Exertion

The RPE was assessed using the Borg 15-point RPE scale [26], ranging from 6 (very light) to 20 (extremely unbearable).

2.5. Statistical Analysis

A normality test was assessed for all variables. ANOVAs were performed, as the F-test remains a valid statistical procedure under non-normality in a variety of conditions [27,28]. A two-way repeated measures analysis of variance (ANOVA) was used to detect the main and interactive effects of treatments (i.e., Control, CHO, and CHO_M) and time (i.e., pretest and posttest) on participants' performance (i.e., vertical jump, sprint performance, RPE level, blood glucose and lactate, muscle pain, and mental fatigue). A one-way repeated ANOVA was used to test the difference of mindfulness state among three groups. For variables that adopted multiple posttests (i.e., sprint), the difference between pretest and each posttest was computed for further analysis. If a significant effect was observed, post hoc tests with Bonferroni correction were conducted. The significance level was set at $\alpha = 0.05$, and effect size was referred to by η^2 (partial eta squared). The analyses were conducted in SPSS 25.0 (SPSS, Inc., Chicago, IL, USA).

3. Results

3.1. Vertical Jump

Table 1 presents the mean (M) and standard deviation (SD) of five indices of vertical jump (i.e., height, flight time, velocity, force, and power). The five indices did not exhibit any interactive and treatment effects. Three indices exhibited significant time differences, with the values of pretest being higher than those of posttest ($p < 0.01$, partial $\eta^2 = 0.65$ for flight time; $p < 0.01$, partial $\eta^2 = 0.65$ for velocity; and $p < 0.01$, partial $\eta^2 = 0.67$ for height).

Table 1. The performance of five dimensions for vertical jump between pre and post-test (M ± SD).

Variable	Pre			Post		
	Control	CHO	CHO_M	Control	CHO	CHO_M
Height (cm)	42.92 (6.93)	42.08 (8.10)	43.27 (8.08)	39.45 (7.48)	40.32 (8.15)	41.84 (8.28)
Flight time (ms)	589.93 (46.81)	583.43 (55.51)	591.71 (54.41)	564.86 (53.42)	570.93 (56.72)	581.64 (56.68)
Velocity (m/s)	1.45 (0.11)	1.43 (0.14)	1.45 (0.13)	1.39 (0.13)	1.40 (0.14)	1.43 (0.14)
Force (N)	1308.92 (139.02)	1365.90 (232.93)	1360.36 (179.85)	1294.10 (188.70)	1376.68 (213.91)	1356.29 (177.09)
Power (W)	1905.58 (337.06)	1976.70 (500.84)	1988.99 (405.81)	1809.15 (396.63)	1945.52 (454.65)	1941.32 (413.26)

3.2. Sprint Performance

3.2.1. Sprint Performance—Difference between Pretest and Each of the Posttests

Table 2 presents the difference of sprint performance between pretest and each of six posttests. A significant interactive effect ($p = 0.02$, partial $\eta^2 = 0.20$) and treatment effect ($p = 0.01$, partial $\eta^2 = 0.30$) was observed. Post hoc analysis revealed that the CHO_M group performed better than the CHO ($p = 0.02$) and Control groups ($p = 0.02$) in post repeated sprint tests. No group differences were detected between CHO and Control groups ($p = 1.00$) (Table 2).

Table 2. The sprint performance—difference between pretest and each of the posttests (M ± SD).

	Post					
	1	2	3	4	5	6
Control	0.10 (0.20)	0.10 (0.26)	0.15 (0.16)	0.19 (0.24)	0.48 (0.14)	0.11 (0.12)
CHO	0.15 (0.20)	0.15 (0.22)	0.13 (0.14)	0.10 (0.17)	0.85 (0.12)	0.07 (0.15)
CHO_M [a,b]	0.14 (0.19)	0.06 (0.23)	0.16 (0.15)	0.05 (0.19)	0.07 (0.12)	−0.01 (0.15)

[a] $p < 0.05$, CHO_M vs. Control; [b] $p < 0.05$, CHO_M vs. CHO.

3.2.2. Sprint Performance—Pretest and First Posttest

No significant interaction effect on sprint performance ($p = 0.12$, partial $\eta^2 = 0.30$) was found. There was no significant treatment effect on sprint performance ($p = 0.60$, partial $\eta^2 = 0.08$), but time had a significant main effect ($p < 0.01$, partial $\eta^2 = 0.50$). Post hoc analysis revealed that sprint performance in the pretest (M = 3.32, SD = 0.03) was significantly better than that in the first posttest (M = 3.42, SD = 0.05; $p < 0.01$).

3.3. Mindfulness State

The mindfulness state of the three groups showed significant differences ($p < 0.01$, partial $\eta^2 = 0.97$). The post hoc tests showed that participants in the CHO_M group had significantly higher mindfulness levels (M = 5.32; SD = 0.15) than those in the Control (M = 2.11; SD = 0.19; $p < 0.01$) and CHO groups (M = 2.43; SD = 0.27; $p < 0.01$). However, the Control and CHO groups showed no significant difference ($p = 1.00$).

3.4. Blood Glucose and Lactate

The interaction effect was not statistically significant in terms of blood glucose ($p = 0.60$, partial $\eta^2 = 0.22$). The treatment had no significant effect ($p = 0.86$, partial $\eta^2 = 0.03$), but there was significant time effect on blood glucose ($p < 0.01$, partial $\eta^2 = 0.60$). Post hoc analysis revealed that the mid-test glucose level (M = 6.61, SD = 0.21) was significantly higher than that of the posttest (M = 5.74, SD = 0.11; $p < 0.01$).

For lactate, there was no interactive effect ($p = 0.31$, partial $\eta^2 = 0.09$). A significant main effect was revealed in terms of time ($p < 0.01$, partial $\eta^2 = 0.96$) but not on treatment ($p = 0.15$, partial $\eta^2 = 0.27$). The post hoc test showed that the mid-test lactate level (M = 6.06, SD = 0.33) was significantly higher than that of the pretest (M = 1.58, SD = 0.16; $p < 0.01$) and posttest (M = 5.82, SD = 0.29; $p < 0.01$). Moreover, the posttest lactate level was higher than that of the pretest ($p < 0.01$).

3.5. Muscle Pain and Mental Fatigue

The interaction effect between treatment and time was not statistically significant in terms of muscle pain ($p = 0.29$, partial $\eta^2 = 0.19$). There was no significant treatment effect ($p = 0.51$, partial $\eta^2 = 0.11$), but time had a significant main effect ($p < 0.01$, partial $\eta^2 = 0.89$). Post hoc analysis revealed that the muscle pain in the pretest (M = 1.93, SD = 0.24) was significantly lower than that in the posttest (M = 4.76, SD = 0.26; $p < 0.01$).

Regarding mental fatigue, a significant interactive effect was observed ($p < 0.01$, partial $\eta^2 = 0.65$). Post hoc analysis showed that there was a significant treatment effect in posttest (Control vs. CHO vs. CHO_M: 52.14 ± 7.43 vs. 67.14 ± 4.25 vs. 28.57 ± 6.10; $p = 0.23$ for Control vs. CHO; $p = 0.05$ for CHO vs. CHO_M and $p < 0.01$ for Control vs. CHO_M). A significant within group difference was also observed in both CHO (pre vs. post: 47.86 ± 23.92 vs. 67.14 ± 15.90, $p < 0.01$) and CHO_M groups (pre vs. post: 59.29 ± 15.92 vs. 28.57 ± 22.82, $p < 0.01$) but not in the control group (pre vs. post: 55.00 ± 14.01 vs. 52.14 ± 27.78, $p = 0.68$) (Figure 2).

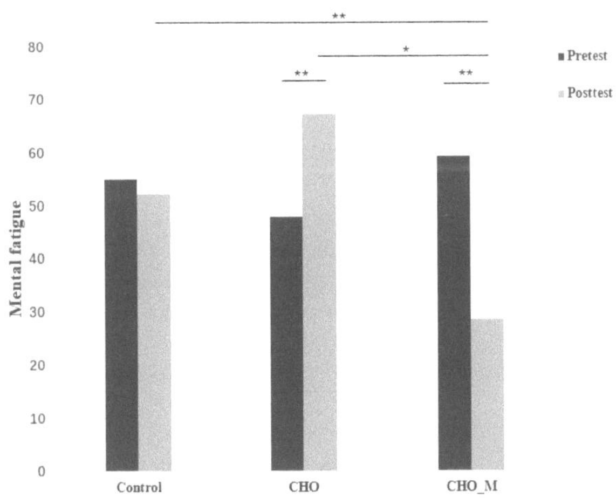

Figure 2. Changes in the 3 groups' mental fatigue through time. * $p = 0.05$; ** $p < 0.01$.

3.6. *Rate of Perceived Exertion*

The interaction was not significant ($p = 0.44$, partial $\eta^2 = 0.07$). No significant treatment effect was detected ($p = 0.77$, partial $\eta^2 = 0.04$), but the main effect of time was significant ($p < 0.01$, partial $\eta^2 = 0.95$). According to the post hoc analysis, the pretest scores (M = 8.33, SD = 0.42) were significantly lower than other following scores. Scores of the third (M = 18.69, SD = 0.41) and fourth tests (M = 19.31, SD = 0.23) were the two highest, followed by the second (M = 16.244, SD = 0.41) and posttest (M = 16.17, SD = 0.27). No difference was found between the third and mid-tests and between the second and posttest.

3.7. *Heart Rate*

Results indicated that no interactive effect was detected ($p = 0.26$, partial $\eta^2 = 0.09$). There was no significant treatment effect ($p = 0.24$, partial $\eta^2 = 0.20$), but a significant time effect ($p < 0.01$, partial $\eta^2 = 0.73$). Post hoc analysis showed that participants' heartrate decreased significantly during the intervention period (pre vs. post: M = 129.14, SD = 11.27; M = 115.19, SD = 11.71, $p < 0.01$).

4. Discussion

To our knowledge, this study is the first field trial that investigated the application of brief MBI coupled with CHO on soccer players' recovery during a half-time break. Applying brief MBI coupled with CHO ingestion during half-time breaks was found to significantly increase athletes' mindfulness levels and decrease athletes' mental fatigue. In addition, compared with the participants in Control and CHO groups, participants in the CHO_M performed better in the repeated sprint tests but not in single measures (e.g., vertical jump, pretest, and first posttest in sprint performance).

As hypothesized, participants who received brief MBI coupled with CHO during the half-time break performed better in some facets when compared with those who received other treatments (e.g., sprint performance). Brief MBI was also helpful for recovery from mental fatigue. As previous literature has demonstrated that both acceptant mood and relaxing breath positively affect the brain, the capacity of mindfulness to improve acceptance and relaxation can affect the biological system that regulates the generation of mental fatigue [29]. With regard to our observations about mental fatigue, three potential mechanisms were raised. First, as Smith [30] pointed out in a review study, the causation of mental fatigue during a soccer games is influenced by the anterior cingulate cortex (i.e., it increases adenosine and decreases dopamine). Given that previous studies have demonstrated stronger subgenual and adjacent ventral anterior cingulate cortex activity, which controls parasympathetic activity, in the MBI condition through imaging data [31], it is possible to restore mental fatigue through MBI. Second, MBI has been proven to improve respiratory sinus arrhythmia [32], a variation of heart rate in synchrony with respiration [33] that increases in the resting state and decreases in conditions of stress or tension. Therefore, possibly, the increase of respiratory sinus arrhythmia is closer to the resting state and thus relieves mental fatigue. Third, respiratory sinus arrhythmia is a valid and reliable biomarker of emotional regulation capacity in humans, and has been frequently used as a noninvasive method for investigating cardiac vagal tone [34,35]. In addition, mindfulness is beneficial to the prefrontal cortex, which can modulate brain activities in multiple emotion-processing systems [36]. Therefore, mindfulness has potential effects on emotional regulation and mental fatigue.

One explanation for the observed improvement in repetitive sprinting is that, in general, the sympathetic nervous system (SNS) and parasympathetic nervous system (PNS) are in equilibrium in the rest state. During exercise, increased levels of SNS activity upsets the balance, leading to biological changes such as pupil dilation, faster heart beats, atelectasis, and blood pressure elevation [37]. After receiving the acceptance hint (i.e., MBI), the activity levels of the PNS are induced, thus promoting the "rest and digest" response that calms the body down [16]. Another reason for the observed improvement in repeated sprinting is that it might be affected by cerebral oxygenation, which is related to the prefrontal cortex [38]. Previous fMRI studies have determined that MBI regulates the activity of the prefrontal cortex [36]. Therefore, we observed an increase in repeated sprinting performance. For vertical jump, three of the five indices exhibited significant pre–post differences, while the other two did not. This is not very surprising, as a previous review study has indicated that compared with other indices, power should be reported with caution [39]. Additionally, one possible explanation is that after half time break, athletes' power and force recovered relatively faster than the other three indices.

Although some previous studies have confirmed the immediate effect of MBI on releasing pathological pain [13], the same results were not observed in the present research. Probably, short-term mindfulness training for acute pain is not always effective [40]. This is because the mechanisms that cause pathological pain and those that cause exercise-induced muscle pain are different from each other [41,42]. As the improved immune system is probably the mediator between MBI and pathological pain [11], such a link may be absent in sports-related muscle damage. Another potential reason might be that there was no effect of mindfulness on adjusting endorphin levels, which can cause muscle pain [43].

Further, although previous studies have asserted that MBI positively affects HR recovery by improving cardiac efficiency [14], no statistically significant group difference was observed in our research. This is probably due to participants in this study being beginners in the use of mindfulness techniques. Another possible reason is that the period of receiving MBI in this study was also the period of a transition from high-intensity exercise to a relaxed state. Therefore, the heart rate changes due to the difference of activity state may buffer the change caused by MBI. Further research on this phenomenon is necessary.

No statistically significant influence was observed on the values of blood glucose and lactate between the Control, CHO, and CHO_M groups. This result is consistent with previous studies in which both ingestion of a CHO beverage before and during a competition had no effect on participants' blood glucose [44]. A possible explanation is that respiratory sinus arrhythmia may have evolved to save energy for both cardiac and respiratory systems by suppressing unnecessary heartbeats during exhalation and ineffective ventilation during the ebb of perfusion (delivery of blood from arteries to capillaries for oxygenation and nutrition) [33,45]. Therefore, MBI practice may delay the effect of CHO digestion and glucose absorption at the capillaries during the test.

Our findings also indicate that the ingestion of CHO during a half-time break may have both positive and negative effects on the initial stage of second-half performance. Although previous review studies have reported that the ingestion of CHO in prolonged exercise can enhance athletes' performance and maintain their endurance [6], this study found CHO to have a significant negative effect on mental fatigue. This is in line with a previous meta-analysis that concluded that CHO ingestion does not have a beneficial effect on mood and may increase fatigue within 30 min post-consumption [46]. In reference to the mentioned results, MBI seems to have the effect of buffering the negative influence of CHO. This point also requires further investigation.

The results of our study have practical implications. It has been confirmed that MBI can be used during half-time breaks of soccer games. Although mindfulness resulted in a significant increase in RSA compared with a relaxation strategy in a nonathletic- or nonexercise-population [32], considering that half-time is short and important, MBI's superiority to other mainstream psychological interventions (e.g., self-talk, goal setting, imagery) needs to be further investigated. The current study was a field test that could simulate exercise intensity but not athletes' moods during the game. Future studies should be conducted in real games.

This study has several limitations. First, although the current trial simulated the exercise intensity of half of a soccer match, the atmosphere of competition was not simulated. As previous studies have suggested, athletes' moods could affect their performance [47], and it is possible that the atmosphere of real competition may affect the physiological and psychological measurements in the current study. Future studies may consider conducting trials in a real soccer competition. Second, although ingesting CHO is a convenient and common recovery strategy during the half-time break, no control group with MBI alone was involved in the current study. Future research may consider investigating the unique effect of brief MBI alone on soccer players.

5. Conclusions

In conclusion, our field experiment provides preliminary evidence of the positive effects of brief MBI coupled with ingestion of CHO on athletes' recovery from fatigue in the initial stage of the second half of a game.

Author Contributions: Conceptualization, Y.Z., F.S., C.L. and D.H.K.C.; Formal analysis, Y.Z. and C.L.; Funding acquisition, F.S., Methodology, Y.Z., F.S., C.L. and D.H.K.C.; Resources, F.S.; Supervision, F.S.; Writing—original draft, Y.Z.; Writing—review and editing, F.S., C.L. and D.H.K.C. All authors have read and agreed to the published version of the manuscript.

Funding: The work was partly supported by Internal Research Grant of Education University of Hong Kong (RG91/17-18R).

Conflicts of Interest: The authors declare no conflict of interest. The funders had no role in the design of the study; in the collection, analyses, or interpretation of data; in the writing of the manuscript; or in the decision to publish the results.

References

1. Mohr, M.; Krustrup, P.; Bangsbo, J. Fatigue in soccer: A brief review. *J. Sports Sci.* **2005**, *23*, 593–599. [CrossRef]
2. Ispirlidis, I.; Fatouros, I.G.; Jamurtas, A.Z.; Nikolaidis, M.G.; Michailidis, I.; Douroudos, I.; Margonis, K.; Chatzinikolaou, A.; Kalistratos, E.; Katrabasas, I.; et al. Time-course of changes in inflammatory and performance responses following a soccer game. *Clin. J. Sport Med.* **2008**, *18*, 423–431. [CrossRef]
3. Boksem, M.A.S.; Meijman, T.F.; Lorist, M.M. Effects of mental fatigue on attention: An ERP study. *Cogn. Brain Res.* **2005**, *25*, 107–116. [CrossRef] [PubMed]
4. Russell, M.; West, D.J.; Harper, L.D.; Cook, C.J.; Kilduff, L.P. Half-time strategies to enhance second-half performance in team-sports players: A review and recommendations. *Sport. Med.* **2015**, *45*, 353–364. [CrossRef] [PubMed]
5. Holway, F.E.; Spriet, L.L. Sport-specific nutrition: Practical strategies for team sports. *J. Sports Sci.* **2011**, *29*, S115–S125. [CrossRef] [PubMed]

6. Pöchmüller, M.; Schwingshackl, L.; Colombani, P.C.; Hoffmann, G. A systematic review and meta-analysis of carbohydrate benefits associated with randomized controlled competition-based performance trials. *J. Int. Soc. Sports Nutr.* **2016**, *13*, 27. [CrossRef] [PubMed]
7. Li, C.; Kee, Y.H.; Lam, L.S. Effect of brief mindfulness induction on university athletes' sleep quality following night training. *Front. Psychol.* **2018**, *9*, 508. [CrossRef]
8. Li, C.; Zhu, Y.; Zhang, M.; Gustafsson, H.; Chen, T. Mindfulness and athlete burnout: A systematic review and meta-analysis. *Int. J. Environ. Res. Public Health* **2019**, *16*, 449. [CrossRef]
9. Kee, Y.H.; Li, C.; Kong, L.C.; Tang, C.J.; Chuang, K.-L. Scoping review of mindfulness research: A topic modelling approach. *Mindfulness* **2019**, *10*, 1474–1488. [CrossRef]
10. Kabat-Zinn, J. Mindfulness-based interventions in context: Past, present, and future. *Clin. Psychol. Sci. Pract.* **2003**, *10*, 144–156. [CrossRef]
11. Creswell, J.D. Mindfulness Interventions. *Annu. Rev. Psychol.* **2017**, *68*, 491–516. [CrossRef] [PubMed]
12. Sollgruber, A.; Bornemann-Cimenti, H.; Szilagyi, I.S.; Sandner-Kiesling, A. Spirituality in pain medicine: A randomized experiment of pain perception, heart rate and religious spiritual well-being by using a single session meditation methodology. *PLoS ONE* **2018**, *13*, e0203336. [CrossRef] [PubMed]
13. Ussher, M.; Spatz, A.; Copland, C.; Nicolaou, A.; Cargill, A.; Amini-Tabrizi, N.; McCracken, L.M. Immediate effects of a brief mindfulness-based body scan on patients with chronic pain. *J. Behav. Med.* **2014**, *37*, 127–134. [CrossRef] [PubMed]
14. May, R.W.; Bamber, M.; Seibert, G.S.; Sanchez-Gonzalez, M.A.; Leonard, J.T.; Salsbury, R.A.; Fincham, F.D. Understanding the physiology of mindfulness: Aortic hemodynamics and heart rate variability. *Stress* **2016**, *19*, 168–174. [CrossRef]
15. Singh, Y.; Sharma, R.; Talwar, A. Immediate and long-term effects of meditation on acute stress reactivity, cognitive functions, and intelligence. *Altern. Ther. Health Med.* **2012**, *18*, 46–53.
16. Soni, R.; Muniyandi, M. Breath rate variability: Anovel measure to study the meditation effects. *Int. J. Yoga* **2019**, *12*, 45. [CrossRef]
17. Zhu, Y.; Sun, F.; Li, C.; Chow, D.H.K.; Wang, K. Acute effect of brief mindfulness-based intervention coupled with fluid intake on athletes' cognitive function. *J. Sports Sci. Med.* **2020**, *19*, 753–760.
18. Léger, L.; Gadoury, C. Validity of the 20 m shuttle run test with 1 min stages to predict VO_{2max} in adults. *Can. J. Sport Sci.* **1989**, *14*, 21–26.
19. Sun, F.-H.; Cooper, S.B.; Chak-Fung Tse, F. Effects of different solutions consumed during exercise on cognitive function of male college soccer players. *J. Exerc. Sci. Fit.* **2020**, *18*, 155–161. [CrossRef]
20. Nicholas, C.W.; Nuttall, F.E.; Williams, C. The loughborough intermittent shuttle test: A field test that simulates the activity pattern of soccer. *J. Sports Sci.* **2000**, *18*, 97–104. [CrossRef]
21. Smith, M.R.; Coutts, A.J.; Merlini, M.; Deprez, D.; Lenoir, M.; Marcora, S.M. Mental fatigue impairs soccer-specific physical and technical performance. *Med. Sci. Sports Exerc.* **2016**, *48*, 267–276. [CrossRef] [PubMed]
22. Foskett, A.; Ali, A.; Gant, N. Caffeine enhances cognitive function and skill performance during simulated soccer activity. *Int. J. Sport Nutr. Exerc. Metab.* **2009**, *19*, 410–423. [CrossRef] [PubMed]
23. Bosco, C.; Luhtanen, P.; Komi, P.V. A simple method for measurement of mechanical power in jumping. *Eur. J. Appl. Physiol. Occup. Physiol.* **1983**, *50*, 273–282. [CrossRef] [PubMed]
24. Balsalobre-Fernández, C.; Glaister, M.; Lockey, R.A. The validity and reliability of an iPhone app for measuring vertical jump performance. *J. Sports Sci.* **2015**, *33*, 1574–1579. [CrossRef]
25. Qin, L.; Wong, S.H.S.; Sun, F.H.; Huang, Y.; Sheridan, S.; Sit, C.H.P. Effects of alpha-lactalbumin or whey protein isolate on muscle damage, muscle pain, and mood states following prolonged strenuous endurance exercise. *Front. Physiol.* **2017**, *8*, 754. [CrossRef]
26. Borg, G.A.V. Psychophysical bases of perceived exertion. *Plast. Reconstr. Surg.* **1954**, *14*, 377–381. [CrossRef]
27. Schmider, E.; Ziegler, M.; Danay, E.; Beyer, L.; Bühner, M. Is it really robust? Reinvestigating the robustness of ANOVA against violations of the normal distribution assumption. *Methodology* **2010**, *6*, 147–151. [CrossRef]
28. Blanca, M.J.; Alarcón, R.; Arnau, J.; Bono, R.; Bendayan, R. Non-normal data: Is ANOVA still a valid option? *Psicothema* **2017**, *29*, 552–557.
29. Creswell, J.D. Chapter: Biological pathways linking mindfulness with health. In *Handbook of Mindfulness: Theory, Research, and Practice*; The Guilford Press: New York, NY, USA, 2015; pp. 426–440.
30. Smith, M.R.; Thompson, C.; Marcora, S.M.; Skorski, S.; Meyer, T.; Coutts, A.J. Mental fatigue and soccer: Current knowledge and future directions. *Sport. Med.* **2018**, *48*, 1525–1532. [CrossRef]

31. Tang, Y.Y.; Ma, Y.; Fan, Y.; Feng, H.; Wang, J.; Feng, S.; Lu, Q.; Hu, B.; Lin, Y.; Li, J.; et al. Central and autonomic nervous system interaction is altered by short-term meditation. *Proc. Natl. Acad. Sci. USA* **2009**, *106*, 8865–8870. [CrossRef]
32. Ditto, B.; Eclache, M.; Goldman, N. Short-term autonomic and cardiovascular effects of mindfulness body scan meditation. *Ann. Behav. Med.* **2006**, *32*, 227–234. [CrossRef] [PubMed]
33. Ben-Tal, A.; Shamailov, S.S.; Paton, J.F.R. Evaluating the physiological significance of respiratory sinus arrhythmia: Looking beyond ventilation-perfusion efficiency. *J. Physiol.* **2012**, *590*, 1989–2008. [CrossRef] [PubMed]
34. Grossman, P.; Taylor, E.W. Toward understanding respiratory sinus arrhythmia: Relations to cardiac vagal tone, evolution and biobehavioral functions. *Biol. Psychol.* **2007**, *74*, 263–285. [CrossRef] [PubMed]
35. Porges, S.W.; Doussard-Roosevelt, J.A.; Maiti, A.K. Vagal tone and the physiological regulation of emotion. *Monogr. Soc. Res. Child Dev.* **1994**, *59*, 167–186. [CrossRef] [PubMed]
36. Chen, F.; Lv, X.; Fang, J.; Yu, S.; Sui, J.; Fan, L.; Li, T.; Hong, Y.; Wang, X.L.; Wang, W.; et al. The effect of body-mind relaxation meditation induction on major depressive disorder: A resting-state fMRI study. *J. Affect. Disord.* **2015**, *183*, 75–82. [CrossRef]
37. Fisher, J.P.; Young, C.N.; Fadel, P.J. Autonomic adjustments to exercise in humans. *Compr. Physiol.* **2015**, *5*, 475–512. [CrossRef]
38. Smith, K.J.; Billaut, F. Influence of cerebral and muscle oxygenation on repeated-sprint ability. *Eur. J. Appl. Physiol.* **2010**, *109*, 989–999. [CrossRef]
39. Sharp, A.; Cronin, J.; Neville, J. Using smartphones for jump diagnostics: A brief review of the validity and reliability of the my jump app. *Strength Cond. J.* **2019**, *41*, 96–107. [CrossRef]
40. Evans, D.R.; Eisenlohr-Moul, T.A.; Button, D.F.; Baer, R.A.; Segerstrom, S.C. Self-regulatory deficits associated with unpracticed mindfulness strategies for coping with acute pain. *J. Appl. Soc. Psychol.* **2014**, *44*, 23–30. [CrossRef]
41. Grace, P.M.; Gaudet, A.D.; Staikopoulos, V.; Maier, S.F.; Hutchinson, M.R.; Salvemini, D.; Watkins, L.R. Nitroxidative signaling mechanisms in pathological pain. *Trends Neurosci.* **2016**, *39*, 862–879. [CrossRef]
42. Smith, B.E.; Hendrick, P.; Bateman, M.; Holden, S.; Littlewood, C.; Smith, T.O.; Logan, P. Musculoskeletal pain and exercise—Challenging existing paradigms and introducing new. *Br. J. Sports Med.* **2019**, *53*, 907–912. [CrossRef] [PubMed]
43. Maybery, D.J.; Graham, D. The influence of physical and mental training on plasma beta-endorphin level and pain perception after intensive physical exercise. *Stress Health* **2001**, *17*, 121–127. [CrossRef]
44. Russell, M.; Benton, D.; Kingsley, M. Carbohydrate ingestion before and during soccer match play and blood glucose and lactate concentrations. *J. Athl. Train.* **2014**, *49*, 447–453. [CrossRef] [PubMed]
45. Hayano, J.; Yasuma, F.; Okada, A.; Mukai, S.; Fujinami, T. Respiratory sinus arrhythmia: A phenomenon improving pulmonary gas exchange and circulatory efficiency. *Circulation* **1996**, *94*, 842–847. [CrossRef] [PubMed]
46. Mantantzis, K.; Schlaghecken, F.; Sünram-Lea, S.I.; Maylor, E.A. Sugar rush or sugar crash? A meta-analysis of carbohydrate effects on mood. *Neurosci. Biobehav. Rev.* **2019**, *101*, 45–67. [CrossRef] [PubMed]
47. Hassmén, P.; Blomstrand, E. Mood state relationships and soccer team performance. *Sport Psychol.* **1995**, *9*, 297–308. [CrossRef]

Publisher's Note: MDPI stays neutral with regard to jurisdictional claims in published maps and institutional affiliations.

International Journal of
Environmental Research and Public Health

MDPI

Article

Shared Situational Awareness in a Professional Soccer Team: An Explorative Analysis of Post-Performance Interviews

Gaute S. Schei [1,*] and Rune Giske [2]

1 Department of Sports Science and Physical Education, University of Agder, 4630 Kristiansand, Norway
2 Department of Education and Sports Science, University of Stavanger, 4021 Stavanger, Norway; rune.giske@uis.no
* Correspondence: gaute.s.schei@uia.no; Tel.: +47-416-85-870

Received: 5 November 2020; Accepted: 7 December 2020; Published: 9 December 2020

Abstract: Sport science research has done little to elaborate on the cognitive factors that turn a collection of individual players into a coordinated elite team. The purpose of this paper is to clarify if the players and coach of an elite soccer team express shared situational awareness. Ten players and one coach were exposed to twelve video pictures from a previous soccer match, and their statements for each picture were recorded and analyzed using a qualitative approach. Two of five game situations were with ball possession and three out of seven were without ball possession; the player statements are contradictory, with a high threat for inadequate coordination. In seven of the twelve game situations, the players' statements coincided and expressed a shared situational awareness, with good opportunities for adequate defensive and offensive coordination. In two of the game situations, there was a high threat for inadequate coordination. There was consensus among 9 out of 10 players, but the player with the divergent statement was central in the situation. The procedure followed in the study could be used to elucidate if a team has shared situational awareness and clarify in which situations there exists discrepancies and data that can be used to improve team coordination on and off the field.

Keywords: team performance; coordination; situational assessment; qualitative interview

1. Introduction

Soccer teams can be described as action teams, where performance is characterized by rapid, complex, and coordinated task behavior [1], and where the team dynamically adapts proactively and reactively to the environments within which they operate [2]. The players' actions create a continuous stream of playing situations, where the effect of an action depends on the actions of other actors. Coordination between team members becomes therefore critical, considering how the team as an entity dynamically solves defensive and offensive tasks, where different team members primarily undertake different tasks [3]. Hence, team cognitive properties were considered by several authors to be a team performance prerequisite [4,5]. Therefore, elite soccer players must acquire team competencies that include requisite knowledge, principles, and concepts underlying the team's performance [6]. Collective guidelines of the players' perception, what Collins and Collins [7] refer to as the master plan of the coach, are task-solving cursors that can be conceptualized as a shared mental model (SMM). Cannon-Bowers, Salas, and Converse [8] describe the SMM as knowledge structures held by members of a team that enable them to form accurate explanations and expectations of the task by coordinating their actions and adapting their behavior to the demands of the task and other team members. In basketball, Phil Jackson, the legendary coach of the Chicago Bulls and Los Angeles Lakers, has an offensive system named "the triangle", which can be considered as a shared mental model of task sharing. Jackson describes the "triangle" as "five-man tai chi", because it involves the players moving together in response to the way the defense players position themselves [9]. In other words, the shared knowledge makes it possible for the players to move together in unison so they can take advantage of openings the other team's defense offers. The purpose of the SMM is to permit team members to draw their own structured knowledge as a source for choosing actions that are consistent and coordinated with those of their teammates, and as the level of task interdependence increases, teams rely more on team member coordination as a central process for effective functioning [10].

Shared cognitions have primarily been studied outside of sports, and a review of the literature has shown that there is a strong, positive relationship between team cognition and behavioral process, motivational state, and performance in military, educational, medicine, industrial, and high-tech settings [11]. In the last two decades, there has been emerging interest in sport science, and the SMM has been explored in collegiate basketball teams [12], soccer teams [13,14], rugby officials [15], ice hockey, and handball teams [16,17]. Research shows further that a lack of shared knowledge could lead to weak coordination and reduce the team's ability to adapt to changing environmental demands [8], and teams experiencing communication breakdown are more likely to experience difficulties with coordination [18]. In an elite team sport setting, Apitzsch [19] showed that two out of five major factors that lead to a collective collapse in handball were failure of the role system and negative communication within the team. Reimer, Park, and Hinsz [20] propose that assigning players to particular roles should enhance coordination and team performance, because the ambiguity concerning who is doing what is reduced. Giske and colleagues [17] underpinned this assumption when they demonstrated a strong positive relationship between role clarity and the SMM in elite team handball and ice hockey. Moreover, an understanding of what to do and when to do it are a precursor to a mental model of task sharing.

To date, SMM research on interactional team sports has shown that shared knowledge among players could probably promote better understanding of players' synchronized actions during the game. Salas, Stout, and Cannon-Bowers [21] suggest that there is a positive relationship between shared knowledge and team situational awareness, and propose that information that is shared in strategic models allows members to have common explanations of the meaning of the task cues, as well as make compatible assessments of the situation and form common expectations. Endsley [22] simply states that individual situational awareness is knowing what is going on around the individual, whereas Wellens [23] expands the definition to group situational awareness, defining it as "the sharing of a common perspective between two or more individuals regarding current environmental events, their meaning and projected future status" (p. 272). In other words, what to do and when to do it in unison in interactional team sports presuppose shared situational awareness. In sports, however, Eccles and Tenenbaum [5] develop a "flower" model illustrating knowledge unique to each team member and general and specific knowledge shared by multiple team members. Bourbousson, R'Kiouak, and Eccles [24] adapt and refine this model to cover situational awareness, and suggest that team members' connections are numerous and local, indicating that dyadic or triadic arrangements of players are well-connected, where one player heeds the other's actions. In a team setting, common interpretation of cues or overlap of each member's individual level of situational awareness allow for action that is both accurate and expected by teammates [21,22,25]. On the other hand, insufficient shared awareness could lead to weak coordination, and reduce the team's ability to adapt to changing environmental demands. It was further suggested that repeated experience in an environment allows one to develop expectations about future events, and introduces immediate pattern-matching mechanisms as fundamental for developing situational awareness [22]. Klein [26] claims that once a situation is assessed, the appropriate course of action will usually be apparent without deliberation, indicating that assessing a situation and retrieving information on how to deal with it are part of the same process, something known as recognition-primed decision-making. In line with this idea, Eccles and Tran [27] suggest that practice sessions and games in sports provide opportunities for team members to acquire situational probability related to their own team and individual teammates.

To our knowledge, few studies have been empirically concerned about the players' shared situational awareness, which in SMM theory is considered essential to establish synchronized team behavior. Bourbousson, Poizat, Saury, and Sève [28] interviewed five basketball players when they viewed a videotape of a previous 10 min real match. The results from the post-match interviews show that the same typical concerns were relatively rare, but partial sharedness occurred more frequently and the same typical concern was evoked when they all recognized the same situation type. Bourbousson, Kiouak, and Eccles [24] revealed in a similar basketball research design using a social network analysis that team members had a low level of awareness of their teammates, and that one team member in each team often heeded or was heeded by his teammate, indicating that some players appear more important in coordinating the team. Therefore, several authors argue that descriptive and empirical studies are needed to improve our understanding of how team sports function [4,29,30]. However, most of the research on SMMs has been non-empirical [5,20,31], or done by questionnaires [16,17] and interviews [13]. Previous post-performance interviews with video exposure are primarily conducted in youth basketball [24,28]. Therefore, the purpose of the present study is to gain insight into the shared situational awareness of a professional soccer team and their coach by exposing them to a video from a real match where all participant players were in the line-up.

2. Materials and Methods

2.1. Research Design

Yin [32] argues that the case study is an especially appropriate research strategy if the researcher wants to understand a phenomenon in depth and within its real context. Investigating a professional soccer team can be considered an extreme case, which is a research strategy that generally follows an idiographic approach [33], and often reveals more information and more basic mechanisms in situation studies [34]. Classical case studies usually focus on an individual person as the case, but the research methodology is also applicable to small groups [32]. The research design is exploratory, and two types of data were gathered: (a) video recordings of the team performance of a real match, and (b) verbalizations during post-performance interviews. Cook and colleagues [35] recommend process tracing techniques, which are methods for collecting data concurrently with task performance, as an approach to gather data about knowledge underlying task performance. Thinking aloud during performance was considered as a methodology for gathering process data, but it strongly interferes with the players' task completion. Direct access to process data that reveal something about knowledge heterogeneity in an elite soccer team is therefore challenging, indicating that the research design in the present study is probably the most appropriate knowledge elicitation method.

Based on primary aircraft studies, Endsley [22] developed the situational awareness concept, suggesting different zones extending outward in time and space from the individual (i.e., immediate, intermediate, and long-term), where the immediate surroundings seem to be the most relevant for synchronized group behavior in soccer. Yin´s [32] argument is that a real-world case study assumes that important contextual conditions are pertinent in the case. Since context-dependent knowledge appears as the heart of expert activity [34], professional soccer players' verbalization of given game situations could reveal the degree of shared awareness in the team. Therefore, participants in this study were exposed to twelve video situations from a previous match and were questioned about those situations. Based on the individual player's and the coach's statements, the analysis intended to explore shared cognition in selected game situations, and this procedure was inspired by the suggestions of Eccles and Tenenbaum [5] related to the measurement of shared knowledge in sports, and Bourbousson, Kiouak, and Eccles' [24] study of a basketball team. Furthermore, Cooke and colleagues [35] argue that a holistic approach to team knowledge measurement requires new methods; for example, interviewing the team as a whole. A basic assumption in this holistic approach is that team knowledge is more than a collection of aggregated individual team member knowledge. Cooke with colleagues [35] argue that we need knowledge elicitation methodologies that address a more fleeting, context-specific understanding of a situation.

2.2. Participants

An elite professional soccer team consisting of 10 players and their head coach volunteered to participate in the present study. The participants were 26.1 (SD = 4.7) years old, with playing experience on the same team of 4.27 (SD = 4.3) years. Eight players were in the line-up most of the games in the season. A criterion for inclusion was that the players were in the starting line-up in the match where the exposed video sequences were recorded. The study was conducted according to the Helsinki Declaration and the Norwegian National Committees for Research Ethics. This study is approved by the Norwegian Center for Research Data (id: 738807). Table 1 shows the participants´ characteristics in detail.

Table 1. Participants' experience, number of national and youth matches, interview length, and number of transcriptase pages.

ID	Elite Player Experience in Norway (Years) [1]	National Matches	Youth National Matches	Number of Matches [2]	Interview Length Time (min)	Transcript Pages
Player 1	13	No	Yes	120+	35	11
Player 2	3	No	Yes	40+	28	8
Player 3	7	No	No	140+	35	10
Player 4	3	Yes	Yes	70+	30	10
Player 5	5	No	Yes	100+	27	7
Player 6	15	Yes	Yes	300+	35	10
Player 7	6	Yes	Yes	70+	28	7
Player 8	4	No	Yes	20+	28	10
Player 9	2	No	No	30+	31	8
Player 10	3	No	No	70+	42	14
Coach					38	12

[1] Years of experience in the premier league in Norway. [2] Exact information about the number of matches is not given due to the possibility of identifying the player.

2.3. Video

Soccer is an intermitted game where the ball is in and out of play, and research has shown that effective playing time in the World Cup final is decreasing. In 2010, it was approximately 52% of match time [36]. The game dynamically changes, and situations grow and disappear continuously, primarily because of the distribution of ball possession between the opponents. Twelve videos out of this stream of situations were selected from a match, seven situations while the team was not in possession of the ball and five situations while in possession of the ball. Bergo, Johansen, Larsen, and Morisbak's [37] categorization of playing situations formed the basis of the selected situations. Therefore, there were four situations in established defense (when the team has balance, is in control of threatening spaces, and has enough players on the right side of the ball); three situations in defensive transition (the team has lost the ball, there is an imbalance between the ball and the team's own goal, and the players are not in control of threatening spaces); four situations in established attack (the attacks start with ball possession in the rear or central parts against a team with good defense balance); and one situation in offensive transition (the team captures the ball and the opponent is in defensive imbalance). All situations were taken from the first half of the game, and the score was 1–1. One of the three defensive transition situations resulted in a goal against the examined team.

2.4. Procedure

A video camera (Canon XA20, Tokyo, Japan) was used to record participants' statements and, in addition, a tape recorder was used to ensure voice documentation. The playing situations were exposed by a projector (NEC np-m300w projector, Tokyo, Japan) on a canvas. All technical equipment and appropriate facilities were made available for the research team from the club at the club stadium. After each exposed video picture, the player was simply asked: "Describe what you perceive in this situation?" Depending on the player's answer, different follow-up questions were utilized to add nuance to, concretize, and explore all (newly) mentioned sources of information in the players' statements [38]. In addition to these questions, probes were made to create a natural and effortless conversation with the subjects [39]. After video sequences, the players were asked if they perceived that the team in general was guided by a shared understanding during matches, and if so, in what way. The interview length among the players varied between 27–42 min or 7–14 transcribed pages (Table 1). A basic assumption in this study was that elite soccer players are experts that are able to verbalize their continuing thoughts [40] when exposed to the video of their team in a game situation where they might be centrally or peripherally localized. A similar research design was used in basketball [4], soccer, and team handball [41]. However, there is most likely unconscious information from the game situation encounters with teammates that the player is unable to verbalize that might be crucial in co-acting. These elements are left unaddressed in the analysis.

2.5. Data Analysis

Endsley [22] and Bourbousson and colleagues [24] suggest that team situational awareness can be visually illustrated by overlapping circles between individual team members' situational awareness, and they propose that this knowledge state may serve as an index of team coordination. According to Eccles and Tran [27], team coordination is the process of arranging team members' actions (type of action, timing, and location) so that, when combined, they are in a suitable relation for the most effective result. The data corpus was therefore analyzed to reveal similarity or differences between players' perception of each of the twelve videos. Contradictory statements between players are considered a threat for inadequate coordination, while similarity provides good possibilities for adequate coordination. The criteria used were the situational description (theme—terminology—playing area—positions) and situational solution (e.g., "We have complete control in this situation. They have one player in the box and one that is on his way to the box. We have 5–6 players located in the situation, so we are playing six against three. We should have complete control, but player 4 has the totally wrong position."). This situational description and solution stating that player 4 has the wrong position and that the team is in the numeric majority were held by eight of the respondents. An example of contradictory statements is the following: "we shall defend in zones" and "we shall defend man–man". The number of players with contradictory statements was considered a greater threat for coordination. The location (central or peripheral) of the player in the situation and coordinative solution were also emphasized in the analysis (e.g., in situation 9, the player with the ball had a deviant statement compared with the others, and because he is in possession of the ball (central), it became a threat for inadequate coordination). All transcripts were conducted using NVivo software (version 11.1.0.411) (QSR International, Burlington, NJ, USA) for organizing the qualitative data. The analysis was organized based on defensive pictures (the opponent has the ball in possession) and offensive pictures (investigated team in possession of the ball), and to avoid subjectivity, all authors were involved in the analysis.

3. Results

Table 1 shows that the length of interviews diverged considerably, and this may reflect different abilities to articulate answers or verbalized meaningful information when the players are exposed to the videos. Years of experience, number of matches, and experience from national matches seem to be unrelated to the quantity and quality of the interviews.

When the respondents were asked if they experienced that the team was influenced by a shared mental model, some of the players were unsure about the question. However, most of the players and coach argued that the defensive part (pressure on the player with the ball and right positioning) was more pertinent and somehow easier, and it was more challenging to create a shared understanding in the offensive part of the teams' behavior. Interestingly, one of the players specified changes in position, playing formation, and turnovers as obstacles to building shared cognition in the team.

The results displayed in Figure 1 show the compliance of the players' (and coach's) statements in seven game situations where the opponent had ball possession. In three of the situations, the players' statements were contradictory, with a high threat of inadequate coordination. There was a consensus among 9 out of 10 players in situation number three, but there was still a high threat of inadequate coordination because the player with the divergent statement was central in the situation. In four of the exposed defensive situations, the statements expressed shared situational awareness and good opportunities for adequate coordination.

Situation 1

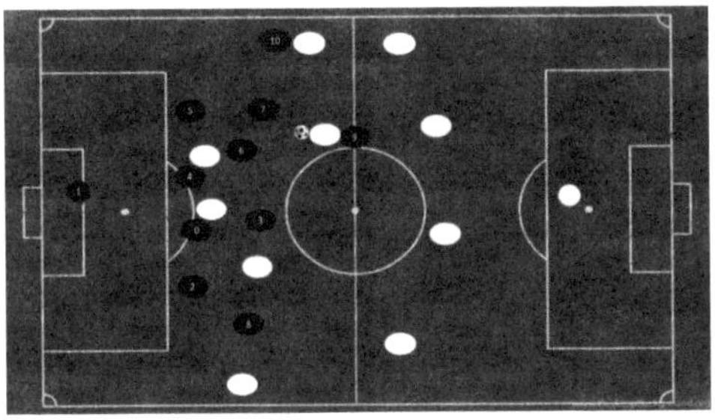

Nine players: We are well-organized

—Five players: Number 7 is supposed to press the ball.

—Two players: Number 9 is supposed to press the ball.

—One player: The team should be a bit lower

—Coach: We are well-organized, and Number 7 is supposed to press the ball keeper.

—Shared situational awareness and good opportunities for adequate coordination.

Situation 2

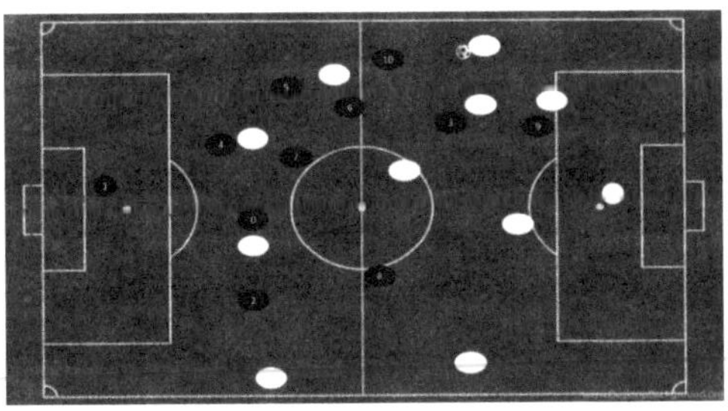

—Six players: We have full control.

—Four players: Too much space between our players.

—Coach: Too much space between our players.

—Contradictory statement. High threat for inadequate coordination because of conflicting situational awareness between the players.

Figure 1. *Cont.*

Situation 3

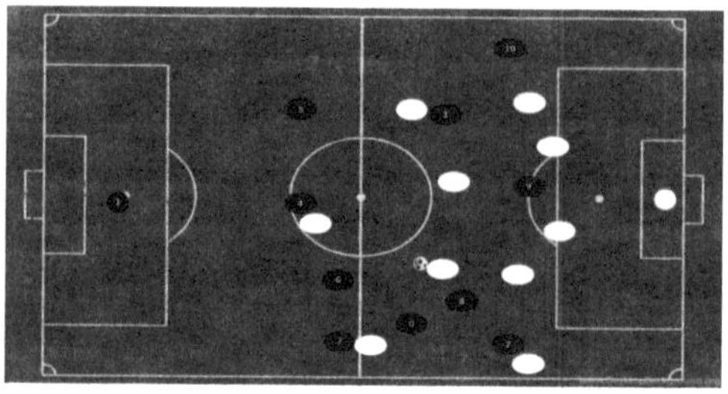

—Nine players: The team should drop lower.

—One player: The team should stand higher.

—Coach: The team should drop lower.

—Contradictory statement. High threat for inadequate coordination because the contradictory player is central in the situation (player number 7).

Situation 4

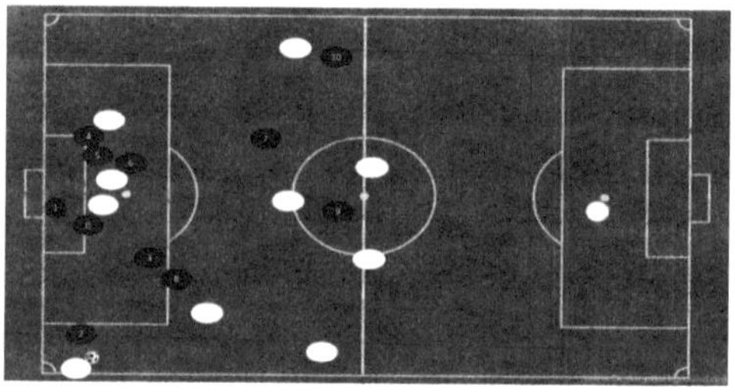

—Six players: We shall defend in zones.

—Four players: We shall defend man–man.

—Coach: We shall defend in zones.

—Contradictory statement. Critical threat for inadequate coordination. Contradictory responses in the back four.

Situation 5

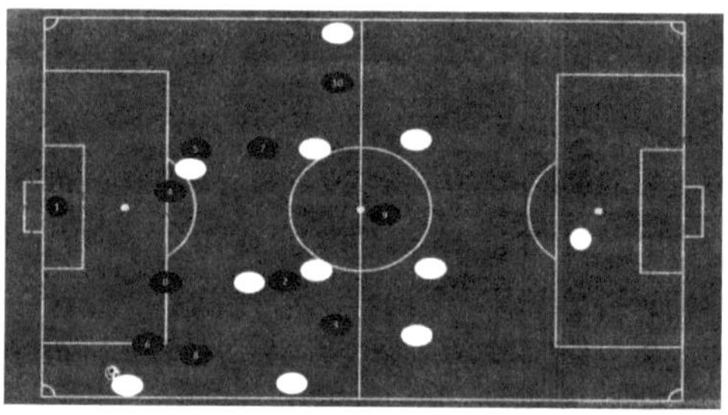

—Nine players: Cover dangerous space in front of goal.

—One player: Irrelevant statement.

—Coach: Cover dangerous space in front of goal.

—Shared situational awareness and good opportunities for adequate coordination. The player with an irrelevant statement is peripheral in the situation.

Figure 1. *Cont.*

Situation 6

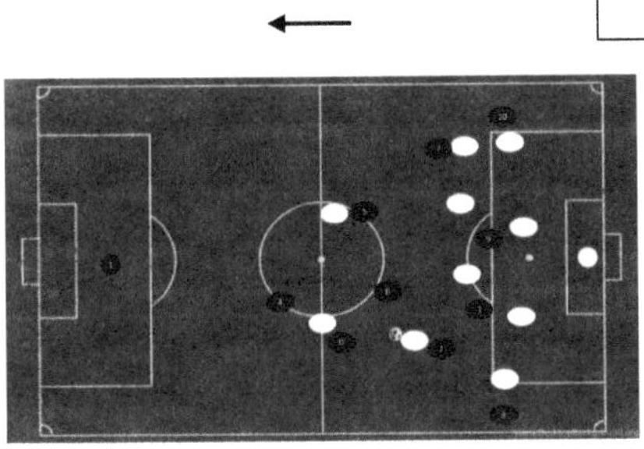

—Eight players: The team should drop lower.

—Two players: Make a free kick.

—Coach: The team should drop lower.

—Shared situational awareness and good opportunities for adequate coordination. Supplemental solution where a free kick will remove the need to drop lower.

Situation 7

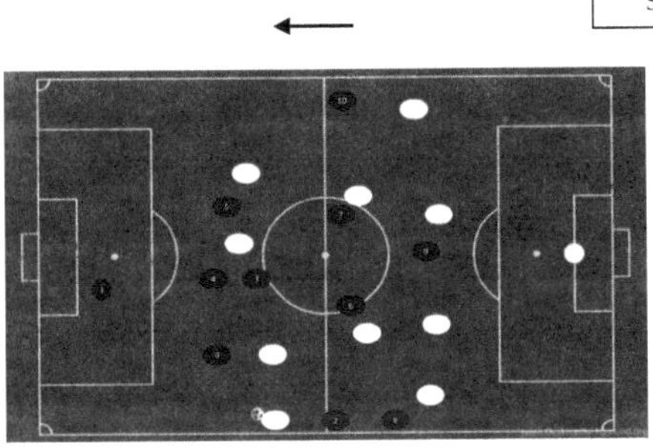

—10 players: Lead the opposition out.

—Coach: Lead the opposition out.

—Shared situational awareness and good opportunities for adequate coordination.

Figure 1. Defensive situations and the distribution of player responses in categories. Players with numbers represent the inquired team and the arrow specifies the attacking direction. Player 0 is the player that did not participate in the study.

The results displayed in Figure 2 show the compliance of the players' (and coach's) statements in five game situations where the examined team had ball possession. In three of the situations, the players' statements coincided and expressed a shared situational awareness and good opportunities for adequate coordination. In two of the situations, where the team was in possession of the ball, the player statements were contradictory with a high threat of inadequate coordination. There was a consensus among 9 out of 10 players in situation number nine, which should indicate sufficiently shared situational awareness, but there was still a high threat of inadequate coordination because the player with the divergent statement was central in the situation.

Situation 8

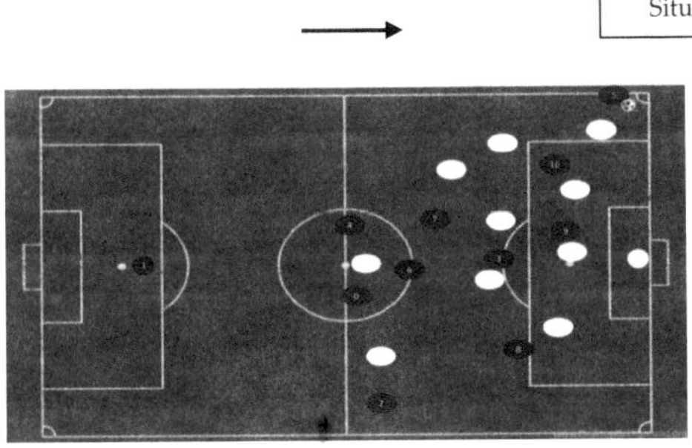

—10 players: Winger attacks first post, striker attacks second post.

—Coach: Winger attacks first post, striker attacks second post.

—Shared situational awareness and good opportunities for adequate coordination.

Figure 2. *Cont.*

Situation 9

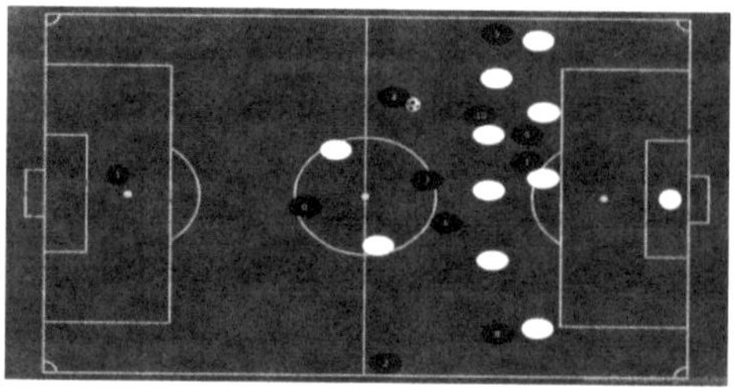

—Nine players: Switch play to the other side.

—One player: Play between the opposition, or behind the opposition.

—Coach: Switch play to the other side and create two against one against the fullback.

—The player with the divergent perspective is in possession of the ball (Player 4). Critical threat for inadequate coordination.

Situation 10

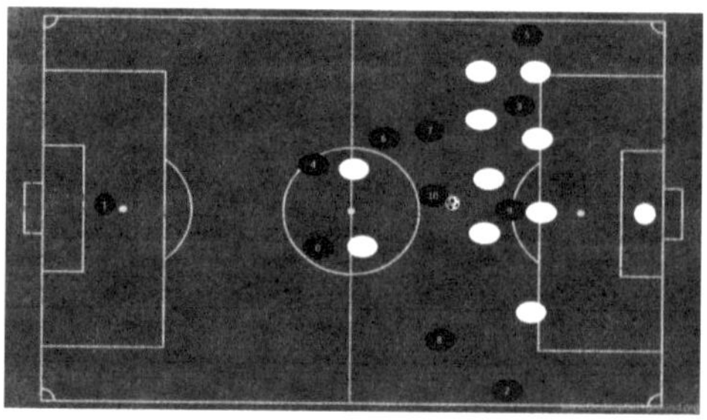

—Five players: Create two against one against the fullback (A).

—Two players: Threaten the space behind the opposition.

—One player: Passing combination to create something (B).

—One player: Keep the ball, no good options.

—One player: Suggest two solutions (A, B)

—Coach: Create two against one against the fullback.

—Contradictory statement and limited shared situational awareness.

Situation 11

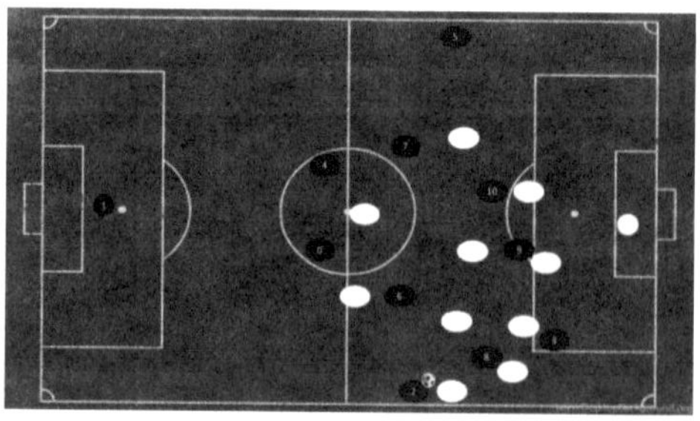

—Eight players: Play number six and switch play.

—Two players: Passing combination to create something.

—Coach: Play number six and switch play.

—Shared situational awareness and good opportunities for adequate coordination. The majority had a more specific solution than the minority.

Figure 2. *Cont.*

Situation 12

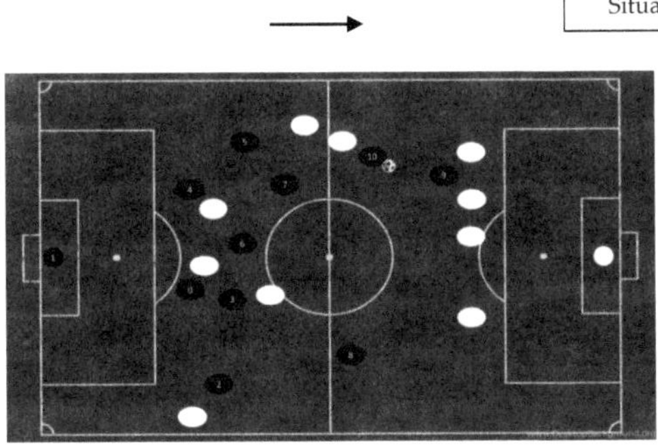

—Eight players: Player eight has to sprint forward to help Number 10.

—Two players: Keep the ball, no good solutions.

—Coach: Player eight has to sprint forward to help Number 10.

—Shared situation awareness and good opportunities for adequate coordination. The majority gave a specific co-active solution, while the minority didn't see an obvious solution other than keeping the ball.

Figure 2. Offensive situations and the distribution of player responses in categories. Players with numbers represent the inquired team and the arrow specifies the attacking direction. Player 0 is the player that did not participate in the study.

4. Discussion

The purpose of presenting an empirical study is to gain insight into the shared situational awareness of an elite soccer team and their correspondent coach by exposing them to videos from a previous match. Endsley [22] argues that there is evidence that a person's manner of characterizing a situation will determine the decision process of solving a problem, and that every team member must have situational awareness for all of his or her requirements or will risk becoming the proverbial chain's weakest link, independent of overlap demands. Eccles and Tenenbaum [5] claim that similar knowledge is required to establish team coordination, and an increased number of equivalent player statements related to the individual exposed video should therefore be desirable. The results from Figures 1 and 2 reveal variegated depictions, and show that the verbal statements from the players in seven of the exposed game situations correspond in such a way that the team has sufficient shared situational awareness and therefore good opportunities for adequate coordination. Interestingly, Bourbousson with colleagues [4] argue that the coordinated network was quite hetrogenus, and essentially built on local coordination where one player heeds the co-action in such a way that the team does not necessarily form a single unit. However, to have knowledge and to understand that the players' task in this situation is not to move or make an initiative is also a vital part in the process of appearing as a unit. Local coordination on this performance level presupposes that the players that are not directly involved do not interfere.

In five of the exposed game situations, the comparison of the verbal statements reveals contradictory situational awareness, and there is a critical threat for inadequate coordination. The players' responses in situations two, four, and 10 reveal a minority group of four players or five players, and in situations three and nine, one centrally located player expresses a contradictory point of view compared with the rest of the group. Based on Eccles and Tenenbaum's [5] assumption that similar knowledge is required when establishing team coordination, an increased number of deviant statements are undesirable, and it becomes more critical if the players are central in the coordination solution. Salas et al. [25] argues that a complete overlap is probably not the most expedient, because it is time-consuming to establish and preservative in the sense that it reduces the availability of solutions. They suggest that each member is required to have sufficient similar and compatible mental models guiding them towards team objectives. These five situations, which are assessed with a high threat for inadequate coordination, have contradictory verbal statements and incompatible solutions from relevant players in the game situation. In the remaining seven exposed videos, the players' statements and their localization reveal sufficient overlap, and their shared awareness of the situation might influence their individual decision process in such a way that it enables efficient team coordination.

The analysis also has considered the players' locations in the game situation when the threat for inadequate coordination is assessed. Since previous findings have primarily been obtained in basketball, such as Bourbousson with colleagues [4,24,28], where the playing area is smaller and the number of players fewer, the localization of the player in game situations appears more significant in coordination in soccer. In situation three, the player that held a contradictory point of view compared with the rest of the team members could lead to coordinative difficulties because he has a central position in that situation. This is not the case in situation five, where the statement from the deviant player is characterized as irrelevant because he is localized as peripheral in the situation. Even though there is only one player in both of these situations who has a statement that deviates from the rest of the team, this deviation could have a negative effect on team coordination [20]. Contradictory statements among players that are central in the situation are considered by far more devastating for team coordination than a blurred statement from a peripherally located player.

The findings underpin the dynamics of shared situation awareness among team members, and designate great demands on continuously monitoring and updating the situation to enable the players' coaction. Previous observational research on elite soccer players shows that higher frequencies of head movements (explorative actions) are positively related to the individual player's game performance [42–45]. The shared situational awareness perspective in the present study complements this individually player-oriented research avenue, and points out that perception in elite soccer also has an essentially collective dimension and how the team as an entity dynamically solves defensive and offensive tasks [3]. However, these overarching de-contextual defensive and offensive tasks must be further elaborated on by establishing mutual expectations in different offensive and defensive game situations before they can promote internal predictability, which is critical in co-acting [8]. Because the behavioral expectations are so closely related to game situations (the players' task is more or less continuously defined by the situation), providing equal or approximately identical situational assessments becomes an important prerequisite for coordinated player behavior in an elite soccer team.

Previous research on team coordination has not been particularly concerned with the distinction between defensive and offensive situations, despite the fact that the defensive part of the game (the team is not in the possession of the ball) seems to be more reactive, while the offensive part can be considered more proactive. Comparing the results displayed in Figures 1 and 2, both offensive and defensive situations reveal comparable statements with good opportunities for adequate coordination and contradictory statements that pose a high threat of inadequate coordination. This finding indicates that shared situational awareness in an elite soccer team is a coaching issue for both offensive and defensive situations. However, the answers from the open questions and responses from the exposed videos reveal that there are differences between the players' responses comparing offensive and defensive situations. The defensive situation evoked more contradictory statements, while differences in offensive situations seem to be more aimed at the degree of specificity (e.g., situations 11 and 12). Established attack and offensive transition situations may reduce available solutions with a detailed coordination plan that impairs team effectiveness, because the idea is often to take the opponent by surprise, which means a higher risk [37]. Defending against established attack and offensive transitions may be considered as more reactive with fewer solutions, lower risk, and defined backup behavior. Shared coordinated solutions in defensive situations thus become more expedient.

Cannon-Bowers and Salas [46] categorized the content of shared mental models in task and team member knowledge, and previous qualitative research among elite soccer players reveals that knowledge about teammates' strengths, weaknesses, and preferences in specific situations are important as a source in the decision-making process during the game [20,47]. The exposure of one of the offensive videos (12) awoke a response among seven of the respondents related to team member knowledge. Player three expressed: "We know that player 10 is extreme in the one against one situations", and player five said: "Then he will be set up in situations where we know that he is good".

There are several aspects of the responses worth commenting on. First, player three uses the plural pronoun "we", which indicates that this knowledge is shared in the team. Secondly, player five's responses show that the team endeavors to create situations where Number 10 can display his special skills. This finding seems to be in line with Giske et al. [47], suggesting that in games like soccer, it is possible to create a situational development that gives team members an opportunity for pattern recognition. Furthermore, it shows how interviewed team member knowledge is in specific game situations. Previous research has primarily been concerned with situational awareness, more like monitoring or visual search [42,48], but, in elite team sports, it is also about creating situational conditions that provide a chance for pattern recognition, preferably without disclosing the intention to the opponent [47]. This is about the difference between the ability to see opportunities and the ability to create opportunities in the game.

Video number four is a cross-defensive situation, and the responses reveal the most conflicting viewpoints among the players in the squad. Most of the players and the coach say that the team shall defend cross situations by zone organization. However, four of the players express that the team shall defend these situations by man-to-man marking. Two of these four players are defenders, where one of their primary tasks is to solve these situations. One of the players (number four) stated: "We haven't discussed so carefully if we are organized in zone or man-to-man marking. I think zone, but obviously you attack the ball and mark the man in your zone." The quote is complex, and can be interpreted in several different ways, but in this context, the most obvious is that he is unsure of the solution because it has not been accentuated in the coaching process. In other words, he makes a reservation before he states his point of view. This reservation supports the findings by showing conflicting differences between the players' points of view, and indicates that there is no accurate shared knowledge in the team concerning how this situation should be solved [8]. This finding reveals a potential for a coordination breakdown [27], and should therefore be accommodated by a teaching sequence.

Mutual performance monitoring has been defined as the ability to keep track of fellow members' work to ensure that everything is running as expected and, in addition, ensure that they are following procedures correctly [49]. According to Eccles and Tran [27], effective mutual performance monitoring requires shared knowledge of the task responsibility, and they suggest that if the team does not share the same mental model for how the team should appear, performance monitoring becomes ineffective. The findings when the players were exposed to video number five show a high degree of agreement about the major task in the situation (cover dangerous space in front of goal), but a closer inspection of the data also reveals that six of the respondents claim that the team has a feeble marking in a cross situation, and that there is a shared understanding among them that the team has not perceived the situation well enough. These six players also share a common monitoring of team coordination in the situation, which presupposes a shared knowledge of an ideal coordinative solution. The players' responses to video eight show that all of the respondents (the coach included) monitored the situation in the same manner, and they suggest the same team solution to solve the situation. According to Salas et al. [25], the SMM is important for mutual performance monitoring, as it provides co-players with an understanding of what team members are supposed to be doing in a given situation and also acts as an anchor for feedback. Exposing players to previous team action with videos may make performance monitoring expedient through precise feedback, which, in the next step, may make team member models more accurate.

The team leader's failure to guide and structure team experiences to facilitate coordinative and adaptive action can be a key factor in ineffective team performance [50]. Deviant situational awareness between the majority of the players and the coach may be a major leadership threat, because it places greater demands on communication. Clarity in these expectations in specific game situations enables the team to adapt, and might increase leadership trust [25]. McComb [51] suggests that mental model convergence may be the key to understanding how individuals are transformed into team members, and the results show that the coach is on the same page as the majority of the players in all of the exposed videos, except video number two. To our knowledge, these facets of leadership in elite team ball games have not been considered in the literature and should be further elaborated on. This finding indicates that the coach and the players have similar preconditions to form accurate expectations for the task. Giving feedback and supervising players' decisions in the game presuppose approximately identical situational awareness, otherwise coaching is about bringing similar situational awareness. By influencing situational awareness, the coach may also impact the players' decision-making process [22]. This can be done, for example, by illuminating different options in the situations and clarifying priorities. To disclose players' situational awareness, one should presume a dialogical coaching approach, where the players are invited to explore and verbalize their experiences from the game. Such a coaching practice seems to be in line with Salas et al. [25], who argue that team leadership affects team effectiveness, not by handing down solutions to the team, but by joint problem solving.

5. Conclusions and Practical Implications

The results from the present study reveal situations that point to the existence of shared situational awareness, whereas others display contradictory perceptions. However, being central or peripheral in the situation are conditions that also determine the possibility for adequate team coordination in soccer. According to Salas with colleagues [52], team training should only prioritize team competencies that yield the greatest impact on performance, and a major coaching task is therefore to uncover contradictory perceptions among the players in the most critical game situations. Exposing teams to videos from previous games, where the players individually express their opinion, may both improve their skills in monitoring team performance and strengthen their shared knowledge. The opinions from the players can uncover if the team has shared knowledge and in which situations there might exist discrepancies. Such information makes it possible to tailor teaching sequences directly towards situations where there are coordinative challenges. Furthermore, this approach gives information about each individual player's cognition, and can therefore generate knowledge, which in the next step can be used to facilitate individual player development. Such a procedure is probably especially important with new players in the squad. However, further research is needed to confirm the usefulness of this approach. We encourage other researchers to investigate if our findings are comparable to other professional soccer teams. We would suggest a longitudinal approach to explore how teams develop and maintain shared situational awareness, and which methods in team training yield the best result. A main challenge in research with professional teams is getting access to do in-depth studies. Overcoming this obstacle would help expand our knowledge of cognitive factors in professional teams that are central in team coordination.

This study is not without its limitations, and these issues should be considered when the findings are interpreted. First, decision-making and situational awareness in sports is understood in a completely different way than in an ecological dynamics approach, where there is a direct link between perception and action [53]. This paper is, however, based on team literature, where knowledge or cognition is considered as essential, guiding players' actions in some game situations. Second, the players and coach responded to twelve videos from one match. The selection of videos was based on the research group's subjective perception of relevance. Other pictures from the match or other matches might have given a different result. However, the first author has been working as a professional with the responsibility of match analysis in a premier league club for several years, which should ensure both the relevance of the videos and trustworthiness in the interpretation of the data. In our opinion, the empirical material does "saturate" the phenomenon.

Author Contributions: Conceptualization, G.S.S. and R.G.; methodology, G.S.S. and R.G.; software, G.S.S.; validation, G.S.S. and R.G.; formal analysis, G.S.S. and R.G.; investigation, G.S.S. and R.G.; resources, G.S.S. and R.G.; data curation, G.S.S. and R.G.; writing—original draft preparation, G.S.S. and R.G.; writing—review and editing, G.S.S. and R.G.; visualization, G.S.S. and R.G.; supervision, R.G.; project administration, R.G.; funding acquisition, G.S.S. and R.G. All authors have read and agreed to the published version of the manuscript.

Funding: This research received no external funding.

Conflicts of Interest: The authors declare no conflict of interest.

References

1. Kozlowski, S.W.J.; Gully, S.M.; Salas, E.; Cannon-Bowers, J.A. Team leadership and development: Theory, principles, and guidelines for training leaders and teams. In *Advances in Interdisciplinary Studies of Work Teams: Team Leadership*; Beyerlein, M.M., Johnson, D.A., Beyerlein, S.T., Eds.; Emerald Group: Bingley, UK, 1996; pp. 253–292.
2. Marks, M.A.; Zaccaro, S.J.; Mathieu, J.E. Performance implications of leader briefings and team-interaction training for team adaptation to novel environments. *J. Appl. Psychol.* **2000**, *85*, 971–986. [CrossRef] [PubMed]
3. Eccles, D. The coordination of labour in sports teams. *Int. Rev. Sport Exerc. Psychol.* **2010**, *3*, 154–170. [CrossRef]
4. Bourbousson, J.; Poizat, G.; Saury, J.; Seve, C. Team Coordination in Basketball: Description of the Cognitive Connections among Teammates. *J. Appl. Sport Psychol.* **2010**, *22*, 150–166. [CrossRef]
5. Eccles, D.W.; Tenenbaum, G. Why an Expert Team is More Than a Team of Experts: A Social-Cognitive Conceptualization of Team Coordination and Communication in Sport. *J. Sport Exerc. Psychol.* **2004**, *26*, 542–560. [CrossRef]
6. Cannon-Bowers, J.A.; Tannenbaum, S.I.; Salas, E.; Volpe, C.E. Defining competencies and establishing team training requirements. In *Team Effectiveness and Decision Making in Organizations*; Guzzo, R., Salas, E., Eds.; Jossey-Bass: San Francisco, CA, USA, 1995; pp. 333–380.
7. Collins, D.; Collins, J. Putting them together: Skill packages to optimize team/group performance. In *Performance Psychology: A Practitioner's Guide*; Collins, D., Angela, A., Richards, H., Eds.; Churchill Livingstone: London, UK, 2011; pp. 361–391.
8. Cannon-Bowers, J.A.; Salas, E.; Converse, S.A. Shared mental models in expert team decision-making. In *Individual and Group Decision Making: Current Issues*; Castellan, N.J., Ed.; Hillsdale: Erlbaum, NJ, USA, 1993; pp. 221–246.
9. Jackson, P.; Delehanty, H. *Eleven Rings. The Soul of Success*; Penguin Books: New York, NY, USA, 2013.
10. Tesluk, P.; Mathieu, J.E.; Zaccaro, S.J.; Marks, M. Task and aggregation issues in the analysis and assessment of team performance. In *Team Performance Assessment and Measurement: Theory, Methods, and Applications (pp. 197–224). Mahwah: Erlbaum*; Brannick, M.T., Salas, E., Prince, C., Eds.; Lawrence Erlbaum Associates: Mahwah, NJ, USA, 1997; pp. 197–224.
11. DeChurch, L.A.; Mesmer-Magnus, J.R. The cognitive underpinnings of effective teamwork: A meta-analysis. *J. Appl. Psychol.* **2010**, *95*, 32–53. [CrossRef]
12. Webber, S.S.; Chen, G.; Payne, S.C.; Marsh, S.M.; Zaccaro, S.J. Enhancing team mental model measurement with performance appraisal practices. *Organ. Res. Methods* **2000**, *3*, 307–322. [CrossRef]
13. Gershgoren, L.; Basevitch, I.; Filho, E.; Gershgoren, A.; Brill, Y.S.; Schinke, R.J.; Tenenbaum, G. Expertise in soccer teams: A thematic inquiry into the role of Shared Mental Models within team chemistry. *Psychol. Sport Exerc.* **2016**, *24*, 128–139. [CrossRef]
14. Gershgoren, L.; Filho, E.M.; Tenenbaum, G.; Schinke, R.J. Coaching Shared Mental Models in Soccer: A Longitudinal Case Study. *J. Clin. Sport Psychol.* **2013**, *7*, 293–312. [CrossRef]
15. Mascarenhas, D.R.D.; Collins, D.; Mortimer, P.W.; Morris, B. Training Accurate and Coherent Decision Making in Rugby Union Referees. *Sport Psychol.* **2005**, *19*, 131–147. [CrossRef]
16. Giske, R.; Rodahl, S.E.; Haugen, T.; Høigaard, R. Shared mental models, role ambiguity, team identification and social loafing in elite sports groups: A mediation analysis. *Sport Exerc. Psychol. Rev.* **2017**, *13*, 2–12.
17. Giske, R.; Rodahl, S.E.; Høigaard, R. Shared Mental Task Models in Elite Ice Hockey and Handball Teams: Does It Exist and How Does the Coach Intervene to Make an Impact? *J. Appl. Sport Psychol.* **2015**, *27*, 20–34. [CrossRef]
18. Marks, M.A.; Sabella, M.J.; Burke, C.S.; Zaccaro, S.J. The impact of cross-training on team effectiveness. *J. Appl. Psychol.* **2002**, *87*, 3–13. [CrossRef] [PubMed]
19. Apitzsch, E. Coaches' and elite team players' perception and experiencing of collective collapse. *Athl. Insight* **2009**, *11*, 57–74.

20. Reimer, T.; Park, E.S.; Hinsz, V.B. Shared and Coordinated Cognition in Competitive and Dynamic Task Environments: An Information-Processing Perspective for Team Sports. *Int. J. Sport Exerc. Psychol.* **2006**, *4*, 376–400. [CrossRef]
21. Salas, E.; Stout, R.J.; Cannon-Bowers, J.A. The role of shared mental models in developing shared situational awareness. In *Situational Awareness in Complex Systems. Proceedinp of a CAHFA Conference*; Gilson, R., Garland, D., Koonce, J., Eds.; Embry-Riddle Aeronautical University Press: Daytona Beach, FL, USA, 1994; pp. 297–304.
22. Endsley, M.R. Toward a Theory of Situation Awareness in Dynamic Systems. *Hum. Factors: J. Hum. Factors Ergon. Soc.* **1995**, *37*, 32–64. [CrossRef]
23. Wellens, A.R. Group situation awareness and distributed decision making: From military to civilian applications. In *Individual and Group Decision Making: Current Issues*; Castellan, N.J., Jr., Ed.; Lawrence Erlbaum: Hillsdale, NJ, USA, 1993; pp. 267–291.
24. Bourbousson, J.; R'Kiouak, M.; Eccles, D.W. The dynamics of team coordination: A social network analysis as a window to shared awareness. *Eur. J. Work Organ. Psychol.* **2015**, *24*, 742–760. [CrossRef]
25. Salas, E.; Sims, D.E.; Burke, C.S. Is there a "Big Five" in Teamwork? *Small Group Res.* **2005**, *36*, 555–599. [CrossRef]
26. Klein, G. *Streetlights and Shadows: Searching for the Keys to Adaptive Decision Making*; MIT Press: Cambridge, MA, USA, 2009.
27. Eccles, D.W.; Tran, K.B. Getting Them on the Same Page: Strategies for Enhancing Coordination and Communication in Sports Teams. *J. Sport Psychol. Action* **2012**, *3*, 30–40. [CrossRef]
28. Bourbousson, J.; Poizat, G.; Saury, J.; Seve, C. Temporal Aspects of Team Cognition: A Case Study on Concerns Sharing Within Basketball. *J. Appl. Sport Psychol.* **2012**, *24*, 224–241. [CrossRef]
29. Cannon-Bowers, J.A.; Bowers, C. Applying work team results to sports teams: Opportunities and cautions. *Int. J. Sport Exerc. Psychol.* **2006**, *4*, 447–462. [CrossRef]
30. Ward, P.; Eccles, D.W. A commentary on "team cognition and expert teams: Emerging insights into performance for exceptional teams". *Int. J. Sport Exerc. Psychol.* **2006**, *4*, 463–483. [CrossRef]
31. Gréhaigne, J.F. Jean-Paul Sartre and Team Dynamics in Collective Sport. *Sport Ethics Philos.* **2011**, *5*, 34–45. [CrossRef]
32. Yin, R.K. *Case Study Research: Design and Methods*, 5th ed.; Saga Publications: London, UK, 2014.
33. Robson, C.; McCartan, K. *Real World Research*, 4th ed.; John Wiley: Chichester, UK, 2016.
34. Flyvbjerg, B. Five Misunderstandings about Case-Study Research. *Qual. Inq.* **2006**, *12*, 219–245. [CrossRef]
35. Cooke, N.J.; Salas, E.; Cannon-Bowers, J.A.; Stout, R.J. Measuring team knowledge. *Hum. Factors* **2000**, *42*, 151–173. [CrossRef] [PubMed]
36. Wallace, J.L.; Norton, K.I. Evolution of World Cup soccer final games 1966–2010: Game structure, speed and play patterns. *J. Sci. Med. Sport* **2014**, *17*, 223–228. [CrossRef] [PubMed]
37. Bergo, A.; Johansen, P.A.; Larsen, Ø.; Morisbak, A. *Ferdighetsutvikling i Fotball: Handlingsvalg og Handling. [Skills Development in Football: Action Choices and Actions]*; Akilles: Oslo, Norway, 2002.
38. Patton, M.Q. Qualitative interviewing. In *Qualitative Research and Evaluation Methods*, 3rd ed.; Saga Publications: Thousand Oaks, CA, USA, 2002; pp. 339–344.
39. Rubin, H.J.; Rubin, I.S. *Qualitative Interviewing: The Art of Hearing Data*; Saga Publications: Thousand Oaks, CA, USA, 2012.
40. Ericsson, K.A.; Simon, H.A. Verbal reports as data. *Psychol. Rev.* **1980**, *87*, 215–251. [CrossRef]
41. Giske, R. *Individuelle Handlingsvalg i Lagballspill: En Teoretisk og Empirisk Analyse. [Individual Decisions in Team Ball Games. A Theoretical and Emprical Analysis]*; Norwegian School of Sport Sciences: Oslo, Norway, 2001.
42. Jordet, G. Perceptual Training in Soccer: An Imagery Intervention Study with Elite Players. *J. Appl. Sport Psychol.* **2005**, *17*, 140–156. [CrossRef]
43. Eldridge, D.; Pulling, C.; Robins, M.T. Visual exploratory activity and resultant behavioural analysis of youth midfield soccer players. *J. Hum. Sport Exerc.* **2013**, *8*, 560–577. [CrossRef]
44. McGuckian, T.B.; Cole, M.H.; Jordet, G.; Chalkey, D.; Pepping, G.J. Don't turn blind! The relationship between exploration before ball posession and on-ball performance in association football. *Front. Psychol.* **2018**, *9*, 2520. [CrossRef]
45. Phatak, A.; Gruber, M. Keep your head up–correlation between visual exploration frequency, passing percentage and turnover rate in elite football midfielders. *Sports* **2019**, *7*, 139. [CrossRef]

46. Cannon-Bowers, J.A.; Salas, E. Reflections on shared cognition. *Hum. Resour. Abstr.* **2001**, *36*, 309–456. [CrossRef]
47. Giske, R.; Gaard, H.S.; Gjerde, J. Felles mentale modeller i elitelagballspill: En kvalitativ analyse av spilleres opplevelse av medspillerkunnskap i fotball og håndball. [Shared mental models in elite team ball games. A qualitative analysis of the players' experience in team member knowledge in football and handball]. In *Trender i Idrettspsykologisk Forskning i Skandinavia. [Trends in Sports Psychological Research in Skandinavia]*; Haugen, T., Høigaard, R., Eds.; Cappelen: Oslo, Norway, 2018; pp. 163–185.
48. Williams, A.M.; Davids, K. Visual search strategy, selective attention, and expertise in soccer. *Res. Q. Exerc. Sport* **1998**, *69*, 111–128. [CrossRef] [PubMed]
49. McIntyre, R.M.; Salas, E. Measuring and managing for team performance: Emerging principles from complex environments. In *Team Effectiveness and Decision Making in Organizations*; Guzzo, R.A., Salas, E., Eds.; Jossey-Bass: San Francisco, CA, USA, 1995; pp. 9–45.
50. Stewart, G.L.; Manz, C.C. Leadership for Self-Managing Work Teams: A typology and Integrative Model. *Hum. Relat.* **1995**, *48*, 747–770. [CrossRef]
51. McComb, S.A. Mental Model Convergence: The Shift from being an Individual to being a Team Member. In *Multi-Level Issues in Organizations and Time*; Dansereau, F., Yammarino, F.J., Eds.; Emerald Group Publishing Limited: Bingley, UK, 2007; Volume 6, pp. 95–147.
52. Salas, E.; Benishek, L.; Coultas, C.; Dietz, A.; Grossman, R.; Lazzara, E.; Oglesby, J. *Team Training Essentials: A Research-Based Guide*; Routledge: New York, NY, USA, 2015.
53. Araújo, D.; Davids, K.; Hristovski, R. The ecological dynamics of decision making in sport. *Psychol. Sport Exerc.* **2006**, *7*, 653–676. [CrossRef]

International Journal of
Environmental Research and Public Health

MDPI

Article

The Effects of Green and Urban Walking in Different Time Frames on Physio-Psychological Responses of Middle-Aged and Older People in Chengdu, China

Hansen Li [1], Haowei Liu [1], Zongqian Yang [1], Shilin Bi [2], Yang Cao [3,4,*] and Guodong Zhang [1,*]

1 Institute of Sports Science, Key Lab of Physical Fitness Evaluation and Motor Function Monitoring of General Administration of Sports of China, College of Physical Education, Southwest University, Chongqing 400715, China; lhs510416413@email.swu.edu.cn (H.L.); haoweiliu@email.swu.edu.cn (H.L.); Yzq000133@email.swu.edu.cn (Z.Y.)
2 National Institute of Education, Nanyang Technological University, Singapore 637616, Singapore; NIE20.BS@E.NTU.EDU.SG
3 Clinical Epidemiology and Biostatistics, School of Medical Sciences, Örebro University, 70182 Örebro, Sweden
4 Unit of Integrative Epidemiology, Institute of Environmental Medicine, Karolinska Institutet, 17177 Stockholm, Sweden
* Correspondence: yang.cao@oru.se (Y.C.); lygd777@swu.edu.cn (G.Z.); Tel.: +46-19-602-6236 (Y.C.); +86-15730267257 (G.Z.)

Abstract: Nighttime walking is becoming a popular exercise for many middle-aged and older people in Asian countries. However, the health benefits of nighttime walking in urban areas and green spaces are still unclear. This study evaluated the physiological and psychological responses of 48 middle-aged and older people who walked 1.6 km through a green space and an urban area during daytime and nighttime. The Positive and Negative Affect Schedule (PANAS), Profile of Mood States (POMS), Perceived Restorativeness Scale (PRS), and Restorative Outcome Scale (ROS) were employed to measure the psychological responses, and pulse rate and blood pressure (SBP, DBP and MAP) were measured to evaluate the physiological responses. The results showed that the daytime green walking induced psychological improvements and lowered blood pressure ($p < 0.05$), while the daytime urban walking resulted in slight deterioration of all the measured parameters ($p > 0.05$). On the other hand, the nighttime green walking induced lowered blood pressure ($p < 0.05$), whilst the nighttime urban walking resulted in psychological improvements and lowered blood pressure ($p < 0.05$), and no significant difference was found in any measured parameter between the two nighttime walking groups. In conclusion, urban areas are noisy and irritating in the daytime, and not suitable for walking, but may become pleasurable and attractive at night. The psychological benefits of green walking may decrease at night, and nighttime walking in either an urban area or a green space may achieve similar health benefits. Therefore, we recommend that urban citizens start nighttime walking in a green space or an urban area to keep fit when the air is less polluted.

Keywords: walking; green space; urban; nighttime; blood pressure; physiological; psychological

Citation: Li, H.; Liu, H.; Yang, Z.; Bi, S.; Cao, Y.; Zhang, G. The Effects of Green and Urban Walking in Different Time Frames on Physio-Psychological Responses of Middle-Aged and Older People in Chengdu, China. *Int. J. Environ. Res. Public Health* **2021**, *18*, 90. https://dx.doi.org/10.3390/ijerph18010090

Received: 23 November 2020
Accepted: 22 December 2020
Published: 24 December 2020

1. Introduction

As populations become increasingly urbanized, urban living is associated with a series of stressors, including noise, air pollution, and crowding [1–3], which have resulted in a range of negative effects on public health, such as the increased risk of cardiovascular diseases and mental problems [4,5]. In response, various attempts have been made to relieve stress and maintain health, and green walking is one of the important solutions, which refers to walking in forests or other natural environments with plants [6]. As both natural settings and physical activities have been considered to benefit physical and mental health [7–10], the green walking has thus been expected to bring additional health benefits [11].

Numerous studies have found that walking in forests or urban parks could lower blood pressure, increase parasympathetic activities, and improve emotional outcomes [12–15]. On the contrary, walking in urban areas seems to be less attractive and lack health benefits [16–18]. However, there was evidence that the physical and psychological responses could be related to the characteristics of environments, and some urban scenes may also exert positive effects on physical exercise [19], which has implied the possibility of urban surroundings in improving physio-psychological health. For instance, potential health benefits derive from walking through a clean and orderly street, or exercise in a city with less air pollution. Although the importance of nature is irrefutable, the worldwide urbanization makes it harder for people to reach forests or other completely natural environments, and there is thus a rising demand to explore places with restorativeness and positive effects among cities [20].

In recent years, more and more urban citizens choose walking as their daily exercise, especially those middle-aged and older people, who prefer moderate exercises without technical difficulty [21,22]. For most citizens who are employed, nighttime walking is one of their best options. For one, a few hours after dinner are their only time available to exercise. For another, the nighttime exercise may be more effective in lowering blood pressure [23], and may also help to moderate nocturnal blood pressure in active people [24]. Besides, mild exercise, like walking, is unlikely to be a threat to sleep quality [25]. In fact, nighttime exercises are popular in many Asian countries due to the local cultures, and a vast number of people have already got involved in the nighttime walking [26,27], which may be considered as an easy and safe exercise owing to the bright urban illumination, the fine walking facilities, and the good public order. Many middle-aged and older people in China usually go on nighttime walking together, which not only meets their needs of keeping fit, but also provides opportunities for social communication, thus make them adhere to long-term physical exercise. In terms of nighttime walking environment, the urban citizens today can easily access to various green spaces owing to the advanced urban greening [28,29]. Nevertheless, there are quite a few people who tend to carry out nighttime walking in urban areas instead of green spaces, and the reasons were unknown. Whereas the daytime green walking and urban walking have been well studied, less attention has been paid to the cases in the nighttime, and the characteristics of the two nighttime environments remain to be further investigated.

Theoretically, visual experience plays an important role in green walking [30], and greenness of plants can help to achieve positive changes in physical and mental indices [31]. Therefore, improper lighting at night may interfere with the cognition of greenness and thus reduce the effects from natural elements. Moreover, plants are the key for carbon sequestration and oxygen generation [32], which may exert positive impacts on the respiratory and related nervous system. However, the photosynthesis is becoming inactive at night, and plants' respiration may even lead to higher carbon dioxide concentration, which may also reduce the health benefits brought by the green walking. On the other hand, urban areas have better illumination, the artificial lights in cities may improve the scenic experience and sense of safety [33], and further add joy to nighttime recreations. Besides, the traffic emission, one of the main street air pollutants that prevent people from urban activities, may reduce at night, and so do the noise and crowding, which may make nighttime urban walking more comfortable and enjoyable. Thereby, our experimental study was aimed to assess the effects of green walking and urban walking in daytime and nighttime, and further reveal the differences between the nighttime walking in green space and urban area. The specific hypotheses were:

(1) The daytime urban walking has negative effects while the nighttime urban walking has positive effects on the investigated psychological and physiological responses;
(2) The daytime green walking has positive effects while the nighttime green walking has negative effects;
(3) Compared to the nighttime green walking, the urban walking has greater positive effects and is more attractive to urban citizens.

2. Materials and Methods

2.1. Participants

The inclusion criteria for recruiting the middle-aged and older people who were eligible for the study are:

(1) Aged between 40 and 75 years.
(2) Absence of serious cardiovascular disease.
(3) Absence of chronic symptoms causing walking problems.
(4) Absence of cognitive impairment and mental disorders.

As a result, 48 people (40–71 years old) were recruited from a community in Chengdu, Sichuan Province, China. Participants were informed of experimental procedures and the possible risks and benefits of their participation. All participants were randomly divided into the following four groups by computer (Table 1). There was no statistically significant difference in age or BMI index among the different groups (analyzed using Kruska–Wallis test).

(1) Daytime green walking (**DG**).
(2) Nighttime green walking (**NG**).
(3) Daytime urban walking (**DU**).
(4) Nighttime urban walking (**NU**).

Table 1. Basic information of participants from each group.

Groups	Number	Age	BMI Index
Group1 (DG)	12 (5 males)	56.92 ± 2.29	36.30 ± 0.98
Group2 (NG)	12 (4 males)	51.50 ± 2.61	36.16 ± 1.16
Group3 (DU)	12 (3 males)	56.41 ± 2.79	34.79 ± 1.55
Group3 (NU)	12 (4 males)	53.42 ± 2.60	35.95 ± 1.31

Note: Data are expressed as mean ± stand error (N = 12).

As analyzed in a previous study, a sample size between 9 and 19 participants is enough to achieve acceptable statistical power for the predefined hypotheses [12], therefore our sample size is appropriate. All experimental procedures undertaken in the present study were under regulations of and approved by the Ethics Committee of the Physical Education College of Southwest University, China.

2.2. Study Sites

After a field investigation, a green space and an urban area in Wenjing District, Chengdu, were selected for walking (Figure 1). Both sites are flat without slope, and less than half a kilometer from the participants' community. The green space is located in the middle of two residential zones, decorated with trees, shrubs, and grass, and close to a river. The urban area contains a street among commercial and residential zones, decorated with a few trees, and there are wide pedestrian areas on both sides of the street.

In order to ensure the safety of the participants, two circular routes (1.6 km each) were set up in flat and illuminated walkways among the green space and urban area, respectively, which need approximately 20 min to finish (Figure 1). Besides, three staff were arranged to stay in the routes to monitor the whole walking program, and a community doctor was also hired to stay at the check point to provide medical attention. The main views of the two routes in daytime and nighttime are demonstrated in Figure 2. An indoor check point was established in each route for measurements of pre-tests and post-tests.

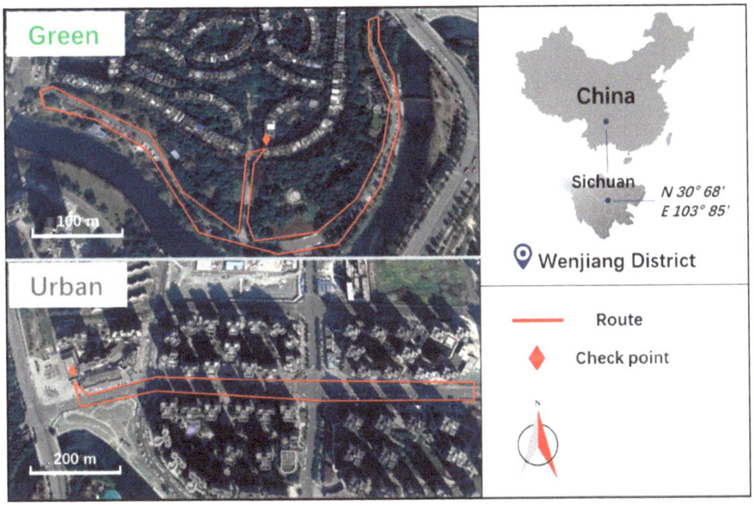

Figure 1. Location of the study area and the two walking routes in the green space and urban area.

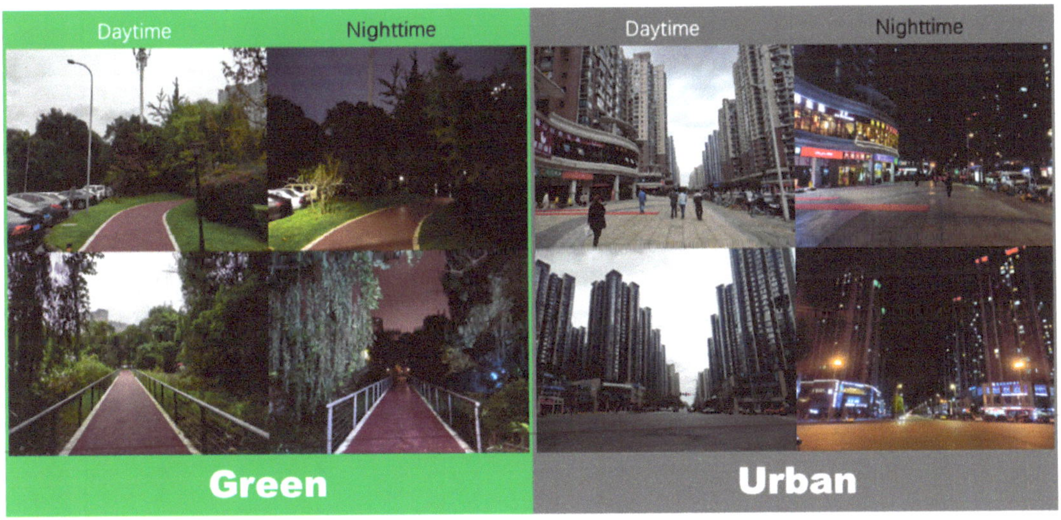

Figure 2. The main views of the two walking routes in daytime and nighttime.

2.3. Process and Contents of Walking Experiment

The experiment was carried out in October. As the experiment sites were in the participants' neighborhoods, the participants were asked to reach the check points on their own before the beginning of the experiment. Thereafter, all the participants were seated in the waiting rooms for a half-hour rest. During the rest, the participants were provided with route maps and informed of walking and measurement details by the research staff. The experiment was introduced as self-paced walking, and the participants were asked to walk alone at their easy and comfortable speeds. Psychological questionnaires, measurements of blood pressure, and measurement of pulse rate were completed before and after the walking (Table 2).

Table 2. Process and test contents of the experiment.

Time	Daytime Walking (3:30–5:00 PM)		Nighttime Walking (8:30–10:00 PM)	
Day 1	Green Walking		Green Walking	
Day 2	Urban Walking		Urban Walking	
Test	**Psychological Item**	**Measuring Time**	**Physiological Item**	**Measuring Time**
Pre-test	PANAS, POMS	15 min before walk	SBP, DBP, Pulse rate	Just before walk
Post-test	PANAS, POMS, PRS, ROS	Immediately after walk	SBP, DBP, Pulse rate	15 min after walk

The data of illumination, temperature, and noise were collected every 300 m of the routes using a light detector (Suwei-SW6013), an ambient thermometer (SmartSensor-AS817), and a cell-phone noise detection software, respectively. In addition, the real-time air quality index was also obtained from the website of the Chengdu Meteorological Bureau. The relevant data are shown in Table 3.

Table 3. The environmental parameters in the experiment.

Group	Illumination (lx)	Humidity (%)	Temperature (°C)	Noise (dB)	AQI
DG	3510.67 ± 192.21b	63.27 ± 1.4a	21.73 ± 0.21a	46.33 ± 1.23a	18
NG	8 ± 3.64a	71.07 ± 1.46b	19.02 ± 0.21c	45.33 ± 1.87a	23
DU	7982.5 ± 1642.74c	67.83 ± 1.16b	19.6 ± 0.13b	60.83 ± 2.12c	19
NU	29.5 ± 7.41a	78.25 ± 0.73c	17.5 ± 0.14d	52.17 ± 0.54b	25

Note: The DG, NG, DU, and NU represent daytime green walking, nighttime green walking, daytime urban walking, and nighttime urban walking, respectively. AQI represents Air Quality Index, and AQI < 50 means excellent air quality. Data are expressed as mean ± stand error. Different lowercase letters after the numbers represent statistically significant differences in different trials ($p < 0.05$), analyzed using one-way ANOVA and Duncan's multiple range test ($N = 6$).

After the walk, an interview was conducted to evaluate the preference of participants. After confirming that all the participants were familiar with the nighttime and daytime images of the study area, the participants were required to make two choices, one was to choose between the daytime urban area and daytime green space, another was to choose between the nighttime urban area and nighttime green space, and the reasons for their like or dislike were also asked and recorded.

2.4. Measurement of the Outcomes

2.4.1. Physiological Parameters

Systolic blood pressure (SBP), diastolic blood pressure (DBP), and pulse rate were measured using portable electronic sphygmomanometers (OMRON HEM-7211) at the check points before and after the walk. Measurements were performed in a relaxed sitting position and the instrument was placed at heart height. The mean arterial pressure (MAP) was calculated as $((\text{DBP} \times 2) + \text{SBP})/3$.

2.4.2. Psychological Parameters

Four psychological scales were employed to measure the emotional outcomes and restorative effects.

The Positive and Negative Affect Schedule (PANAS), which consists of 20 items and is evaluated by a Likert five-point scale, is widely used to evaluate changes in positive and negative emotions [34,35]. The reliability and validity of PANAS were tested in previous studies [36,37]. A validated Chinese version of PANAS scale was employed in this study [38].

A simplified Chinese version of Mood States questionnaire (POMS), which contains 40 items and is evaluated by a four-point Likert scale, was employed to measure personal moods. The Chinese version has been proved to be suitable for the Chinese population, and has been widely used [39,40]. Results of the POMS scale can help to explain six subscales of mood: Tension or anxiety (T), anger or hostility (A), fatigue (F), depression or dejection (D), vigor (V), and confusion or bewilderment (C). Besides, the Chinese POMS contains 5 items (items 7, 14, 27, 34, and 40) that are related to self-esteem. Meanwhile, the total mood disturbance (TMD) can be evaluated from the subscales (TMD = the sum of negative emotions − the sum of positive emotions + 100).

Restorativeness is defined as the potential of certain surroundings for restoring certain cognitive capacities related to human information [41]. Two relevant scales were used in the present study to observe the restorative effects of environments.

A shortened version of the Perceived Restorativeness Scale (PRS) was used to measure perceived restorativeness of environment based on the Attention Restoration Theory [42–44]. The reliability and validity of the short scale were tested previously [45]. The scale consists of five items with a 10-point Likert scale.

The Restorative Outcome Scale (ROS), which contains six items and is evaluated by a seven-point Likert scale, was used to evaluate properties of the environments that contributed to the restorative outcomes. According to previous research, the scale has been confirmed with high reliability and validity. [46,47].

As there are no Chinese version of the short PRS and ROS, they were translated into Chinese, and checked by back-and-forth translation in our study.

2.5. Statistical Methods

All the data were processed via SPSS 25.0 (SPSS Inc., Chicago, IL, USA). Given our sample size, the Shapiro–Wilk test was employed to determine the distribution of all data. Due to some data that were hard to normalize, the nonparametric test was employed for non-normal data. When comparing the difference between pre- and post-test, the paired t-test was employed to compare normal data, and the Wilcoxon signed-rank test was employed to compare non-normal data. When comparing the difference between multiple scenarios, if normal distribution and variance homogeneity were confirmed, then the one-way ANOVA was employed, and followed with post hoc comparisons using the Duncan's multiple range test. On the other hand, the Kruskal–Wallis test was employed for comparisons of non-normal data between different groups. When determining the effects of time and sites, if the data were normally distributed and consistent with homogeneity of variance, the two-way ANOVA was performed. If there was a significant interaction, the simple effect was tested using the post hoc LSD method. The Fisher's exact test was performed to check the difference in the proportion of participants with a positive response between different groups, and followed with post hoc multiple tests adjusted with Bonferroni correction. The Chi-squared test was employed to check the difference in participants' preference between the two walking environments. A p-value < 0.05 was considered statistically significant in the present study.

3. Results

3.1. Validation of the Psychological Measurements

The Cronbach's α showed good internal consistency (>0.7) for the PANAS and PRS in the all scenarios (Table 4). In the case of the POMS, though good reliabilities were found in nighttime green walking, daytime urban walking, and nighttime urban walking, the coherence in daytime green walking did not meet a satisfactory level (Cronbach's $\alpha = 0.56$). Moreover, the reliabilities of ROS in daytime green walking (Cronbach's $\alpha = 0.62$) and nighttime green walking (Cronbach's $\alpha = 0.69$) were barely within the acceptable level (Cronbach's α between 0.6 and 0.7).

Table 4. Internal consistency of the scales in each scenario.

Parameter	Cronbach's α			
	DG	NG	DU	NU
PANAS	0.76	0.77	0.82	0.73
POMS	0.56	0.86	0.94	0.84
PRS	0.95	0.88	0.96	0.80
ROS	0.62	0.69	0.78	0.93

Note: The DG, NG, DU, and NU represent daytime green walking, nighttime green walking, daytime urban walking, and nighttime urban walking, respectively.

3.2. Pyschological Outcomes of Walking in Different Scenarios

The median score of PANAS-positive significantly increased after daytime green walking ($p = 0.03$) and nighttime urban walking ($p = 0.046$), and the value after nighttime green walking also increased but not statistically significantly ($p > 0.05$) (Figure 3). However, no statistically significant change was found in PANAS-negative score of any scenario (Figure 3).

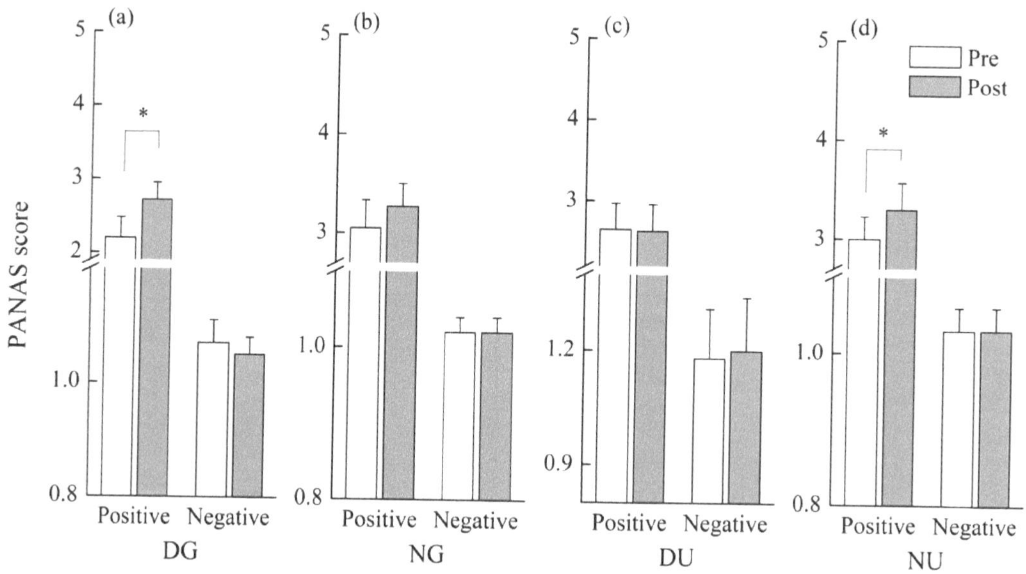

Figure 3. Outcomes of Positive and Negative Affect Schedule (PANAS) in: (**a**) daytime green walking; (**b**) nighttime green walking; (**c**) daytime urban walking; and (**d**) nighttime urban walking. The error bar represents standard error, and * represents $p < 0.05$. Analyzed using Wilcoxon signed-rank test ($N = 12$).

In terms of the POMS subscales, the median scores of tension-anxiety, anger-hostility, fatigue, depression-dejection, and confusion-bewilderment slightly decreased after walking in all scenarios without statistical significance ($p > 0.05$). The median score of vigor significantly increased after daytime green walking ($p = 0.034$) and nighttime urban walking ($p = 0.024$) (Figure 4a,d).

The median score of TMD decreased in all scenarios, but only the decreases after daytime green walking ($p = 0.018$) and nighttime urban walking ($p = 0.003$) were statistically significant (Figure 5a,d).

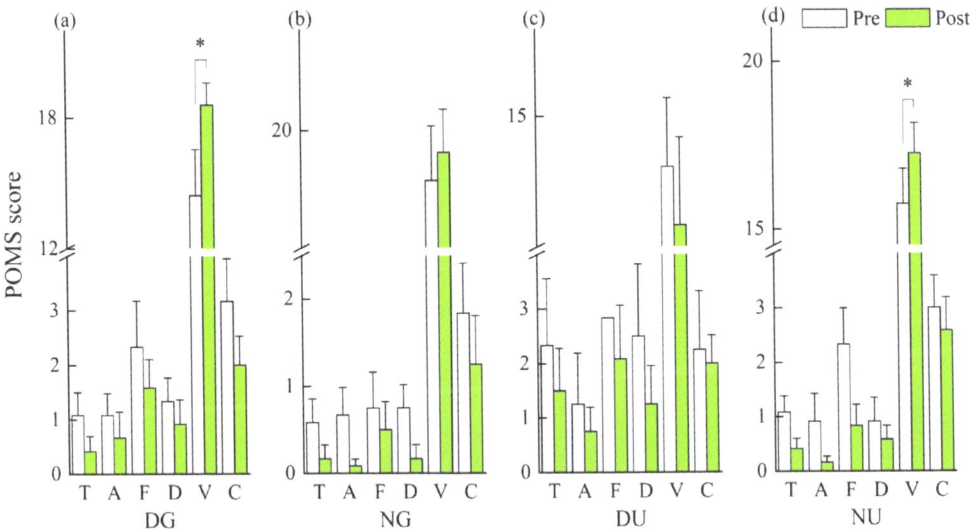

Figure 4. Outcomes of Profile of Mood States (POMS) subscales in: (**a**) daytime green walking; (**b**) nighttime green walking; (**c**) daytime urban walking; and (**d**) nighttime urban walking. T: Tension or anxiety; A: Anger or hostility; F: Fatigue; D: Depression or dejection; V: Vigor; C: Confusion or bewilderment. The error bar represents standard error, and * represents $p < 0.05$. Analyzed using Wilcoxon signed-rank test ($N = 12$).

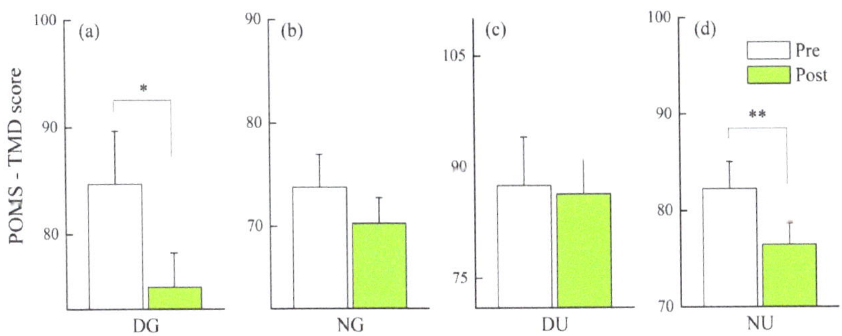

Figure 5. Outcomes of POMS-total mood disturbance (TMD) in: (**a**) daytime green walking; (**b**) nighttime green walking; (**c**) daytime urban walking; and (**d**) nighttime urban walking. The error bar represents standard error, and * represents $p < 0.05$, ** represent $p < 0.01$. Analyzed using Wilcoxon signed-rank test ($N = 12$).

Due to the non-normal psychological data, the mean changes of measured parameters were calculated to reveal the differences of walking in different scenarios. The psychological changes demonstrated that the increase in score of PANAS-positive in daytime green walking was significantly greater than that in daytime urban walking ($p = 0.032$) (Figure 6a). The decrease in score of POMS-TMD in nighttime urban walking was significantly greater than that in daytime urban walking ($p = 0.02$) (Figure 6c). No statistically significant difference was found in the psychological changes between nighttime green walking and nighttime urban walking.

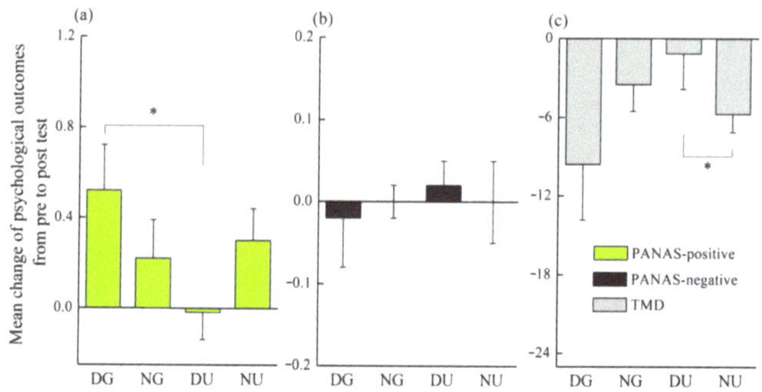

Figure 6. The psychological changes of walking in different scenarios. The (**a**), (**b**), and (**c**) represent changes in scores of PANAS-positive, PANAS-negative, and POMS-TMD respectively. The DG, NG, DU, and NU represent daytime green walking, nighttime green walking, daytime urban walking, and nighttime urban walking respectively. The error bar represents standard error, and * represents $p < 0.05$. Analyzed using the Kruskal–Wallis test ($N = 12$).

The proportions of participants who exhibited positive responses were also calculated to reveal the difference among different walking scenarios. However, no statistically significant difference was found among the scenarios (Table 5).

Table 5. Proportions of participants with positive responses in psychological parameters after walking in different scenarios.

Psychological Parameter	DG	NG	DU	NU	p
PANAS-Positive	9 (75%)	7 (58.3%)	3 (25%)	7 (58.3%)	$p = 0.084$
PANAS-Negative	3 (25%)	1 (8.3%)	1 (8.3%)	1 (8.3%)	$p = 0.693$
POMS-TMD	8 (66.7%)	8 (66.7%)	3 (25%)	11 (91.7%)	$p = 0.10$

Note: The DG, NG, DU, and NU represent daytime green walking, nighttime green walking, daytime urban walking, and nighttime urban walking respectively. Analyzed using the Fisher's exact test.

3.3. Restorativeness of Different Walking Environments

The restorativeness of the environments was assessed using the PRS and ROS scales after the walks. Similar results were observed in the two scales, and a significant correlation was found between the two measurements (Pearson's r = 0.834, $p < 0.001$). Due to the non-normal distribution of ROS outcomes, the Kruskal–Wallis test was performed and revealed a statistically significant difference between nighttime green walking and daytime urban walking ($p = 0.022$) (Figure 7).

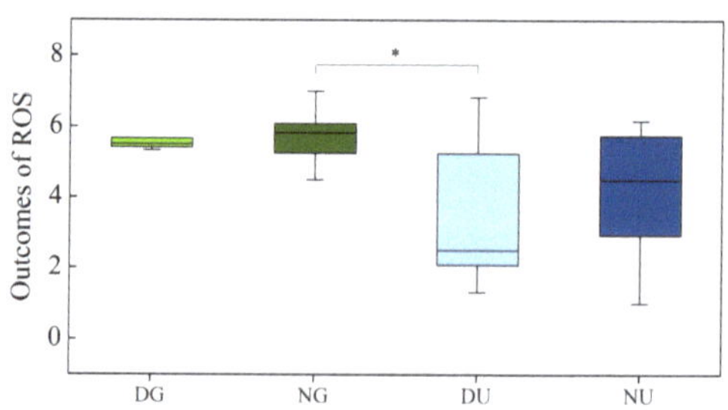

Figure 7. Restorative outcomes of Restorative Outcome Scale (ROS) in different scenarios. The DG, NG, DU, and NU represent daytime green walking, nighttime green walking, daytime urban walking, and nighttime urban walking, respectively. The * represents significant differences ($p < 0.05$). Analyzed using the Kruskal–Wallis test ($N = 12$).

In the case of PRS, the two-way ANOVA revealed that there was a statistically significant difference between sites, but no significant difference between time frames (Table 6). A significant interaction between time frames and sites was also observed (Table 6).

Table 6. Results of two-way ANOVA for ROS outcomes.

	df	F	*p*
Site	1	16.418	<0.001
Time	1	0.701	0.407
Site × Time	1	4.885	0.032

The analysis of simple effects revealed that during the daytime, the score of PRS in green walking was significantly higher than that in urban walking ($p < 0.001$) (Figure 8a), but no statistically significant difference was found between them during nighttime (Figure 8b). In the urban walking, the score of PRS in nighttime walking was significantly higher than that in daytime walking ($p = 0.037$) (Figure 8d), but no significant difference was found between the time frames in green walking (Figure 8c).

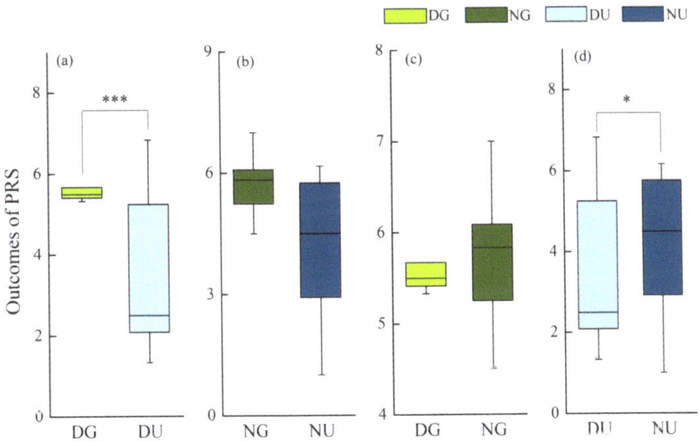

Figure 8. Restorative outcomes of Perceived Restorativeness Scale (PRS) in: (**a**) daytime walking; (**b**) nighttime walking; (**c**) green walking; and (**d**) urban walking. The * represents $p < 0.05$, and *** represents $p < 0.001$. Compared using Post Hoc Multiple comparisons (LSD method) ($N = 12$).

3.4. Physiological Outcomes of Walking in Different Scenarios

The SBP significantly decreased after daytime green walking ($p = 0.038$), nighttime green walking ($p = 0.005$), and nighttime urban walking ($p = 0.006$). The DBP significantly decreased after daytime green walking ($p = 0.006$) and nighttime green walking ($p = 0.009$). The MAP significantly decreased after daytime green walking ($p = 0.008$), nighttime green walking ($p = 0.005$), and nighttime urban walking ($p = 0.045$). However, no statistically significant change difference was found in the pulse rate in any scenario (Figure 9).

Due to the diurnal variation of physiological parameters, the mean changes of physiological outcomes were calculated to reveal the differences in walking in different scenarios. The physiological changes demonstrated that the decreases of SBP in both nighttime green walking ($p = 0.04$) and nighttime urban walking ($p = 0.048$) were significantly greater than that in daytime urban walking (Figure 10a). The decreases of DBP in both daytime green walking ($p = 0.06$) and nighttime green walking ($p = 0.03$) were significantly greater than that in daytime urban walking (Figure 10b). The decrease of MAP in nighttime urban walking was significantly greater than that in daytime urban walking ($p = 0.033$) (Figure 10c). No statistically significant difference was found in the physiological changes between nighttime green walking and nighttime urban walking.

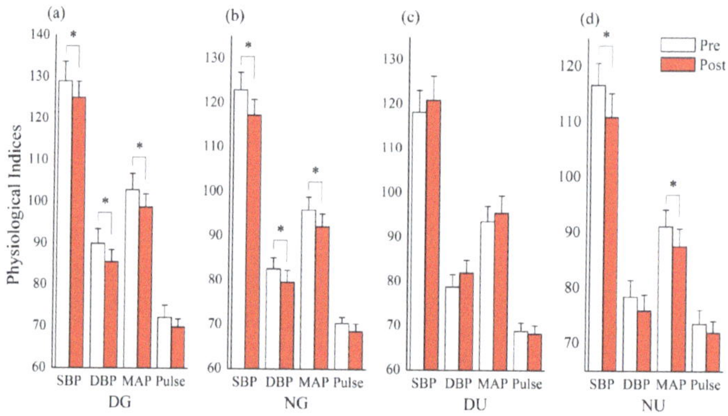

Figure 9. Outcomes of physiological measurements in: (**a**) daytime green walking; (**b**) nighttime green walking; (**c**) daytime urban walking; and (**d**) nighttime urban walking. The error bar represents standard error, and * represent $p < 0.05$. Analyzed using Paired t-test ($N = 12$).

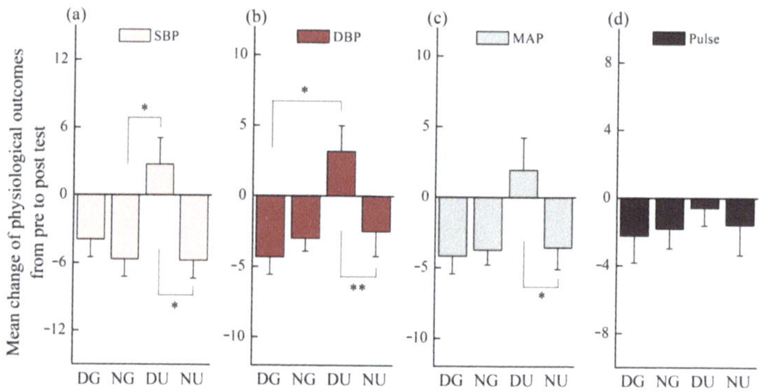

Figure 10. The physiological changes of walking in different scenarios. The (**a**), (**b**), (**c**), and (**d**) represent changes in SBP, DBP, MAP, and pulse rate respectively. The DG, NG, DU, and NU represent daytime green walking, nighttime green walking, daytime urban walking, and nighttime urban walking, respectively. The error bar represents standard error, * represents $p < 0.05$, and ** represents $p < 0.01$. Analyzed using the Kruskal–Wallis test ($N = 12$).

The Fisher's Exact Test revealed statistically significant differences in proportions of participants with positive responses in SBP ($p = 0.002$), DBP ($p = 0.005$), and MAP ($p = 0.004$) among different scenarios (Table 7).

Table 7. Proportions of participants with positive responses in measured parameters after walking in different scenarios.

Physiological Parameter	DG	NG	DU	NU	p
SBP	11 (91.7%) a	11 (91.7%) a	4 (33.3%) b	9 (75%) ab	$p = 0.002$
DBP	11 (91.7%) a	11 (91.7%) a	5 (41.7%) a	11 (91.7%) a	$p = 0.005$
MAP	11 (91.7%) a	11 (91.7%) a	4 (33.3%) b	10 (83.3%) ab	$p = 0.004$
Pulse rate	6 (50%) a	8 (66.7%) a	7 (58.3%) a	9 (75%) a	$p = 0.753$

Note: The DG, NG, DU, and NU represent daytime green walking, nighttime green walking, daytime urban walking, and nighttime urban walking, respectively. Lowercase letters indicate significant difference ($p < 0.05$). Analyzed using the Fisher's exact test.

3.5. Walking Environment Preference of Participants

In terms of daytime walking environments, 93.7% of the participants preferred the daytime green space (Figure 11a). However, in terms of nighttime walking environments, only 52.1% of participants chose the nighttime green space (Figure 11b). In the interview, only some participants could give explicit reasons for their options, and these reasons could be classified into several points (Figure 11).

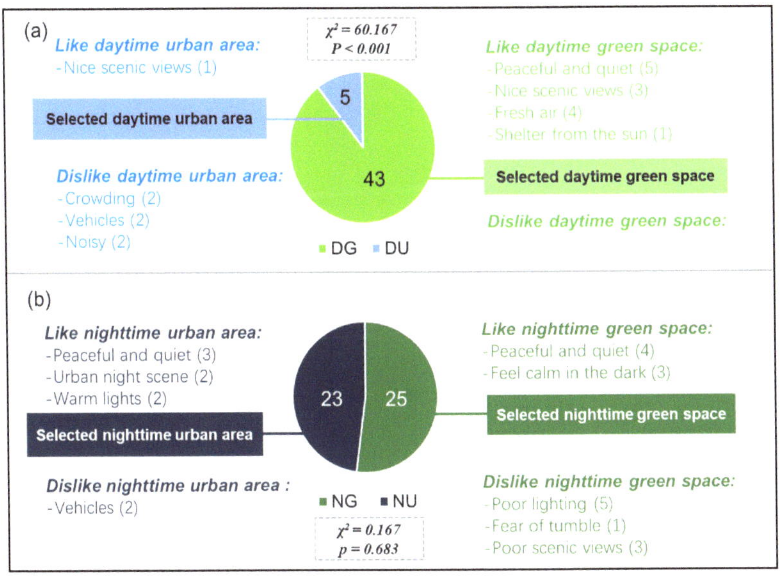

Figure 11. Preferences of participants towards different walking environments. The (**a**) and (**b**) represent daytime walking environments and nighttime walking environments respectively. The DG, NG, DU, and NU represent daytime green space, nighttime green space, daytime urban area, and nighttime urban area, respectively. Analyzed using Chi square test (N = 48).

4. Discussion

The present study aimed to check how green walking and urban walking in different time frames affect the physiological and psychological characteristics of the participants. The main findings indicated that both the daytime green walking and nighttime urban walking induced significant positive changes in blood pressure and psychological outcomes, and the nighttime green walking also induced lowered blood pressure. The daytime urban walking was inferior to the other three scenarios in psychological or physiological improvements, but no significant difference was found among the daytime green walking, nighttime green walking, and nighttime urban walking.

4.1. Urban Walking

In the present experimental study, blood pressure (SBP, DBP, and MAP), and some psychological parameters (PANAS-positive and POMS-Vigor) demonstrated reduction after the daytime urban walking. In contrast, the nighttime urban walking was associated with significant improvements in moods (PANAS-positive, POMS-vigor, and POMS-TMD) and blood pressure (SBP and MAP). In addition, the nighttime PRS score of the urban area was significantly higher than the daytime counterpart. These findings supported our first hypothesis that the daytime urban walking has negative effects while the nighttime urban walking has positive effects. Since the two walking options were carried out in the same area, these differences might be due to the change of the properties of the urban environment at night.

Compared with previous works, our results of daytime urban walking agreed with the finding of Ji, et al. [14], Hassan, et al. [48], and Song, et al. [49], who have also reported negative effects of urban environments on blood pressure as well as some psychological outcomes. However, there is a difference between the participants: Our study only included middle-aged and older people, while the above studies only included young participants, which indicates that the daytime urban environment may have negative impacts on people of different ages. Besides, these negative impacts, according to Ji, et al. [14], and Hassan, et al. [48], were caused by increased stress levels in urban surroundings, and the stress responses were detected in the test of amylase and brain wave. Theoretically, physical activity can benefit physiological and psychological health [10,50,51], and walking, the basic exercise that we were concerned with, has been proved to lower blood pressure and improve moods [50,51]. However, the health benefits of physical activity may be counteracted by urban stressors such as noise, crowding, and pollution [52,53]. For example, the autonomic nervous system, an important regulator for peripheral resistance and cardiac outputs [54], can be inhibited by certain traffic noise, and thus increase blood pressure [55–57]. In the following interview of the present study, these urban conditions were also considered as unpleasant factors by some participants (Figure 11). Therefore, the poorer effects observed in the daytime urban walking suggest that the daytime urban environment exerts a dominant influence, which might attenuate or even mask the benefits of walking.

In terms of the nighttime urban walking, responses were found more positive. In a relevant study, Fullick, et al. [24] found that a night exercise carried out indoors resulted in postexercise hypotension, which was similar to our results, indicating that the effects of physical activity remained in the outdoor urban environment. Based on the field investigation, a significant decrease in noise was observed in the nighttime urban area (Table 3). Meanwhile, according to our observation during the experiment, the pedestrians were obviously fewer at night, which could also reduce feelings of being exposed and make participants feel safe and comfortable [58]. Besides, some participants in our study also mentioned that the urban area was quiet and peaceful at night (Figure 11). These changes might partly explain the better responses at night. Moreover, another important reason might be the enhanced safety and visuality owing to artificial lighting [33]. Despite current concerns over light pollution, artificial lights do bring convenience to the urban citizen's nighttime activities. Cajochen, et al. [59] has reported that exposure to commercial light at 6500K resulted in enhanced subjective alertness, well-being, and visual comfort. Another study further emphasized the psychological experiences affected by light properties, and reported that the exposure to an artificial morning dawn simulation light improved participants' well-being, mood, and cognitive performance [60]. Our data showed that the urban street had the best illumination in all scenarios (Table 3), and the lights from streetlights and shops were generally warm, which made some participants feel warm and comfortable (Figure 11). Overall, our findings confirm the negative impacts of the daytime urban area, but indicate that nighttime urban walking may have positive effects. Given that many cities have pedestrian streets or areas that are open and free of vehicles, these places at night, especially the quiet ones, are probably suitable places for nighttime walking after work.

4.2. Green Walking

In the present study, the daytime green walking has resulted in significant improvements in psychological (PANAS-positive, POMS-vigor, and POMS-TMD) and physiological (SBP, DBP, and MAP) parameters. By comparison, though the psychological improvements were not statistically significant at night, similar positive trends were found, and decreases in blood pressure (SBP, DBP, and MAP) were statistically significant. In terms of the PRS and ROS, both scenarios received similar good scores. These results do not support our second hypothesis that the daytime green walking has positive while the nighttime green walking has negative effects.

In the published literature, the benefits of green walking in lowering blood pressure and improving psychological outcomes have been recorded [12,13,61]. Our findings of daytime green walking have reconfirmed the effects of lowering blood pressure and improving moods. However, there is still a notable difference, the green environments in previous studies were forests or urban parks, in contrast to the urban greenway in our study. Unlike forests or parks with relatively independent large areas, urban green spaces are usually distributed in cities, close to the building area, have smaller green coverage, and may be parked with cars like the present study area (Figure 2). This difference suggests that small-scale or incomplete natural green environments in cities may also exert positive effects on walking exercise. The finding is similar to that by Janeczko, et al. [62] who also concluded that walking in an urban environment with greenery and walking in a forest environment induced similar effects on physiological and psychological relaxation. Taken together, these results further confirm the positive roles of urban green space in stress relief and health improvement.

In terms of the nighttime green walking, the reasons for the non-significant psychological improvements and the decreased blood pressure were still unclear. As speculated previously, visual experience might play an important role in green walking [30]. A simulation by Briki and Majed [31] has confirmed the calming and relaxing effect of the color green on the human organism, which further implied the importance of visual interacting with plants during green walking. As the night went on, though considerable lights were placed in the green space, the illumination situation was still the worst due to the shading of tree crowns (Table 3). Theoretically, the color vision and foveal acuity seriously reduced in nighttime due to characteristics of human rod-mediated vision. Reeves, et al. [63] found that human night vision is very slow to adapt to changes in light levels. Therefore, in addition to insufficient illumination, uneven illumination caused by plant shading may also interfere with visual interacting when walking through the green space. In a similar study, Horiuchi et al. (2014) found that staying in a forest without visual interacting had led to lowered blood pressure, but the outcomes of POMS were not affected. Our findings were very similar to those recorded by Horiuchi et al. (2014), which indicate that visual interacting may play a key role in psychological responses. Considering that some participants disliked the nighttime green space for its poor scenic views (Figure 11), the non-significant psychological responses in nighttime green walking could be partly explained by the insufficient visual interacting with green elements. Moreover, the lowered blood pressure, according to Horiuchi et al. (2014), was possibly induced by other environmental factors such as smell and sound. In the present study, the green space had the lowest noise level (Table 3), which might help participants to stay calm and lower their blood pressure [64]. Besides, some studies have found that smell materials produced by trees may increase parasympathetic activity, thereby lowering blood pressure [65,66]. However, these mechanisms are not confirmed in the present study. Our findings suggest that nighttime green walking may not effectively improve moods, but it is still effective in lowering blood pressure. The green space in cities is still a feasible option for daytime and nighttime walking.

4.3. Nighttime Walking

In the present study, nighttime walking in both the green space and urban area induced positive changes, but no statistically significant differences were found in the post-test or the proportion of participants with positive responses. In terms of the PRS and ROS, though the green space scored a little higher than the urban area, the difference is not statistically significant. These results do not support our third hypothesis that urban walking has more positive and is more attractive than green walking at nighttime.

In recent years, green environments have been widely recognized to be more advantageous to human health than urban environments [67,68]. Pratiwi, et al. [12] have found greater improvements in blood pressure (SBP and DBP) and psychological parameters (POMS-TMD and STAI) after walking in an urban park than walking in the city. Likewise, similar results were also reported in other walking studies [49,69]. However, these differences were not seen in the nighttime green walking, which might be explained by the changes in environmental properties as we discussed above. These results indicate the similar benefits of nighttime walking in urban areas and green spaces.

In addition, the results of restorativeness were not in accordance with the findings by Sonntag-Öström, et al. [58], who reported that four types of green environments all scored much higher than a city environment. There was an assumption that urban environments were inherently lacking stress-reducing and mood-enhancing functions [18], and the restorative effects of urban areas were possibly associated with urban greening [45]. However, in the present study, only a few plants were observed in the urban area, and the restorativeness of the nighttime urban environment did not seem to be strongly associated with plants. Han [70] reported that in addition to the scenic beauty, the restorativeness was also related to viewers' preference, which may help to understand our results. Our interview results showed that nearly half of the participants preferred the urban environment in the nighttime walking (Figure 11), which might be the reason for the similar restorative effects in the urban area and green space. Overall, our findings imply that in addition to natural environments, other artificial environments may also be positive and restorative in a specific population or under certain conditions.

4.4. Limitations

With intriguing findings in the present study, there are still some limitations. Firstly, because of the non-normally distributed data, the diurnal variation of measured physiological parameters, we could not explore the interaction between time and sites. Secondly, detailed physiological responses such as stress hormones and brain waves were not investigated due to the limited experimental conditions. Therefore, the mechanisms of benefits in in different walking scenarios were not further discussed. Thirdly, the main reason to walk in green environments is the air purification function of trees [71,72]. However, the experiment was carried out in October, which is just in the rainy season of Chengdu Plain, and the air pollution was at very low levels during the whole experiment (Table 3), so the influences of air pollution were not investigated, which limits us to generalize our findings to less polluted periods or areas. Besides, the impact of air pollution on the nighttime walking and whether a small green space such as a greenway can purify air need to be verified in future studies. Lastly, we ran the physiological and psychological tests immediately after the walking program, therefore only the acute effects were considered, and the long-term effects may remain a future topic.

5. Conclusions

This study provided scientific evidence for the physiological and psychological effects of walking in urban areas and green spaces. Our findings suggest that the daytime green environments are advantageous to mental relaxation and can help to lower blood pressure, while the urban environments are negatively associated with walking exercise and may attenuate positive effects of physical activities. However, the urban area may become attractive and show positive effects in nighttime walking, while the psychological influences may be subtle during the nighttime green walking, and nighttime walking in both urban areas and green spaces may provide similar benefits. Taking into account the limitations of the present study, we would recommend the urban citizens start nighttime green walking after work, and nighttime urban walking is also advisable when the air is less polluted.

Author Contributions: Conceptualization, H.L. (Hansen Li) and G.Z.; methodology, H.L. (Hansen Li) and G.Z.; validation, H.L. (Hansen Li); formal analysis, H.L. (Hansen Li); investigation, H.L. (Hansen Li), H.L. (Haowei Liu), and Z.Y.; resources, G.Z.; data curation, H.L. (Hansen Li); writing—original draft preparation, H.L. (Hansen Li); writing—review and editing, H.L. (Hansen Li), S.B., G.Z., and Y.C.; visualization, H.L. (Hansen Li); supervision, G.Z., and Y.C.; project administration, G.Z., and Y.C.; funding acquisition, G.Z. All authors have read and agreed to the published version of the manuscript.

Funding: This research was founded by the Fundamental Research Funds for the Central Universities (SWU1909105).

Institutional Review Board Statement: The study was conducted according to the guidelines of the Declaration of Helsinki, and approved by the Ethics Committee of the Physical Education College of Southwest University, China (protocol code 2020307005; 20 September 2020).

Informed Consent Statement: Informed consent was obtained from all subjects involved in the study.

Data Availability Statement: The data presented in this study are available on request from the corresponding author. The data are not publicly available due to privacy.

Acknowledgments: We would like to express appreciation to the Senyu community members who participated in the experiment, also to local residential property agency who provide the measurement facilities.

Conflicts of Interest: The authors declare no conflict of interest.

References

1. Okkels, N.; Kristiansen, C.B.; Munk-Jørgensen, P.; Sartorius, N. Urban mental health: Challenges and perspectives. *Curr. Opin. Psychiatry* **2018**, *31*, 258–264. [CrossRef] [PubMed]
2. Ulrich, R.S.; Simons, R.F.; Losito, B.D.; Fiorito, E.; Zelson, M. Stress recovery during exposure to natural and urban environments. *J. Environ. Psychol.* **1991**, *11*, 201–230. [CrossRef]
3. Hahad, O.; Kröller-Schön, S.; Daiber, A.; Münzel, T. The Cardiovascular Effects of Noise. *Dtsch. Arztebl. Int.* **2019**, *116*, 245–250. [CrossRef] [PubMed]
4. Armstrong, A.D.C.; Ladeia, A.M.T.; Marques, J.; Armstrong, D.; Silva, A.; Morais Junior, J.C.; Barral, A.; Correia, L.C.L.; Barral-Netto, M.; Lima, J.A.C. Urbanization is Associated with Increased Trends in Cardiovascular Mortality Among Indigenous Populations: The PAI Study. *Arq. Bras. Cardiol.* **2018**, *110*, 240–245. [CrossRef] [PubMed]
5. Wang, R.; Xue, D.; Liu, Y.; Chen, H.; Qiu, Y. The relationship between urbanization and depression in China: The mediating role of neighborhood social capital. *Int. J. Equity Health* **2018**, *17*, 105. [CrossRef] [PubMed]
6. Koselka, E.P.D.; Weidner, L.C.; Minasov, A.; Berman, M.G.; Leonard, W.R.; Santoso, M.V.; de Brito, J.N.; Pope, Z.C.; Pereira, M.A.; Horton, T.H. Walking Green: Developing an Evidence Base for Nature Prescriptions. *Int. J. Environ. Res. Public Health* **2019**, *16*, 4338. [CrossRef]
7. Trøstrup, C.H.; Christiansen, A.B.; Stølen, K.S.; Nielsen, P.K.; Stelter, R. The effect of nature exposure on the mental health of patients: A systematic review. *Qual. Life Res.* **2019**, *28*, 1695–1703. [CrossRef]
8. Repke, M.A.; Berry, M.S.; Conway, L.G., 3rd; Metcalf, A.; Hensen, R.M.; Phelan, C. How does nature exposure make people healthier?: Evidence for the role of impulsivity and expanded space perception. *PLoS ONE* **2018**, *13*, e0202216. [CrossRef]
9. Agüera Sánchez, M.; Barbancho Ma, M.; García-Casares, N. Effect of physical exercise on Alzheimer's disease. A sistematic review. *Aten. Primaria* **2020**, *52*, 307–318. [CrossRef]
10. Marker, A.M.; Steele, R.G.; Noser, A.E. Physical activity and health-related quality of life in children and adolescents: A systematic review and meta-analysis. *Health Psychol.* **2018**, *37*, 893–903. [CrossRef]
11. Shanahan, D.F.; Franco, L.; Lin, B.B.; Gaston, K.J.; Fuller, R.A. The Benefits of Natural Environments for Physical Activity. *Sports Med.* **2016**, *46*, 989–995. [CrossRef] [PubMed]
12. Pratiwi, P.I.; Xiang, Q.; Furuya, K. Physiological and Psychological Effects of Walking in Urban Parks and Its Imagery in Different Seasons in Middle-Aged and Older Adults: Evidence from Matsudo City, Japan. *Sustainability* **2020**, *12*, 4003. [CrossRef]
13. Song, C.; Joung, D.; Ikei, H.; Igarashi, M.; Aga, M.; Park, B.-J.; Miwa, M.; Takagaki, M.; Miyazaki, Y. Physiological and psychological effects of walking on young males in urban parks in winter. *J. Physiol. Anthropol.* **2013**, *32*, 18. [CrossRef] [PubMed]
14. Ji, G.; Kim, K.; Han, G.-S. Physiological and Psychological Effects of Viewing and Walking in Forest and Urban Area. *J. Environ. Sci.* **2012**, *21*, 605–611. [CrossRef]
15. Kobayashi, H.; Song, C.; Ikei, H.; Park, B.J.; Lee, J.; Kagawa, T.; Miyazaki, Y. Forest Walking Affects Autonomic Nervous Activity: A Population-Based Study. *Front. Public Health* **2018**, *6*, 278. [CrossRef]
16. Li, Q.; Otsuka, T.; Kobayashi, M.; Wakayama, Y.; Inagaki, H.; Katsumata, M.; Hirata, Y.; Li, Y.; Hirata, K.; Shimizu, T.; et al. Acute effects of walking in forest environments on cardiovascular and metabolic parameters. *Eur. J. Appl. Physiol.* **2011**, *111*, 2845–2853. [CrossRef] [PubMed]
17. Lee, J.Y.; Lee, D.C. Cardiac and pulmonary benefits of forest walking versus city walking in elderly women: A randomised, controlled, open-label trial. *Eur. J. Integr. Med.* **2014**, *6*, 5–11. [CrossRef]
18. Karmanov, D.; Hamel, R. Assessing the restorative potential of contemporary urban environment(s): Beyond the nature versus urban dichotomy. *Landsc. Urban Plan.* **2008**, *86*, 115–125. [CrossRef]
19. Pretty, J.; Peacock, J.; Sellens, M.; Griffin, M. The mental and physical health outcomes of green exercise. *Int. J. Environ. Health Res.* **2005**, *15*, 319–337. [CrossRef]

20. Paulina, K.; Katarzyna, B. Restorative Qualities of and Preference for Natural and Urban Soundscapes. *Front. Psychol.* **2017**, *8*, 1705.
21. Yang, M. A study on characteristics of middle and advanced-aged people's exercise in scenic resorts. *J. Beijing Sport Univ.* **2009**, *32*, 54–56.
22. Pang, Y.N.; He, J.W. Sports participation of Chinese people of different ages. *China Sport Sci.* **2000**, *20*, 23–25.
23. Brito, L.C.; Peçanha, T.; Fecchio, R.Y.; Rezende, R.A.; Sousa, P.; Silva-Júnior, N.D.; Abreu, A.; Silva, G.; Mion-Junior, D.; Halliwill, J.R.; et al. Morning versus Evening Aerobic Training Effects on Blood Pressure in Treated Hypertension. *Med. Sci. Sports Exerc.* **2019**, *51*, 653–662. [CrossRef] [PubMed]
24. Fullick, S.; Morris, C.; Jones, H.; Atkinson, G. Prior exercise lowers blood pressure during simulated night-work with different meal schedules. *Am. J. Hypertens.* **2009**, *22*, 835–841. [CrossRef] [PubMed]
25. Miller, D.J.; Sargent, C.; Roach, G.D.; Scanlan, A.T.; Vincent, G.E.; Lastella, M. Moderate-intensity exercise performed in the evening does not impair sleep in healthy males. *Eur. J. Sport Sci.* **2020**, *20*, 80–89. [CrossRef] [PubMed]
26. Li, Z.Q.; Dai, X.; Guo, L. Investigation and reflection on morning and evening exercise groups in Guangzhou. *J. Phys. Educ.* **1998**, *1*, 23–25.
27. Gong, J.W. Investigation on Present Situation and Analysis on Main Factors Affecting Activity2takers in the Morning and Evening Exercise Spots in Nanjing City. *J. Shenyang Sport Univ.* **2008**, *27*, 83–86.
28. Larkin, A.; Hystad, P. Evaluating street view exposure measures of visible green space for health research. *J. Expo. Sci. Environ. Epidemiol.* **2019**, *29*, 447–456. [CrossRef]
29. Hunter, R.F.; Cleland, C.; Cleary, A.; Droomers, M.; Wheeler, B.W.; Sinnett, D.; Nieuwenhuijsen, M.J.; Braubach, M. Environmental, health, wellbeing, social and equity effects of urban green space interventions: A meta-narrative evidence synthesis. *Environ. Int.* **2019**, *130*, 104923. [CrossRef]
30. Wooller, J.J.; Rogerson, M.; Barton, J.; Micklewright, D.; Gladwell, V. Can Simulated Green Exercise Improve Recovery From Acute Mental Stress? *Front. Psychol.* **2018**, *9*, 2167. [CrossRef]
31. Briki, W.; Majed, L. Adaptive Effects of Seeing Green Environment on Psychophysiological Parameters When Walking or Running. *Front. Psychol.* **2019**, *10*, 252. [CrossRef] [PubMed]
32. Devi, B.; Bhardwaj, D.R.; Panwar, P.; Pal, S.; Gupta, N.K.; Thakur, C.L. Carbon allocation, sequestration and carbon dioxide mitigation under plantation forests of north western Himalaya, India. *Ann. For. Res.* **2013**, *56*, 44–50.
33. Tähkämö, L.; Partonen, T.; Pesonen, A.K. Systematic review of light exposure impact on human circadian rhythm. *Chronobiol. Int.* **2019**, *36*, 151–170. [CrossRef] [PubMed]
34. Tang, Y.Y.; Tang, R.; Posner, M.I. Mindfulness meditation improves emotion regulation and reduces drug abuse. *Drug Alcohol Depend.* **2016**, *163* (Suppl. 1), S13–S18. [CrossRef]
35. Saxon, L.; Henriksson, S.; Kvarnström, A.; Hiltunen, A.J. Affective Changes During Cognitive Behavioural Therapy-As Measured by PANAS. *Clin. Pract. Epidemiol. Ment. Health CP EMH* **2017**, *13*, 115–124. [CrossRef]
36. Watson, D.; Clark, L.A.; Tellegen, A. Development and validation of brief measures of positive and negative affect: The PANAS scales. *J. Personal. Soc. Psychol.* **1988**, *54*, 1063–1070. [CrossRef]
37. Crawford, J.R.; Henry, J.D. The positive and negative affect schedule (PANAS): Construct validity, measurement properties and normative data in a large non-clinical sample. *Br. J. Clin. Psychol.* **2004**, *43*, 245–265. [CrossRef]
38. Huang, L.; Yang, T.Z.; Ji, Z.M. Applicability of positive and negative scale in Chinese population. *Chin. J. Ment. Health* **2003**, *17*, 54–56.
39. Wang, J.P.; Lin, W.J.; Chen, J.G.; Cui, J.N.; Liu, J. A trial report of the brief mood scale (POMS) in China. *J. Psychol.* **2000**, *32*, 110–114.
40. Zhang, W.Y. Applicability of POMS scale on mood state of female college students during physical entertainment. *J. Xian Phys. Educ. Univ.* **2009**, *26*, 508–512.
41. Berto, R. The role of familiarity on the restorative value of a place. Research on a Spanish sample. *IAPS Bull.* **2001**, *18*, 22–24.
42. Ruiz, C.; Hernandez, B. Emotions and coping strategies during an episode of volcanic activity and their relations to place attachment. *J. Environ. Psychol.* **2014**, *38*, 279–287. [CrossRef]
43. Hartig, T.; Korpela, K.; Evans, G.W. A measure of restorative quality in environments: Scandinavian Housing and Planning Research. *Scand. Hous. Plan. Res.* **1997**, *14*, 175–194. [CrossRef]
44. Hartig, T.; Korpela, K.; Evans, G.W.; Gärling, T. Validation of a measure of perceived environmental restorativeness. *Göteborg Psychol. Rep.* **1997**, *26*, 1–64.
45. Fátima, N.; Estefanía, H.F.; Stephany, H.; Bernardo, H. Discrimination of Urban Spaces with Different Level of Restorativeness Based on the Original and on a Shorter Version of Hartig et al.'s Perceived Restorativeness Scale. *Front. Psychol.* **2017**, *8*, 1735.
46. Silvennoinen, H. Favorite green, waterside and urban environments, restorative experiences and perceived health in Finland. *Health Promot. Int.* **2010**, *25*, 200–209.
47. Korpela, K.M.; Ylén, M.; Tyrväinen, L.; Silvennoinen, H. Determinants of restorative experiences in everyday favorite places. *Health Place* **2008**, *14*, 636–652. [CrossRef]
48. Hassan, A.; Tao, J.; Li, G.; Jiang, M.; Aii, L.; Jiang, Z.; Liu, Z.; Chen, Q. Effects of Walking in Bamboo Forest and City Environments on Brainwave Activity in Young Adults. *Evid. Based Complement. Altern. Med.* **2018**, *2018*, 9653857. [CrossRef]

49. Song, C.; Ikei, H.; Kagawa, T.; Miyazaki, Y. Effects of Walking in a Forest on Young Women. *Int. J. Environ. Res. Public Health* **2019**, *16*, 229. [CrossRef]
50. Lee, L.L.; Watson, M.C.; Mulvaney, C.A.; Tsai, C.C.; Lo, S.F. The effect of walking intervention on blood pressure control: A systematic review. *Int. J. Nurs. Stud.* **2010**, *47*, 1545–1561. [CrossRef]
51. Kelly, P.; Williamson, C.; Niven, A.G.; Hunter, R.; Mutrie, N.; Richards, J. Walking on sunshine: Scoping review of the evidence for walking and mental health. *Br. J. Sports Med.* **2018**, *52*, 800–806. [CrossRef]
52. Kuehn, B.M. Pollution Exposure Counteracts Exercise Benefits: Exercise in Green Spaces, Pollution Reductions Recommended. *Circulation* **2018**, *137*, 1516–1517. [CrossRef]
53. Dzhambov, A.; Tilov, B.; Markevych, I.; Dimitrova, D. Residential road traffic noise and general mental health in youth: The role of noise annoyance, neighborhood restorative quality, physical activity, and social cohesion as potential mediators. *Environ. Int.* **2017**, *109*, 1–9. [CrossRef]
54. Piepoli, M.; Coats, A.J.; Adamopoulos, S.; Bernardi, L.; Feng, Y.H.; Conway, J.; Sleight, P. Persistent peripheral vasodilation and sympathetic activity in hypotension after maximal exercise. *J. Appl. Physiol.* **1993**, *75*, 1807–1814. [CrossRef]
55. Regecová, V.; Kellerová, E. Effects of urban noise pollution on blood pressure and heart rate in preschool children. *J. Hypertens.* **1995**, *13*, 405–412. [CrossRef]
56. Moshammer, H.; Panholzer, J.; Ulbing, L.; Udvarhelyi, E.; Ebenbauer, B.; Peter, S. Acute Effects of Air Pollution and Noise from Road Traffic in a Panel of Young Healthy Adults. *Int. J. Environ. Res. Public Health* **2019**, *16*, 778. [CrossRef]
57. Graham, J.M.; Janssen, S.A.; Vos, H.; Miedema, H.M. Habitual traffic noise at home reduces cardiac parasympathetic tone during sleep. *Int. J. Psychophysiol.* **2009**, *72*, 179–186. [CrossRef]
58. Sonntag-Öström, E.; Nordin, M.; Lundell, Y.; Dolling, A.; Wiklund, U.; Karlsson, M.; Carlberg, B.; Järvholm, L.S. Restorative effects of visits to urban and forest environments in patients with exhaustion disorder. *Urban For. Urban Green.* **2014**, *13*, 344–354. [CrossRef]
59. Cajochen, C.; Frey, S.; Anders, D.; Späti, J.; Bues, M.; Pross, A.; Mager, R.; Wirz-Justice, A.; Stefani, O. Evening exposure to a light-emitting diodes (LED)-backlit computer screen affects circadian physiology and cognitive performance. *J. Appl. Physiol.* **2011**, *110*, 1432–1438. [CrossRef]
60. Gabel, V.; Maire, M.; Reichert, C.F.; Chellappa, S.L.; Schmidt, C.; Hommes, V.; Viola, A.U.; Cajochen, C. Effects of artificial dawn and morning blue light on daytime cognitive performance, well-being, cortisol and melatonin levels. *Chronobiol. Int.* **2013**, *30*, 988–997. [CrossRef]
61. Song, C.; Ikei, H.; Igarashi, M.; Takagaki, M.; Miyazaki, Y. Physiological and Psychological Effects of a Walk in Urban Parks in Fall. *Int. J. Env. Res. Public Health* **2015**, *12*, 14216–14228. [CrossRef]
62. Janeczko, E.; Bielinis, E.; Wójcik, R.; Woźnicka, M.; Kędziora, W.; Łukowski, A.; Elsadek, M.; Szyc, K.; Janeczko, K. When Urban Environment Is Restorative: The Effect of Walking in Suburbs and Forests on Psychological and Physiological Relaxation of Young Polish Adults. *Forests* **2020**, *11*, 591. [CrossRef]
63. Reeves, A.; Grayhem, R.; Hwang, A.D. Rapid Adaptation of Night Vision. *Front. Psychol.* **2018**, *9*, 8. [CrossRef] [PubMed]
64. Nserat, S.; Al-Musa, A.; Khader, Y.S.; Abu Slaih, A.; Iblan, I. Blood Pressure of Jordanian Workers Chronically Exposed to Noise in Industrial Plants. *Int. J. Occup. Environ. Med.* **2017**, *8*, 217–223. [CrossRef] [PubMed]
65. Dayawansa, S.; Umeno, K.; Takakura, H.; Hori, E.; Tabuchi, E.; Nagashima, Y.; Oosu, H.; Yada, Y.; Suzuki, T.; Ono, T.; et al. Autonomic responses during inhalation of natural fragrance of Cedrol in humans. *Auton. Neurosci. Basic Clin.* **2003**, *108*, 79–86. [CrossRef] [PubMed]
66. Li, Q.; Kobayashi, M.; Inagaki, H.; Hirata, Y.; Li, Y.J.; Hirata, K.; Shimizu, T.; Suzuki, H.; Katsumata, M.; Wakayama, Y.; et al. A day trip to a forest park increases human natural killer activity and the expression of anti-cancer proteins in male subjects. *J. Biol. Regul. Homeost. Agents* **2010**, *24*, 157–165.
67. Tischer, C.; Gascon, M.; Fernández-Somoano, A.; Tardón, A.; Lertxundi Materola, A.; Ibarluzea, J.; Ferrero, A.; Estarlich, M.; Cirach, M.; Vrijheid, M.; et al. Urban green and grey space in relation to respiratory health in children. *Eur. Respir. J.* **2017**, *49*, 1502112. [CrossRef]
68. Morita, E.; Fukuda, S.; Nagano, J.; Hamajima, N.; Yamamoto, H.; Iwai, Y.; Nakashima, T.; Ohira, H.; Shirakawa, T. Psychological effects of forest environments on healthy adults: Shinrin-yoku (forest-air bathing, walking) as a possible method of stress reduction. *Public Health* **2007**, *121*, 54–63. [CrossRef]
69. Shin, J.-W.; Choi, J.-H. The Effects of Single Session Forest Walking on Physiological and Psychological State of Myocardial Infarction Patients. *J. People Plants Environ.* **2019**, *22*, 109–118. [CrossRef]
70. Han, K.T. An Exploration of Relationships Among the Responses to Natural Scenes: Scenic Beauty, Preference, and Restoration. *Environ. Behav.* **2010**, *42*, 243–270. [CrossRef]
71. Buccolieri, R.; Gromke, C.; Sabatino, S.D.; Ruck, B. Aerodynamic effects of trees on pollutant concentration in street canyons. *Sci. Total Environ.* **2009**, *407*, 5247–5256. [CrossRef]
72. Nowak, D.J.; Greenfield, E.J.; Hoehn, R.E.; Lapoint, E. Carbon storage and sequestration by trees in urban and community areas of the United States. *Environ. Pollut.* **2013**, *178*, 229–236. [CrossRef] [PubMed]

International Journal of
Environmental Research and Public Health

MDPI

Article

Development and Investigation of a New Model Explaining Job Performance and Uncertainty among Nurses and Physicians

Espen Olsen [1,*] and Aslaug Mikkelsen [1,2]

1 Department of Innovation, Leadership and Marketing, UiS Business School, University of Stavanger, 4036 Stavanger, Norway; aslaug.mikkelsen@uis.no
2 Stavanger University Hospital, 4011 Stavanger, Norway
* Correspondence: espen.olsen@uis.no

Abstract: The purpose of this paper is to develop and investigate a new theoretical model explaining variance in job performance and uncertainty among nurses and physicians. The study adopted a cross-sectional survey. Data was collected from 2946 nurses and 556 physicians employed at four public hospitals in Norway. We analysed data using descriptive statistics, correlations, Cronbach's alpha, confirmatory factor analyses and structural equation modelling. To explain job performance and uncertainty, two sets of explanatory variables were used: first, satisfactions of three psychological needs—namely autonomy, social support and competence development—and second, employee perceptions of hospital management quality (HMQ) and local leadership quality (LLQ). The results supported the theoretical model among nurses and physicians; (1) HMQ was positively associated with LLQ; (2) LLQ was positively associated with psychological needs; (3) the majority of psychological needs were positively associated with job performance and negatively associated with uncertainty, but more of these relations were significant among nurses than physicians. The results suggest that job performance and uncertainty among nurses and physicians can be improved by helping personnel meet their psychological needs. Improving job design and staff involvement will be important to strengthen need satisfaction. Results suggest enhancement of HMQ and LLQ will be positively related to need satisfaction among nurses and physicians and will strengthen job performance and reduce uncertainty.

Keywords: management; leadership; psychological needs; healthcare services; job performance; uncertainty; job resources

Citation: Olsen, E.; Mikkelsen, A. Development and Investigation of a New Model Explaining Job Performance and Uncertainty among Nurses and Physicians. *Int. J. Environ. Res. Public Health* **2021**, *18*, 164. https://doi.org/10.3390/ijerph18010164

Received: 10 December 2020
Accepted: 22 December 2020
Published: 28 December 2020

1. Introduction

The complexity of healthcare systems, tasks and patient care can develop high levels of uncertainty among healthcare workers. In virtually all clinical situations experienced by patients and health professionals, uncertainty is interwoven on a daily basis. Uncertainty is influenced by numerous unknowns. Will a patient develop a particular condition? How will that condition evolve? Is the treatment beneficial? Is the patient receiving the right care at the right time, in the right place, and from the right people? Hence, the variety of these unknowns, behaviours and feelings, reflects the concept of uncertainty and "make uncertainty a ubiquitous problem in health care" [1]. Uncertainty influences how people think, feel or behave [1]. Moreover, based on the rapid emergence and development of new medical technologies, uncertainty is a growing problem in healthcare. Uncertainty has many potential psychological effects and is a critical phenomenon in healthcare. Uncertainty can provoke fear, worry, anxiety and avoidance of decision-making. Individuals will, therefore, engage in a variety of different responses to minimise the negative effects of uncertainty. Some will try to avoid uncertainty, while others will seek information to reduce uncertainty. The responses to uncertainty will also depend on the specific context [1,2]. Given the increasing exposure of health providers to uncertain situations and information, researchers should develop knowledge that can be used to reduce uncertainty and improve uncertainty tolerance in healthcare. For this to happen, we need research that can increase the general understanding of uncertainty in healthcare settings [1], a clearer understanding of the causes of uncertainty, and new response strategies [3].

Many factors are related to uncertainty among clinicians, and this study aims to develop a taxonomy explaining direct and indirect causes of uncertainty and job performance among nurses and physicians. Since many factors at different levels influence clinicians, both micro- and macro-organisational factors will be included in the development of a theoretical model. First, we assume that both managers and leaders influence the work setting and psychological need satisfaction among clinicians. Moreover, we assume that psychological need satisfaction significantly influences uncertainty and job performance. In summary, we use these assumptions to develop a new taxonomy linking hospital management quality (HMQ), local leadership quality (LLQ), psychological need satisfaction, uncertainty and job performance. This new taxonomy is to be tested among nurses and physicians. The study provides new insights into the system dynamics of hospitals, starting from the top management down to each individual worker who treats patients in clinical settings. Furthermore, the study aims to contribute new knowledge that can be used to understand clinical mechanisms and to improve hospital performance and delivery of care in various settings. To cross-validate the research findings and potentially explore unique findings across different groups, hypothesis testing will be conducted separately for nurses and physicians.

Psychological health has a moderate to strong correlation with job performance across scientific studies [4]. Indisputably, healthcare institutions aim to avoid burnout of staff and develop healthy working conditions that support job performance. Unfortunately, healthcare institutions are often characterised as the opposite, with working conditions poorer than other sectors' increasing the likelihood of burnout and reduced quality of care [5].

Many factors influence system outcomes and quality of care. Hence, it may be necessary to integrate individual factors with micro- and macro-organisational factors when trying to understand systems' dynamics [6]. Both managers and leaders influence the work context of healthcare staff [7], and research suggests that the work environment significantly influences patient care [8–10]. In the current study, we take these principles into account. Therefore, we develop and present a new theoretical model illustrating how hospital management quality (HMQ) is positively related to local leadership quality (LLQ) Furthermore, LLQ of hospital wards is expected to be positively related to the satisfaction of employees' important psychological needs, namely autonomy, competence development and colleague support [11]. Since delivery of care is mediated by the performance of each individual healthcare worker, we also suggest that fulfilling the psychological needs of hospital employees has the potential to improve job performance and reduce uncertainty among staff. Hence, the current study focuses on incorporating and integrating important system components influencing healthcare workers' delivery of care. A new holistic framework is developed which integrates HMQ and LLQ with the level of need satisfaction, which in turn is expected to improve job performance and reduce uncertainty. This framework will be tested with survey data collected from nurses and physicians. Furthermore, we will test the validity of a structural model reflecting the theoretical framework, validating this model based on data.

1.1. Theoretical Framework and Hypotheses

This study draws upon theories originating from various bodies of literature. First, using knowledge from leadership and management literature, HMQ and LLQ are conceptualised and theoretically linked to each other. Next, insights from self-determination literature are used to conceptualise how HMQ and LLQ are linked to the satisfaction of psychological needs of healthcare personnel. Finally, theoretical arguments are built to hypothesise two model outcomes: uncertainty and job performance (Figure 1). Hence, we combine insights from management and leadership theory with organisational psychology and apply these sources to study uncertainty and job performance among physicians and nurses in a hospital context.

1.1.1. Managers' Influence on Leaders

Management and leadership have been substantially studied for decades, have multiple approaches and definitions [12], and have been empirically linked to outcomes both in healthcare [8,13,14] and other industries, e.g., [15].In the current study, we focus on core areas of leadership and management: HMQ and LLQ. Hospital management must cope with financial pressures and conflicting demands while dealing with pressure from the board. Research suggests that managers select different coping strategies to handle conflicting values and that these mechanisms challenge the integrity of managers [16] as well as their choices and priorities. Furthermore, to correctly prioritise, hospital managers need to have knowledge at both the institutional and regional levels. Hence, we suggest that HMQ consists of the following managerial skills: (1) correct prioritisation, (2) adequate knowledge at the institutional level, and (3) knowledge at the regional level which constitutes the hospital context.

Hospital managers define a large share of hospital agendas and implement prioritisations top-down in hospital organisations [17]. On the other hand, leaders at lower levels must potentially handle pressure from staff, patients and next of kin. In the daily care of patients; therefore, it is likely that the perception of HMQ and LLQ will vary across staff. Specifically, we include three leadership elements we regard as most important related to LLQ: (1) relational skills to retain workers, (2) overview and knowledge at the local hospital level, and (3) the ability to develop employees. Summarised, we expect HMQ to strengthen LLQ, which leads to the following hypothesis:

H1: *HMQ will be positively related to LLQ.*

1.1.2. Leadership Is Related to Psychological Needs

Next, we consider the potential positive influence LLQ has on the satisfaction of hospital staff's psychological needs. According to the self-determination theory, relatedness and inclusion in social groups constitute an important psychological need [18]. Leaders have the potential to build, develop and influence the social relationships in wards and units. Developing relationships is a potential way in which managers can influence perceived social belonging among employees. Healthcare professionals need to interact with one another as well as with professionals in other fields, developing mutual respect that will positively affect the work environment and social support [18].

Another topic concerns the potential influence leaders have on the need for autonomy. Research suggests the leaders have the potential to empower employees [19]. We, therefore, expect that managers can have a great effect on the autonomy of workers by either restricting or increasing it. The control that local managers have over different aspects of the workplace considerably influences the ways in which the employees perceive their work environment as controlling versus autonomous, which, according to self-determination theory, is important for motivation [20]. An independent and autonomous employee will have the opportunity to express what needs to be done, how and when. An employee may still autonomously complete a task that has been assigned by a supervisor as long as the employee believes that the nature of the task is inherently interesting and congruent with his or her values [21]. A leader may support autonomy through empowerment strategies, through sharing control over how the work gets done, and through trying to understand employees' perspectives on the work [19,22].

The need for and development of competence is the third important psychological need, according to Deci and Ryan [20]. We expect that managers have the capability to satisfy the need for competence by delegating tasks that fit well with individual employees' skills and abilities and by developing such skills and abilities according to goals, tasks and patient treatment challenges. Earlier research suggests that a transformational leadership style is positively related to competence, while management by exception is negatively related to competence [11].

Baard et al. [22] found that leadership behaviours that promote the satisfaction of employees' basic psychological needs produced positive outcomes, such as motivation, whereas behaviours that prevented need satisfaction led to negative outcomes. In summary, we expect LLQ to be positively related to employees' need satisfaction of autonomy, competence development and support [20]. Accordingly, the following hypothesis was formulated:

H2: *LLQ is positively related to psychological need (competence development, colleague support and autonomy) satisfaction.*

1.1.3. Psychological Needs Are Related to Uncertainty and Job Performance

Next, we will examine the potential outcomes of satisfying employees' psychological needs. Various studies have indicated that when people's basic psychological needs are satisfied, they behave with a sense of willingness and choice, e.g., [23]. Such positivity and engagement among staff have the potential to improve patient care [24–26]. On the contrary, lower engagement reflected in burnout is expected to be negatively related to patient safety and satisfaction outcomes [27–29].

Satisfaction of the three basic psychological needs is expected to positively influence health and well-being [30,31] as well as performance [22,32]. Individual job performance consists of distinct sets of activities that contribute to an organisation's output. When employees have satisfied their needs for competence, autonomy and social support, they will be motivated to invest their physical, cognitive and emotional energies into their work, e.g., [20,33–35]. This, again, may enhance job performance among hospital staff. Furthermore, by satisfying employees' need for autonomy, competence and relatedness, leaders are creating an environment where all employees can perform better, with positive emotions and higher engagement levels [36]. The research connecting need satisfaction to well-being and high-quality performance has been demonstrated in many fields [35], including healthcare [34].

Meta-analyses [37] of organisational studies suggest that poor worker health, e.g., as exemplified by burnout, is positively associated with adverse events and accidents. On the other hand, job resources, such as autonomy and social support, are related to less burnout and higher job engagement [37]. Transferring findings from the meta-analysis, we expect need satisfaction to be positively related to job performance and negatively related to uncertainty. Therefore, we expect that the fulfilment of psychological needs will be negatively related to uncertainty and positively related to job performance. This leads to the following hypothesis:

H3: *Satisfaction of psychological needs are (a) negatively related to uncertainty and (b) positively related to job performance.*

1.1.4. Final Model to Be Tested

This study contributes to the development and testing of a theoretical framework illustrated in Figure 1. This framework explains the direct and indirect links from hospital top management (HMQ) and local leadership (LLQ) to psychological need satisfaction, which is related to two outcomes in hospitals: uncertainty and job performance. A multilevel organisational perspective is integrated into the model, suggesting that managers indirectly influence the psychological needs of hospital employees and that local leaders directly influence need satisfaction. To cross-validate the research findings and potentially explore unique findings across different groups, hypothesis testing is conducted separately for nurses and physicians.

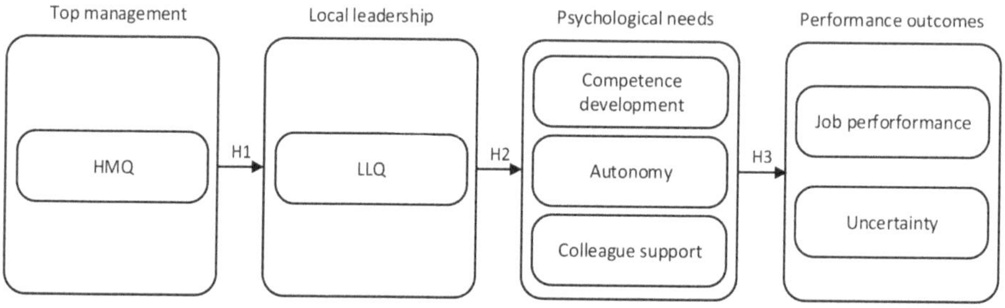

Figure 1. Research model. HMQ: Hospital management quality; LLQ: Local leadership quality.

2. Material and Methods

2.1. Sample and Data Collection

The current study was carried out in a Norwegian health region providing services to a population of 1.1 million citizens. The human resource departments across the hospitals generated employee email listings. A cross-sectional web-based survey design was employed, and 22,883 employees working across four hospitals in the health region were engaged. The overall response rate was 40% (N = 9162). For the purpose of this study, physicians (N = 556) and nurses (N = 2946) were selected from the total sample. Hence, 3502 respondents were included in the current study.

2.2. Measures

All study variables were based on employees' perception, with the use of Likert type scales. All measurement concepts were operationalised with the use of multi-item measures.

Hospital management quality (HMQ) and local leadership quality (LLQ) were adopted and developed based on earlier studies using the Work Research and Quality Improvement Questionnaire [38–40].

HMQ was measured with three items using a five-point scale (1 = not correct, 5 = totally correct). The items assessed whether hospital management had knowledge about departments, whether management priorities were correctly based on holistic understanding, and whether regional management possessed strong knowledge about the hospital. An example item reads, "The hospital management has good knowledge about the work in the different departments." Cronbach's alpha was 0.84.

LLQ was measured using three items on a five-point scale (1 = not correct, 5 = totally correct). The items assessed the leaders' ability to retain workers, to possess general knowledge, and to develop employees. An example item reads, "My closest leader has good knowledge about my working situation." Cronbach's alpha was 0.86.

Autonomy [41] was based on an index consisting of four items measured on a five-point scale (1 = to a very small extent, 5 = to a great extent). An example item reads, "Employees have good opportunities to influence how work is carried out." Cronbach's alpha was 0.91.

Competence development [42] was assessed with four items on a five-point scale (1 = to a very small extent, 5 = to a great extent). An example item reads, "Do you have the opportunity to learn new things through your work?". Cronbach's alpha was 0.76.

Colleague support [43] was assessed with three items on a five-point scale (1 = never, 5 = very often). An example item being "Are your colleagues able to appreciate the value of your work and see the results of it?". Cronbach's alpha was 0.74.

Job performance [44] comprised four items measured on a five-point scale (1 = very seldom/never, 5 = very often/always). An example item reads, "Are you satisfied with the quality of the work you carry out?". The other items concerned their ability to solve problems at work, capacity to maintain good working relationships with colleagues, and satisfaction related to the amount of work conducted. Cronbach's alpha was 0.77.

Uncertainty comprised six items measuring job-related situations associated with uncertainty on a four-point scale (1 = never, 4 = very often). Perception of uncertainty was, for instance, related to insufficient information and doubt regarding whether patients' relatives should be informed of patients' medical condition and treatment. The items were adopted from the Nurses Early Exit Study (http://www.next-study.net). An example item reads, "Uncertainty regarding the use and function of special equipment." Cronbach's alpha was 0.65.

2.3. Data Analysis

Descriptive statistics and multivariate analysis of variance (MANOVA) were performed with SPSS 26.0, while the remaining assessments were performed using AMOS 25.0. Pearson's correlations indicated some overlap between concepts. Since social phenomena were expected to vary across groups, MANOVA (Wilks' lambda) was conducted to test differences between the means of identified groups of subjects on a combination of variables. Variance across demographic variables should be expected and should support the discriminant validity of the study.

Confirmatory factor analyses (CFA) with the use of maximum likelihood estimation (MLE) was performed to test the validity of constructs. All the latent variables and observed variables were entered simultaneously to assess the construct validity. CFA is important since survey instruments are evolving, and the validity of measurements may differ across contexts. Second, structural equation modelling (SEM) with the use of MLE was performed to test the hypothetical model developed. The following indicators and thresholds were used to evaluate the fit: the root mean square error of approximation (RMSEA), Tucker–Lewis Index (TLI), incremental fit index (IFI > 0.90) and comparative fit index (CFI > 0.90). An RMSEA of less than 0.05 indicates a "good" fit, and an RMSEA of less than 0.08 corresponds to an "acceptable" fit [45]. Values of 0.90 or greater for other indicators indicate a "good" fit [45,46]. Chi-square is normally not recommended to evaluate fit for larger samples and was, therefore, not employed [47].

Based on the two target groups selected for the current study, descriptive statistics, CFA and structural modelling were run separately for nurses and physicians to cross-validate findings.

3. Results

3.1. Demographics

A total of 2946 nurses and 556 physicians participated in the study. Among nurses, 2661 were female (90.3%), 636 were less than 31 years old (21.6%), 316 were short-term employees (10.7%), 1572 were full-time employees (53.4%), 1576 had specialisation or further education (53.5%) and 508 had less than 4 years of experience (17.2%). Among physicians, 287 were female (51.6%), 57 were less than 31 years old (10.3%), 244 were short-term employees (43.9%), 509 were full-time employees (91.5%), 351 had specialisation or further education (63.1%) and 112 had less than 4 years of experience (20.1%). Other demographic data are presented in Table 1.

Table 1. Participants in the study.

Demographic Variables		Physicians (N = 556)		Nurses (N = 2946)		Total Sample (N = 3502)	
		n	%	n	%	n	%
Gender							
	Female	287	51.6	2661	90.3	2948	84.2
	Male	269	48.4	285	9.7	554	15.8
Age							
	<31	57	10.3	636	21.6	693	19.8
	31–40	243	43.7	753	25.6	996	28.4
	41–50	130	23.4	749	25.4	879	25.1
	51–60	80	14.4	651	22.1	731	20.9
	>60	46	8.3	157	5.3	203	5.8
Employment (long-/short-term)							
	Long-term employee	312	56.1	2630	89.3	2942	84.0
	Short-term employee	244	43.9	316	10.7	560	16.0
Employment (full-/part-time)							
	Full-time employee	509	91.5	1572	53.4	2081	59.4
	Part-time employee	47	8.5	1374	46.6	1421	40.6
Specialisation/further education							
	Yes	351	63.1	1576	53.5	1927	55.0
	No	205	36.9	1370	46.5	1575	45.0
Years of experience							
	≤4	112	20.1	508	17.2	620	21.7
	5–10	140	25.2	512	17.4	652	22.8
	11–20	117	21.0	709	24.1	826	28.9
	≥21	95	17.1	668	22.7	763	26.7

3.2. Descriptive Statistics

Descriptive statistics for the different target groups are presented in Table 2. Competence development had the highest score among physicians (mean = 4.47, SD = 0.55) and nurses (mean = 4.45, SD = 0.53). Job performance had the second highest scores among physicians (mean = 4.05, SD = 0.46) and nurses (mean = 4.07, SD = 0.45). Uncertainty in patient treatment had the lowest score among physicians (mean = 1.84, SD = 0.40) and nurses (mean = 1.80, SD = 0.36). The statistical variation on the different indicators was generally considered satisfactory.

Table 2. Descriptive statistics.

	Physicians		Nurses		Total	
	Mean	SD	Mean	SD	Mean	SD
Hospital management quality (HMQ)	3.00	0.87	3.11	0.79	3.10	0.80
Local leadership quality (LLQ)	3.75	1.01	3.75	0.97	3.75	0.97
Autonomy	3.07	0.87	3.24	0.79	3.21	0.81
Competence development	4.47	0.55	4.45	0.53	4.45	0.53
Colleague support	3.52	0.70	3.47	0.67	3.48	0.67
Job performance	4.05	0.46	4.07	0.45	4.07	0.46
Uncertainty	1.84	0.40	1.80	0.36	1.81	0.37

3.3. Variance across Sub-Groups

The results of MANOVA (Wilks' lambda) indicated that age, gender and personnel category (physician or nurse) were significantly ($p < 0.05$) related to the variance of the seven dimensions included in Table 1. Hence, results generally indicated different scorings based on age, gender and personnel category. This indicates statistical variance and distribution, which is in accordance with expectancies in social science studies [48,49].

3.4. Correlations

In general, HMQ, LLQ, competence development, autonomy, colleague support and job performance were positively correlated with one another. On the other hand, uncertainty was negatively correlated with all the other dimensions, which is not unexpected. All correlations and Cronbach's alpha can be seen in Table 3. Generally, all correlations were significant ($p < 0.01$), and the level of overlaps between concepts and internal consistency (Cronbach's alpha) are considered satisfactory.

Table 3. Cronbach's alpha (total sample in parentheses) and correlations among nurses (below diagonal) and physicians (above diagonal).

	1	2	3	4	5	6	7
1. Hospital management quality (HMQ)	(0.84)	0.42	0.23	0.48	0.11	0.19	−0.54
2. Local leadership quality (LLQ)	0.52	(0.86)	0.39	0.67	0.22	0.24	−0.44
3. Competence development	0.18	0.33	(0.70)	0.35	0.23	0.30	−0.20
4. Autonomy	0.43	0.66	0.32	(0.91)	0.27	0.18	−0.49
5. Colleague support	0.12	0.18	0.32	0.24	(0.74)	0.25	−0.14
6. Job performance	0.21	0.21	0.29	0.22	0.28	(0.77)	−0.30
7. Uncertainty	−0.43	−0.39	−0.12	−0.36	−0.06	−0.29	(0.65)

Note: All correlations are significant at $p < 0.001$ (two-tailed test).

Ad hoc assessments were conducted to control for the different demographic variables listed in Table 1. Among the demographic variables, age had the strongest correlation with the concepts included in the study, and uncertainty was most strongly correlated with age among nurses ($r = -0.23$, $p < 0.01$) and physicians ($r = -0.19$, $p < 0.01$).

3.5. Confirmatory Factor Analyses

Confirmatory factor analyses (CFA) was performed using maximum likelihood extraction (MLE) to assess the validity of all concepts among nurses and physicians. All dimensions with associated items were included in the assessments (Table 4). CFA supported the use of the measurement concepts among nurses (IFI = 0.93, TLI = 0.91, CFI = 0.93, RMSEA = 0.049, 90% confidence interval = 0.047–0.051) and physicians (IFI = 0.93, TLI = 0.91, CFI = 0.93, RMSEA = 0.050, 90% confidence interval = 0.046–0.055). Among nurses, the standardised factor to item loadings ranged from 0.34–0.90, and among physicians loading ranged from 0.33–0.90. Uncertainty had the lowest loadings on "uncertainty regarding the use and function of special equipment", which was 0.34 and 0.33 among nurses and physicians, respectively. Additionally, the loading on the items "Doubt if a patient's relatives should get informed about the patient's medical condition and treatment" was 0.37 among physicians. Even though two items had factor loading below 0.44, these items were not removed because the content of the items was relevant for capturing the theoretical domains they measure. Moreover, the theoretical concepts were operationalised with relatively few items, and none of the items were, therefore, considered redundant. Based on the fit indices and the overall results, the factor-to-item relations were considered satisfactory, indicating robust and valid measures. Thus, the structural model could be tested with the use of validated measurement concepts.

Table 4. Standardised factor loadings based on confirmatory factor analyses (CFA).

Dimension/Item	Standardised Factor Loadings Nurses	Physicians
Competence development		
Does your work require you to change?	0.63	0.55
Does your work require you to take initiative?	0.64	0.60
Can you use your skills and your expertise in your job?	0.68	0.76
Do you have the opportunity to learn new things through your work?	0.68	0.75
Autonomy		
In my department, we often influence goals or measures	0.87	0.86
Employees have the possibility to influence the work situations	0.89	0.90
All of the employees in my department are involved in important decisions that affect them	0.85	0.87
In my department, we can influence requirements associated with doing a good job	0.80	0.78
Colleague support		
Give your colleagues constructive advice	0.74	0.72
Do your colleagues express their opinions about your work?	0.81	0.79
Are your colleagues able to appreciate the value of your work and see the results of it?	0.58	0.57
Local leadership quality (LLQ)		
The leader of my unit emphasises the development of employees	0.84	0.90
My nearest leader has good knowledge about my work situation	0.71	0.67
The leader of my unit emphasises keeping employees	0.86	0.89
Hospital management quality (HMQ)		
The hospital management has good knowledge about the situation in the departments	0.79	0.85
In my hospital, the management priorities are correctly based on a holistic understanding	0.90	0.88
The regional hospital management has good knowledge of our hospital	0.73	0.73
Uncertainty		
Insufficient information from other healthcare professionals regarding a patient's medical condition	0.52	0.42
Providing wrong treatment to a patient	0.54	0.43
No doctor present at a medical emergency	0.46	0.44
Too few personnel to provide reasonable treatment	0.58	0.65
Doubt if a patient's relatives should be informed about the patient's medical condition and treatment	0.48	0.37
Uncertainty regarding the use and function of special equipment	0.34	0.33
Job performance		
Are you satisfied with the quality of the work you perform?	0.80	0.70
Are you satisfied with the amount of work you get done?	0.78	0.60
Are you satisfied with your ability to resolve problems that pop up during your work?	0.70	0.79
Are you satisfied with your ability to have a good relationship with your work colleagues?	0.48	0.54

3.6. Results of Structural Equation Modelling (SEM)

The full structural model was tested (MLE) with all the latent and manifest variables. Among nurses, all fit indicators (Figure 2) were acceptable and above recommended thresholds. All beta coefficients were in the expected directions. HMQ was positively related to LLQ (b = 0.54, $p < 0.001$), supporting hypothesis 1. Further, LLQ was significantly related to competence development (b = 0.36, $p < 0.001$), colleague support (b = 0.21, $p < 0.001$) and autonomy (b = 0.68), supporting hypothesis 2. Additionally, job performance was significantly related to competence development (b = 0.21, $p < 0.001$), colleague support (b = 0.20, $p < 0.001$) and autonomy (b = 0.12, $p < 0.001$), as specified in hypothesis 3. Lastly, also supporting hypothesis 3, uncertainty was related to competence development (b = −0.05, $p < 0.05$) and autonomy (b = −0.35, $p < 0.001$), but not with colleague support (b = 0.02, p = not significant). Hence, the majority of the relations were significant and in expected directions, supporting the theoretical model among nurses. In total, the model explained 12% of the variance related to job performance, and 14% of the variance related to uncertainty among nurses.

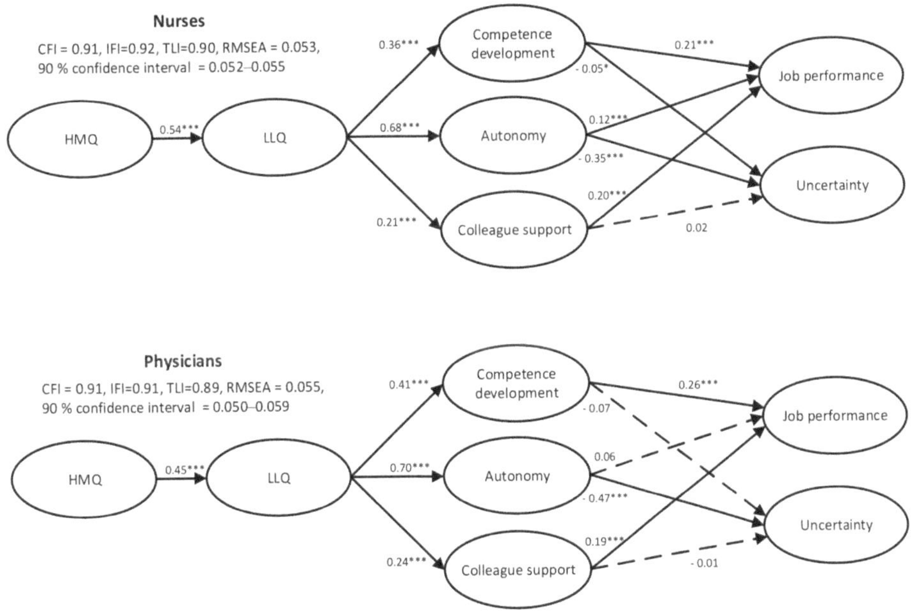

Figure 2. Structural modelling conducted on nurses and physicians. Note: * $p < 0.05$, *** $p < 0.001$. HMQ: Hospital management quality; LLQ: Local leadership quality.

The model fit was also considered adequate among physicians (Figure 2) even though TLI (0.89) was marginally below the 0.90 threshold. Further, all beta coefficients were in the expected directions. HMQ was positively related to LLQ (b = 0.45, < 0.001), supporting hypothesis 1. LLQ was significantly related to competence development (b = 0.41, $p < 0.001$), colleague support (b = 0.24, $p < 0.001$) and autonomy (b = 0.70, < 0.001), supporting hypothesis 2. According to hypothesis 3, psychological needs should be positively related to job performance and negatively related to uncertainty. Findings revealed that colleague support (b = 0.19, $p < 0.001$) and competence development (b = 0.26, $p < 0.001$) were positively related to job performance. Furthermore, autonomy was negatively related to uncertainty (b = −0.47, $p < 0.001$). Some non-significant results were also revealed among physicians. Autonomy was not significantly related to job performance, and uncertainty was not significantly related to competence development and colleague support. Among physicians, the model explained 13% of the variance related to job performance and 24% of the uncertainty.

Ad hoc assessments were conducted to control for the influence of age on uncertainty and job performance. Results revealed that age was significantly and negatively related to uncertainty both among nurses (b = −0.13, $p < 0.001$) and physicians (b = −0.13, $p < 0.05$) but did not influence job performance. However, the inclusion of age in the model reduced the model fit below the recommended thresholds and was, therefore, not included in the final model and presentation of the results (Figure 2).

4. Discussion

Overall, the majority of the results supported the theoretical framework proposed in this study: (1) HMQ is positively related to the quality of local leadership; (2) LLQ is positively related to psychological needs; (3) the majority of the psychological needs are positively related to job performance and negatively related to uncertainty. Moreover, the model is relevant and explains a substantial portion of variance related to uncertainty and job performance among nurses and physicians.

4.1. Theoretical and Practical Implications

Daily care of patients in hospital wards, typically provided by physicians, nurses and other hospital staff, depends on many factors that constitute the microsystems in hospitals. The working conditions of these employees, as well as their needs satisfaction in hospital microsystems are influenced by local managers, as suggested by the theoretical model developed in the current study. Furthermore, the model developed and tested in this study illustrates how HMQ can positively influence LLQ. Sometimes, this perspective is referred to as a multilevel organisational approach since top-level management has a responsibility to define organisational goals and strategies [50,51], which, in turn, influence local leaders and staff. In summary, this study suggests that line management, including both the hospital top-management and local leaders, have a significant and positive influence on psychological need satisfaction of both nurses and physicians. Moreover, the theoretical model developed in this study demonstrates that increased psychological need satisfaction will improve job performance and reduce uncertainty among nurses and physicians.

Managers develop and influence budgets, staff-to-patient ratios and opportunities for staff to develop competence through courses, learning activities and other initiatives. The approach used in the current study suggests multilevel organisational paths, indicating that managers indirectly influence the psychological needs of hospital employees while local leaders influence these needs directly. Since the fulfilment of psychological needs is expected to have a direct influence on both job performance and uncertainty, hospital top managers and local leaders play important roles in developing well-functioning and efficient microsystems, which take into consideration the psychological needs of physicians and nurses.

Hospital systems are hierarchical and complex structures comprising separate but interconnected components. The components of organisations are supposed to play complementary roles to accomplish their joint tasks [52–54]. However, shifts and different working hours make hospital teams and systems less stable, with the rotation of staff, individuals and patients [55]. Other barriers and challenges can be related to temporal resources, negative peer opinion, legislative hindrances and reimbursement shortfalls [56]. Additionally, complex organisations usually have competing agendas, values and goals [57,58] that may lead to fragmentation, competition and malpractice instead of integration, collaboration and cooperation between different actors of the system [58].

With different challenges and barriers towards providing quality care [56], the results of the current study suggest that hospital top-management and local leaders play crucial roles in adequately meeting the psychological needs of staff. Across sub-samples consisting of nurses and physicians, this finding is substantial. Local leaders strongly influence the competence development, autonomy and colleague support, although autonomy appears to have the strongest relation with LLQ across the sub-groups. Interestingly, the relation between autonomy and job performance is not significant among physicians. Autonomy might be related to more advanced and difficult tasks, which may explain why colleague support and competence development are generally more significantly related to job performance. Hence, local leaders and work process designers should be aware that higher levels of autonomy do not necessarily provide higher levels of job performance among physicians. Moreover, competence development and support from colleagues might have a more positive influence on job performance, which implies that local leaders should emphasise competence development and support from colleagues to improve wards and clinical working conditions. However, nurses' autonomy significantly influences job performance. As a general approach, increasing autonomy among nurses seems to be an adequate strategy. However, the results suggest that colleague support and competence development are more important when trying to improve job performance among physicians.

Research and literature [55,59,60] emphasise that managers and leaders need to establish integrated care and address other challenges, such as the development of strong patient safety cultures [61]. According to the theoretical model developed and examined in the current study, the fulfilment of the psychological needs of nurses and physicians may be more important in the development of integrated care and patient safety cultures than earlier assumed and emphasised in research. As such, the findings suggest that attention to psychological need satisfaction among hospital staff can or should be higher on the agenda when developing leadership development programs in hospitals. Further, the fulfilment of psychological needs should be incorporated and emphasised in hospital improvement programs and the design of the working conditions for hospital staff.

4.2. Research Limitations

The findings of this study should be considered in view of the following limitations. The sample size comprising nurses (N = 2946) was much greater compared to that of physicians (N = 556). Nevertheless, the statistical power should be considered relatively robust in the physician sample. Future studies, however, should aim at using large samples to reduce the likelihood of type II error. Moreover, this study is conducted using a sample of physicians and nurses in a single country, and more studies should be conducted in other cultures and contexts before the generalisation of the results. The cross-sectional design incorporates staff perception and does not establish evidence of causal relationships. Hence, other types of research design, analysing multiple time periods, are suggested for follow-up studies. In addition, future studies can consider the use of different types of job performance indicators, as job performance is a difficult concept to measure [62].

5. Conclusions

The results suggest hospitals and their line managers should aim at increasing job performance and reducing uncertainty by fulfilling the psychological needs of their employees. The results suggest that psychological needs perspectives should be integrated into quality-improvement interventions and strategies for nurses and physicians. The findings illustrate how hospital line managers need to address the psychological needs of nurses and physicians in hospital settings. For health professionals to be efficient and confident in what they do, the social environment must provide experiences that will satisfy their basic psychological needs [63]. The results of the current study suggest that the job performance of hospital staff will suffer without psychological nutrients, and because of this, patients are likely to suffer as well. The hospitals' HR practices should incorporate perspectives related to the satisfaction of workers' psychological needs in the development of managers while considering job characteristics and organisational systems. To be able to deliver high quality care, the psychological needs of nurses and physicians must be met. Achieving a fit between individuals and their jobs is an important approach to increase psychological need satisfaction.

Author Contributions: Conceptualisation, E.O.; methodology, E.O. and A.M.; software, E.O.; validation, E.O. and A.M.; formal analysis, E.O.; investigation, E.O.; resources, E.O.; data curation, E.O.; writing—original draft preparation, E.O.; writing—review and editing, E.O.; visualisation, E.O.; project administration, A.M.; funding acquisition, A.M. All authors have read and agreed to the published version of the manuscript.

Funding: This research is funded by then Western Norway Regional Health Authority.

Institutional Review Board Statement: The Norwegian Centre for Research Data approved the study's procedures, project number 33,311.

Informed Consent Statement: Informed consent was obtained from all subjects involved in the study.

Data Availability Statement: Not applicable or agreed with the Western Norway Regional Health Authority.

Acknowledgments: This study has been supported by the Western Norway Regional Health Authority, Stavanger University Hospital, and the University of Stavanger. The authors would like to thank the personnel who participated in the study and all administrative personnel who supported survey procedures.

Conflicts of Interest: The authors declare no conflict of interest. The funders had no role in the design of the study; in the collection, analyses, or interpretation of data; in the writing of the manuscript; or in the decision to publish the results.

References

1. Hillen, M.A.; Gutheil, C.M.; Strout, T.D.; Smets, E.M.; Han, P.K. Tolerance of uncertainty: Conceptual analysis, integrative model, and implications for healthcare. *Soc. Sci. Med.* **2017**, *180*, 62–75. [CrossRef] [PubMed]
2. Durrheim, K.; Foster, D. Tolerance of ambiguity as a content specific construct. *Personal. Individ. Differ.* **1997**, *22*, 741–750. [CrossRef]
3. Logan, R.; Scott, P. Uncertainty in clinical practice: Implications for quality and costs of health care. *Lancet* **1996**, *347*, 595–598. [CrossRef]
4. Ford, M.T.; Cerasoli, C.P.; Higgins, J.A.; Decesare, A.L. Relationships between psychological, physical, and behavioural health and work performance: A review and meta-analysis. *Work Stress* **2011**, *25*, 185–204. [CrossRef]
5. Gaba, D.M.; Howard, S.K. Fatigue among clinicians and the safety of patients. *N. Engl. J. Med.* **2002**, *347*, 1249–1255. [CrossRef]
6. Hofmann, D.A.; Jacobs, R.; Landy, F. High reliability process industries: Individual, micro, and macro organizational influences on safety performance. *J. Saf. Res.* **1995**, *26*, 131–149. [CrossRef]
7. Tomey, A. Nursing leadership and management effects work environments. *J. Nurs. Manag.* **2009**, *17*, 15–25. [CrossRef] [PubMed]
8. Cummings, G.G.; MacGregor, T.; Davey, M.; Lee, H.; Wong, C.A.; Lo, E.; Muise, M.; Stafford, E. Leadership styles and outcome patterns for the nursing workforce and work environment: A systematic review. *Int. J. Nurs. Stud.* **2010**, *47*, 363–385. [CrossRef] [PubMed]
9. Duffield, C.; Diers, D.; O'Brien-Pallas, L.; Aisbett, C.; Roche, M.; King, M.; Aisbett, K. Nursing staffing, nursing workload, the work environment and patient outcomes. *Appl. Nurs. Res.* **2011**, *24*, 244–255. [CrossRef] [PubMed]
10. Laschinger, H.K.S.; Leiter, M.P. The impact of nursing work environments on patient safety outcomes: The mediating role of burnout engagement. *J. Nurs. Adm.* **2006**, *36*, 259–267. [CrossRef] [PubMed]
11. Hetland, H.; Hetland, J.; Schou Andreassen, C.; Pallesen, S.; Notelaers, G. Leadership and fulfillment of the three basic psychological needs at work. *Career Dev. Int.* **2011**, *16*, 507–523. [CrossRef]
12. Ronald, B. Comprehensive leadership review-literature, theories and research. *Adv. In Manag.* **2014**, *7*, 52.
13. Wong, C.A.; Cummings, G.G. The relationship between nursing leadership and patient outcomes: A systematic review. *J. Nurs. Manag.* **2007**, *15*, 508–521. [CrossRef] [PubMed]
14. Cummings, G.; MacGregor, T.; Davey, M.; Wong, C.; Paul, L.; Stafford, E. Factors contributing to nursing leadership: A systematic review. *J. Health Serv. Res. Policy* **2008**, *13*, 240–248. [CrossRef] [PubMed]
15. Kuoppala, J.; Lamminpää, A.; Liira, J.; Vainio, H. Leadership, job well-being, and health effects—A systematic review and a meta-analysis. *J. Occup. Environ. Med.* **2008**, *50*, 904–915. [CrossRef]
16. Orvik, A.; Vågen, S.R.; Axelsson, S.B.; Axelsson, R. Quality, efficiency and integrity: Value squeezes in management of hospital wards. *J. Nurs. Manag.* **2015**, *23*, 65–74. [CrossRef]
17. Von Krogh, G.; Nonaka, I.; Rechsteiner, L. Leadership in organizational knowledge creation: A review and framework. *J. Manag. Stud.* **2012**, *49*, 240–277. [CrossRef]
18. Reeves, S.; Lewin, S. Interprofessional collaboration in the hospital: Strategies and meanings. *J. Health Serv. Res. Policy* **2004**, *9*, 218–225. [CrossRef]
19. Dewettinck, K.; van Ameijde, M. Linking leadership empowerment behaviour to employee attitudes and behavioural intentions: Testing the mediating role of psychological empowerment. *Pers. Rev.* **2011**, *40*, 284–305. [CrossRef]
20. Deci, E.L.; Ryan, R.M. The "what" and "why" of goal pursuits: Human needs and the self-determination of behavior. *Psychol. Inq.* **2000**, *11*, 227–268. [CrossRef]
21. Paarlberg, L.E.; Perry, J.L. Values management aligning employee values and organization goals. *Am. Rev. Public Adm.* **2007**, *37*, 387–408. [CrossRef]
22. Baard, P.P.; Deci, E.L.; Ryan, R.M. Intrinsic Need Satisfaction: A Motivational Basis of Performance and Weil-Being in Two Work Settings1. *J. Appl. Soc. Psychol.* **2004**, *34*, 2045–2068. [CrossRef]
23. Lynch Jr, M.F.; Plant, R.W.; Ryan, R.M. Psychological needs and threat to safety: Implications for staff and patients in a psychiatric hospital for youth. *Prof. Psychol. Res. Pract.* **2005**, *36*, 415. [CrossRef]
24. Abdelhadi, N.; Drach-Zahavy, A. Promoting patient care: Work engagement as a mediator between ward service climate and patient-centred care. *J. Adv. Nurs.* **2012**, *68*, 1276–1287. [CrossRef]
25. Simpson, M.R. Engagement at work: A review of the literature. *Int. J. Nurs. Stud.* **2009**, *46*, 1012–1024. [CrossRef]
26. Antoinette Bargagliotti, L. Work engagement in nursing: A concept analysis. *J. Adv. Nurs.* **2012**, *68*, 1414–1428. [CrossRef]
27. Halbesleben, J.R.; Rathert, C. Linking physician burnout and patient outcomes: Exploring the dyadic relationship between physicians and patients. *Health Care Manag. Rev.* **2008**, *33*, 29–39. [CrossRef]

28. Scheepers, R.A.; Boerebach, B.C.; Arah, O.A.; Heineman, M.J.; Lombarts, K.M. A systematic review of the impact of physicians' occupational well-being on the quality of patient care. *Int. J. Behav. Med.* **2015**, *22*, 683–698. [CrossRef]
29. Wallace, J.E.; Lemaire, J.B.; Ghali, W.A. Physician wellness: A missing quality indicator. *Lancet* **2009**, *374*, 1714–1721. [CrossRef]
30. Reis, H.T.; Sheldon, K.M.; Gable, S.L.; Roscoe, J.; Ryan, R.M. Daily well-being: The role of autonomy, competence, and relatedness. *Personal. Soc. Psychol. Bull.* **2000**, *26*, 419–435. [CrossRef]
31. Ryan, R. Self determination theory and well being. *Soc. Psychol.* **2009**, *84*, e848.
32. Rich, B.L.; Lepine, J.A.; Crawford, E.R. Job engagement: Antecedents and effects on job performance. *Acad. Manag. J.* **2010**, *53*, 617–635. [CrossRef]
33. Van den Broeck, A.; Ferris, D.L.; Chang, C.-H.; Rosen, C.C. A review of self-determination theory's basic psychological needs at work. *J. Manag.* **2016**, *42*, 1195–1229. [CrossRef]
34. Ng, J.Y.; Ntoumanis, N.; Thøgersen-Ntoumani, C.; Deci, E.L.; Ryan, R.M.; Duda, J.L.; Williams, G.C. Self-determination theory applied to health contexts: A meta-analysis. *Perspect. Psychol. Sci.* **2012**, *7*, 325–340. [CrossRef]
35. Deci, E.L.; Ryan, R.M. *Self-Determination*; Wiley Online Library: New York, NY, USA, 2010.
36. Trépanier, S.-G.; Fernet, C.; Austin, S.; Forest, J.; Vallerand, R.J. Linking job demands and resources to burnout and work engagement: Does passion underlie these differential relationships? *Motiv. Emot.* **2014**, *38*, 353–366. [CrossRef]
37. Nahrgang, J.D.; Morgeson, F.P.; Hofmann, D.A. Safety at work: A meta-analytic investigation of the link between job demands, job resources, burnout, engagement, and safety outcomes. *J. Appl. Psychol.* **2011**, *96*, 71. [CrossRef]
38. Aasland, O. Study on physicians' conditions in Norway. *Nord. Med.* **1994**, *110*, 65–67.
39. Karasek, R.A.; Theorell, T.; Schwartz, J.; Pieper, C.; Alfredsson, L. Job, psychological factors and coronary heart disease. In *Psychological Problems before and after Myocardial Infarction*; Karger Publishers: Basel, Switzerland, 1982; pp. 62–67.
40. Krogstad, U.; Hofoss, D.; Hjortdahl, P. Doctor and nurse perception of inter-professional co-operation in hospitals. *Int. J. Qual. Health Care* **2004**, *16*, 491–497. [CrossRef]
41. Dye, D.A. *Organizational Assessment Survey*; Office of Personnel Management: Washington, DC, USA, 1996.
42. Kristensen, T. *A New Tool for Assessing Psychosocial Factors at Work: The Copenhagen Psychosocial Questionnaire*; National Institute of Health: Copenhagen, Denmark, 2000.
43. Van der Heijden, B.I. The Measurement and Development of Professional Expertise Throughout the Career. A Retrospective Study among Higher Level Dutch Professionals. Ph.D. Thesis, University of Twente, Enschede, The Netherlands, 1998.
44. Ørhede, E.; Hottinen, V.; Skogstad, A.; Knardahl, S.; Elo, A.-L.; Dallner, M.; Gamberale, F. *User's Guide for the QPSNordic: General Nordic Questionnaire for Psychological and Social Factors at Work*; Nordic Council of Ministers: Copenhagen, Denmark, 2000.
45. McDonald, R.P.; Ho, M.-H.R. Principles and practice in reporting structural equation analyses. *Psychol. Methods* **2002**, *7*, 64. [CrossRef]
46. Hoyle, R.H. *Structural Equation Modeling: Concepts, Issues, and Applications*; Sage Publications: New York, NY, USA, 1995.
47. Bentler, P.M.; Bonett, D.G. Significance tests and goodness of fit in the analysis of covariance structures. *Psychol. Bull.* **1980**, *88*, 588. [CrossRef]
48. DeVillis, R.F. *Scale Development: Theory and Application*; Sage Publications: Thousands Oaks, CA, USA, 2003.
49. Netemeyer, R.G.; Bearden, W.O.; Sharma, S. *Scaling Procedures: Issues and Application*; SAGE Publications Ltd.: London, UK, 2003.
50. Olsen, E. Exploring the possibility of a common structural model measuring associations between safety climate factors and safety behaviour in health care and the petroleum sectors. *Accid. Anal. Prev.* **2010**, *42*, 1507–1516. [CrossRef] [PubMed]
51. Zohar, D.; Luria, G. A Multilevel Model of Safety Climate: Cross-Level Relationships Between Organization and Group-Level Climates. *J. Appl. Psychol.* **2005**, *90*, 616. [CrossRef] [PubMed]
52. Plsek, P.E.; Wilson, T. Complexity, leadership, and management in healthcare organisations. *BMJ Br. Med. J.* **2001**, *323*, 746. [CrossRef] [PubMed]
53. Singer, S.J.; Burgers, J.; Friedberg, M.; Rosenthal, M.B.; Leape, L.; Schneider, E. Defining and measuring integrated patient care: Promoting the next frontier in health care delivery. *Med. Care Res. Rev.* **2011**, *68*, 112–127. [CrossRef] [PubMed]
54. Stokes, J.; Checkland, K.; Kristensen, S.R. Integrated care: Theory to practice. *J. Health Serv. Res. Policy* **2016**, *21*, 282–285. [CrossRef]
55. Krogstad, U.; Hofoss, D.; Veenstra, M.; Hjortdahl, P. Predictors of job satisfaction among doctors, nurses and auxiliaries in Norwegian hospitals: Relevance for micro unit culture. *Hum. Resour. Health* **2006**, *4*, 3. [CrossRef]
56. Mann, D.; Gaylord, S.; Norton, S. Moving toward integrative care: Rationales, models, and steps for conventional-care providers. *Complementary Health Pract. Rev.* **2004**, *9*, 155–172. [CrossRef]
57. Cameron, K.S.; Quinn, R.E. *Diagnosing and Changing Organizational Culture: Based on the Competing Values Framework*; Addison-Wesley Publishing Company, Inc.: Boston, MA, USA, 1999.
58. Richter, A.; Koch, C. Integration, differentation and ambiguity in safety cultures. *Saf. Sci.* **2004**, *42*, 703–722. [CrossRef]
59. Grol, R.; Wensing, M.; Eccles, M.; Davis, D. *Improving Patient Care: The Implementation of Change in Health Care*; John Wiley & Sons: Hoboken, NJ, USA, 2013.
60. Headrick, L.A.; Wilcock, P.M.; Batalden, P.B. Interprofessional working and continuing medical education. *BMJ Br. Med. J.* **1998**, *316*, 771. [CrossRef]

61. Morello, R.T.; Lowthian, J.A.; Barker, A.L.; McGinnes, R.; Dunt, D.; Brand, C. Strategies for improving patient safety culture in hospitals: A systematic review. *BMJ Qual. Saf.* **2013**, *22*, 11–18. [CrossRef]
62. Matilu, C.M.; K'Obonyo, P. The Relationship Between Job Characteristics and Employee Performance: A Review. *Int. J. Bus. Law Res.* **2018**, *6*, 44–59.
63. Deci, E.L.; Ryan, R.M. Facilitating optimal motivation and psychological well-being across life's domains. *Can. Psychol. Psychol. Can.* **2008**, *49*, 14. [CrossRef]

International Journal of
Environmental Research and Public Health

MDPI

Article

High Level of Physical Activity Reduces the Risk of Renal Progression in Hypertensive Patients

Po-Ya Chang [1], Shu-Yu Lyu [1], Yuh-Feng Lin [2] and Chun-Ching Huang [3,*]

1 Department of Leisure Industry and Health Promotion, National Taipei University of Nursing and Health Sciences, Taipei City 11219, Taiwan; pychang@ntunhs.edu.tw (P.-Y.C.); sylyu2016@ntunhs.edu.tw (S.-Y.L.)

2 Graduate Institute of Clinical Medicine, Taipei Medical University, Taipei City 11031, Taiwan; linyf@shh.org.tw

3 Department of Exercise and Health Science, National Taipei University of Nursing and Health Sciences, Taipei City 11219, Taiwan

* Correspondence: cchuang@ntunhs.edu.tw

Received: 30 January 2020; Accepted: 1 March 2020; Published: 4 March 2020

Abstract: Physical activity has long been associated with chronic diseases. However, the association between physical activity and renal progression in hypertensive patients remains unclear. This study investigated the relationship between the level of physical activity and renal function in hypertensive patients. We analyzed 3543 patients with hypertension. Data on patients' demographic characteristics, comorbidities, physical activity, and lifestyle characteristics were collected via questionnaires. An estimated glomerular filtration rate (eGFR) that was reduced by more than 25% from the baseline eGFR was defined as renal progression. This study divided physical activity into three levels (low, moderate, and high) based on their metabolic equivalent of tasks (METs) levels. The mean age was 63.32 ± 12.29 years. After we adjusted for covariates, renal progression was significantly higher among patients with low levels of physical activity (odds ratio (OR), 1.39; 95% confidence interval (CI), 1.01–1.90)) and moderate levels of physical activity (OR, 1.39; 95% CI, 1.04–1.86) than among patients with high levels of physical activity. We found a significant association between physical activity and renal progression in hypertensive patients, especially in elderly patients and men. Therefore, to reduce the risk of renal progression, we recommend that clinicians should encourage patients to improve their physical activity.

Keywords: physical activity; renal progression; hypertension

1. Introduction

Hypertension is a tremendous global public health threat. It contributes to the burden of coronary artery disease, heart attack, and stroke, as well as chronic kidney disease (CKD) and end-stage renal disease (ESRD) [1,2]. Hypertension is closely related to renal progression and nondiabetic CKD [3,4]. According to the United States Renal Data System (USRDS) reports, 28% of newly diagnosed ESRD is the result of hypertension [5]. It has been reported that the prevalence of ESRD in Taiwan is the highest in the world [5]. In Taiwan, the three most common comorbidities among ESRD patients were hypertension, cardiovascular disease, and diabetes, which were present in 82%, 56.2%, and 49.3%, respectively [6]. Patients with hypertension gradually develop ischemic glomeruli owing to vascular injury [7]. Hypertension that is inadequately or inappropriately treated could progress rapidly to renal failure [7]. In summary, patients with hypertension may experience a decline in renal function and develop renal dysfunction throughout their lives.

Previous studies have proposed that physical exercise has a protective effect against a number of chronic diseases [8,9]. According to World Health Organization (WHO) recommendations, adults should perform at least 150 min of moderate-intensity aerobic physical activity per week, at least 75 min of vigorous-intensity aerobic physical activity per week, or an equivalent combination of moderate- and vigorous-intensity activity [10]. Previous meta-analyses showed that people who reached an overall level of physical exercise that was several times higher than the currently recommended minimum amount of exercise had significantly lower risks of breast cancer, colon cancer, diabetes, ischemic heart disease, and ischemic stroke events [8]. The Kidney Disease Outcomes Quality Initiative (K/DOQI) Clinical Practice Guidelines suggest that increased physical function and a higher level of physical activity could reduce the risk of cardiovascular disease in dialysis patients [11]. Additional benefits may improve patents' ability to perform basic activities of daily living and quality of life [12]. Among patients with diabetes, not only leisure-time physical activity, but also daily commuting and occupational activity can reduce the risk of cardiovascular disease mortality [13]. Non-vigorous activity as well as vigorous physical activity was associated with insulin sensitivity [14].

Despite the causal relationships between physical inactivity and chronic diseases [15], there is a lack of data regarding the association between the risk of renal progression in hypertensive patients and the level of total physical activity. Therefore, we examined the relationship between the level of physical activity and changes in renal function in hypertensive patients. This analysis will help future interventions to prevent renal progression in high-risk populations.

2. Materials and Methods

2.1. Study Population

The study data were obtained from the Epidemiology and Risk Factors Surveillance of CKD database (2008–2016); these data were collected at 14 medical centers and communities in Taiwan from October 2008 to February 2016. In this study, we identified data from at least two serum creatinine measurements in patients aged ≥18 years, with a total of 10,823 participants. Patients were excluded from the analysis based on the following criteria: follow-up periods were less than 12 months, missing data on the level of physical activity, and inability to assess renal function. Our study used a self-report questionnaire to define patients with hypertension. The diagnosis question was "Have you ever been diagnosed with hypertension by a doctor"? (Answer: "Yes/No"). If the patient answered yes, the patient was defined as having hypertension. In total, 3543 patients with hypertension were enrolled; Figure 1.

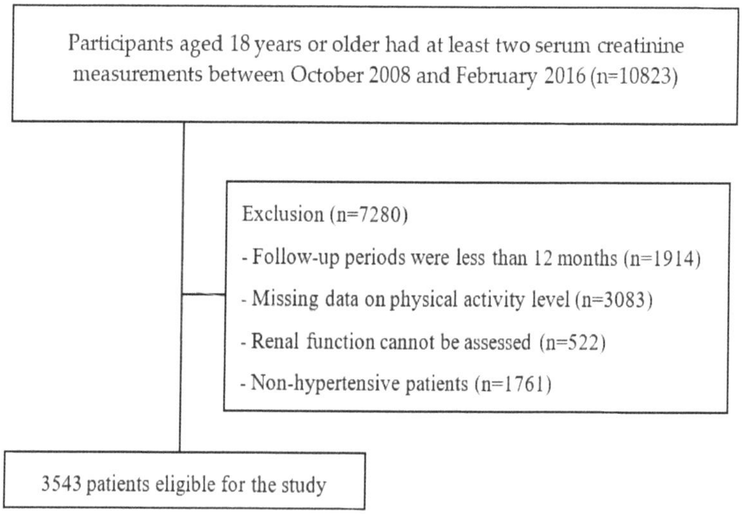

Figure 1. Flowchart of participant analyzed in this study.

2.2. Study Variables and Definitions

Data on patients' demographic characteristics, comorbidities, physical activity, and lifestyle were collected via self-report questionnaires, including sex, age, hypertension, CKD, diabetes mellitus, dyslipidemia, stroke, gout, cigarette smoking, alcohol consumption, sitting time, and levels of physical activity. Patients' physical examination data were obtained via clinical chart review, including serum creatinine, baseline estimated glomerular filtration rate (eGFR), height, weight, body mass index (BMI), fasting glucose, systolic blood pressure (SBP), diastolic blood pressure (DBP), and total cholesterol.

The definition of CKD was determined according to the Kidney Disease Outcomes Quality Initiative guidelines [16]. The eGFR was calculated using the Chronic Kidney Epidemiology Collaboration (CKD-EPI) The Taiwan equation is as follows: eGFR (mL/min/1.73 m^2) = 1.262 × (141 × min (serum creatinine (SCr)/κ, 1)$^{\alpha}$ × max (SCr/κ, 1)$^{-1.209}$ × 0.993^{age} × 1.018 (if female) × 1.159 (if black))$^{0.914}$, κ = 0.7 (for female) and 0.9 (for male), α = −0.329 (female), and −0.411 (male); min denotes the minimum of SCr/κ or 1, and max denotes the maximum of SCr/κ or 1 [17].

An eGFR that was reduced by more than 25% from the baseline eGFR was defined as renal progression [18]. Each patients' renal function was evaluated at the same medical center to reduce variability. Cigarette smoking was classified as smoking or never smoking. Smoking was defined as at least 100 cigarettes in a lifetime [19]. Alcohol consumption was classified as current alcohol consumption or never.

Because all of the participating research medical centers and communities used the same medical laboratory standards and protocols, research serum creatinine values from the different contributing research units can be compared and standardized with each other. This study was approved by the Joint Institutional Review Board of Tri-Service General Hospital (TSGHIRB 100-05-197), Kaohsiung Medical University Chung-Ho Memorial Hospital (KMUHIRB 20120019), Taipei Medical University (TMU-JIRB 20124036), National Cheng Kung University Hospital (A-ER-101-117), Kaohsiung Chang Gung Memorial Hospital (101-1096B), Cardinal Tien Hospital (TMU-JIRB 201204035), Changhua Christian Hospital (CCHIRB 120405), and China Medical University Hospital (DMR101-IRB2-273(CR-1). Written informed consent was obtained from the study participants before any data collection occurred.

2.3. Physical Activities Definitions

This study used the Taiwan version of the International Physical Activity Questionnaire (IPAQ), a short, last-seven-day self-administered format, to measure physical activity (http://www.ipaq.ki.se). The IPAQ is a validated instrument used to assess cross-national physical activity. It is a validated questionnaire that has been translated into multiple languages and has been extensively tested in many countries around the world [20–22]. The questionnaire collected information on the frequency of physical activity and measured vigorous-intensity activity, moderate-intensity activity, and walking activities in the past seven days. The IPAQ asks participants to report physical activities performed for more than 10 continuous minutes [23].

The metabolic equivalent of tasks (METs) represents the amount of oxygen consumed while sitting at rest and is equal to 3.5 mL/kg/min of VO2 Max [24]. METs were calculated based on the IPAQ questions in this study by assigning standard MET values for walking as well as moderate- and vigorous-intensity activity: 3.3 METs, 4.0 METs, and 8.0 METs, respectively (http://www.ipaq.ki.se). These values were used to calculate vigorous-intensity activity, moderate-intensity activity, and walking activity METs (minutes per week) as follows: walking activity METs = 3.3 × walking minutes × walking days; moderate-intensity activity METs = 4.0 × moderate-intensity activity minutes × moderate days; and vigorous activity METs = 8.0 × vigorous-intensity activity minutes × vigorous-intensity days. Total physical activity = sum of walking + moderate + vigorous MET minutes/week scores [23,25].

This study divided physical activity into three levels (low, moderate, and high) based on the following criteria: low physical activity was defined as not meeting the criteria of the moderate or high category; moderate physical activity was defined as meeting any of the following three conditions: (a) three or more days of vigorous-intensity activity of at least 20 min/day; (b) five or more days of moderate-intensity activity and/or walking of at least 30 min/day; or (c) five or more days of any combination of walking, moderate-intensity, or vigorous-intensity activities achieving at least 600 MET-minutes/week. High physical activity was defined as meeting any of the following two conditions: (a) vigorous-intensity activity on at least three days/week and accumulating at least 1500 MET-minutes/week; (b) seven or more days of any combination of walking, moderate-intensity, or vigorous-intensity activities achieving at least 3000 MET-minutes/week [23,25].

2.4. Statistical Analysis

The patient characteristics data were analyzed by descriptive statistics. The chi-square test and Student's t test were used to determine the significant differences between patients with and without renal progression. The chi-square test and one-way analysis of variance test were used to determine the significant differences between levels of physical activity. The odds ratio (OR) and 95% confidence interval (CI) for the risk of renal progression were calculated for the levels of physical activity. After adjusting for all covariates, we used multivariate logistic regression models to evaluate the relationship between the level of physical activity and risk of renal progression. Covariates included sex, age, CKD, diabetes mellitus, dyslipidemia, stroke, gout, body mass index (BMI), serum creatinine, cigarette smoking, and alcohol consumption. We further performed a stratified analysis by sex and age to assess the association between levels of physical activity and renal progression. All analyses and calculations were performed using Statistical Analysis System (SAS) software (SAS Institute), version 9.4. The results were considered statistically significant at $p < 0.05$.

3. Results

A total of 30.29% of patients with hypertension revealed renal progression. The average follow-up time was 35.42 (SD ±16.13) months. Table 1 lists the baseline demographic and clinical characteristics of renal non-progression and renal progression among hypertensive patients. The mean age was 63.32 (SD ±12.29) years, and males accounted for 2043 (57.66%) of the hypertensive patients. The patients with renal progression had a higher prevalence of CKD (1016 (94.69%)), diabetes mellitus (573 (53.40%)), stroke (124 (11.56%)), and gout (409 (38.12%)), as well as lower levels of physical activity than those without renal progression.

Table 1. The baseline characteristics subjects.

Characteristic	Overall (*n* = 3543)	Renal Non-Progression (*n* = 2470)	Renal Progression (*n* = 1073)	*p*-Value
Sex, %				0.052
Female	1500 (42.34)	1019 (41.26)	481 (44.83)	
Male	2043 (57.66)	1451 (58.74)	592 (55.17)	
Age (years), mean ± SD	63.32 ± 12.29	63.02 ± 12.21	63.99 ± 12.45	0.031
Comorbidities, %				
CKD	2771 (78.21)	1755 (71.05)	1016 (94.69)	<0.001
Diabetes mellitus	1642 (46.34)	1069 (43.28)	573 (53.40)	<0.001
Dyslipidemia	1428 (40.30)	992 (40.16)	436 (40.63)	0.821
Stroke	330 (9.31)	206 (8.34)	124 (11.56)	0.003
Gout	1005 (28.37)	596 (24.13)	409 (38.12)	<0.001
Physical examination, mean ± SD				
Serum creatinine (mg/dL)	1.58 ± 1.22	1.29 ± 0.98	2.25 ± 1.44	<0.001
Baseline eGFR (mL/min per 1.73 m^2)	52.70 ± 24.66	59.27 ± 22.43	37.57 ± 22.86	<0.001
Height (cm)	161.39 ± 8.28	161.71 ± 8.32	160.65 ± 8.12	<0.001
Weight (kg)	67.58 ± 12.91	68.03 ± 13.03	66.55 ± 12.58	0.002
BMI (kg/m^2)	25.87 ± 4.11	25.93 ± 4.10	25.73 ± 4.14	0.181
Fasting glucose (mg/dL)	115.63 ± 36.33	113.54 ± 33.92	120.32 ± 40.87	<0.001
SBP (mmHg)	133.88 ± 16.70	133.07 ± 16.64	135.73 ± 16.70	<0.001
DBP (mmHg)	77.33 ± 11.61	77.63 ± 11.35	76.62 ± 12.17	0.022
Total cholesterol (mg/dL)	181.91 ± 38.58	181.45 ± 37.02	182.96 ± 41.88	0.332
Lifestyle, %				
Cigarette smoking	919 (25.95)	630 (25.51)	289 (26.96)	0.387
Alcohol consumption	423 (11.94)	304 (12.31)	119 (11.09)	0.332
Sitting Time (HR/per day), mean ± SD	242.84 ± 136.91	241.90 ± 137.36	244.53 ± 136.20	0.717
Levels of Physical Activity, %				<0.001
Low	2235 (63.08)	1519 (61.50)	716 (66.73)	
Moderate	926 (26.14)	653 (26.44)	273 (25.44)	
High	382 (10.78)	298 (12.06)	84 (7.83)	

Data expressed as percentage or mean ± SD. Abbreviations: CKD, chronic kidney disease; BMI, body mass index; SBP, systolic blood pressure; DBP, diastolic blood pressure; HR, heart rate; eGFR, estimated glomerular filtration rate.

Table 2 presents the baseline characteristics and level of physical activity of the study hypertensive patients. Among the 3543 patients in the overall cohort, 2235 (63.08%), 926 (26.14%), and 382 (10.78%) were in the low, moderate, and high level of physical activity, respectively. The patients in the low level of physical activity were older (63.29 (SD ±12.70)) than those in the moderate (64.19 [(SD ±11.33)) and high level (61.34 (SD ±11.86)). The low level of physical activity also had higher proportions of diabetes mellitus (1085 (48.55%)). Compared with the moderate and high level of physical activity, the low level of physical activity had a higher serum creatinine (0.73 (SD ±0.15)), BMI (25.98 (SD ±4.26)), and fasting glucose (116.90 (SD ±38.76)).

Table 2. Levels of physical activity by patient characteristics.

Characteristic	Low	Moderate	High	p-Value
	$n = 2235$	$n = 926$	$n = 382$	
Sex, %				<0.001
Female	1021 (45.68)	380 (41.04)	99 (25.92)	
Male	1214 (54.32)	546 (58.96)	283 (74.08)	
Age (years), mean ± SD	63.29 ± 12.70	64.19 ± 11.33	61.34 ± 11.86	<0.001
Comorbidities, %				
CKD	1765 (78.97)	725 (78.29)	281 (73.56)	0.061
Diabetes mellitus	1085 (48.55)	404 (43.63)	153 (40.05)	0.001
Dyslipidemia	881 (39.42)	375 (40.50)	172 (45.03)	0.118
Stroke	214 (9.57)	83 (8.96)	33 (8.64)	0.771
Gout	619 (27.70)	262 (28.29)	124 (32.46)	0.161
Physical examination, mean ± SD				
Serum creatinine (mg/dL)	1.63 ± 1.28	1.52 ± 1.16	1.46 ± 1.02	0.010
Baseline eGFR (mL/min per 1.73 m^2)	51.89 ± 25.26	53.31 ± 23.77	55.90 ± 22.97	0.009
Height (cm)	161.14 ± 8.34	161.23 ± 8.17	163.16 ± 7.96	<0.001
Weight (kg)	67.66 ± 13.31	66.64 ± 11.87	69.37 ± 12.84	0.002
BMI (kg/m^2)	25.98 ± 4.26	25.58 ± 3.85	25.96 ± 3.80	0.044
Fasting glucose (mg/dL)	116.90 ± 38.76	114.31 ± 32.27	111.53 ± 30.44	0.016
SBP (mmHg)	133.94 ± 16.82	133.81 ± 16.63	133.67 ± 16.18	0.948
DBP (mmHg)	77.18 ± 11.35	77.61 ± 12.22	77.51 ± 11.58	0.609
Total cholesterol (mg/dL)	181.97 ± 39.65	182.32 ± 38.26	180.59 ± 32.74	0.777
Lifestyle, %				
Cigarette smoking	561 (25.10)	237 (25.62)	121 (31.68)	0.025
Alcohol consumption	261 (11.68)	102 (11.02)	60 (15.71)	0.048
Sitting time, mean ± SD	246.43 ± 139.73	240.75 ± 135.73	232.71 ± 127.43	0.396

Abbreviations: CKD, chronic kidney disease; BMI, body mass index; SBP, systolic blood pressure; DBP, diastolic blood pressure.

Table 3 shows the crude and adjusted odds ratio (OR) of the risk of renal progression across different levels of physical activity in hypertensive patients, calculated using the logistic regression model. The crude OR of renal progression was 1.67 (1.29–2.16) for low levels of physical activity and 1.48 (1.12–1.96) for moderate levels of physical activity compared with high levels of physical activity. After we adjusted for covariates, a higher risk of renal progression was still significantly associated with a low level of physical activity (OR, 1.39; 95% CI, 1.01–1.90) and a moderate level of physical activity (OR, 1.39; 95% CI, 1.04–1.86) compared with a high level of physical activity.

Table 3. Risk of renal progression across different levels of physical activity.

Variable	Crude Odds Ratio (95% CI)	Adjusted Odds Ratio (95% CI)
Levels of Physical Activity		
High	Reference	Reference
Moderate	1.48 (1.12–1.96)	1.39 (1.01–1.90)
Low	1.67 (1.29–2.16)	1.39 (1.04–1.86)
Sex		
Male	Reference	Reference
Female	1.16 (1.00–1.33)	1.16 (1.00–1.33)
Age (years)	1.01 (1.00–1.01)	1.00 (0.99–1.00)
Comorbidities, %		
CKD	7.26 (5.48–9.61)	3.87 (2.86–5.24)
Diabetes mellitus	1.50 (1.30–1.73)	1.75 (1.48–2.08)
Dyslipidemia	1.02 (0.88–1.18)	1.01 (0.85–1.19)
Stroke	1.44 (1.14–1.82)	1.30 (1.00–1.70)
Gout	1.94 (1.66–2.26)	1.47 (1.23–1.77)
BMI (kg/m^2)	0.99 (0.97–1.01)	0.99 (0.97–1.01)
Serum creatinine (mg/dL)	2.05 (1.90–2.21)	2.00 (1.83–2.18)
Cigarette smoking	1.08 (0.92–1.27)	1.09 (0.88–1.35)
Alcohol consumption	0.87 (0.71–1.11)	0.98 (0.76–1.28)

Abbreviations: CI, confidence interval; CKD, chronic kidney disease; BMI, body mass index; SBP, systolic blood pressure; DBP, diastolic blood pressure; OR, odds ratio.

Table 4 lists the OR for the risk of renal progression across different levels of physical activity in hypertensive patients stratified by sex and age group. In males, the multivariate adjustment for age, CKD, diabetes mellitus, dyslipidemia, stroke, gout, BMI, serum creatinine, cigarette smoking, and alcohol consumption resulted in an OR for renal progression that was significantly associated with a low level of physical activity (OR, 1.56; 95% CI, 1.10–2.20) relative to the high level of physical activity (p for trend is <0.020). In females, there was no association between levels of physical activity and developing renal progression. In patients aged ≥60 years, after we adjusted for covariates, the resulting OR for renal progression was significantly associated with a low level of physical activity (OR, 1.54; 95% CI, 1.08–2.22) and a moderate level of physical activity (OR, 1.50; 95% CI, 1.02–2.21) relative to the high level of physical activity (p for trend is 0.052). The results for patients aged <60 years were not significant.

Table 4. Risk of renal progression across different levels of physical activity by gender and age.

Subgroups	High	Moderate Odds Ratio (95% CI)	Low Odds Ratio (95% CI)	p for Trend
Male	Reference	1.45 (0.99–2.12)	1.56 (1.10–2.20)	<0.020
Female	Reference	1.20 (0.63–1.87)	1.09 (0.67–2.12)	0.866
Age ≥ 60	Reference	1.50 (1.02–2.21)	1.54 (1.08–2.22)	0.052
Age < 60	Reference	1.52 (0.87–2.64)	1.51 (0.92–2.48)	0.191

Reference group is high. Odds ratio were adjusted for covariate factors, including age, CKD, diabetes mellitus, dyslipidemia, stroke, gout, BMI, serum creatinine, cigarette smoking, and alcohol consumption.

4. Discussion

This multicenter prospective cohort study enrolled subjects with hypertension to demonstrate that the level of physical activity was an independent predictor of renal progression. We found that a low level of physical activity and a moderate level of physical activity were associated with an increased risk of renal progression compared with a high level of physical activity. In particular, in male or elderly patients, different levels of physical activity were significantly associated with renal function. To our knowledge, this is the first prospective cohort study to elucidate the effects of physical activity differences on kidney damage in patients with hypertension.

Low levels of physical activity and low physical function are associated with adverse clinical outcomes [12]. A previous study indicated that higher levels of physical activity are attributed to a lower prevalence of CKD, which is broadly consistent with this study [26]. Insufficient physical activity is associated with increased morbidity and mortality, both in the general population and in patients with noncommunicable diseases [27,28]. Therefore, physical activity is related to primary prevention in the general population and the secondary and tertiary care of the patient population [29]. Many scientific studies indicate that most physiological systems can be positively altered by physical activity [30–32]. Participation also plays a role in the prevention and treatment of chronic diseases [33]. Therefore, physical activity could be a natural treatment for many diseases [34].

Our results indicated a trend toward men having a higher risk of renal progression with lower levels of physical activity than women. Previous studies have proposed that men show a lower risk of CKD with higher levels of vigorous intensity physical activity compared with women, while shorter sitting times are associated with CKD in women, but not in men [26]. A possible explanation for this finding is that cultural and social environmental differences and biological effects have caused sex differences [35–37]. It has been reported that estrogens may bring into play potent antioxidant action and may have protective effects on renal progression in women [38]. A previous study also shows sex steroids and sex chromosomes play a mediating role in causing kidney disease [39].

Our findings suggest that the level of physical activity is related to renal progression in older patients, but not in younger patients. These findings are consistent with those of previous studies that show that exercising with sufficient intensity and frequency can improve health in older adults [40,41]. The meta-analysis also reported that increased physical activity could prevent and slow down the onset of dysfunction and the progression of functional decline in the elderly [42]. However, with increasing age, the prevalence of physical exercise decreases [43]. In addition, our research shows that hypertensive patients with CKD, diabetes, stroke, or gout were associated with kidney function decline, which is consistent with previous studies. Diabetes mellitus, CKD, stroke, and gout are independent risk factors for renal disease [35,44–46].

Our study uses the IPAQ questionnaire to assess physical activity and calculate the level of physical activity (low, medium, and high) through MET. The IPAQ questionnaire has been validated and widely used in other studies [20–22,26]. MET is defined as the ratio of working metabolic rate to resting metabolic rate, and is usually used to indicate the intensity of physical activity [26]. According to the World Health Organization guidelines, four METs are assigned to the time spent doing moderate activities, and eight METs to the time spent doing vigorous activities [47].

Our study has advantages. First, our study provided evidence in a large cohort study showing that a low level of physical activity was an independent predictor of kidney function decline in patients with hypertension. Second, data on patient demographics, comorbidities, physical activity, and lifestyle were collected through face-to-face interviews. To ensure the quality of our data, our interviewers were given in-depth training. However, the authors acknowledge some limitations. First, voluntary participation in research may lead to selection bias. Second, misclassification of physical activity, which was recorded from the self-report questionnaires at baseline, is possible. However, this misclassification may be non-differential, thus leading to an underestimation of certain test results. Third, because the participants' physical examination data were collected from multiple centers, equipment variations may affect the test results. Nonetheless, all supervisors tried to minimize measurement errors.

5. Conclusions

This study offers evidence demonstrating that physical activity is related to renal progression among patients with hypertension. We observed that a low level of physical activity had significant adverse effects, especially in male and elderly patients. Therefore, to reduce the risk of renal progression, we recommend that clinicians should encourage patients to improve physical activity. In addition, we recommend that healthcare providers develop strategies and clinical interventions to increase patients' motivation for exercise.

Author Contributions: Conceptualization, P.-Y.C. and C.-C.H.; methodology, P.-Y.C.; software, P.-Y.C.; validation, S.-Y.L. and C.-C.H.; formal analysis, P.-Y.C.; investigation, P.-Y.C. and Y.-F.L.; writing—original draft preparation, P.-Y.C. and C.-C.H.; writing—review and editing, P.-Y.C.; supervision, S.-Y.L. and C.-C.H.; funding acquisition, Y.-F.L. and C.-C.H. All authors have read and agreed to the published version of the manuscript.

Funding: This study was funded by a grant from the Health Promotion Administration, Ministry of Health and Welfare, Taiwan, Republic of China (DOH101-HP-1103, DOH102-HP-1103, MOHW103-HPA-H-114-134101, MOHW104-HPA-H-114-134101).

Conflicts of Interest: The authors declare no conflict of interest.

References

1. Whelton, P.K. Epidemiology of hypertension. *Lancet* **1994**, *344*, 101–106. [CrossRef]
2. Horowitz, B.; Miskulin, D.; Zager, P. Epidemiology of Hypertension in CKD. *Adv. Chronic Kidney Dis.* **2015**, *22*, 88–95. [CrossRef]
3. Tsai, W.C.; Wu, H.Y.; Peng, Y.S.; Yang, J.Y.; Chen, H.Y.; Chiu, Y.L.; Hsu, S.P.; Ko, M.J.; Pai, M.F.; Tu, Y.K.; et al. Association of Intensive Blood Pressure Control and Kidney Disease Progression in Nondiabetic Patients with Chronic Kidney Disease: A Systematic Review and Meta-analysis. *JAMA Int. Med.* **2017**, *177*, 792–799. [CrossRef]
4. Ku, E.; Lee, B.J.; Wei, J.; Weir, M.R. Hypertension in CKD: Core Curriculum 2019. *Am. J. Kidney Dis.* **2019**, *74*, 120–131. [CrossRef]
5. U.S. Renal Data System. *USRDS 2013 Annual Data Report: Atlas of Chronic Kidney Disease and End-Stage Renal Disease in the United States*; USRDS: Bethesda, MD, USA, 2013.
6. National Health Research Institutes. *Annual Report on Kidney Disease in Taiwan*; National Health Research Institutes: Zhunan, Taiwan, 2017.
7. Bidani, A.K.; Griffin, K.A. Pathophysiology of hypertensive renal damage: Implications for therapy. *Hypertension* **2004**, *44*, 595–601. [CrossRef]
8. Kyu, H.H.; Bachman, V.F.; Alexander, L.T.; Mumford, J.E.; Afshin, A.; Estep, K.; Veerman, J.L.; Delwiche, K.; Iannarone, M.L.; Moyer, M.L.; et al. Physical activity and risk of breast cancer, colon cancer, diabetes, ischemic heart disease, and ischemic stroke events: Systematic review and dose-response meta-analysis for the Global Burden of Disease Study 2013. *BMJ* **2016**, *354*, 1–10. [CrossRef]
9. Howden, E.J.; Coombes, J.S.; Strand, H.; Douglas, B.; Campbell, K.L.; Isbel, N.M. Exercise Training in CKD: Efficacy, Adherence, and Safety. *Am. J. Kidney Dis.* **2015**, *56*, 583–591. [CrossRef]
10. World Health Organization. Physical Activity and Adults-Recommended Levels of Physical Activity for Adults Aged 18–64 Years. Available online: https://www.who.int/dietphysicalactivity/factsheet_adults/en/ (accessed on 19 January 2020).
11. National Kidney Foundation. K/DOQI clinical practice guidelines for cardiovascular disease in dialysis patients. *Am. J. Kidney Dis.* **2005**, *45*, S1–S154.
12. Painter, P.; Roshanravan, B. The association of physical activity and physical function with clinical outcomes in adults with chronic kidney disease. *Curr. Opin. Nephrol. Hypertens.* **2013**, *22*, 615–623. [CrossRef]
13. Hu, G.; Eriksson, J.; Barengo, N.C.; Lakka, T.A.; Valle, T.T.; Nissinen, A.; Jousilahti, P.; Tuomilehto, J. Occupational, commuting, and leisure-time physical activity in relation to total and cardiovascular mortality among Finnish subjects with type 2 diabetes. *Circulation* **2004**, *110*, 666–673. [CrossRef]
14. Mayer-Davis, E.J.; D'Agostino, R., Jr.; Karter, A.J.; Haffner, S.M.; Rewers, M.J.; Saad, M.; Bergman, R.N. Intensity and amount of physical activity in relation to insulin sensitivity: The Insulin Resistance Atherosclerosis Study. *JAMA* **1998**, *279*, 669–674. [CrossRef]
15. Booth, F.W.; Roberts, C.K.; Laye, M.J. Lack of exercise is a major cause of chronic diseases. *Compr. Physiol.* **2012**, *2*, 1143–1211.
16. Levey, A.S.; Coresh, J.; Bolton, K.; Culleton, B.; Harvey, K.S.; Ikizler, T.A.; Johnson, C.A.; Kausz, A.; Kimmel, P.L.; Kusek, J.; et al. K/DOQI clinical practice guidelines for chronic kidney disease: Evaluation, classification, and stratification. *Am. J. Kidney Dis.* **2002**, *39*, S1–S266.
17. Chen, L.I.; Guh, J.Y.; Wu, K.D.; Chen, Y.M.; Kuo, M.C.; Hwang, S.J.; Chen, T.H.; Chen, H.C. Modification of diet in renal disease (MDRD) study and CKD epidemiology collaboration (CKD-EPI) equations for Taiwanese adults. *PLoS ONE* **2014**, *9*, e99645. [CrossRef]

18. Kidney Disease: Improving Global Outcomes (KDIGO) CKD Work Group. KDIGO 2012 clinical practice guideline for the evaluation and management of chronic kidney disease. *Kidney Int. Suppl.* **2013**, *3*, 1–150.
19. Vupputuri, S.; Sandler, D.P. Lifestyle risk factors and chronic kidney disease. *Ann. Epidemiol.* **2003**, *13*, 712–720. [CrossRef]
20. Bauman, A.; Bull, F.; Chey, T.; Craig, C.L.; Ainsworth, B.E.; Sallis, J.F.; Bowles, H.R.; Hagstromer, M.; Sjostrom, M.; Pratt, M. The International Prevalence Study on Physical Activity: Results from 20 countries. *Int. J. Behav. Nutr. Phys. Act.* **2009**, *6*, 1–11. [CrossRef]
21. Oyeyemi, A.L.; Oyeyemi, A.Y.; Adegoke, B.O.; Oyetoke, F.O.; Aliyu, H.N.; Aliyu, S.U.; Rufai, A.A. The Short International Physical Activity Questionnaire: Cross-cultural adaptation, validation and reliability of the Hausa language version in Nigeria. *BMC Med. Res. Methodol.* **2011**, *11*, 1–11. [CrossRef]
22. Liou, Y.M.; Jwo, C.J.; Yao, K.G.; Chiang, L.C.; Huang, L.H. Selection of appropriate Chinese terms to represent intensity and types of physical activity terms for use in the Taiwan version of IPAQ. *J. Nurs. Res.* **2008**, *16*, 252–263. [CrossRef]
23. Craig, C.L.; Marshall, A.L.; Sjostrom, M.; Bauman, A.E.; Booth, M.L.; Ainsworth, B.E.; Pratt, M.; Ekelund, U.; Yngve, A.; Sallis, J.F.; et al. International physical activity questionnaire: 12-country reliability and validity. *Med. Sci. Sports. Exerc.* **2003**, *35*, 1381–1395. [CrossRef]
24. Jette, M.; Sidney, K.; Blumchen, G. Metabolic equivalents (METS) in exercise testing, exercise prescription, and evaluation of functional capacity. *Clin. Cardiol.* **1990**, *13*, 555–565. [CrossRef]
25. International Physical Activity Questionnaires (IPAQ). IPAQ Scoring Protocol. Available online: http://www.ipaq.ki.se (accessed on 12 January 2020).
26. Bharakhada, N.; Yates, T.; Davies, M.J.; Wilmot, E.G.; Edwardson, C.; Henson, J.; Webb, D.; Khunti, K. Association of sitting time and physical activity with CKD: A cross-sectional study in family practices. *Am. J. Kidney Dis.* **2012**, *60*, 583–590. [CrossRef]
27. World Health Organization. *Global Recommendations on Physical Activity for Health*; WHO: Geneva, Switzerland, 2010.
28. Kohl, H.W., 3rd; Craig, C.L.; Lambert, E.V.; Inoue, S.; Alkandari, J.R.; Leetongin, G.; Kahlmeier, S. The pandemic of physical inactivity: Global action for public health. *Lancet* **2012**, *380*, 294–305. [CrossRef]
29. Zelle, D.M.; Klaassen, G.; van Adrichem, E.; Bakker, S.J.; Corpeleijn, E.; Navis, G. Physical inactivity: A risk factor and target for intervention in renal care. *Nat. Rev. Nephrol.* **2017**, *13*, 152–168. [CrossRef]
30. Warburton, D.E.; Nicol, C.W.; Bredin, S.S. Health benefits of physical activity: The evidence. *Cmaj* **2006**, *174*, 801–809. [CrossRef]
31. Neufer, P.D.; Bamman, M.M.; Muoio, D.M.; Bouchard, C.; Cooper, D.M.; Goodpaster, B.H.; Booth, F.W.; Kohrt, W.M.; Gerszten, R.E.; Mattson, M.P.; et al. Understanding the Cellular and Molecular Mechanisms of Physical Activity-Induced Health Benefits. *Cell Metab.* **2015**, *22*, 4–11. [CrossRef]
32. Ruegsegger, G.N.; Booth, F.W. Health Benefits of Exercise. *Cold Spring Harb. Perspect. Med.* **2018**, *8*, 1–16. [CrossRef]
33. Nunan, D.; Mahtani, K.R.; Roberts, N.; Heneghan, C. Physical activity for the prevention and treatment of major chronic disease: An overview of systematic reviews. *Syst. Rev.* **2013**, *2*, 1–6. [CrossRef]
34. Anderson, E.; Durstine, J.L. Physical activity, exercise, and chronic diseases: A brief review. *Sports Med. Health Sci.* **2019**, *1*, 3–10. [CrossRef]
35. Chang, P.Y.; Chien, L.N.; Lin, Y.F.; Wu, M.S.; Chiu, W.T.; Chiou, H.Y. Risk factors of gender for renal progression in patients with early chronic kidney disease. *Medicine* **2016**, *95*, 1–7. [CrossRef]
36. Sabolic, I.; Asif, A.R.; Budach, W.E.; Wanke, C.; Bahn, A.; Burckhardt, G. Gender differences in kidney function. *Pflugers Archiv: Eur. J. Physiol.* **2007**, *455*, 397–429. [CrossRef]
37. Iseki, K. Gender differences in chronic kidney disease. *Kidney Int.* **2008**, *74*, 415–417. [CrossRef]
38. Silbiger, S.R.; Neugarten, J. The impact of gender on the progression of chronic renal disease. *Am. J. Kidney Dis.* **1995**, *25*, 515–533. [CrossRef]
39. Reckelhoff, J.F.; Samson, W.K. Sex and gender differences in cardiovascular, renal and metabolic diseases. *Am. J. Physiol. Regul. Integr. Comp. Physiol.* **2015**, *309*, R1057–R1059. [CrossRef]
40. Taylor, D. Physical activity is medicine for older adults. *Postgrad. Med. J.* **2014**, *90*, 26–32. [CrossRef]
41. Paterson, D.H.; Warburton, D.E. Physical activity and functional limitations in older adults: A systematic review related to Canada's Physical Activity Guidelines. *Int. J. Behav. Nutr. Phys. Act.* **2010**, *7*, 1–22. [CrossRef]

42. Tak, E.; Kuiper, R.; Chorus, A.; Hopman-Rock, M. Prevention of onset and progression of basic ADL disability by physical activity in community dwelling older adults: A meta-analysis. *Ageing Res. Rev.* **2013**, *12*, 329–338. [CrossRef]
43. Spittaels, H.; Van Cauwenberghe, E.; Verbestel, V.; De Meester, F.; van Dyck, D.; Verloigne, M.; Haerens, L.; Deforche, B.; Cardon, G.; De Bourdeaudhuij, I. Objectively measured sedentary time and physical activity time across the lifespan: A cross-sectional study in four age groups. *Int. J. Behav. Nutr. Phys. Act.* **2012**, *9*, 1–12. [CrossRef]
44. Najafi, I.; Attari, F.; Islami, F.; Shakeri, R.; Malekzadeh, F.; Salahi, R.; Gharavi, M.Y.; Hosseini, M.; Broumand, B.; Haghighi, A.N.; et al. Renal function and risk factors of moderate to severe chronic kidney disease in Golestan Province, northeast of Iran. *PLoS ONE* **2010**, *5*, e14216. [CrossRef]
45. Weiner, D.E.; Tighiouart, H.; Elsayed, E.F.; Griffith, J.L.; Salem, D.N.; Levey, A.S. Uric acid and incident kidney disease in the community. *J. Am. Soc. Nephrol.* **2008**, *19*, 1204–1211. [CrossRef]
46. Fandler-Hofler, S.; Enzinger, C.; Kneihsl, M.; Pinter, D.; Eppinger, S.; Obermayer-Pietsch, B.; Goritschan, A.; Hafner-Giessauf, H.; Rosenkranz, A.R.; Fazekas, F.; et al. Early renal dysfunction and fibroblast growth factor-23 in patients with small vessel disease-related stroke. *Sci. Rep.* **2019**, *9*, 15410. [CrossRef]
47. World Health Organization. Global Physical Activity Questionnaire (GPAQ) Analysis Guide. Available online: https://www.who.int/ncds/surveillance/steps/resources/GPAQ_Analysis_Guide.pdf (accessed on 19 February 2020).

MDPI AG
Grosspeteranlage 5
4052 Basel
Switzerland
Tel.: +41 61 683 77 34

International Journal of Environmental Research and Public Health Editorial Office
E-mail: ijerph@mdpi.com
www.mdpi.com/journal/ijerph

www.ingramcontent.com/pod-product-compliance
Lightning Source LLC
Chambersburg PA
CBHW041431210926
51850CB00013B/3399